Medicine in Ancient Assur

Ancient Magic and Divination

VOLUME 18

The titles published in this series are listed at *brill.com/amd*

Medicine in Ancient Assur

A Microhistorical Study of the Neo-Assyrian Healer Kiṣir-Aššur

By

Troels Pank Arbøll

BRILL

LEIDEN | BOSTON

Cover image by Troels Pank Arbøll, 2019.

The publication of this book was supported by The Edubba Foundation, The Elisabeth Munksgaard Foundation and The Augustinus Foundation.

Library of Congress Cataloging-in-Publication Data

Names: Arbøll, Troels Pank, author.
Title: Medicine in ancient Assur : a microhistorical study of the Neo-Assyrian healer Kiṣir-Aššur / Troels Pank Arbøll.
Description: Leiden ; Boston : Brill, [2021] | Series: Ancient magic and divination, 15667952 ; vol. 18 | Includes bibliographical references and index.
Identifiers: LCCN 2020029398 (print) | LCCN 2020029399 (ebook) | ISBN 9789004436077 (hardback) | ISBN 9789004436084 (ebook)
Subjects: LCSH: Medicine, Assyro-Babylonian. | Medicine, Ancient.
Classification: LCC R135.3 .A73 2021 (print) | LCC R135.3 (ebook) | DDC 610.938—dc23
LC record available at https://lccn.loc.gov/2020029398
LC ebook record available at https://lccn.loc.gov/2020029399

Typeface for the Latin, Greek, and Cyrillic scripts: "Brill". See and download: brill.com/brill-typeface.

ISSN 1566-7952
ISBN 978-90-04-43607-7 (hardback)
ISBN 978-90-04-43608-4 (e-book)

This book is printed on acid-free paper and produced in a sustainable manner.

Contents

Acknowledgements

This book is based on my PhD dissertation, which was successfully defended in December 2017. It gives me great pleasure to publicly thank the foundations and people who have supported and helped me throughout the process. I gratefully acknowledge the generous financial support of the Edubba Foundation, the Carlsberg Foundation and the Augustinus Foundation, which allowed me to revise and prepare the manuscript for this book. The Edubba Foundation, the Elisabeth Munksgaard Foundation and the Augustinus Foundation kindly granted the funds to publish the volume with Open Access. Additionally, grants from the Elisabeth Munksgaard Foundation, the Augustinus Foundation and the Danish Institute in Damascus enabled me to conduct research stays in Berlin and Würzbrug during 2015 and 2016. Finally, the research was made possible by a PhD stipend from the Department of Cross-Cultural and Regional Studies at the University of Copenhagen.

I am eternally grateful to Nicole Brisch, whose continuous encouragement and meticulous feedback as my supervisor helped me write the foundation for this book. Words cannot express my gratitude for the academic generosity and personal support she has shown me. Furthermore, I would like to express my deepest gratitude to Barbara Böck and Daniel Schwemer, who were not only inspiring co-supervisors throughout my time as a PhD student, but also continue to encourage and support my academic interests. Furthermore, Barbara Böck generously offered me the original impetus for using Kiṣir-Aššur's tablets as the focus for my study. Daniel Schwemer collated several of Kiṣir-Aššur's tablets in Istanbul and kindly shared the results with me on several occasions with characteristic generosity. Additionally, I am indebted to Nils Heeßel, Stefan Maul and Daniel Schwemer who allowed me to include information about several unpublished Kiṣir-Aššur tablets kept in Istanbul. My gratitude furthermore extends to Andrew George and Nils Heeßel who – in the role of opponents – meticulously read through my PhD dissertation and provided me with much valuable feedback and criticism. Their generous support is sincerely appreciated and acknowledged here. In addition, it is a pleasure to thank Claus Ambos who kindly agreed to be my pre-defence examiner and provided me with valuable comments before handing in my dissertation.

I am particularly thankful to Aage Westenholz and Inger Jentoft for their friendship, hospitality and profound interest in my work. Westenholz tirelessly discussed countless points and arguments with me on several occasions, and he took it upon himself to read through the entire manuscript and provide me with much appreciated comments and corrections. I am sincerely grateful for our friendship and the kindness he has shown me these past years. Among my Egyptological colleagues in Copenhagen, I am truly indebted to Kim Ryholt for all his thoughtful help and support in many forms from my time as a student to the present day. Furthermore, Fredrik Hagen has kindly helped me in countless academic matters these past years, and as chairman of my dissertation examination committee he raised several important points, for which I am thankful.

It gives me great pleasure to thank the Vorderasiatisches Museum zu Berlin for permission to study several of Kiṣir-Aššur's tablets discussed in this volume. Especially Lutz Martin deserves special recognition for his assistance in helping me arrange visits to the VAM during the summer of 2015 and 2016. I am also indebted to Erica Couto-Ferreira, Eckart Frahm, Irene Sibbing-Plantholt and the BabMed project for kindly sharing forthcoming works with me prior to their publication. I am also thankful to Jacob Dahl for an invitation to present my research under stimulating circumstances in Oxford during May 2019. Additionally, I am grateful to researchers and students at the Würzburg Lehrstuhl für Altorientalistik for three inspiring months I spent there in 2016, and I am particularly thankful to the Würzburg *CMAwR* research group for their friendship and interest in my work. My thanks furthermore extend to my two anonymous peer-reviewers who provided helpful comments and criticism.

Jennifer Cromwell and Seraina Nett deserve special recognition and profound thanks for diligently reading through my drafts with great attention, addressing various issues and correcting my English. To Ulla Koch, I am grateful for her interest in my research and an invitation to discuss certain issues relating to my work. Mogens Trolle Larsen and Thomas Hertel are also recognized for their support and for helpful discussions about my work. It is a pleasure to also thank paediatrician Elisabeth Lund and biologist Sophie Lund Rasmussen for numerous discussions of the modern veterinary and human medical aspects of ancient medicine. Their inputs and suggestions greatly helped me shape the ideas formulated in this volume. Additionally, I am grateful to Katelyn Chin, Erika Mandarino and Kristen Chevalier at Brill for all their assistance during the process of publishing this book.

For their help in various matters throughout the years, it is a pleasure to acknowledge the following people: Jakob Andersson, Paul Delnero, Mark Geller, İlgi Gerçek, Manfred Krebernik, Piotr Michalowski, Matthias Müller, Strahil Panayotov, Hratch Papazian, JoAnn Scurlock, Kathryn Stevens, Ingolf Thuesen, Martin Worthington, and Kenneth Zysk. Among my current and former colleagues and friends at the University of Copenhagen, I would also like to thank: Rasmus Aarslev, Gojko Barjamovic, Agnieszka Bystron, Thomas Christiansen, Ole Herslund, Amanda Sass Hertel, Amber Jacob, Susanne

Kerner, Bjarne Lodahl, Rune Olsen, Jes Heise Rasmussen, Rune Rattenborg, Tobias Richter, Sofie Schiødt, Rana Sérida and Daniel Soliman. Furthermore, several of my friends outside the narrow confines of the Ancient Near East deserve to be mentioned for their patience and support, especially: Kim Bavnild, Peter Engkjær, Rasmus Jensen, Christian Johansen, Daniel Theis Lund, Dennis Tougaard, Daniel Sønder, and Mikkel Zimakoff. Finally, I am grateful to my primary school teacher Erik Ingemann Sørensen for showing me that it is possible to make history come alive.

Most importantly, this work would not have been possible without the encouragement and loving support of my family, namely my beloved son Theodor, my wife, Sophie Lund Rasmussen, and my mother, Birgitte Pank Arbøll. I only wish my father, Kurt Arbøl, was alive to see this book in print. With admiration and appreciation, I lovingly dedicate this work to them.

Copenhagen, May 2020

Figures and Tables

Figures

Tables

Abbreviations and Symbols

Bibliographical Abbreviations

See generally <http://cdli.ox.ac.uk/wiki/doku.php?id=abbreviations_for_assyriology> (accessed 12/05/2020). For abbreviations of lexical lists, see Veldhuis (2014: 430–41). In addition, the following abbreviations are used:

AbB 1 — *Altbabylonische Briefe in Umschrift und Übersetzung 1. Briefe aus dem British Museum* (*CT 43 und 44*), F. R. Kraus 1964 (Leiden: Brill).

AHw — *Akkadisches Handwörterbuch* (Wiesbaden: Otto Harrassowitz).

AMC — Assur Medical Catalogue (see references in Section 9.3.2).

AMT — *Assyrian Medical Texts from the Originals in the British Museum* (see Thompson 1923).

BabMed — *Babylonische Medizin* (see online ⟨https://www.geschkult.fu-berlin.de/e/babmed/Corpora/index.html⟩ (accessed 12/09/2019)).

BAK — *Babylonische und assyrische Kolophone* (see Hunger 1968).

BAM — *Die babylonisch-assyrische Medizin in Texten und Untersuchungen* (see Köcher 1963a–1971; Köcher 1980a–1980b; Geller 2005; Geller 2016; Steinert 2018e; Geller and Panayotov in press; Johnson in press).

CAD — *The Assyrian Dictionary of the Oriental Institute of the University of Chicago* (Illinois and Glückstadt / Illionois: The Oriental Institute and J. J. Augustin Verlagsbuchhandlung / The Oriental Institute).

CCP — *Cuneiform Commentaries Project* (see online ⟨http://ccp.yale.edu⟩ (accessed 12/05/2020)).

CDA — *A Concise Dictionary of Akkadian*, ed. J. Black, A. R. George and N. Postgate 2000 [Second (corrected) printing] (Wiesbaden: Harrassowitz Verlag).

CDLI — *Cuneiform Digital Library Initiative* (see online ⟨http://cdli.ucla.edu⟩ (accessed 14/05/2020)).

CMAwR — *Corpus of Mesopotamian Anti-Witchcraft Rituals* (see Abusch and Schwemer 2011; Abusch, Schwemer, Luukko and van Buylaere 2016).

CT — *Cuneiform Texts from Babylonian Tablets, &c., in the British Museum / Cuneiform Texts from Babylonian Tablets in the British Museum* (London: The Trustees of the British Museum).

CTN 4 — *Cuneiform Texts from Nimrud 4. Literary Texts from the Temple of Nabû*, D. J. Wiseman and J. A. Black 1996 (London: British School of Archaeology in Iraq).

EM — Exorcist's Manual (see references in Section 9.4).

KADP	*Keilschrifttexte zur assyrisch-babylonischen Drogen- und Pflanzenkunde* (see Köcher 1955).
KAH	*Keilschrifttexte aus Assur historischen Inhalts* (Leipzig: J. C. Hinrichs'sche Buchhandlung)
KAL	*Keilschrifttexte aus Assur literarischen Inhalts* (see Heeßel 2007a; Schwemer 2007b; Maul and Strauß 2011; Heeßel 2012; Meinhold 2017; Jakob 2018; Maul 2019).
KAR	*Keilschrifttexte aus Assur religiösen Inhalts* (see Ebeling 1919a; Ebeling 1920–23).
KAV	*Keilschrifttexte aus Assur verschiedenen Inhalts* (see Schroeder 1920).
LKA	*Literarische Keilschrifttexte aus Assur* (see Ebeling 1953a).
LKU	*Literarische Keilschrifttexte aus Uruk*, A. Falkenstein 1979 (Hildesheim and New York: Georg Olms Verlag).
MSL	*Materialien zum Sumerischen Lexikon / Materials for the Sumerian Lexicon* (see Landsberger 1960; Landsberger 1962; Landsberger 1967; Civil 1969; Civil 2004).
RA	*Revue d'assyriologie et d'archéologie orientale* (Paris: Ernest Leroux / Presses universitaires de France).
SAA	*State Archives of Assyria* (Helsinki: Helsinki University Press / The Neo-Assyrian Text Corpus Project).
SAAS	*State Archives of Assyria Studies* (see Millard 1994; Radner 1997; Pongratz-Leisten 1999; Annus 2002; Lenzi 2008a; Macgregor 2012; Kolev 2013).
Sa-gig	The diagnostic-prognostic omen series *Sakikkû* (see references in Sections 3.1 and 3.6.1).
SEAL	*Sources of Early Akkadian Literature. A Text Corpus of Babylonian and Assyrian Literary Texts from the 3rd and 2nd Millennia BCE* (see online ⟨http://www.seal.uni-leipzig.de⟩ (accessed 10/12/2019)).
SpTU	*Spätbabylonische Texte aus Uruk / Uruk. Spätbabylonische Texte aus dem Planquadrat U 18* (Berlin / Mainz: Gebr. Mann Verlag / Verlag Philipp von Zabern).
STT	*The Sultantepe Tablets* (London: The British Institute of Archaeology at Ankara).
UET 5	*Ur Excavations Texts 5. Letters and Documents of the Old-Babylonian Period*, H. H. Figulla and W. J. Martin 1953 (London and Philadelphia: The Trustees of the British Museum and the University Museum, University of Pennsylvania).
Ugu	The therapeutic series "If the crown of a man's head is feverish", *šumma amēlu muḫḫašu umma ukāl* (see references in Section 9.3.1).
YOS	*Yale Oriental Series* (see van Dijk, Goetze and Hussey 1985).

Symbols and Further Abbreviations

šu$^{!}$	emended, but certain reading (against unidentifiable or irregular sign on tablet)
šu$^{!?}$	emended, but uncertain reading of a sign
šu$^{?}$	uncertain reading of a sign
x	undeciphered sign
:	cuneiform division mark
[ ]	break
[x]	indicates space available in break
[...]	indicates a break of uncertain length
⸢ ⸣	partially broken sign(s)
< >	sign(s) to be added to the text
{ }	sign(s) to be deleted from the text
* *	sign(s) written over erasure
{ }	erased sign(s) to be removed from the text
...	untranscribed, untranslated sign(s), word(s) or passage(s) of text
\	indented line
→	indicates the continuation of a line if one line in a given manuscript is spread over more than one line in the edition
+	joined to
(+)	indirectly joined to
BCE	Before Common Era, the equivalent of BC
CE	Common Era, the equivalent of AD
LB	Late Babylonian
lo.e.	lower edge
MA	Middle Assyrian
MB	Middle Babylonian
ms(s)	manuscript(s) (cuneiform tablet or fragment)
n', n"	line number (n) with a number of broken lines (x) preceding it (x+n, x+y+n, etc.)
NA	Neo-Assyrian
NB	Neo-Babylonian
OB	Old Babylonian
obv.	obverse
rev.	reverse

CHAPTER 1

Introduction

This monograph approaches ancient medicine through the study of a single individual who practiced magico-medical healing in ancient Mesopotamia. The healer's name was Kiṣir-Aššur and he was the grandson of Bāba-šuma-ibni, the patronymic ancestor of a family of exorcists. We know nothing about Kiṣir-Aššur's birth and death, except that he lived around the middle of the 7th century BCE in the ancient city of Assur, located some 100 kilometres south of Nineveh, present-day Mosul. Here he resided in the family home, the so-called "N4 house", and practiced the family trade, namely the exorcist's craft. Little is known about his personal life, but due to an abundance of textual sources relating to his profession it is possible to reconstruct and evaluate aspects of his education, career and practice as an exorcist (Akkadian *āšipu*/*mašmaššu*).

By the 7th century BCE, Assur was the religious centre of the Neo-Assyrian (NA) Empire whereas Nineveh was the political and intellectual capital. Although Assur had earlier been the political capital as well, it retained a special position, as it was still home to the temple of the national deity Aššur and the burial site of the NA kings. It was within this old city that Kiṣir-Aššur and his family practiced their trade as exorcists for private individuals and possibly also for official institutions. Here, the Bāba-šuma-ibni family assembled a large and private text collection pertaining to their profession as *āšipu*s, which provides information about their education, practice, and professional interests. In particular, the texts from this collection provide information regarding Kiṣir-Aššur's career.

This study focuses on how the Mesopotamian healer Kiṣir-Aššur was educated, how he practiced his craft, and how he produced and organized his knowledge, as revealed by his texts. Although some information is now lost, and although the N4 collection spans several generations and does not only contain texts that exclusively concern Kiṣir-Aššur's training and practice, the texts assigned to him can be allocated to specific phases of his career. They therefore provide information about his education and practice that can be used to discuss his production and use of scholarly texts. Through this mode of investigation, this study provides a rounded analysis of all aspects of an ancient healer's profession, and in turn assesses the socio-cultural aspects of healing in combination with analysing the magico-medical content. The monograph will thus improve our understanding of the functional aspects of texts in their specialist environment. The microhistorical description of Kiṣir-Aššur's education and career offered here is the first analysis with this level of detail of a single Mesopotamian healer's training and practice. Furthermore, to my knowledge, this work situates Kiṣir-Aššur as the earliest healer in world history for whom we have such details pertaining to his training and practice, which originates from his own time.

1.1 Colophons

Before examining the Mesopotamian magico-medical sources, practices and beliefs, as well as the problems related to studying Mesopotamian scholarship, it is necessary to understand how Kiṣir-Aššur is identified as a copyist and owner of the source material. Kiṣir-Aššur's cuneiform tablets can be identified through a subscript at the end of the texts called a colophon.[1] Colophons consisted of more or less formulaic elements describing from what manuscript the text was copied,[2] who copied, checked or owned the tablet, and what titles these individuals held at the time.[3] It is assumed that the copyists themselves wrote them.

Colophons from private text collections tend to be less formulaic than their official counterparts, for example, from the library of Assurbanipal, even though they do in some cases employ somewhat formulaic expressions.[4] As Kiṣir-Aššur is the subject of this study, the elements of his colophons are investigated throughout this work. The colophons enable us to examine the knowledge that was part of Kiṣir-Aššur's education and career and are therefore the basis for this work. For the purpose of this study, I use the terms "education", "training", and "career". The first two terms are used interchangeably to refer to Kiṣir-Aššur's written and practical schooling. The term "career" is used to designate progression in Kiṣir-Aššur's titles.

1.2 Mesopotamian Medicine

Any history of ancient medicine must be written on the basis of surviving manuscripts. Ancient Mesopotamia has left us a large corpus of medical and

1 For colophons in general, see Hunger 1968 and Leichty 1964.
2 Colophons can also provide a fictional history of a text, see Heeßel 2011: 171–76.
3 For the elements in colophons, see George 2010; Cavigneaux 1996; Pearce 1993; Cavigneaux 1981: 37; Borger 1970b; Hunger 1968: 1–15; Leichty 1964. See also Maul 2010a: 215; Gesche 2001: 153–66; Foster 1991: 18.
4 Stevens 2013: 212; Hunger 1968: 1, 15; Leichty 1964: 147.

magical literature, mostly dating to the first millennium BCE (Pedersén 1998). In general, studies in Mesopotamian medicine have increased since the early publications by Küchler (1904), Thompson (1923), Labat (1951), and Köcher (1955),[5] and the previous decades have seen a growth in publications on Mesopotamian medicine, healing practices, and professions.[6] Although many texts related to Mesopotamian healing have been passed down to us, these manuscripts are snapshots of specific times and particular places (Nutton 2004: 12). Therefore, tendencies to write overarching histories of medicine on the basis of preserved manuscripts must be nuanced with localized studies such as the present one. Furthermore, considerable information is lost today. Manuscripts have perished, oral traditions disappeared, and some knowledge was never committed to writing. Furthermore, specialist knowledge was not necessarily widely available, political upheaval could result in the disappearance of entire libraries, and the written medium and primary vernacular changed in the first millennium BCE (see Robson 2011a; Nutton 2004: 5–7). It is therefore necessary to consider when and where individual sources were copied, as well as what purpose the knowledge may have served to the copyist.

Another problem relates to the temporal distance. Over two and a half millennia separates the knowledge preserved in the surviving texts from the present day. In Assyriology, Landsberger's understanding of the "Eigenbegrifflichkeit" of Mesopotamian cultures, namely that Mesopotamian cultures cannot be adequately described by western terminology and definitions based on the Greek understanding of our world, is still justifiably discussed as a sound approach for examining the ancient texts.[7] In order to bridge the gap between the medicine of the modern and ancient world, this study draws on the works of Unschuld (2009: 2–6; ibid. 1980: 13–16), who saw illness as a subjective assessment of poor health influenced by a socio-political context. Yet, a society can operate with multiple explanatory models, of which some may have an objective medical factor defined by the respective culture. In some areas of medical anthropology, the term "disease" implies a biological understanding of the cause of illness and carries connotations of modern Western medicine.[8] However, Eisenberg (1977: 13) stressed "the discrepancy between disease as it is conceptualized by the physician and illness as it is experienced by the patient", and such a division of "disease" and "illness" may exist regardless of the culture in question (see also Kleinman 1980: 72–80). This view on the term "disease"

5 Also, e.g., Köcher 1963a–1971; Kinnier Wilson 1965; Biggs 1967; Golz 1974; Herrero 1984; van der Toorn 1985.

6 E.g., Böck 2014a; Scurlock 2014; Geller 2010; Scurlock and Andersen 2005; Heeßel 2000; Stol 1993. See the bibliography in Verderame 2012.

7 Landsberger 1926 and 1976; see Sallaberger 2007.

8 Kottak 2010: 63; see also Avalos 1995: 27.

is not completely anachronistic in regard to ancient Mesopotamia, seeing as cuneiform medical texts can contain traits of professional conceptualisations, which designate states of poor health. Another term useful for describing poor health is "sickness", describing "the process through which worrisome behavioural and biological signs, particularly ones originating in disease, are given socially recognizable meanings, i.e. they are made into symptoms and socially significant outcomes" (Young 1982: 270). Furthermore, terms such as "disorder" (e.g., Kleinman 1998: 389, 393) and possibly "syndrome" (e.g., Arbøll 2018a: 278–279) may be applied carefully to some aspects of ancient Mesopotamian medicine. Nonetheless, the words "illness" or "malady" are preferred throughout the present study, although I acknowledge that other terms concerning poor health can be applied to ancient Mesopotamian medicine.

1.2.1 *Magico-medical Healing*

The Mesopotamians did not distinguish between what we today label as "magic" and "medicine", instead believing that illnesses were caused by supernatural forces, such as gods or demons.[9] Once a patient was seized by an illness, healing could be achieved through identifying the ailment and the agent causing the malady and subsequently applying therapeutic or ritual treatments to cure the illness and its symptoms, as well as ritual actions to appease the god in question.[10] Some terms for ancient illnesses could refer to both the malady and the demon believed to be responsible for the affliction.[11] Mesopotamian healing therefore consisted of both magical and medical treatments, and some texts that researchers label "medical" contain a mix of diagnoses, symptom descriptions, prescriptions, incantations, and prayers, as well as religious

9 Scurlock 2014: 7; Böck 2009b; Scurlock 2006: 5–20; Heeßel 2000: 11–12, 49–53, 81–90, 94–96; Stol 1991–92: 42; Biggs 1995; Biggs 1987–90; van der Toorn 1985: 68–70. The body could perhaps malfunction on its own, see Scurlock 2014: 7. On the question of "natural" illnesses, see Collins 1999.

10 Koch unpublished; Heeßel 2000: 81–87, 94–96; see Böck 2014a: 3, 165, 171–72, 180; *CMAwR* 1: 1–2; Geller 2010: 9, 24–42; Stol 1991–92: 44–46. For therapeutic treatments, see Böck 2009a; Herrero 1984: 43–114; Golz 1974: 1–95. Note that the symptoms specified in such texts as appearing on the left/right side of the patient may have been described from the perspective of the healer, as suggested by Scurlock and Andersen (2005: xxii–xxiii). However, this suggestion remains a hypothesis.

11 Böck 2014a: 179. Few ancient illnesses can with certainty be identified as a modern disease, and applying retrospective diagnoses to ancient Mesopotamian medicine is generally problematic (see Arbøll 2018a: 261). Caution is therefore advised when drawing on studies of Mesopotamian medicine primarily employing retrospective diagnoses.

rituals.[12] Among the reasons for falling ill were sins committed in the past or witchcraft performed against the patient.[13] Illness, however, was not the only type of divine punishment and other examples include economic ruin or social ostracism.[14] All of these problems could be diagnosed and healed by the *āšipu*.[15]

Three generalized subcategories of texts are often recognized within the magico-medical corpus, namely diagnostic, therapeutic, and pharmaceutical texts (e.g., *CMAwR* 1: 8–9). There are no theoretical works on healing from ancient Mesopotamia (Geller 2010: 11; see Section 3.2). Diagnostic texts usually contain a symptom description, formulated as a conditional "if"-clause (*Šumma*-clause), and an illness diagnosis or information on the cause of the illness and occasionally a prognosis.[16] The therapeutic texts typically contain prescriptions with lists of ingredients for, e.g., potions, poultices, enemas, or amulets, and occasionally ritual instructions as well as incantations. Some prescriptions open with a symptom description or a diagnosis formulated as a *Šumma*-clause and others end with the name of the symptom or illness against which the prescription is considered useful (see, e.g., Johnson 2015: 308; Wee 2012: 198–200). The pharmaceutical texts provide information about individual plants or other ingredients against certain symptoms or illnesses, how they are administered, their appearance, or alternative names.[17] It is often unknown how much of the written material related to the *āšipu* was actually put to use.[18] Although the above grouping of magico-medical texts places manuscripts with magical and medical content together, it is clear that these could serve specific purposes as approaches to achieve healing.[19]

---

12 See references in Ch. 1 note 10. A prime example combining both approaches remains the "rubbing" *muššu'u* ritual (Böck 2007; Böck 2003).

13 Böck 2014a: 193; *CMAwR* 1: 2–8; Maul 2004: 93; Stol 1991–92: 46–47; van der Toorn 1985. A proper study of what it meant to be ill (*marāṣu*) is still a *desideratum*; for now, see Stol 2009b.

14 This is described alongside various other maladies in *Ludlul bēl nēmeqi* (Lambert 1996: 32–36; see Annus and Lenzi 2010: 31–33). See also *CMAwR* 1: 3, 5; Schwemer 2007a: 132, 147, 168, 170, 178, 181–82, 252, 279.

15 The *āšipu* is occasionally advised not to provide a prognosis of the patient's illness in Sa-gig (Scurlock 2014: 188, 208). In the literary text *Ludlul bēl nēmeqi*, the exorcist cannot diagnose the patient's illness, and, thus, he cannot bring about its cure (Lambert 1996: 38–39, 44–45; Annus and Lenzi 2010: 35, 37).

16 E.g., Heeßel 2000; Labat 1951.

17 E.g., Attia and Buisson 2012; Böck 2011; Kinnier Wilson 2005; Köcher 1955.

18 Robson 2008: 474; Heeßel 2000: 92–4; for a discussion of the astrological-astronomical literature used in practice, see Veldhuis 2010.

19 Geller (2016: 30) saw these approaches as complementary, in which medicine could "alleviate the symptoms and distress of disease", whereas "magic was required to elucidate

The term "healing" is used here to describe the ancient magico-medical approaches for diagnosing and treating illness as well as ensuring social, physical, or mental wellbeing.[20] This provides us with a holistic term that can account for the incongruous, but practical, division of healing into "magical" and "medical" practices, as long as we disregard any loaded meaning of the term.[21] Nonetheless, the analytical terms "medicine" and "magic" are unavoidable when analysing Mesopotamian healing practices,[22] although they have several connotations. Medicine implies rationality and an empirically based Western medical science (Heeßel 2009: 13–14; Scurlock 1999: 69), whereas the term "magic" is a polemic concept with connotations of irrational and superstitious ritual practices.[23] However, there is no equivalent to the term "magic" native to Mesopotamia.

In the early days of studying Mesopotamian medicine, this dichotomous division of the healing arts was transferred diachronically onto two main healing disciplines: the craft of the "physician" (*asû*) and the "exorcist" (*āšipu*, Ritter 1965; see Section 1.2.3). Today, it is clear that medicine and magic in the first millennium cannot be assigned to either profession exclusively (see recently May 2018). Yet, magico-medical material is still occasionally assigned to these disciplines according to various principles.[24] However, such divisions are rarely reflected in the context of the manuscripts investigated.[25] Medical and magical approaches to healing in ancient Mesopotamia are therefore still discussed as separate entities, although the abandonment of such a distinction has been recommended (Robson 2008: 476–477). Though the form and content of these approaches may have differed, they were clearly intertwined

the nature and cause of illness", i.e., it functioned as theory (see also Geller 2007b; Geller 1999). However, the view on magic's role in healing differs between researchers (see, e.g., Böck 2014a: 185–186).

20 A concise definition can be found in Ember and Ember 2004: xxxi. See Unschuld 2009: 6–7; Robson 2008: 276–77; see also Koch unpublished.

21 See discussion with references in Koch unpublished.

22 Geller 2016: 33; Böck 2014a: 176–85; Schwemer 2011: 419; Geller 2010: 8–10; Heeßel 2009: 13–14; Geller 2007b: 389.

23 Schwemer 2015: 17; Sørensen 2013: 230–32; see Böck 2014a: 176–78; Sørensen 2007: 32.

24 E.g., in discussions of Mesopotamian magic, high-prose incantations have been suggested to belong to the lore of the *āšipu*, while crude spells belong to the lore of the *asû* (van Binsbergen and Wiggermann 1999: 29–30; cf. Böck 2014a: 186ff.). Johnson (2018) recently suggested a difference in disease aetiologies between the two disciplines.

25 Although the AMC may have been linked to the craft of the *asû* (see Steinert 2018c: 178ff.), it included many magical elements (see Section 9.3.2). Furthermore, May (2018: 71) has suggested that the copyist of the AMC was related to Kiṣir-Aššur.

approaches for healing in Kiṣir-Aššur's texts. Thus, at his time we may see them as part of a healing system with a fusion of views (Böck 2014a: 180).

As a result of the inherent biases, some researchers consider the term "magic" best abandoned (e.g., Smith 2004: 218), while others have argued for the validity of "magic" as a scientific concept,[26] also within Assyriology (e.g., Schwemer 2011: 419–420). In relation to Mesopotamia, magical acts are part of rituals, which in turn are cultural practices often considered to be part of the religious sphere.[27] Although magic is often considered to be something predating or operating between religion and science, resembling as well as contrasting elements of both (Smith 2004: 215–18; see Sørensen 2013: 242), magic must be considered as being linked to ritual and thereby to religion in Mesopotamia (Farber 1995: 1895–96). However, medicine in Mesopotamia must also be considered interrelated with both religion and magic (Böck 2014a: 176).

Magic and medicine were intermingled in NA healing. They are useful terms for discussing Kiṣir-Aššur's manuscripts, although they should not be used to force unwarranted meanings of efficacy or rationality onto the texts. Both types of treatments were clearly considered legitimate approaches to healing by the ancient practitioners. This monograph therefore draws on the terms "magic", "medicine" and "ritual", while always being conscious of their inherent connotations. Throughout this work, the term "ritual" is mainly used as an analytical category to distinguish between different texts, thereby analytically identifying their content based on primarily "magical" components.[28]

1.2.2 *The* āšipu-/mašmaššu-*exorcist*

The *āšipu*, also transcribed as *mašmaššu*, was one of five main scholarly professions throughout the NA period alongside the *asû* "physician", *ṭupšarru* "scribe" or *ṭupšar Enūma Anu Enlil* "astrologer", *kalû* "lamentation priest", and *bārû* "diviner".[29] The *āšipu* was primarily concerned with magico-medical healing and diagnosing causes of problems for clients, and he could perform rituals for the city, the cults, and the court.[30] Among his tools were numerous rituals, medical remedies, prayers, and incantations (Schwemer 2011: 423–26). His duties overlapped with the *asû* and *bārû* in terms of medical treatments and

26 See, e.g., Sørensen 2013; Sørensen 2007; cf. Smith 2004: 218.

27 See Bell 1997: 20–21, 80, 164, 267. For a definition of religion, see Lincoln 2003: 5–8; Boyer 2002.

28 See Section 1.2.3. For the term "magic" used in Assyriology, see, e.g., Geller 2016: 27–32; Schwemer 2015: 19; Böck 2014a: 178; Schwemer 2011: 420; Geller 1999; van Binsbergen and Wiggermann 1999; cf. Robson 2008: 476; Scurlock 2002b.

29 Parpola 1993: XIII–XIV.

30 Koch 2015: 20–21; Schwemer 2011: 421–23; Jean 2006: 83–143, 183–84.

diagnostic-prognostic practice.[31] In accordance with his duties, the *āšipu* is ordinarily translated as, e.g., "exorcist, conjurer" or "Beschwörungspriester".[32] Although such translations are inadequate and often incorrect in describing his competences and duties, this study adopts the translation "exorcist" for the sake of convenience.

The exorcist is typically referred to by the Sumerogram MAŠ.MAŠ in first millennium BCE sources. Yet, it is often uncertain whether MAŠ.MAŠ should be transcribed as *āšipu* or *mašmaššu*.[33] Various texts equate the Sumerogram lúMAŠ.MAŠ with *āšipu* or *mašmaššu*,[34] but it is largely unclear if these readings differed or could be used interchangeably.[35] Throughout this study, the transcriptions *āšipu* and *mašmaššu* are used interchangeably because the secondary literature uses both.

1.2.3 *Genres of Texts*

The ancient Mesopotamians did not group their texts according to modern taxonomies of genres. As a result, modern genres are often applied anachronistically to group the magico-medical texts and rituals studied here.[36] Such an approach runs the risk of decontextualizing the formal labels used within the ancient texts to categorize the content, such as incantations or prayers introduced by ÉN (Lambert 2008), ritual instructions introduced by DÙ.DÙ.BI (Maul 2009), remedies as well as some ritual procedures labelled as *bulṭu* (Steinert 2018c: 179 note 112), or particular types of texts such as *namburbi*-rituals.[37] Earlier studies divided magico-medical texts into dichotomous groups of knowledge in which the *āšipu* was interpreted as practicing magic to cure "supernatural" causes of illness and the *asû* practiced "rational" medicine to "natural" causes of illness (Ritter 1965; see Herrero 1984: 22–24, 38). This dichotomy was continuously discussed[38] and Scurlock (1999: 78–79) suggested the *asû* and *āšipu* could have functioned respectively as pharmacist and physician. Scurlock's suggestion has been criticized in various recent studies,[39] and

31 Koch 2015: 20–21; see Heeßel 2009: 14 and note 6; Robson 2008: 472–74.

32 E.g., Schwemer 2011: 418; Geller 2010: 45ff.; Maul 2010a; Stol 1991–92: 42, 62; Lambert 1967: 107; cf. Jean 2006: 22, 52; Sallaberger and Vulliet 2005. See Koch unpublished.

33 For possible etymologies, see Geller 2010: 43–44; Jean 2006: 19–21.

34 Jean 2006: 22–31; see Geller 2010: 43–50.

35 Geller 2010: 48–50; Attinger 2008: 76; Geller 2007c: 1–4, 8; Jean 2006: 17, 23–24, 35–37.

36 See Michalowski 1999; Vanstiphout 1999; Röllig 1987–90: 48ff.; Vanstiphout 1986.

37 Maul 1994; see *CMAwR* 1: 9–10; Rochberg 2010: 23–24.

38 E.g., Biggs 1995: 1914, 1918–20; Stol 1991–92: 49, 58–62 and note 103; Golz 1974: 9–14; Labat 1952.

39 E.g., Heeßel 2009; Geller 2007c; Zucconi 2007: 19. See also Geller 2010: 43, 50–52; Robson 2008: 475; Jean 2006: 14–15. For recent discussions of magico-medical scholarly knowledge

during Kiṣir-Aššur's time these professions must have overlapped and functioned complementary.[40] In Assur at Kiṣir-Aššur's time the craft of the *āšipu* was a healing art drawing on a multitude of magical and medical approaches, including those of the *asû*, for averting disaster, removing ill omens as well as sickness, and preserving health (Maul 2019: 26 note 3).

Grouping texts according to modern principles is never straightforward. Nevertheless, I assign Kiṣir-Aššur's manuscripts to groups of texts with "medical", "ritual", or "other" content: medical texts consist of diagnoses, symptom descriptions, prescriptions, ritual instructions and incantations intended to soothe an affliction of the body or the mind; the ritual texts contain incantations, prayers, and ritual instructions for appeasing causes of illness, removing negative omens, and other purposes; and the "other" group comprises texts that do not fit into either of these categories. The terms are solely intended to divide Kiṣir-Aššur's texts roughly according to content for the reader's convenience. The categories are admittedly problematic, seeing as texts labelled as "medical" can also include incantations and ritual instructions, and texts labelled as "ritual" could in some cases be used to appease the divine cause of an illness or remove omens leading to sickness. Thus, texts in both categories would have been part of a shared framework of healing, although they are grouped differently.

1.3 Authorship

A number of problems associated with the study of Mesopotamian scholarly knowledge concern the lack of known authorship and the anonymity of cuneiform literature. Furthermore, the textual traditions of scholarly knowledge have in recent decades been shown to be more diverse and individually founded than previously imagined. The question is, of course, whether Kiṣir-Aššur was really the author or merely the copyist of the texts that bear his colophons. We know that Mesopotamian literature was by and large anonymous (Lambert 1957: 1). Authors can rarely be identified (cf. Foster 1996: 20 and note 2), and there are few text-internal references to composers[41] or to a specific editor (George 2003: 28–33; Lambert 1962: 66–67, 77). Catalogues of texts

---

in relation to *āšipūtu* and *asûtu*, see Geller 2018b; Johnson 2018; Panayotov 2018b: 90–91; Steinert 2018a: 90ff.; Steinert 2018b: 13; Steinert 2018c: 187, 189 and note 165, 190–191.

40 A N4 text (*BAM* 199 obv. 10) describes the production of a medical "ointment" that is later classified as (rev. 14): "a [sec]ret of the *mašmaššu*". See also Johnson 2018: 56–57; Panayotov 2018b: 90 and note 18; Böck 2014a: 28; Schwemer 2011: 423; Robson 2008: 472–76.

41 Lambert 1996: 63; Foster 1991: 17; see Hecker 1977: 248–49; Lambert 1967; Hallo 1962: 14–15.

and authors show that Mesopotamian scholars of the NA period were concerned with tracing certain texts or text series back to gods, sages and legendary scholars (Lambert 1962), although this information must be considered unrealistic (Foster 1991: 18, 31). Cuneiform scholarship depended on textual transmission through education (Robson 2011a: 562), and evidence of changes occurs regularly as a result (Worthington 2012: 5–7, 16–28). It is possible that oral traditions also played a substantial role in the transmission of knowledge.[42] A single author of scholarly texts therefore rarely existed and many "authors" were often involved in forming a certain composition (Foster 1991: 17–19 and note 7). Several individuals attributed with "authorship" were probably authors, editors, redactors, or something in between.[43]

Throughout this work, the words "written" and "copied" are used interchangeably to describe Kiṣir-Aššur and other scholars' act of copying and writing a text from, e.g., another manuscript, memory, or dictation onto the cuneiform tablet investigated. Therefore, this monograph explicitly notes whenever questions of authorship, redaction, or creativity are addressed.

1.4 Proof and Possibility

The present study presupposes the existence of a correlation between content and purpose at the point when texts were copied.[44] To clarify, I do not propose a direct correlation between writing a text and acquiring medical expertise in the relevant area or applying the text directly in practice. The function of a text could vary. As I argue throughout this study, Kiṣir-Aššur's texts may generally have been related to practicing the knowledge found therein, as part of a training curriculum he needed to learn regardless of applicability, to improve his understanding of what was described in the text, or a combination of these areas. The purpose has to be evaluated through careful analyses of individual manuscripts and their colophons. Admittedly, only texts with so-called "purpose statements" (Section 7.4) can be directly related to practice. Still, the Bāba-šuma-ibni family were *āšipu*s, who must have been engaged in healing activities. Therefore, it is justifiable to presuppose that texts copied

42 See Worthington 2012: 7–13; Frahm 2011a: 43–45, 87, 322; Foster 1991: 31; Elman 1975; Læssøe 1953: 212–13.

43 Frahm 2011a: 334–32; Rutz 2011: 299 and note 21; George 2003: 32–33; Finkel 1988: 144–45; Hallo 1962: 14–15; see Geller 1990.

44 See, e.g., Section 7.4; cf. Couto-Ferreira 2018: 163. Although the purposes of texts may be elusive, they are important for reconstructing the context and use of ancient knowledge (see Rochberg 2016: 32).

during their training must have served educational purposes with a practical dimension (see Maul 2010a: 216). Each text likely provided concrete knowledge, which could be considered useful in some form for their practice.

A microhistoric approach is employed for investigating Kiṣir-Aššur's texts (Section 2.1). In microhistory, gaps in the evidence are welcomed as part of the account, by accepting the limitations while exploring the inherent implications (Ginzburg 2012: 208–209). Some microhistorians therefore allow the conditional and the speculative in order to go beyond the information obtained from a given source (Tivellato 2015: 128). By researching sources from similar or contemporary geographical, social and cultural domains to illuminate the subject's world, it is therefore possible to carefully combine "proof" with "possibility" (Ginzburg 2012: 57; Davis 1985: 5).

As outlined in Section 2.3.1, the N4 text collection consists of limited and incomplete textual evidence. Furthermore, the magico-medical corpus of Mesopotamian healing generally comprises prescriptions, diagnoses, rituals and recitations, which are mainly anonymously authored, stylistically locked in rhetoric, and seemingly detached from theory and practice (Sections 1.2.3 and 1.3). Due to the nature of the material, my approach combines "proofs", i.e., information provided by a source alone, with "possibility", i.e., rigorously researched hypotheses and carefully argued speculations, in order to outline the otherwise inaccessible contours of an ancient healer's training and practice. Such a method is sure to raise objections in Assyriology, although I hold a distinct line between argumentation and meticulously reasoned hypotheses on the one hand, and wild and free guesswork on the other. Therefore, what some readers may mistake for straightforward conclusions or equivocations are in fact carefully formulated hypotheses and suggestions. As a result of this approach and its caveats, the impact that the identified individual magico-medical focuses might have had on Kiṣir-Aššur's training and practice is likely to be subject to interpretation in future studies, regardless of how probable specific assessments may be.

1.5 Scope and Structure

This study comprises ten chapters, which are structured around the various phases of Kiṣir-Aššur's career and the groups of texts assigned to each phase. Where there are relatively few texts assigned to a phase, several phases have been grouped together in a single chapter.

Chapter 2 provides the framework for the study by defining the microhistorical approach and its applicability here. It furthermore offers an overview of the previous research on and a description of Kiṣir-Aššur and the Bāba-šuma-ibni family. This chapter sets the stage for the analysis of Kiṣir-Aššur's texts within the N4 collection.

Chapter 3 focuses on Kiṣir-Aššur's earliest attested career phase, the *šamallû ṣeḫru*-phase. Kiṣir-Aššur copied a number of medical texts during this period, and the chapter discusses their diagnoses in relation to Kiṣir-Aššur's medical proficiency. It is proposed here that Kiṣir-Aššur's anatomical and physiological understanding, as well as his diagnostic capabilities, were trained during this phase.

In chapter 4, I discuss physiological aspects of Kiṣir-Aššur's training as *šamallû ṣeḫru* by contextualizing the snakebites, scorpion stings, and horse illnesses treated in *RA* 15 pl. 76. I explore the role of venom in Kiṣir-Aššur's anatomical understanding by proposing a new framework for the cultural and scholarly understanding of venom in relation to symptoms and illnesses, according to which venom, bile, and saliva may have provided an interspecies conceptual framework for understanding human physiology. Here, I also address the role of veterinarian knowledge in Kiṣir-Aššur's education.

Kiṣir-Aššur's *šamallû-*, *šamallû mašmaššu ṣeḫru-*, and *mašmaššu ṣeḫru*-phases, for which only a few texts are attested, are studied in chapter 5. The texts from these phases indicate that Kiṣir-Aššur copied rituals connected to private religion and a text to calm a child. On the basis of the child treatment, the chapter contextualizes the text by discussing paediatricians in Mesopotamia and provides a hypothesis suggesting that Kiṣir-Aššur may have worked with greater autonomy on animals first and children secondarily, before moving on to adults later.

Chapter 6 scrutinizes the texts from Kiṣir-Aššur's *mašmaššu*-phase and I argue that he began conducting house calls and organizing healing rituals during this phase. Furthermore, contemporary evidence indicates that he protected households prophylactically from illness and epidemics and that such rituals may have functioned as quarantine measures. Additionally, a number of *namburbi*-rituals from this and Kiṣir-Aššur's later *mašmaš bīt Aššur*-phase may relate to conducting house calls and supervising rituals. Furthermore, a single lexical text possibly attests to Kiṣir-Aššur's scholarly training during this phase.

Chapter 7 studies a number of texts with colophons that do not contain titles or are broken, which are relevant for an understanding of Kiṣir-Aššur's career. On the basis of text-internal features, this chapter argues that a number of texts should be assigned to the *mašmaššu-* and *mašmaš bīt Aššur*-phases of Kiṣir-Aššur's career. In particular, the addition of so-called "purpose statements", i.e., statements designating the tablet as produced for preparing a ritual, are argued to stem from his *mašmaššu*-phase and later. The chapter also discusses two texts possibly consisting of commentaries.

Chapter 8 investigates the texts from Kiṣir-Aššur's final career phase, the *mašmaš bīt Aššur*-phase. The content of three large groups of medical, ritual, and other texts, of which the last group was associated with the Aššur temple, are investigated. In connection with the medical texts, the chapter offers a case study of the prescriptions labelled as "tested". This chapter also discusses a text labelled as a panacea, i.e., a universal prescription, as well as Kiṣir-Aššur's use of medical incantations.

Chapter 9 provides a general outlook on Kiṣir-Aššur's overall knowledge production. It is argued that Kiṣir-Aššur may have focused on certain areas of medicine during his career. This chapter also addresses the question of numbered extract texts and their interpretation, as well as the catch-lines and their relationship to the therapeutic series Ugu and the Assur Medical Compendium. I further examine the relationship between Kiṣir-Aššur's career and the Exorcist's Manual, which is considered to be a list comprising major works of the *āšipu*'s knowledge base. These preliminary results are contextualized within the larger framework of local knowledge in Assur and Nineveh.

A summary and synthesis of the most important results is presented in chapter 10.

CHAPTER 2

Framework and Background

On the 31st of August 658 BCE Kisir-Aššur quickly extracted select parts of a ritual to remove a ghost and copied them onto a manuscript.[1] On this day, he may have been sitting in the paved courtyard outside the scholarly library of his family home in the middle of Assur (Section 2.3). Let us imagine him sitting on the ground in the sunny yard, holding a moist clay tablet in one hand and a stylus in the other, ready to imprint the clay with cuneiform signs reproducing the original manuscript in front of him containing a complex ritual text.[2] As Kisir-Aššur scans the longer cuneiform tablet, which was a copy of knowledge transmitted for generations by scholarly families in the city of Assur, his eyes fall on the first incantation he needs on this very day, and he drafts this and related paragraphs onto the excerpt manuscript in hand. Having quickly copied all the required sections, Kisir-Aššur checks his copy against the original, he writes a colophon stating that the text is a hastily produced extract copied from and checked against its original, and finally he inscribes his name and records the date.

The narrative above is fiction, although the discussed text is not. Known today as *KAR* 267, this manuscript's text and colophon provide us with information about the tablet's content and context (see Appendix 2). But how is it possible to use such information for analyzing Kiṣir-Aššur's education and career? This chapter provides the framework for conducting a microhistorical study of Kiṣir-Aššur as an *āšipu*-exorcist in a specific context at a certain place during a particular period. The study draws on the theory of microhistory as an analytical approach for studying smaller and select groups of texts to access previously unseen or otherwise unattainable information. Although there are inherent dangers of circular arguments within this analytical approach, ways of safeguarding such pitfalls are explored in the first section. The second section explores the methodological tools used, thereby providing an outline of how Kiṣir-Aššur's material is dissected throughout the following chapters.

1 The manuscript is *KAR* 267, and it was dated to the 9th of the month *Ulūlu*, see Section 7.5 and Appendix 1. The date above is calculated on the basis of Parpola's table for converting Assyrian dates into Julian ones (Parpola 1983a: 382). He states the 1st of *Ulūlu* corresponds to the 23rd of August in the year 658 BCE. The 9th must therefore correspond to the 31st.

2 The manuscripts investigated in this study consist of clay tablets with cuneiform writing. The texts are composed in the artificial literary dialect Standard Babylonian, which was based on the Old Babylonian dialect of the Semitic language Akkadian.

Finally, this chapter provides a detailed discussion of the previous research on Kiṣir-Aššur, the Bāba-šuma-ibni family and their tablet collection.

2.1 Microhistory

Microhistory is an analytical approach employing a reduced scale of observation for the intensive study of select texts to reveal information previously unseen or considered unattainable. This approach primarily uses philology to investigate the (extraordinary) documentation of a clearly defined small-scale area of interest, e.g., an event, a community, a family, or an individual person, and thereby illuminate the underlying structures of the subject.[3] Therefore, microhistory challenges and contrasts quantitative datasets by analysing structures that are not reflected in the main bulk of historic documentation and cannot be recovered through conventional approaches.[4] The method therefore allows "concrete individual or local experience to re-enter history" (Burke 2008: 45).

Microhistory became well-known throughout the late 1970s and 1980s (Muir 1991: vii). Several of the most influential researchers of this period were affiliated with the so-called "Italian school" of microhistory, and one of the foremost works produced during this time remains the pioneering work *The Cheese and the Worms* by Carlo Ginzburg (1980).[5] Broadly, the Italian school of microhistory searches for information concerning particular beliefs or behaviour among social groups or milieus that may seem exceptional in relation to the contemporary political or religious norms.[6] In several ways, microhistory draws indirectly on anthropology by employing an emic approach seeking to understand and describe the people and cultures investigated on their own terms (Muir 1991: xi, xiii-xiv; Levi 1991: 98).[7]

Microhistory is rarely considered a theory as such, but rather a "historiographical practice" that draws on theoretical references in an eclectic manner

3 Szijártó 2013a: 4–5; Ginzburg 2012: 203, 213; Ginzburg and Poni 1991: 3–4, 5, 8–9; Levi 1991: 95, 97, 107, 109; Muir 1991: ix–x; Ginzburg 1990: ix–x, 164; Ginzburg 1980: xiii–xiv, xx, 126.

4 Ginzburg 2012: 212–13; Gregory 1999: 102; Ginzburg and Poni 1991: 7–8; Levi 1991: 105; Ginzburg 1980: xiii, xv.

5 For a discussion of the history of the term "microhistory", see Ginzburg 2012; Muir 1991. For an overview of Ginzburg's impact and criticism of his work, see Szijártó 2013a: 3–4; Schutte 1976.

6 Ginzburg and Poni 1991: 8; Muir 1991: xiv; Levi 1991: 94–95; see Ginzburg 2012: 202; Szijártó 2013a: 5.

7 The term "culture" is here loosely defined. I realize that the term has problematic implications, but as it is not employed as a fundamental term in this study I refer the reader to Burke (2008).

(Levi 1991: 93, 99–101). Giovanni Levi, another pioneer of the Italian school of microhistory, describes it as follows:

> Microhistory, in common with all experimental work, has no body of established orthodoxy to draw on.
>
> LEVI 1991: 93

As a result of microhistory's theoretical eclecticism, this methodological approach contains some inherent problems. One problem concerns "selectivity and significance" (Muir 1991: xiv). Due to the focus on qualitative over quantitative documentation, it is the historian's responsibility to avoid overemphasizing particular details when forming arguments. Another problem relates to the significance of spectacular observations within the select and often limited empirical basis for broader social groups or macrohistorical arguments.[8] As a result, conclusions reached through microhistorical studies cannot automatically be transferred to a general historic sphere (see Ginzburg 2012: 207; Levi 1991: 109; Ginzburg 1980: xx–xxi). Yet, a certain interdependence must be accepted. Muir (1991: xix) noted that "microhistorical arguments, especially those devoted to some form of cultural interpretation, are vulnerable to circularity", because the interpretations presuppose, in Ginzburg's words, "a reciprocal interchange between the whole and the parts" (Ginzburg 1985: 21; see also Simon 2015: 237).

Therefore, microhistory can provide nuanced and extraordinary information about aspects of society, its cultures, as well as individual persons, although it risks producing idiosyncratic and even trivial results. This needs to be evaluated in each specific case. Furthermore, microhistory cannot be produced devoid of general historical context, and the influence of the two upon each other risks creating circular arguments (Ginzburg 1985: 21). Two means, both of which are employed throughout this study, serve to safeguard against such circular arguments: 1) the combination of exposing formal analogies within a limited dataset with verifying these through external evidence, and 2) the use of Occam's Razor to evaluate the interpretation with minimal hypotheses or variables as the most probable (Muir 1991: xix; see Ginzburg 1985: 21).

2.2 Framework

In order to properly analyse Kiṣir-Aššur's texts via the microhistorical approach and extract useful information, it is necessary to establish a methodological

8 Muir 1991: xiv; see also Gregory 1999: 106, 108–109; Levi 1991: 95.

framework. Using the archaeological information available, Kiṣir-Aššur's cuneiform tablets are investigated as part of a specific collection, as groups, as individual manuscripts, and in relation to their content to gain information about the use and functions of Kiṣir-Aššur's tablets in relation to his training and career.[9] This study primarily uses philology to investigate Kiṣir-Aššur's manuscripts by providing thorough readings of texts or select passages to scrutinize particular vocabulary and investigate grammatical features and syntax in order to understand a text and outline its meaning (George 2007: 37). This approach is combined with recent advancements in Mesopotamian textual criticism (e.g., Delnero 2012; Worthington 2012). In relation to NA texts, textual criticism broadly involves studying minute textual changes in duplicate manuscripts and the mechanisms behind these, e.g., by identifying errors of transmission, to gain information about the methods and competences of the transmitters of the texts.[10]

One premise of this study is that Kiṣir-Aššur's surviving cuneiform tablets with colophons can be used as the basis for partially reconstructing the content and structure of his education, training, and career, thereby improving our understanding of Kiṣir-Aššur's career development. Three methodological issues related to this problem must be considered: 1) the danger of assigning too much significance to individual pieces of surviving evidence and observations acquired through studying the texts, 2) the unknown impact of oral training, which could account for knowledge taught to Kiṣir-Aššur by his father or other practitioners, which is not preserved in the surviving evidence, and 3) the nature of the N4 cuneiform tablet collection compared to other contemporary collections. The first issue relates to the general problem of microhistorical studies, whereas the second issue is difficult to account for. The third issue is discussed below to provide the background necessary for studying Kiṣir-Aššur (see Section 2.3.1). Throughout this work, these issues are addressed in order to contextualize specific findings.

Kiṣir-Aššur was part of the scholarly elite in Assur, although Robson (2019: 256) describes his family as part of "the urban middle classes". Still, subjects of microhistorical studies need not necessarily consist of common people (Lepore 2001: 131). Therefore, microhistory can also be an effective tool when

9 For contextualizing texts in relation to their collections, see, e.g., Robson 2013; du Toit 1998: 392; Veenhof 1986a: 35–36; Reade 1986: 222. For specific studies, see, e.g., Tanret 2011; Maul 2010a; Heeßel 2009; Frahm 1999; Radner 1999b. According to Robson, we should move from studying "tablets as witnesses of scholarly compositions" to analysing them as artefacts derived from "historically situated individuals" (Robson 2011a: 572–73).

10 Worthington 2012: 38–40. It should be emphasized that textual criticism can be problematic in relation to the evaluation of ancient textual variation or mistakes (Brisch 2015; see also Delnero 2012: 179–80; Worthington 2012: 41ff.).

studying individuals situated within spheres of power (e.g., Ginzburg 2015). Kiṣir-Aššur is interesting because he was not attached to the royal court, but part of a local scholarly elite situated outside the seat of power. Furthermore, his family's text collection is the largest assembly of magico-medical cuneiform texts excavated outside of the royal libraries, and it is crucial for our reconstruction of Mesopotamian healing.

Microhistory often approaches "through the anomalous, not the analogous" (Ginzburg 2012: 212–213), and thereby it attempts to solve small mysteries to elucidate broader historical questions (e.g., Lepore 2001: 133; Joyner 1999: 1). This is mirrored in my examinations of Kiṣir-Aššur's texts within the broader context of, e.g., anatomical and physiological knowledge as well as veterinarian medicine in Chapter 4, and paediatricians in Section 5.2.2. As the subjects of microhistorical studies are often devices for answering larger questions, the approach differs from biography (Lepore 2001). Therefore, this focus on hitherto unexplored avenues for reconstructing the education, practice and knowledge of a Mesopotamian healing professional establishes a foundation for future inquiries into these areas.

2.3 Background for Studying Kiṣir-Aššur

The so-called "N4 library" or "Haus des Beschwörungspriesters" consisted of a private house located to the east or southeast of the original city centre in Assur (see Frahm 2011a: 268; Pedersén 1986: 41ff.). This building was home to the Bāba-šuma-ibni family and it contained their tablet collection.[11] The structure was partly uncovered during the German excavations from 1903–1914, and the Iraqi excavations during the 1970s and 1980s continued to investigate the area.[12] However, the complete layout of the N4 house remains unknown.

11 Maul 2010a: 190–92, 224; Pedersén 1998: 135–36; Pedersén 1986: 41–76.

12 The house was excavated in the areas hC8I, hD8I, and hE8I (Miglus 1996: 236–37 and pls. 40–41, 132; see Maul 2010a: 224 figure 3; Pedersén 1985: 41; Jordan 1908: 40; cf. ibid.: 38, 43; Andrae 1910: 35). The German expediton, however, did not expose the entire house. As a result, the original interpretation did not link the areas hC-hE8I as a single home (cf. Preusser 1954: 58, pl. 27a). Parts of N4 were excavated during the Iraqi excavations in the 1970s and 80s (Jean 2006: 147; Pedersén 1998: 136 note 11; Ismail 1982). However, it remains unclear during which years the Iraqis excavated in which parts of the house (cf. Anonymous 1981: 173; see Miglus 2006: 146). Radner (1997: 290 and notes 1591–92) stated that the entire house was unearthed during the Iraqi excavations and refered to Finkbeiner and Pongratz-Leisten (1992). However, this map shows an out-dated layout of N4 (see Cavigneaux and Ismail 1998: 1). See Fadhil (2018: 192) for an overview of the excavated tablets and future publications.

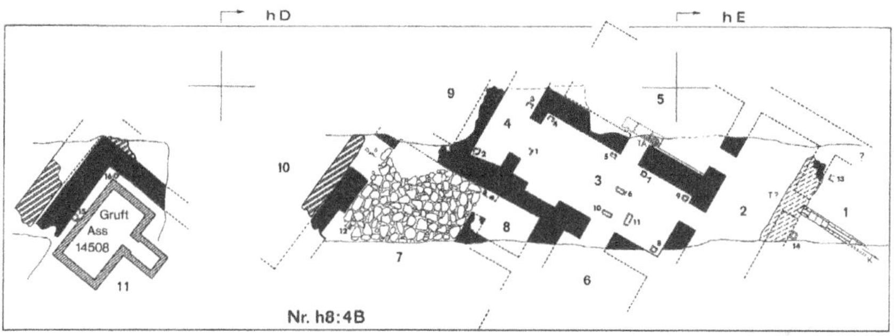

FIGURE 1 The N4 house (Miglus 1996: pl. 132d, reproduced with permission)

Figure 1 shows the layout of the building from the time of the Bāba-šuma-ibni family. Below I will summarize the most important features of the home before discussing the family's tablet collection.

According to Miglus (1996: 237–38) and Pedersén (1986: 41–43 and note 2), the unexcavated entrance of the house probably lay to the southeast. Presumably, the red painted room 3 was once the main room of the house.[13] To the south, room 6 must have led northwest through the unexcavated room(s) to the inner courtyard 7, which contained stone paving.[14] This inner courtyard led to room 10 in its northernmost part. It was in room 10 that the majority of cuneiform tablets were discovered.[15] Further west, the excavators found a

13 This room contained a niche to the left of the entrance from room 6 and another door between room 3 and 5 contained stone covered pivots (Pedersén 1986: 41; see Miglus 1996: 238). May (2018: 64 and notes 4–5) interprets the layout of rooms 3–4 as a "bent axis", largely similar to those found in temples, some palaces or state buildings. Many magical figurines were found underneath the floors of these rooms. Perhaps the family performed rituals here for themselves or clients (Robson 2019: 130; May 2018: 64).

14 Between room 10 and courtyard 7 excavators found two parallel foundations of walls (Miglus 1996: 238). The northwest one was 0,3 m deeper than the southeast one (ibid.; cf. Maul 2010a: 190–92; Pedersén 1986: 41, note 4). Miglus suggested that the northwest foundation was the remains of an older wall separating room 10 and courtyard 7 (Miglus 1996: 238). Pedersén used the excavation report stating that the tablets were found underneath a house to suggest this "house" may have been the northwest wall (Pedersén 1986: 42 and note 4). This remains unclear. Note that the N4 house may have been sold during Sîn-šar-iškun's reign (Böhme 2010). The N4 house was possibly destroyed in a fire, most likely during the (partial) destruction of Assur in 614 BCE (Maul 2010a: 190–92). Therefore, the house was mostly empty. It has been presumed that original shelves for storing tablets, household goods, furniture, and other equipment were burned in antiquity or destroyed (Maul 2003: 176; see Miglus 1996: 236–41).

15 Room 10 was probably the "library room". Pedersén (1986: 42 and note 6) states that his text groups C, D, G, L, M and perhaps including H, I, N, O, and Q are all from room 10 (see

vaulted underground grave in room 11, which unfortunately had been robbed in antiquity (see Haller 1954: 163 no. 67 = Ass. 14508). Room 11 contained the outer wall of the western part of the N4 house, as well as a small group of administrative tablets and an ivory writing-board.[16] A relatively large number of apotropaic figurines and clay plaques depicting various protective beings were found beneath the floors and thresholds of rooms 1, 3, 4, 7, 10 and 11 in clay brick boxes, jars and small clay pods.[17]

2.3.1 *The N4 Tablet Collection*

The tablets excavated in N4 constitute the largest text collection from the city of Assur, and so far, 1,242 cuneiform tablets and fragments have been identified as coming from the N4 house.[18] The majority of the tablets were found broken and had been sundried in antiquity (Maul 2010a: 191; Maul 2003: 175; Pedersén 1986: 42). Based on the archaeological context, it is reasonable to assume that they were stored in room 10 of the N4 house (Pedersén 1998: 135). Unfortunately, it remains uncertain where in room 10 the texts were discovered (Maul 2010a: 192 note 14, 217–18; cf. Robson 2019: 129). The colophons mainly refer to the

also Ismail 1982: 199; cf. Maul 2010a: 192 note 14). Maul (2010a: 191 note 13) emphasizes that at least 150 tablets and fragments were discovered in N4 by the Iraqis, not 50 as described by Ismail. Miglus (1996: 238) states that the groups of tablets labelled Ass. 13955 and 13956 and perhaps also Ass. 17721 and 17722 likely came from room 10. The number of tablets and fragments from N4 continue to increase with every additional fragment assigned to this collection (see the development of numbers in Maul 2010a: 194; Maul 2003: 178; Pedersén 1998: 135; Pedersén 1986: 42).

16 Miglus 1996: 236–37, 240–41; Pedersén 1986: 42–43 group K; Klengel-Brandt 1975; see Faist 2007: 3; Donbaz and Parpola 2001: 11–13. Interestingly, Pedersén (1987: 44, 47) noted that almost half of the archives excavated in Assur were found in inner rooms with tombs underneath. Around 10 further tablets were found scattered throughout the eastern parts of the house (Pedersén 1986: 42–43 groups A, B, E, F).

17 Maul 2010: 191 note 12; Maul 2003: 180; Miglus 1996: 236–37, 240–41; Wiggermann 1992: 99–100; Pedersén 1986: 43 and notes 9–15; Ismail 1982: 199; Rittig 1977; Klengel-Brandt 1968; Andrae 1938: 13; see also Feldt 2015. Several figurines were painted and some contain inscriptions, e.g., *ṣī mūtu erba balāṭu*: "Go out death; come in life!" (Ismail 1982: 199; see Pedersén 1986: 43 note 9). Some vessels contained traces of copper (Wiggermann 1992: 99–100).

18 Maul 2010a: 194–95; Pedersén 1998: 135; Pedersén 1986: 44. Approximately one-quarter of the original number of texts likely contained colophons. Because the German excavations from 1903–1914 were conducted under Ottoman rule, the collective sum of tablets were divided between Berlin and Istanbul, whereas the tablets later excavated by the Iraqi expeditions are presumably kept in Baghdad (Maul 2010: 193 and notes 16–17; see Kraus 1947: 94, 101–104). Some tablets probably went to other collections or private collectors (e.g., Scheil 1918). The whereabouts of certain tablets, such as *RA* 15 pl. 76, are unknown today (see Appendix 2).

Bāba-šuma-ibni family members, especially Kiṣir-Aššur and Kiṣir-Nabû (Maul 2010a: 196, 203, 208–10; see below).

The N4 collection held a variety of texts, many of which relate to various forms of healing.[19] A large group contains diagnoses, prescriptions, recipes, and instructions for applying treatments for various medical symptoms and illnesses, as well as pharmacological texts for identifying and applying medical substances (Maul 2010a: 198). Another large group consists of rituals, incantations, and prayers for treating and removing demons, evils, witchcraft, and bad omens, as well as for influencing and restoring the human relationships with various gods (see Schwemer 2011). Additional texts relate to aggressive magic to gain control over other individuals (ibid.: 431–32).

Other texts include lexical lists, god lists, hemerological texts, various literary texts such as the Erra Epic, and a text on metrology (Maul 2010a: 198–99; Pedersén 1986: 55–56; see Veldhuis 2014: 367–72). Yet another group of texts relate to the Aššur temple, the Marduk statue's captivity in Assyria, the topography of the city of Assur, royal rituals, kings and their scholars, royal decrees, and the Assyrian army (Pedersén 1986: 56–58; Maul 2010a: 198). Finally, a group of textual commentaries, mainly on rituals, also formed part of the discovery (Frahm 2011a: 268–70). It is remarkable that the N4 collection provided relatively few omen texts (Koch 2015: 325–26 and note 894). Besides the collection in room 10, the administrative texts excavated in room 11 may represent an archive. However, the texts relate to, e.g., rations for various persons, such as temple personnel, who are otherwise unattested in N4.[20]

The N4 collection existed within the private confines of the N4 house, which most likely was inhabited by the Bāba-šuma-ibni family (Maul 2010a: 201). However, several individuals who were not members of this family are attested in the N4 collection, albeit frequently only in a single colophon (Fadhil 2012: 36–43). These individuals often belong to the elite of Assur's priesthood or temple administrations and they left tablets in the collection, perhaps as gifts

19 Robson 2019: 129–34; Maul 2010a: 196–99; Jean 2006: 148–53, 165–67; Pedersén 1986: 48–59; Ismail 1982: 199; see also Koch 2015: 325–26; Frahm 2011a: 268–70; Heeßel 2010a; Cavigneaux and Ismail 1998. Robson (2008: 474), Maul (2010a: 199), and Schwemer (2017: 50–51) have recently stressed that the writing-boards presumably missing today from the N4 collection could produce a false impression concerning some aspects of the content. See Section 3.6.1.

20 Maul 2010a: 201 and note 41–42; Pedersén 1998: 136. For an overview of Kiṣir-Aššur's texts in copies and editions, see Appendix 1. The majority of literary and scholarly texts from N4 can be found in handcopies in publications such as *KAR*, *KAH*, *LKA*, *BAM*, and *KAL*. Additionally, many texts are published in individual articles (e.g., Scheil 1918; Labat and Tournay 1945–46; Cavigneaux and Ismail 1998). The N4 archival texts are only partially published, see Ch. 8 note 111.

or through exchange (Maul 2010a: 212 and note 77).[21] Additionally, some young sons of priestly or scholarly families from Assur left tablets in the collection during their time spent there in their *šamallû ṣeḫru-* and *šamalllû*-phases, in the form of an "internship" (Fadhil 2012: 36–43, 50–51; Maul 2010a: 215–17 and notes 93 and 99–101; see also May 2018: 70–77). It is therefore likely that such apprentices in NA Assur spent time studying associated disciplines under the roof of other families (Maul 2010a: 217 and note 102).[22]

It seems that only one family member per generation, most likely the first-born son, was responsible for the continuation of the collection (Maul 2010a: 206–207 and notes 62 and 65–66; see May 2018: 66 note 14). His brothers would probably have moved to other houses and formed new collections there. Maul argued that this could explain why certain works, such as Sa-gig, are missing from N4 (see Section 3.6.1).

Several texts show that the Bāba-šuma-ibni family copied texts from manuscripts, which were not kept in the collection (Maul 2010a: 213; see Section 9.5.1). Maul considered it likely that the family copied tablets from their colleagues' collections (ibid.). This is based on certain protection and curse formulae found in some N4 manuscripts, which may indicate that colleagues had access to N4 texts (ibid.: 214).[23] Therefore, it is possible that N4 should be labelled a "semi-private text collection", although it is unknown to what extent labels such as "private" can be applied to the ancient world.

2.3.2 *Excursus: Discussion of the Term "Library"*

The term "library" is used in studies to refer to the N4 text collection due to its content.[24] However, researchers use the term for lack of a more appropriate alternative.[25] In Assyriology, the term is generally used to designate the content of a given archaeological space in which a number of literary or scholarly texts was excavated. This is regularly contrasted with the term "archive", which

21 There appears to be no evidence for selling or buying texts in Mesopotamia (Maul 2010a: 212).

22 In later periods, the elementary primary education seems to have been connected to temples (see Clancier 2014: 48; Charpin 2010a: 47; Beaulieu 2007a: 475; van der Toorn 2007: 56; Gesche 2001: 6; Cavigneaux 1999a: 385–86).

23 E.g., *RA* 40 pl. 116 rev. 5 from N4: *šà* IR ᵈA[G] ZÀḪ-*šú liq-b*[*i*], "he who removes (the tablet), let Na[bû] orde[r] his disappearance". Maul (2010a: 214 and note 89–91) also compares this to the LB scholarly texts from Uruk, where the colophons contain curses should the loaner not bring back the tablet on the same evening or a specified day.

24 E.g., "Bibliothek", Maul 2010a; "library", Pedersén 1986: 41. Both researchers are aware of the terminological limitations.

25 Groups of texts cannot always be called an "archive" or a "library" conclusively (see Pedersén 1998: 3). See also discussions in du Toit 1998; Black and Tait 1995.

encompasses texts with administrative, economic, epistolary, or legal content.[26] The term "library" can be problematic as it has connotations concerning the form and function of text collections.[27] This is especially a result of the Library of Alexandria's influence on the later ideals of the ancient library as an institution with an all-encompassing and static collection of texts.[28] However, the Mesopotamian scholarly text collections of the first millennium BCE were not institutionalized, static, similar, or all-encompassing, but often shaped by individual needs and interests (Robson 2013: 56).[29] Concerning the N4 collection, Maul (2010a: 215–16 and note 92) has suggested that it was primarily used for professional training and practice, and it can perhaps be regarded as a physical manifestation of the owners' personal qualifications. This study generally refers to the texts from the N4 house as the "N4 (text) collection". Yet, although this work recognizes the problems inherent in the term "library", the Nineveh text collections are referred to as libraries, and in general the terms "library" and "collection" are used interchangeably to broadly designate a collection of literary, historically, or scholarly texts kept in one or more rooms in a building used by learned individuals.

2.3.3 *The Bāba-šuma-ibni Family*

Seven members of the Bāba-šuma-ibni family are known by name, and possibly two additional members should be included in the genealogy, over five generations (cf. Maul 2010a: 203, 206 note 62). The named individuals are Bāba-šuma-ibni (Radner 1999a: 248–49), his sons Nabû-bēssunu (Baker 2001: 814–15) and Abu-erība (Radner 1998: 16), Nabû-bēssunu's sons Kiṣir-Aššur (Baker 2000: 623–24) and Šamaš-ibni (Baker 2011: 1199), Šamaš-ibni's son Kiṣir-Nabû (Baker

26 See Robson 2013: 40–41. For the problems related to the term "archive" in relation to such groups of texts, see the articles in Brosius 2003. See also Maul 2010a: 217 note 104.

27 Robson 2013: 38; see Michalowski 2003 and the articles concerning the term "library" in Veenhof 1986b. For a critique of the term "library" as applied to Assurbanipal's collections, see Robson 2019: 264–265.

28 See, e.g., Too 2010: 1–4, 6, 244; MacLeod 2010; du Toit 1998: 391–92.

29 Two examples of temple libraries with so-called "pigeon holes" for storing tablets on shelves are known from NA Dūr-Šarrukēn (Loud and Altman 1938 pl. 19c; cf. ibid. pl 24d) and the NB Šamaš temple in Sippar in which tablets were found *in situ* on the shelves (Al Jadir 1998; Anonymous 1987: 248–49 and pl. 47; see also for further references Maul 2010a: 217 and note 105; Potts 2010: 28–29; Al-Rawi and George 1994: 135 note 1; Al-Rawi and George 1990: 149 note 1). For other similar NA uses in Nineveh and Kalḫu, see Veenhof 1986a: 2 note 5, 13 and notes 50–51 with further references. Occasionally, the Mesopotamians used the word *gerginakku* to describe a room in which scholarly tablets were placed (Robson 2013: 41). Other problems related to text collections concern accessability and the availability of texts (see, e.g., Robson 2011a).

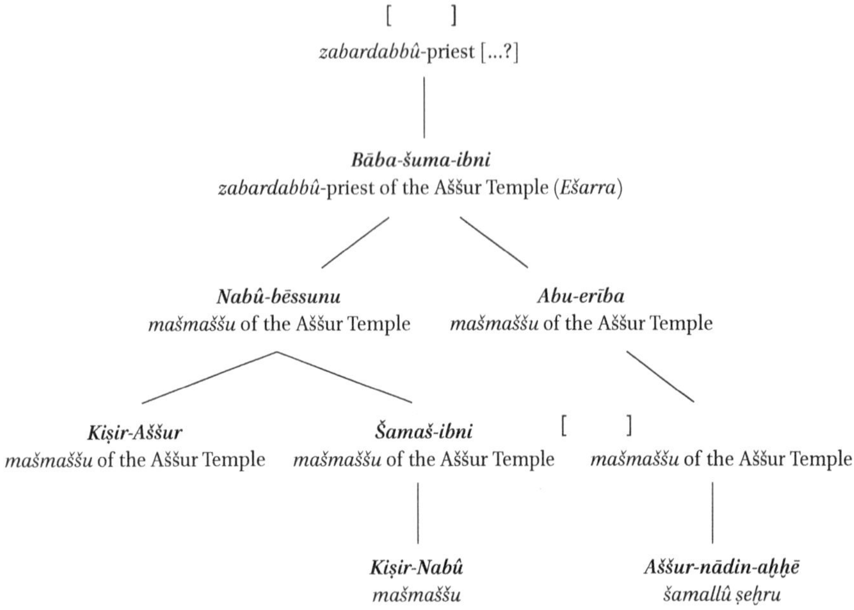

FIGURE 2 The Bāba-šuma-ibni family

2000: 627–28), and Abu-erība's grandson Aššur-nādin-aḫḫē (Radner 1998: 201). Figure 2 represents the Bāba-šuma-ibni family tree.

Several of the individuals are only attested in a single N4 tablet or through genealogies in colophons.[30] Zimmern (1915–16: 184 and note 1) appears to have been the first to comment on the names of the Bāba-šuma-ibni family members found in the colophons (cf. Ebeling 1919a; Ebeling 1920–23). However, it was not until Scheil's treatments of this family's tablets that a genealogy was attempted, albeit with mistakes (Scheil 1918: 77; Scheil 1921: 15–17; see Eilers 1933: 325). Meier later referred to N4 as the "Archiv der Tempelschule in Assur" and provided additional correlations between some tablets and titles within the family (Meier 1937–39: 240 and note 25, 245–46 and notes 33–38; see Weidner 1937–39: 147–48). He also placed the family in the middle of the 7th century BCE. However, Labat and Tournay (1945–46: 121–22) were the first to attempt a reconstruction of a complete family tree. Unfortunately, they misinterpreted

30 Only one tablet has been identified from, e.g., Aššur-nādin-aḫḫē (*PKTA* pl. 19+ = *SAA* 20 no. 17, see also Ch. 2 note 57). The unnamed son of Abu-erība, and father of Aššur-nādin-aḫḫē, is attested only in this text. *BAM* 102 rev. 7: [... ZAB]AR.DAB.B[A ...] may have contained the name of Bāba-šuma-ibni's father. This text is the only one that possibly provides an older ancestor, and it is the basis for an unknown ancestor appearing above Bāba-šuma-ibni in the family tree. However, the evidence remains tenuous.

the phrase *ša Nabû tuklassu* as a name and based an additional name on a problematic copy by Scheil (1918: 77).

It was not until Hunger (1968: 19) corrected the previous genealogies that the Kiṣir-Aššur branch of the family tree and the attested career phases were properly understood.[31] However, Nabû-bēssunu's brother, Abu-erība, remained elusive, and Pedersén (1986: 44–46) only hinted at Abu-erība's grandson, Aššur-nādin-aḫḫe, being part of this family (cf. Pedersén 1998: 135–36). Jean (2006: 189) provided a revised family tree with Abu-erība and Aššur-nādin-aḫḫē whom she believed was Abu-erība's son. However, Maul's recent treatment of the family demonstrated that an unknown individual represents the son of Abu-erība and the father of Aššur-nādin-aḫḫē (Maul 2010a: 203; see Fadhil 2012: 37). Recently, Parpola (2017: 48) has suggested restoring Abu-erība's son's name as [Kiṣi]r-Ašš[ur] in *PKTA* pl. 19+ (= *SAA* 20 no. 17).[32] However, Parpola's collations of the text show that this reconstruction is extremely tenuous (Parpola 2017: 216; see also May 2018: 69 note 61). Furthermore, such a reconstruction would be very problematic for assigning colophons to Nabû-bēssunu's son Kiṣir-Aššur. As a result, this hypothesis is disregarded here and the name of Abu-erība's son remains unknown. Maul's reconstruction of the Bāba-šuma-ibni family genealogy therefore remains authoritative, although this study adds a presumed ancestor of Bāba-šuma-ibni who is possibly mentioned in *BAM* 102.[33]

2.3.4 *The Attested Training and Career Phases*

Kiṣir-Aššur's colophons in particular make it possible to distinguish a set of six consecutive phases with titles that attest to the training and career of the individuals. The titles are: *šamallû ṣeḫru* "junior apprentice", *šamallû* "apprentice", *šamallû mašmaššu ṣeḫru* "junior apprentice exorcist",[34] *mašmaššu ṣeḫru*

31 Many additional texts from this family appeared during these years in Köcher's publications of the N4 medical and pharmacological texts (Köcher 1955, 1963a, 1963b, 1964, 1971).

32 *SAA* 20 no. 17 rev. 15–19: SAR $^{\text{p.d}}$*Aš-šur*-SUM-PAB.ME[Š ^{lú}ŠA]B.TUR TUR ^{16} DUMU ^{p}[*Ki-ṣi*]*r*$^{?}$-⸢$^{\text{d}?}$⸣*Aš-š*[*ur* ^{lú}MAŠ.MAŠ] ^{17} PEŠ ^{p}AD-SU ^{lú}MAŠ.MAŠ É ⸢^{d}⸣[*Aš-šur*] ^{18} A $^{\text{p.d}}$*Ba-ba*$_6$-MU-DÙ ^{lú}ZABAR.DAB.BA ^{19} *ina É-šár-ra*. Cf. Meinhold 2009: pl. 30–31; Menzel 1981: T 103f., T 107f.; Ebeling 1954c: 114–16.

33 Recently, Natalie May has suggested that the ancestor with the broken name is to be identified as Bāba-šuma-iddina, who was also the patronymic ancestor of a family of *asûs* serving as *šangû*-priests of the god Baba in Assur (May 2018: 71–74). This family is also known from manuscripts in the N4 collection (ibid.: 71–72 and note 81). It is possible that the Bāba-šuma-iddina of these families is attested in the N24 archive in Assur (ibid.: 73; Deller et al. 1995: 126–128 no. 136 = N24 no. 11).

34 The normalization of the title $^{(\text{lú})}$ŠÁMAN/DUGUD.LÁ MAŠ.MAŠ TUR varies (e.g., May 2018: 65; Baker 2000: 623; cf. ibid. 2017: 18, 160).

"junior exorcist", *mašmaššu* "exorcist", and *mašmaš bīt Aššur* "exorcist of the Aššur temple".[35] Although *šamallû ṣeḫru* is the earliest attested title, it becomes clear in Chapter 3 that such "junior apprentices" in N4 must have received a basic education in writing and reading cuneiform script beforehand (Maul 2010a: 210 note 74; Gesche 2001; Finkel 2000). Furthermore, from at least the *šamallû ṣeḫru*-phase onwards, it is possible that the father of the apprentice in question or another scholar acted as teacher and instructor.[36] The family members are described in several colophons as connected to the Aššur temple (Maul 2010a: 200–201 and note 40), although it remains uncertain whether these titles designated actual duties (see Sections 8.1 and 8.6). Current research agrees that the six phases attested for Kiṣir-Aššur can be arranged in a sequence that records a progression from junior to senior (Maul 2010a; Baker 2000: 623–24; Pedersén 1986: 45–46; Hunger 1968: 9–11, 19). This hypothesis can therefore be considered uncontroversial, although it is generally unknown how long individual phases lasted, and whether some phases overlapped.[37]

Additional titles are attested for several individuals within the Bāba-šuma-ibni family, and yet other titles are known for individuals outside this family that are also attested in N4 (e.g., "novice *asû*-physician" *asû agašgû*, *BAM* 1 col. iv 27).[38] The text *BAM* 102 may refer to an ancestor of Bāba-šuma-ibni as a *zabardabbû*-priest.[39] Furthermore, Bāba-šuma-ibni is generally referred to as

35 Maul 2010a: 208–11 and notes 67, 70, 74; Hunger 1968: 9–11, 19; see also Baker 2017: 15ff., 18, 160–161. Previous publications reconstructed the phase *šamallû* "apprentice" for Kiṣir-Aššur between his *šamallû ṣeḫru*- and *šamallû mašmaššu ṣeḫru*-phases (e.g., Baker 2017: 160; Maul 2010a: 208) on the basis of information provided in Pedersén's catalogue of tablets from the N4 text collection concerning the texts N4 no. 237, 241 and 289 (Pedersén 1986: 45). However, these previously unpublished texts must now be considered part of Kiṣir-Aššur's *šamallû ṣeḫru*-phase (see Section 3; Arbøll 2018b). *KAL* 10 no. 4 and the newly identified N4 no. 175 belonged to his *šamallû*-phase.

36 Frahm (2011a: 269 note 1277) suggested that Kiṣir-Aššur may have acted as the instructor of Kiṣir-Nabû, but this remains hypothetical.

37 It cannot be excluded that some phases were abbreviations for others, e.g., the title *mašmaššu ṣeḫru* could be an abbreviated form of *šamallû mašmaššu ṣeḫru* (Andrew George, personal communication). Note that there are no attestations where N4 family members employ two titles in a colophon (see May 2018: 65 note 10). However, it remains unclear if a practitioner at the top of his career could yield a title from a previous phase. For example, Kiṣir-Nabû's father Šamaš-ibni was *mašmaš bīt Aššur* when Kiṣir-Nabû was *mašmaššu ṣeḫru* in *AfO* 12 pl. 13–14, but he appears as *mašmaššu* (*BAM* 199) and MAŠ.MAŠ-*ma* (*KAR* 33; *LKA* 93) when Kiṣir-Nabû was *mašmaššu*.

38 For examples of *agašgû* and other NA apprenticeship titles, see Robson 2014: 152; Robson 2011a: 564–65.

39 A literal translation may be "Bronze(-object) holder", although a symbolic meaning had probably lost its value by the first millennium BCE due to changes in the function of the

zabardabbi Ešarra in Kiṣir-Aššur's colophons, except for *LKA* 119.[40] In *LKA* 119, Bāba-šuma-ibni is *mašmaš bīt Aššur*.[41] He is also referred to as the "exorcist of the temple of totality" (*mašmaš bīt kiššūti*) in Nabû-bēssunu's *KAR* 31,[42] which may be a variant of *mašmaš bīt Aššur* (Maul 2010: 200, note 40, 203 note 47).[43]

Nabû-bēssunu, Abu-erība, and Kiṣir-Nabû all held the title "Assur exorcist" (*mašmaššu aššurû*(?), reading uncertain) at some point during their career (Maul 2010a: 209 and note 69).[44] Whether this refers to an exorcist with duties on behalf of the city of Assur or an exorcist defined as a special type from the city of Assur remains uncertain.[45] Additionally, Šamaš-ibni is attested as both

---

title (see *CAD* Z: 6; *CDA*: 442). The title is used infrequently in the NA period, although it is clearly cultic in nature (May 2018: 66–67).

40 The only text currently identified as from Bāba-šuma-ibni is *KAL* 4 no. 36, wherein he was likely *za*[*bardabbi Ešarra*(?)]. Upon collation, this was also his title in Kiṣir-Aššur's *KAR* 230 rev. 15: DUMU $^{\text{p.d}}$*Ba-ba*$_6$-MU-DÙ ⸢ZABAR⸣.DAB.[BA *É-šar-ra*(?)].

41 Two ancestors with fragmentary names are listed as *mašmaš bīt Aššur* in *KAL* 4 no. 37. See the discussion in Ch. 6 note 66 and Maul 2010a: 200 note 40.

42 This title is the Akkadian translation of Sumerian É.ŠÁR.RA.

43 Furthermore, it is possible that Bāba-šuma-ibni was identified as a "senior *šangû*-priest" (*šangû rabû*) of an unknown temple in *BAM* 50, and the text may have been written by Nabû-bēssunu (Maul 2010a: 203 and notes 46–47; Pedersén 1986: 45–46 notes 22–23 and 25; Menzel 1981: 194, 247; Hunger 1968: 67 (= *BAK* no. 191–192); cf. May 2017: 98). If the text was written by Nabû-bēssunu, he misspelled his name, as Köcher's copy rev. 25 reads: DUB-*pi* $^{\text{p.d}}$<PA>-*bi-su-n*[*u* x x x x]. The CDLI picture cannot confirm this reading and further collation is necessary. The picture may agree with the reading SANGA GA[L] in rev. 26, but it shows that only a few signs can be reconstructed before it, and Bāba-šuma-ibni's name may be too long. According to May (2018: 67 note 32, 76 note 110), recent collations of *BAM* 50 show the text should not be attributed to Nabû-bēssunu.

44 For Nabû-bēssunu, see *LKA* 109 rev. 15': [DUB(?)] $^{\text{p!(aš).d}}$ÚMBISAG$^{?}$-*be-sun* ^{lú}MAŠ.MAŠ BAL.TIL^{ki}, as well as Kiṣir-Aššur's N4 no. 289 rev. 3' DUMU $^{\text{p.d}}$AG-*bi-su-nu* ^{lú}MAŠ.MAŠ BAL.TIL^{ki}-*u* (see Ch. 3 note 129). For Abu-erība, see *KAL* 2 no. 34 col. iv 14': ⸢DUB⸣ ^{p}⸢AD⸣-SU ^{lú}MAŠ.MAŠ BAL.TIL^{k}[^{i}] (Schwemer 2007b: 88–89; see Section 9.5.3). For Kiṣir-Nabû, see below. Notably, Nabû-bēssunu is *mašmaš bīt Aššur* in all Kiṣir-Aššur's colophons, although Maul (2010a: 210 and note 70) refers to a tablet from Kiṣir-Aššur in which Nabû-bēssunu was "Assur exorcist" without providing the reference. This text must be unpublished, because there are no indications at present that Nabû-bēssunu's broken title in a number of Kiṣir-Aššur colophons should be reconstructed as "Assur exorcist". For small variations in Nabû-bēssunu's title in Kiṣir-Aššur's tablets, see *KAR* 63 rev. 25': MAŠ.MAŠ É *Aš-šur-ma*, and *KAR* 80 (= *KAL* 2 no. 8) rev. 39: ^{lú}ME.ME É A[N.ŠÁR]. It seems that Kiṣir-Aššur did not supply a title for Nabû-bēssunu in *BAM* 307.

45 Maul (2010a: 209) translates the title "'Beschwörer' von Assur" without transcription. Fadhil (2012: 46) provides a reference to another person claiming the title *mašmaššu aššurû*, which is spelled URU BAL.TIL^{ki}-*u* (see Hunger 1968: 85 no. 256). I disregard the possibility that this title would be a marker of ethnicity, as it is spelled URU and not KUR and that the majority of exorcists within Assur must have been Assyrian (see also Section 9.5.3).

mašmaš bīt Aššur and *mašmaš Ešarra* (Maul 2010a: 209–10 and notes 68 and 73), and he is occasionally provided with the variant MAŠ.MAŠ-*ma* for the title *mašmaššu*.[46] At present, it cannot be established if some of these phases are missing in Kiṣir-Aššur's colophons or if he simply never claimed these titles.

Only one of the Bāba-šuma-ibni family texts contains an exact date, namely Kiṣir-Aššur's *KAR* 267 that is dated to the 9th of *Ulūlu* (August–September) 658 BCE (see Section 7.5; Maul 2010: 205). Maul assumed that each generation preceding and following Kiṣir-Aššur could be dated within approximately 30 year intervals from the year 658 BCE, and he suggested that the middle of Nabû-bēssunu's career should be dated around the year 688 BCE and Bāba-šuma-ibni's around 718 BCE. It seems that the majority of the family's members reached a stage that allowed them to claim the title *mašmaš bīt Aššur*. The only exception appears to be Kiṣir-Nabû, who possibly became only "Assur exorcist", and Aššur-nādin-aḫḫē who is attested in only one text as *šamallû ṣeḫru*.[47] Maul attributed the fragmentary king list *KAV* 182 to Kiṣir-Nabû, even though the copyist's name is broken (Maul 2010a: 204 note 51, 209 note 69). This text ends with the NA king Aššur-etel-ilānī (627–623 BCE), and if the text was copied by Kiṣir-Nabû it would have been copied during this king's reign (ibid.). It is plausible that Kiṣir-Nabû did not reach the stage of *mašmaš bīt Aššur* before the city of Assur fell in 614 BCE (ibid.: 205 note 54, 211; cf. note 595), yet it remains uncertain if Kiṣir-Aššur was still alive and active by this time (cf. ibid.: 205 and note 54).

Maul identified the names of Kiṣir-Aššur and Kiṣir-Nabû in 122 colophons in the N4 collection, which would suggest that the collection had been enlarged during their time, around the middle and the second half of the 7th century BCE (Maul 2010a: 204–205 and notes 49 and 55–56). A few tablets show that the collection was founded around the time of Bāba-šuma-ibni, who was probably a contemporary of Sargon II (722–705 BCE).[48] The evidence from N4 suggests that the male members of the Bāba-šuma-ibni family strove towards claiming the title *mašmaš bīt Aššur* (Maul 2010a: 210–11). However, Maul (ibid.: 206) has argued that several persons within the family could claim the title at the same time. As a result, he refers to this family as a "Kollegium" of *mašmaš bīt Aššur*s (ibid.), which may have had a similar structure as other guilds known from Assur around the same time (see Radner 1999b: 25–33).

46 See *KAR* 33; *LKA* 93.

47 See Ch. 2 note 55, Ch. 8 note 18, Table 1 note h.

48 As argued by Maul (2010a: 206 and note 58) on the basis of two texts dated to 714 BCE (Thureau-Dangin 1912) and 713 BCE (*KAR* 252). He also notes that *LKA* 53 mentions the name of Sargon II. See Maul 1994: 159; Pedersén 1986: 44.

2.3.5 *Other References to Members of the Bāba-šuma-ibni Family*

We know almost nothing about the Bāba-šuma-ibni family members as private individuals. As discussed above in Section 2.3.1, the family must have been affiliated with numerous influential families and, as indicated by their titles, also with the Aššur temple. However, only four documents outside of the N4 collection might mention members of the Bāba-šuma-ibni family. The first one is the letter *SAA* 10 no. 102 from Akkullānu, a prominent *šangû*-priest at the Aššur temple in Assur,[49] which contains a broken passage that describes a certain Kiṣir-Aššur copying tablets for the royal libraries in Nineveh.[50] The second is the letter *SAA* 13 no. 39, perhaps from our Nabû-bēssunu, addressed to a certain Aššur-mudammiq who is to provide silver to the Akkullānu mentioned above for repairing the seats of Aššur and Mullissu.[51] Furthermore, Kiṣir-Aššur of the N4 house is perhaps mentioned alongside other individuals connected to the Aššur temple in *SAA* 13 no. 155.[52] And finally, Šamaš-ibni may have been in charge of offerings at the Aššur temple in *SAA* 7 no. 211.[53] Parpola dated a letter with related content to *SAA* 10 no. 102, namely no. 101, to around the year 655 BCE, which would date no. 102 to the same time (Villard 1998: 19; Parpola 1983a: 347). However, several individuals are known from this period with the name Kiṣir-Aššur (Baker 2000: 623–24), and it remains uncertain if Kiṣir-Aššur actually copied manuscripts for the Nineveh libraries (see Sections 7.6 and 9.5.4; cf. May 2018: 68, 78; Fadhil 2012: 72; Maul 2010a: 205). Nonetheless, the Bāba-šuma-ibni family was connected to families who produced tablets for

49 Akkullānu also reported on astrological matters to the Assyrian king (see Villard 2007: 326–27; Radner 1998: 95ff.; Villard 1998). May (2018: 68 and notes 43–44) regards Akkullānu as an indicator for a connection between the N4 scholarly environment and the royal court based on his astrological reports. However, Akkullānu only wrote 12 out of 243 astrological reports from Assyrian scholars to the NA kings, and none of his texts demonstrate access to the inner circle at Nineveh (*SAA* 8: 60ff.).

50 May 2018: 68; Maul 2010a: 205 and note 53; Villard 1998: 19. *SAA* 10 no. 102 obv. 6'–8': 6' … ^{p}*du-gul*-IGI-[x x x] 7' ^{p}*ki-ṣir-aš-šur ki-lal-le-šú*-[*nu*] 8' UR$_5$.RA : *i-šaṭ-ṭu-r*[*u*], "Dugul-pan-[*ili*] and Kiṣir-Aššur are both copying Ur$_5$-ra". May (2018: 68) provides an overview of Ur$_5$-ra manuscripts and amulet stone lists from N4 and concludes that Kiṣir-Aššur was "a great specialist on stones and lexical lists" (see also ibid.: 78). However, Kiṣir-Aššur's texts with colophons do not substantiate this hypothesis.

51 May 2018: 68 and note 40; Villard 2007: 326. However, this would be the only instance where Nabû-bēssunu's name is written AG-EN-*šú-nu*.

52 May 2018: 69–70. The letter is directed to the king by an anonymous author concerning the future sacrifices in Assur conducted by five individuals, among these a certain Kiṣir-Aššur. However, the letter shows no clear connection to the Nineveh court, and it only shows that a Kiṣir-Aššur was perhaps involved in the Aššur temple cult.

53 May 2018: 69. The text states that a certain Šamaš-ibni was responsible for offerings on the 24th day of an uncertain month.

the Nineveh collections, such as Marduk-šallim-aḫḫē, who is attested in colophons from N4 and Nineveh (Fadhil 2012: 40–41 and note 1; Baker 2001: 726).

2.4 Quantifying and Contextualizing Kiṣir-Aššur's Texts

Kiṣir-Aššur is the N4 individual to whom most colophons can be assigned. Throughout this work I also include other texts from the N4 collection for which text-internal criteria make it likely that they can be assigned to Kiṣir-Aššur. Maul (2010a) has offered the most recent and in-depth treatment of the various phases of the Bāba-šuma-ibni family members' training and careers.[54] In his study, Maul identified and assigned 78 texts to Kiṣir-Aššur and 44 texts to Kiṣir-Nabû, totalling 122 texts.[55] Maul also listed the number of tablets assigned to each of the other Bāba-šuma-ibni family members. Unfortunately, Maul did not provide a full catalogue of these texts, and it is therefore unclear if there are unpublished or fragmentary texts among them. The current study attempts to remedy the situation for Kiṣir-Aššur, although an inherent problem is that many colophons are partly damaged and in several instances it is impossible to identify the name of the owner, copyist, or writer beyond Kiṣir-[…]. Thus, a number of texts may refer to either Kiṣir-Aššur or Kiṣir-Nabû, although genealogies or preserved titles can occasionally aid in the reconstruction. Figure 3 illustrates how many tablets from the available material can be attributed to Kiṣir-Aššur and Kiṣir-Nabû, and how many remain of uncertain attribution.

These numbers do not completely agree with the data collected by Maul.[56] In total, there are 125 texts bearing Kiṣir-Aššur or Kiṣir-Nabû's name, with 73 texts assigned to Kiṣir-Aššur, 39 texts to Kiṣir-Nabû, and 13 texts that cannot be safely assigned to either man. This study therefore provides three additional texts compared to Maul's overview.[57] However, with the continious publication

---

54 Stefan Maul is the principal investigator of the project *Edition literarischer Keilschrifttexte aus Assur*, which aims to publish the literary, historical and scholarly texts excavated during the German excavations from 1903–1914 in Assur.

55 Maul 2010a: 205 note 56, 208–10; see May 2018: 65. Additionally, Maul states that eight tablets were written by Nabû-bēssunu, presumably one by Aššur-nādin-aḫḫē, and one each by Abu-erība and Bāba-šuma-ibni (Maul 2010a: 205–206 note 55 and 60).

56 Adding to the confusion is, e.g., Farber's statement that *LKA* 114 was written in the hand of Kiṣir-Nabû, although no such name is preserved on the colophon (Farber 1989: 23–24). It has not been possible to provide a description of Kiṣir-Aššur's handwriting, although such an attempt is a *desideratum*.

57 Couto-Ferreira (2018: 163) listed *BAM* 232 as one of Kiṣir-Aššur's *šamallû ṣeḫru* manuscripts. However, the collations in *CMAwR* 1: 318–335 and pl. 132 no. 63 show that the colophon in rev. 3' states: [… PA]B??.MEŠ lú⸢ŠÁMAN.LÁ TUR⸣ (cf. ibid.: 322 note 79).

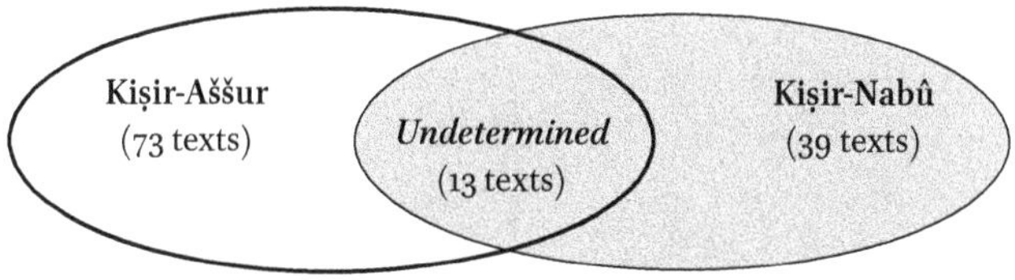

FIGURE 3 Texts assigned to Kiṣir-Aššur and Kiṣir-Nabû

of new texts it is possible additional tablets or new joins may appear in the future that can modify the individual observations made here.[58]

Table 1 divides these 125 tablets according to titles, in accordance with the titles established in Section 2.3.4. The table also notes the differences between this study and the numbers provided by Maul (2010a: 208–209), which are marked separately in parenthesis ($X_{\text{My number}}$ / ($Y_{\text{Maul's number}}$)). I have divided the texts assigned to Kiṣir-Aššur and Kiṣir-Nabû according to what can be read on the collated tablets and published copies, and only in a few individual cases have the titles been reconstructed (see Appendix 1). Additionally, I have included a number of unpublished texts carrying Kiṣir-Aššur's name, and in some instances a title (courtesy of Nils Heeßel, Stefan Maul and Daniel Schwemer; Pedersén 1986: 45–47). However, colophons that have been reconstructed by their editors without sufficient evidence have been disregarded and will be discussed where relevant. I argue for further reconstructions in some colophons and for assigning other texts to specific career phases throughout the following chapters. Consequently, the numbers presented below are not absolute.

Maul has a total of 49 texts with titles from Kiṣir-Aššur and 20 texts with titles from Kiṣir-Nabû, but does not list tablets with broken titles or completely without titles. These texts are added here separately to nuance the study. Furthermore, several of the tablets with and without titles include a phrase stating: "(he) whose trust is Nabû" (*ša Nabû tuklassu*; Section 5.4). Although this is not a title, it is used throughout this study as a criterion for assigning

Accordingly, it is possible the name once read Aššur-nādin-aḫḫē, the grandson of Abu-erība. However, other individuals attested in N4 have names ending in *-aḫḫē* (see Fadhil 2012: 36–42).

58 Other colophons from N4 contain only the purpose for copying the tablet or other information (e.g., *LKA* 88 = N4 no. 162). These are therefore without names and are disregarded here. Note that Anmar Fadhil is currently working with unpublished texts from the Iraqi excavations of N4, among which there are no clear colophons that can be assigned to Bāba-šuma-ibni family members (personal communication).

TABLE 1 Texts assigned to Kiṣir-Aššur's and Kiṣir-Nabû's career phases[a]

Title or Appended Phrase	Kiṣir-Aššur	Kiṣir-Nabû	Undetermined
šamallû ṣeḫru[b]	12 / (10)	–	–
šamallû[c]	2 / (3)	–	–
šamallû mašmaššu ṣeḫru[d]	3 / (2)	–	–
mašmaššu ṣeḫru[e]	1 / (1)	2 / (3)	–
mašmaššu[f]	8 / (8)	12 / (15)	1
mašmaššu + [broken title(?)][g]	–	1	–
mašmaššu aššurû(?)[h]	–	1 / (2)	–
mašmaš bīt Aššur[i]	25 / (25)	–	–
No title[j]	15	16	1
Possibly broken title[k]	7	7	11
In Total	73 Texts	39 Texts	13 Texts

a The totals are listed in Maul 2010: 205 notes 55–56, 209. He lists 123 tablets collectively from Kiṣir-Aššur (78), Kiṣir-Nabû (44), and Aššur-nādin-aḫḫē (1), as well as eight tablets from Nabû-bēssunu, one from Bāba-šuma-ibni, and one from Abu-erība.

b *BAM* 129; *BAM* 201; *KAL* 4 no. 19; *KAL* 4 no. 41; *LKA* 43; N4 A 400; N4 A 2191; N4 no. 237; N4 no. 241; N4 no. 289; *RA* 15 pl. 76; *RA* 40 pl. 116. For the last text as a *šamallû ṣeḫru* text, see Table 2 note b.

c The three manuscripts listed by Maul are presumably the unpublished texts N4 no. 237, 241, and 289 included among Kiṣir-Aššur's *šamallû ṣeḫru*-phase tablets, see Ch. 2 note 35. Only *KAL* 10 no. 4 and the unpublished N4 no. 175 attest to this phase (cf. Arbøll 2018b).

d *LKA* 89+; *LKA* 141; N4 no. 24 (see Section 5.2).

e Kiṣir-Aššur: N4 A 2727. Kiṣir-Nabû: *AfO* 12 pl. 13–14; *BAM* 33.

f Kiṣir-Aššur: *BAM* 81; *BAM* 102; *BAM* 122; *CT* 37 pl. 24f.; *KAL* 4 no. 7; *KAR* 230; *KAR* 298; *LKA* 115. Kiṣir-Nabû: *BAM* 178; *BAM* 199; *KAR* 22; *KAR* 33; *KAR* 56; *LKA* 93; *LKA* 112; *LKA* 143; N4 no. 50; N4 no. 154; N4 no. 247; N4 no. 404. Undetermined: *LKA* 146.

g Kiṣir-Nabû: *KAR* 114. The title should be reconstructed perhaps as MAŠ.MAŠ [TUR] to accommodate Maul's three identified tablets from Kiṣir-Nabû's *mašmaššu ṣeḫru*-phase.

h Kiṣir-Nabû: *KAV* 182(?). As discussed in Section 2.3.4, this tablet is problematic as no names are preserved in the colophon.

i Kiṣir-Aššur: *BAM* 28; *BAM* 99; *BAM* 164; *BAM* 177; *BAM* 186; *BAM* 188; *BAM* 300; *BAM* 303; *BAM* 321; Beckman and Foster 1988 no. 21; *KAR* 38; *KAR* 62; *KAR* 63; *KAR* 80; *KAR* 307; *KAR* 374; *KAV* 42; *LKA* 70+; *LKA* 77; *LKA* 83; *LKA* 113; *LKA* 119; *LKA* 157; N4 no. 110; *PKTA* pl. 10–11.

j Kiṣir-Aššur: *BAM* 9; *BAM* 78; *BAM* 121; *BAM* 131; *BAM* 307; *BAM* 333; *BAM* 351; *KAL* 10 no. 1 (see Section 7.2); *KAL* 10 no. 5; *KAR* 21; *KAR* 171; *KAR* 267; *LKA* 40; N4 no. 224; N4 no. 228. Kiṣir-Nabû: *CMAwR* 1 pl. 25–26; *BAM* 52; *BAM* 106; *BAM* 147; *BAM* 168; *BAM* 191; (*CT* 15 pl. 43f.?); JRL 1053 (Al-Rawi 2000); *KAL* 4 no. 44; *KAR* 72; *KAR* 223; *LKA* 100; *LKA* 118; N4 no. 41; N4 no. 80; N4 no. 163;. Undetermined: *KAL* 4 no. 37.

k Kiṣir-Aššur: *BAM* 40; *KAL* 7 no. 24; *KAL* 10 no. 13; *LKA* 137; N4 A 2362; N4 no. 254; N4 no. 401. Kiṣir-Nabû: *BAM* 101; *KAR* 44; *LKA* 79; *LKA* 81; *LKA* 96; *LKA* 110; N4 no. 220. Undetermined: *ACh Supp.* 2 24; *BAM* 68; *BAM* 202; *BAM* 206; *BAM* 260; *BAM* 311; *BAM* 366; *KAL* 9 no. 41; *KAR* 90; N4 no. 443; *PKTA* pl. 39–40.

certain tablets to phases of Kiṣir-Aššur's career. Several of the tablets including this phrase are for now listed under the title or no title/broken title in Table 1.[59]

From the above numbers, the most significant divergence of my study from Maul's is the number of tablets assigned to Kiṣir-Aššur's *šamallû ṣeḫru-*, *šamallû-* and *šamallû mašmaššu ṣeḫru*-phases.[60] At least one additional tablet without a formal title (*BAM* 9) is argued in Section 5.4.1 as belonging to the *šamallû ṣeḫru*-phase, which would bring the total to 13 tablets. Four tablets with the title *mašmaš bīt Aššur* contain a fragmentary name and cannot be assigned to Kiṣir-Aššur or Kiṣir-Nabû based on genealogy.[61] However, as discussed above, Kiṣir-Nabû may never have reached this phase, and by extension these texts are included as part of Kiṣir-Aššur's *mašmaš bīt Aššur*-phase.[62] The remaining undetermined tablets must have belonged to either Kiṣir-Aššur or Kiṣir-Nabû. Although not all of these texts can be argued to belong to one of them specifically, they still represent knowledge used within this family.

---

59 The texts with this phrase, with or without titles, are *BAM* 9, *BAM* 121, *KAL* 4 no. 37, *LKA* 89+, *LKA* 141, *RA* 15 pl. 76.

60 Maul (2010a: 208) originally listed ten *šamallû ṣeḫru* texts and three *šamallû* texts, but since his study, the three texts identified at the time of Maul's study from Kiṣir-Aššur's *šamallû*-phase have been shown to belong to his *šamallû ṣeḫru*-phase (see Ch. 2 note 35, Table 1 note c).

61 The texts are *BAM* 28, *BAM* 321, *LKA* 157, and *PKTA* pl. 10–11. The last text does not preserve any names, and as such, it is not entirely certain it was copied by either Kiṣir-Aššur or Kiṣir-Nabû, but see Section 8.6.

62 For the colophon of *BAM* 28, see Section 8.2.

CHAPTER 3

Kiṣir-Aššur's Magico-Medical Education as *šamallû ṣeḫru*

Kiṣir-Aššur was likely in his teens when he began his earliest career stage as a "young apprentice" (*šamallû ṣeḫru*). By then, Kiṣir-Aššur is assumed to have completed his primary education and begun a process of specialization (cf. Gesche 2001: 210 and its review in George 2003–04 and Veldhuis 2003). He must therefore already have undergone the education necessary for him to acquire basic reading and writing skills for various subgenres of *āšipūtu*.

Supposedly, students of any craft were not adults (Gesche 2001: 219; Cohen and Kedar 2011: 240; Kedar 2014: 540). We can only estimate the years spent during education through comparative material, and suggestions for the age at which students began their education range from five (Waetzoldt 1974: 9) to 14–15 years of age (Gehlken 2005: 102, 106 and note 25; Cohen and Kedar 2011: 240–41 with further references).[1] The length of a complete education may have been as much as ten years (Wiggermann 2008: 211; Waetzoldt 1989: 38), but in the Book of Daniel the education of an astrologer is three years.[2] In the MA period, two brothers likely had the *ṭupšarru ṣeḫru* title for at least three years (Jakob 2003: 257). Apprentices probably trained through (competitive) teamwork under the tutelage of a senior colleague or family member.[3]

Although the *šamallû ṣeḫru* phase is Kiṣir-Aššur's earliest attested phase, he was already copying complicated medical knowledge. This could indicate that the Bāba-šuma-ibni family did not follow the later Babylonian educational phases established by Gesche, but instead utilized a curriculum targeted at training practical skills. The following table is a list of the texts written by

1 Guinan and Leichty (2008) published an OB school text that had deliberately been bitten into by the student and subsequently broken. The dental marks were identified as belonging to an individual around 12 to 13 years old. The content was the lexical text Proto-Ea, which "was studied toward the end of the first year of scribal training" (ibid.: 50). They conclude, for the OB period: "The beginning of school would have coincided with the reaching of sexual maturity" (ibid.). See Pearce and Doty 2000: 337–38.

2 Book of Daniel chapter 1.3–1.5; cf. Gesche 2001: 219 note 840–42.

3 Radner 2011: 363; *SAA* 10 no. 385 rev. 1–3: [lú]*da-di-bé-*[*e*] [2] *lu-šá-an-ši-*[*lu*] [3] *is-se-šú-nu l*[*i-zi-zu*], "The apprentices should imitate and assist them". See Robson 2011b: 608.

Kiṣir-Aššur as *šamallû ṣeḫru*. I have assigned the texts to three groups, namely, medical texts, ritual texts and other texts, as specified in Section 1.2.3. The text *BAM* 9 is not explicitly supplied with the *šamallû ṣeḫru* title in the colophon, but Section 5.4.1 argues for its place among these tablets. Consequently, it is included in the following table:

TABLE 2 Texts assigned to Kiṣir-Aššur's *šamallû ṣehru*-phase

Area	Text	Content	Format and designation
Medical texts	*BAM* 129	Obverse, col. i–ii: incantations (col. i 1–7, 12–16, 20–23, col. ii 4'–7', 17'?–22', 23'–28') and ritual instructions (col. i 8–11, 18–19, 25–33+[...], col. ii 1'–3'(?), 8'–16', 30'+[...]) against *sagallu* Reverse, col. iii(broken)–iv: six treatments and four diagnoses for *šaššaṭu* in various forms prescribing bandaging (col. iv 1'–2', 3'–5', 6'–13', 14'–17'), washing (col. iv 6'–13') and anointing (col. iv 18') the patient, and possibly fumigating his bed (col. iv 6'–13', 14'–17')	Two-columned on each side; [...]
	BAM 201	Obverse and reverse: five prescriptions for applying bandages (obv. 23'–27', 29'–30') of cloth (obv. 1'–15', 16'–22', rev. 1'–41') with additional instructions, and four preserved symptom descriptions for "ditto" (obv. 16'), a man with swollen insides and fever ill with "Hand of curse" and *kadabbedû* (obv. 23'–25'), a man throwing up blood and pus (obv. 29'), and a man with yellow eyes and "Hand of curse" (rev. 31')	Portrait; *u'iltu*
	KAL 4 no. 41	Obverse: a broken symptom description possibly for *garābu* (obv. 1) and two ritual instructions (obv. 1–8, 9–12+[...]) Reverse: only colophon preserved	(Broken, portrait?); [...]

TABLE 2 Texts assigned to Kiṣir-Aššur's *šamallû ṣehru*-phase (*cont.*)

Area	Text	Content	Format and designation
	N4 A 400	Obverse and reverse: an incantation against *maškadu*-illness followed by instructions	Landscape; *u'iltu*
	N4 no. 237	Obverse and reverse: a prayer to Šamaš (obv. 1–13) followed by a rubrick (obv. 14–15) and two prescriptions directed against a ghost seizing a man. The first prescription recommends the production of an amulet and anointing the patient (obv. 16–rev. 3), and the second recommends anointing the patient (rev. 4–11)	Portrait; *u'iltu*
	RA 15 pl. 76[a]	Obverse: 11 single line prescriptions and one two-line prescription for snakebite (obv. 1–13) prescribing eating (obv. 1') and drinking (obv. 2', 5', 7') substances and fluids, placing plants onto the bite (obv. 2', 3', 4'), placing a certain *ḫimû*-wad on the wound (obv. 8', 9'), placing plants around his neck (obv. 6', 11') and his bed (obv. 10') and anointing the bite (obv. 12'–13'); also 12+[...] single line prescriptions for scorpion stings (obv. 14'–25') prescribing anointing the sting (obv. 14', 17', 18', 22', 23', 24', 25'), drinking a potion (obv. 16', 21', 23', 24', 25'), eating a substance (16', 18'), and covering the sting with flour (obv. 15') Reverse: two broken prescriptions for a horse with an uncertain malady, presumably colic, both are poured into the left nostril of the horse (rev. 1'–4', 5'–8')	Portrait; *ṭuppu*

a Scheil's copy appears to be inaccurate in several places (cf. Stol 2011: 401), and Scheil (1918: 10) misread Kiṣir-Aššur's name and title (cf. Labat and Tournay 1945–46: 121–22). See the new edition in Appendix 2.

TABLE 2 Texts assigned to Kiṣir-Aššur's *šamallû ṣehru*-phase (*cont.*)

Area	Text	Content	Format and designation
	RA 40 pl. 116[b]	Obverse: five prescriptions for a potion (obv. 1–3), to make the patient vomit and eat soup afterwards (obv. 4–7), a potion for tongue and nostrils and drinking beer for vomiting (obv. 8–12), production of seven pills swallowed on an empty stomach (obv. 13–18), a potion to be drunk on an empty stomach with an enema (obv. 19–20), a broken prescription. A diagnosis for *ašû*, *pašittu* and *lubāṭu* (obv. 1), and a symptom description for *suālu*, wind in the windpipe and various coughs with phlegm (obv. 8–9) Reverse: colophon	Portrait; *ṭuppu*
Ritual texts	*KAL* 4 no. 19	Obverse: mainly broken, but may mention Šamaš in an uncertain context Reverse: one fragmentary ritual (rev. 1'–4')	(Broken, portrait?); [...]
	LKA 43	Obverse and reverse: one *šu'illa*-prayer for Madānu (obv. 1–rev. 37)	Portrait; *ṭuppu*
	N4 A 2191	Obverse and reverse: ritual against a ghost	Portrait; [...]
	N4 no. 289	Obverse: ritual instructions for performing the ritual "A substitute for Ereškigal" (obv. 1–15) Reverse: colophon	Portrait(?); *ṭuppu*
Other texts	N4 no. 241	Obverse and reverse: words and phrases in Sumerian and Akkadian (obv. 1–rev. 2) followed by a damaged section (rev. 4–10)	Portrait; *u'iltu*(?)

b Labat and Tournay (1945–46: 114) reconstructed Kiṣir-Aššur's title in the colophon rev. 1 as: lúŠÁ[MAN(?)] (cf. the picture on CDLI (P431342)). The space available on the broken area coupled with the narrow space between the signs in the colophon suggests that ca. two more signs should be reconstructed: lúŠÁ[MAN.LÁ TUR].

TABLE 2 Texts assigned to Kiṣir-Aššur's *šamallû ṣeḫru*-phase (*cont.*)

Area	Text	Content	Format and designation
		Text likely from Kiṣir-Aššur's *šamallû ṣeḫru*-phase	
Medical texts	*BAM* 9	Obverse: 13 prescriptions for applying onto the temple(s) (obv. 1–8, 9–11, 16–17, 23–25(?), 31–32?, 33–34(?), 35–39) and tying on the head(?) (obv. 18–20) against head maladies involving ghost (obv. 1), headache (obv. 16, 18, 21, 40) and *ḫimiṭ ṣēti* (obv. 23) Reverse: eight prescriptions for anointing (rev. 47–50, 51–54), fumigation (rev. 55–57) and applying a bandage (rev. 58–60, 61–63, 64–65(?), 66–68) against *sagkidabbû* (rev. 42), ghost (rev. 47, 51–52, 55), and problems of the temples (rev. 58, 61)	Portrait; *ṭuppu*

Assuming Kiṣir-Aššur accompanied his father when performing his *āšipu* duties during his *šamallû ṣeḫru*-phase, it is plausible that the knowledge Kiṣir-Aššur acquired was for educational reasons with a practical dimension (Maul 2010a: 216).[4] I distinguish three groups of texts among Kiṣir-Aššur's 13 *šamallû ṣeḫru* texts based on whether or not they are related to manipulating the body of the patient. These three groups are: 1) prescriptions and rituals with diagnoses intended to cure symptoms and illnesses affecting a patient's body, 2) rituals and prayers directed towards removing bad omens potentially causing illness(?) or soothing the anger of a cause of affliction,[5] and 3) texts unrealted to healing.

In the first group we find *BAM* 9, which comprises numerous diagnoses and prescriptions for headaches (*sagkidabbû*) and ghost-induced head conditions

4 Finkel (2000: 147) suggested that, for example, dosage measuring was often neglected in the texts because the correct proportions were taught through demonstration. Rote learning was likely also an integral part of copying texts (Clancier 2014: 45–46; Koch 1995: 139; see Maul 2010a: 215 note 215).

5 The evidence presented here does not agree with the general picture presented by Maul (2010a: 216) regarding the early phase tablets from N4: "Fast alle dieser Manuskripte enthalten Gebete oder Beschreibungen von Heilverfahren, die vorwiegend exorzistischer Natur sind."

on both the obverse and reverse. *BAM* 129 is one of the few examples of a library copy (multi-columned tablet) among Kiṣir-Aššur's tablets with colophons. The two obverse columns consist of *abracadabra* incantations and associated rituals intended to cure a patient with *sagallu*-illness. Column three is completely broken, but column four contains diagnoses and complicated prescriptions treating the associated *šaššaṭu*-illness (see Section 3.1).

BAM 201 consists of long prescriptions curing an unknown malady, "Curse" (*māmītu*), and "inability to talk" (*kadabbedû*) and associated symptoms. The unpublished N4 A 400 is a small tablet with a single incantation with accompanying instructions intended to cure *maškadu*-illness. The manuscript N4 no. 237 contains a prayer to Šamaš and two prescriptions for treating the effects of a ghost. The obverse of *RA* 15 pl. 76 concerns brief prescriptions for snakebites and scorpion stings, and the reverse contains two prescriptions likely treating a horse. *RA* 40 pl. 116 comprises prescriptions concerning the illness *ašû*, *pašittu*-bile, *lubāṭu*-sweat and various lung problems related to coughs. The broken *KAL* 4 no. 41 likely treats the skin malady *garābu*.[6] The last example may not have manipulated the patient's body.

In the second group we find the broken ritual *KAL* 4 no. 19[7] and a *šu'illa*-prayer (ŠU.ÍL.LÁ) to the divine judge Madānu, a divine personification of "judgement" related to Marduk.[8] Additionally, N4 A 2191 contains a ritual against a ghost, which duplicates an unspecified part of *BAM* 323 (Daniel Schwemer, personal communication). Kiṣir-Aššur also copied the ritual N4 no. 289 for substituting a patient with a goat kid, which is killed and handed over to Ereškigal, the goddess of the netherworld.[9]

The third group contains the text N4 no. 241 covering words and phrases in Sumerian and Akkadian in individual lines, which are ruled off from one

6 It remains uncertain what the fragment *KAL* 4 no. 41 treated. Maul reconstructs the first line as [*šumma ina zumur amēli pindû peṣû ša garābu i-qa*]*b*-⌜*bu*⌝-*šu* x [x (x)] based on the parallel in *BAM* 580 col. v 17'–20' (= *AMT* 84,4 col. iii 9'–12'), where line 17' reads: *šum*$_4$-*ma ina* SU NA *pi-in-du-ú* BABBAR *ša ga-ra-bu i-qab-bu*-⌜x⌝[…]. While the remaining ritual in *BAM* 580 duplicates *KAL* 4 no. 41, the context differs. Although the ending is not preserved in the first example, the parallel prescriptions in *BAM* 580 contain instructions for "applying" (LÁ) or "anointing" (EŠ.MEŠ), whereas *KAL* 4 no. 41 ends with something being thrown into the river. This action fits the other parallel text, *KAR* 25 col. iii 13'–20', which contains a ritual for a *šu'illa*-prayer to Sîn. As a result, *KAR* 25 makes no mention of *garābu* in col. iii 13', although we know that persons suffering from *garābu* should perform a ritual invoking Sîn possibly due to a connection to epilepsy (Stol 1993: 128 and note 65; cf. *BAM* 580 col. v 20).

7 Maul and Strauß (2011: 49) labelled the text as a *namburbi*-ritual although this remains uncertain. See the discussion in Section 3.7.

8 Krebernik 2007: 356. For *šu'illa*-prayers in general, see Frechette 2012; Lenzi 2011; Zgoll 2004; Mayer 1976.

9 See Ch. 3 note 124.

another. The specific entries were described collectively as *ṣâtu*, a term related to lexical lists and commentaries (see Gabbay 2016: 51–52, 101–103; Frahm 2011a: 48ff.). The tablet was described as copied on behalf of Kiṣir-Aššur.

In general, it is surprising that so few of the surviving colophons from the hand of Kiṣir-Aššur date to this early stage of his career, as we would expect a production of library copies during his early phases of specialization.[10] Several circumstances may explain this situation, such as the chance of survival, very few of his early tablets were provided with colophons, or such tablets were discarded. Individual tablets are discussed in detail below.

3.1 Complex Diagnoses in Kiṣir-Aššur's *šamallû ṣeḫru* Texts

The texts generally imply that Kiṣir-Aššur as a *šamallû ṣeḫru* learned skills related to healing various physiological areas that have the common trait of being influenced by complex illnesses, which are not solely related to a single, easily defined set of symptoms. In what follows, I briefly discuss the various diagnoses copied by Kiṣir-Aššur as *šamallû ṣeḫru* in order to evaluate the difficulties inherent in them. Snakebites and scorpion stings have been excluded from the discussion, although Chapter 4 shows that they were considered to be physiologically complex and intellectually important.

A limited number of diagnoses appear among the earliest tablets from the hand of Kiṣir-Aššur, of which Scurlock and Andersen (2005) classify several as "syndromes".[11] Ghosts (*eṭemmu*) could produce everything from headaches (*sagkidabbû*),[12] ringing ears, bloated and hurting abdomen, and upper abdominal fevers, to various one-sided pains (ibid.: 312, 525–27). *Māmītu* likewise does not always represent a clear-cut set of symptoms (Maul 2010a: 135). This syndrome was frequently connected to or used as an overarching cause of illness related to, e.g., cough or colic.[13] The associated *kadabbedû* (lit.:

10 See Robson 2011a: 562–65; Gesche 2001: 155, 158.

11 The illnesses are *ašû, eṭemmu, māmītu, pašittu, sagallu, šaššaṭu* (Scurlock and Andersen 2005: 505–506, 525). See a discussion of *sagallu* and *šaššaṭu*, as well as a definition and discussion of the term "syndrome", in Arbøll 2018a.

12 For various types of headaches and migraines labelled *sagkidabbû*, see Scurlock and Andersen 2005: 311–12.

13 For *māmītu* and its cures, see Maul 2019: 29–46. For *māmītu* and the associated "witchcraft" *kišpu*, see Schwemer 2015: 33; Schwemer 2007a: 195–96, 235; Maul 2004: 93. The illness *suālu*, a diagnosis as well as a symptom related to coughs (Scurlock and Andersen 2005: 178–79; Cadelli 2000: 313ff.), could turn into *kīs libbi*, a type of colic (see Ch. 9 note 47). A MB letter indicates that a patient with cough (*ganāḫu* and *suālu*) was treated for

'seizing-of-the-mouth') was connected to witchcraft and disabled the proper use of one's mouth and speech (*CMAwR* 2: 398; *CMAwR* 1: 3–4, 16; Kinnier Wilson and Reynolds 2007: 72–76).

The illness *ašû* designated a skin malady, although it also encompassed internal symptoms (Scurlock and Andersen 2005: 74–75, 191, 224; Fincke 2000: 100–3). As such, the illness was not necessarily easily diagnosed. Also a skin ailment, *garābu* produced a certain type of white lesion called *pindû* (*KAL* 4: 91; cf. Scurlock and Andersen 2005: 231–32). It was furthermore connected to epilepsy, and it has been suggested that it designates leprosy.[14]

Sagallu and *šaššaṭu* were two illnesses affecting the (lower) bodily "strings" (*šer'ānu*), here especially the body's muscles and tendons. The two illnesses may have been part of a syndrome beginning with the condition *maškadu* that could progress into *sagallu* and ultimately become *šaššaṭu*. I have studied these three illnesses in a recent article (Arbøll 2018a). These illnesses have traditionally been considered part of the advanced knowledge of the *āšipu*.[15]

A common trait of these diagnoses is that a majority of them are listed as diagnoses of illnesses in the diagnostic-prognostic series Sa-gig.[16] They can therefore be considered complex illness concepts that must have been important for Kiṣir-Aššur to understand in order to provide the right cure. These illnesses can also be considered complex in relation to their symptoms, which inform on the physiological conception of the body. The areas of the body affected by the illnesses in Kiṣir-Aššur's *šamallû ṣeḫru* texts are listed in Table 3.

kīs libbi and was in danger of developing "Hand of curse" *qāt māmīti* (Plantholt 2014: 179; Scurlock and Andersen 2005: 508; Parpola 1983a: 495–96; see Wee 2012: 48–49, 500ff.). It is worth noting that *RA* 40 pl. 116 obv. 8 lists *suālu* as a symptom and the prescriptions on the reverse of *RA* 15 pl. 76 may refer to some sort of colic, perhaps similar to *kīs libbi* (see below). Whether or not Kiṣir-Aššur copied any of his *šamallû ṣeḫru* material with these possible relationships in mind remains uncertain.

14 Scurlock and Andersen 2005: 71, 231–232, 722–724 note 124, 139–140 with discussion and references; Stol 1987–88: 30; Kinnier Wilson 1966: 57–58.

15 *KAR* 44 rev. 32: *ši-pir šim-mat ri-mu-ti u* SA.GAL SA.GIG GIG *ki-sat* ... The hypothesis rests on observing the second part (rev. 28–40) of *KAR* 44 as a more advanced section in relation to the first (obv. 1-rev. 27). See Section 9.4.

16 The associated illness *kadabbedû* is not mentioned in the NA version of Sa-gig, although it was in an earlier version (*CMAwR* 1: 16, 434–443). For the Sa-gig series, see Scurlock 2014: 13–272; Wee 2012; Scurlock and Andersen 2005: 575ff.; Heeßel 2000; Finkel 1988; Labat 1951. Wee (2012: 186) states that it is not clear if the goal of Sa-gig always was to identify cause over illness.

TABLE 3 Illnesses and affected areas of the body

Bodily area	Illness
Head (Headache, etc.)	*sagkidabbû, eṭemmu, (šaššaṭu?)*
(Nose?), Breath	*suālu*
Mouth, (Speech?)	*kadabbedû*
Thorax	*(kīs libbi), māmītu, (pašittu), suālu*
Abdomen	*(ašû), kīs libbi, māmītu, pašittu*
"Strings", Motoric System	*maškadu, sagallu, šaššaṭu*
Skin, Outer Changes	*ašû, garābu*
Sweat(?)	*lubāṭu*

TABLE 4 Types of illness descriptions in Kiṣir-Aššur's *šamallû ṣeḫru* texts

Type of illness description	Preserved entries in text
DIŠ NA (symptom description with or without illness names, and no diagnosis)	*BAM* 9 obv. 1(?); obv. 14; obv. 16; obv. 18; obv. 21; obv. 23–24; obv. 40; rev. 42; rev. 58; rev. 61; *BAM* 201 obv. 29'(?); *RA* 40 pl. 116 obv. 21(?)
DIŠ NA (illness or illnesses name(s)) DAB/GIG/SÌG	*BAM* 9 rev. 47; *BAM* 129 col. iv 19'; N4 no. 237 rev. 4; *RA* 15 pl. 76 obv. 14'; *RA* 40 pl. 116 obv. 1
DIŠ NA (symptom description) NA BI (diagnosis) / (diagnosis) MU.NI	*BAM* 9 rev. 51–52; *BAM* 129 col. iv 3'; col. iv 14'; *BAM* 201 obv. 22'–25'; rev. 31'
DIŠ NA (diagnosis) GIG (additional symptoms)	*BAM* 129 col. iv 6'–7'; *RA* 40 pl. 116 obv. 8–9
KA.INIM.MA (illness name)	*BAM* 129 col. i 6; col. i 17; col. i 24; col. ii 29'(?); N4 no. 237 obv. 14–15(?)
Other	*BAM* 9 rev. 55; *KAL* 4 no. 41(?); *RA* 15 pl. 76 rev. 8'(?)

Clearly, these few illnesses cover a large portion of the body. However, the texts only include a limited number of actual symptom descriptions and diagnoses, a fair amount of "ditto" (KI.MIN) prescriptions, and other prescriptions without listing symptoms or diagnoses altogether. In Table 4 is a schematic overview of the types of symptom descriptions and diagnoses in Kiṣir-Aššur's *šamallû ṣeḫru* texts.

Interestingly, several tablets contain symptom descriptions with or without diagnoses, as well as diagnoses with additional symptom descriptions that were likely directed towards broadening Kiṣir-Aššur's conceptions of how an illness can manifest itself. Other entries simply refer to the name of the illness, presumably because Kiṣir-Aššur already knew (parts of) the illness' manifestations or because his teacher would fill in the gaps during his apprenticeship (see below). I discuss Kiṣir-Aššur's *šamallû ṣeḫru* diagnoses in relation to the diagnostic-prognostic series Sa-gig in Section 3.6.1.

3.1.1 *Earlier Diagnostic Training*

To what extent Kiṣir-Aššur was allowed to engage in actual medical treatments as *šamallû ṣeḫru* is unknown, but, as I argue in Section 6.2.4, he was probably not allowed to "practice" medicine on his own until he was *mašmaššu*. Thus, he may not have studied diagnoses and physiology in depth before becoming a *šamallû ṣeḫru*. However, none of Kiṣir-Aššur's tablets with colophons attest to early-stage educational excerpts with one or two prescriptions.[17] To evaluate Kiṣir-Aššur's prior medical knowledge, Finkel's study of a group of LB school tablets is currently the best comparative material.[18] The majority of the material edited by Finkel consists of single prescriptions, incantations, or small plant lists with no direct duplicates in the therapeutic series Ugu (Finkel 2000: 142). Both the LB school texts, as well as the 24 elementary medical exercises from the N4 collection listed by Finkel (ibid.: 143–44), appear to revolve around relatively simple problems, such as headache, fever (*ummu*),[19] or "Anus illness",[20] of which few are attested in Sa-gig.[21]

17 Although, e.g., *LKA* 43 only contains one text. Some N4 tablets may derive from an earlier education phase. See, e.g., Veldhuis 2014: 369–70; Finkel 2000: 144. In general, the earlier school texts are poorly attested in the NA sources (Veldhuis 2014: 353–72; Gesche 2001: 23–24 and note 113, 41). For LB Uruk, see Clancier 2014: 45 note 16, 48 note 35.

18 See Finkel 2000. The tablets belong to the archive of Bēl-rēmanni. However, Jursa (1999: 1) has stressed that this Bēl-rēmanni was not part of the scribal elite, and the medical texts in this archive may represent certain specific needs related to this family (ibid.: 28–29). Gesche lists medical texts as part of *āšipūtu* specialization, and generally not as part of the NB and LB school texts she investigated (Gesche 2001: 172, 214).

19 *BAM* 10 rev. 18 and 28: SAG.DU-*su* LÁ-*ma*; *BAM* 143 obv. 1: DIŠ NA KÚM DAB-*su*.

20 *BAM* 89 obv. 1: DIŠ NA *k*[*i-iṣ* ŠÀ(?)], and rev. 9: NA BI *qé-reb* DÚR.GIG; *BAM* 98 rev. 2: *nap-šal-ti* ⌜DÚR.GIG⌝. However, a few of the N4 elementary exercises contain more complex diagnoses. *BAM* 183 obv. 19: ... AN.T[A.ŠUB.BA(?)], rev. 23: ... ^{d}DIM$_{11}$.ME, rev. 27: ... AN.TA.ŠUB.BA, rev. 28: ... *mim-ma lem-nu*, etc.; *BAM* 184 col. i 13–14 states: [*n*]*ap-šal-ti* ^{14} [A]N.TA.ŠUB.BA.

21 See references to DÚR.GIG in medical texts in Wee 2012: 226. See Finkel 2000: 203 (text 48), 207 (text 50), 208 (text 51) and 210 (text 52) for more complicated diagnoses.

Drawing on Finkel's findings, the earlier knowledge taught to Kiṣir-Aššur likely consisted of symptoms grouped under less complex illness headings. As a result, the complex diagnoses copied by him as *šamallû ṣeḫru* stand out and attest to the fact that he was taught *āšipūtu*: he needed to learn about the overarching illnesses and causes behind the symptoms. Furthermore, Kiṣir-Aššur's surviving material suggests that he learned about the nature of such illnesses through the therapeutic texts coupled with oral instructions, as discussed in Sections 3.6 and 3.6.1. Although his *šamallû ṣeḫru* texts were not directly related to complex causes of illness, they likely provided prescriptions concerning causes that were illustrative for understanding the human anatomy and physiological processes. Aspects of Kiṣir-Aššur's training in anatomy and physiology are explored in chapter 4. In light of the above evidence, Kiṣir-Aššur appears to have made use of the diagnoses copied as *šamallû ṣeḫru* to learn how to establish a complex diagnosis, and to understand (roughly) how the body functioned and how these treatments were believed to work in relation to symptoms and causes.

3.2 Principles Understood through Examples

Mesopotamian scholarly disciplines likely relied on lists of omens to provide the written, "scientific" background for a principle.[22] Omen series, such as Sa-gig, are therefore often regarded as lists of omens used to establish "theories".[23] But, how would Kiṣir-Aššur have learned the necessary diagnostic principles, if not from Sa-gig? We must assume the Bāba-šuma-ibni family had an extensive oral dimension to their teachings.[24] However, although someone in N4 copied "questions" related to Sa-gig,[25] it still stands to reason that the majority of the written material for Kiṣir-Aššur's diagnostic understanding must have been derived from the therapeutic texts.[26]

22 For discussions with further references, see Rochberg 2016: 140–41; van de Mieroop 2016: 185–93.

23 See Wee 2012: 476–481; Rochberg 2010; Heeßel 2007b: 98, 104, 110–14.

24 Some commentaries exist from the N4 collection, especially from Kiṣir-Nabû, although they do not seem to attest to oral teachings (Frahm 2011a: 268–270).

25 See Ch. 3 note 105.

26 Comparatively, Robson (2013: 49–50) noted that omens account for a small portion of the Ḫuzirina texts and describes the situation as follows: "As its students were not preparing to access the inner circle of the royal court, they had no great need for omens" (ibid.: 50). However, the court scholars rarely quoted Sa-gig (Robson 2008: 474; Heeßel 2000: 93).

Kiṣir-Aššur's therapeutic texts copied as *šamallû ṣeḫru* provided him with the knowledge necessary for producing and providing a therapeutic treatment for the disorders in question (see Section 3.6). While his texts contain some "ditto" (KI.MIN) prescriptions, especially on the obverse of *RA* 15 pl. 76, the majority of entries copied contain at least the name of the illness and a treatment. Finkel's hypothesis that a student would collect (in the KI.MIN format) all the prescriptions that he had learned and copy them onto a large tablet at the end of his studies is therefore not applicable in this context (Finkel 2000: 143).

Instead, as shown in the following sections, Kiṣir-Aššur seems to have copied material related to assignments involving a particular physiological area or malady. However, in order to apply this knowledge, he must also have acquired the necessary abilities for understanding human physiology. While a few useful lists of anatomy from which an abundance of medical knowledge could originate are known,[27] the majority of such knowledge was probably obtained from the principles one could derive from the therapeutic texts with diagnoses and contextualized via the actual praxis of the family. In the following sections, Kiṣir-Aššur's diagnostic-therapeutic texts from the first category of *šamallû ṣeḫru* texts are subjected to a thorough investigation in order to establish what Kiṣir-Aššur may have learned from them and how they were possibly used in his training.

3.3 The Head: *BAM* 9

BAM 9 relates to headaches (*sagkidabbû*; lit.: "affliction of the temple(s)"), the temples, ghosts (*eṭemmu*), and ringing ears. Headaches and pulsating temples are among the most common symptoms of ghostly disorders, although other symptoms were also considered ominous concerning ghostly diagnoses (Scurlock 2006: 12–18).[28] Finally, possibly two entries relate to "burning *ṣētu*-fever" (UD.DA TAB-*ma*) of the head.

In *BAM* 9, Kiṣir-Aššur writes out the diagnosis "[If a man]'s [he]ad burns with *ṣētu* and the hair of his 'head' (*muḫḫu*) falls out, (and) he [(repeatedly?)

---

27 See the list Ugumu and Ur$_5$-ra tablet 15 (Couto Ferreira 2009; Westenholz and Sigrist 2008; *MSL* 9). See also the "List of Diseases", known from Nineveh and Assur, in which a few anatomical features are also described in relation to illnesses (*MSL* 9: 90ff., ms B = VAT 11507).

28 Scurlock 2006; cf. Scurlock and Andersen 2005: 166, 312, 324, 502, 524, 527, 555, 736 note 100.

suff]ers ['rising' (strings of his) temple(s)] ...".[29] This line differs in one significant regard from its four duplicates, namely in the writing of SAG.DU-*šú* in reference to the place wherefrom the hair falls out.[30] Kiṣir-Aššur writes *muḫḫišu* (UGU-*šú*), which Worthington translated "crown (of his head)" (Worthington 2005: 19).[31] However, the other duplicates preserve *qaqqadišu* (SAG.DU-*šú*). According to Westenholz and Sigrist (2006: 4, 8), the first subseries of Ugu contains a distinction between the use of *qaqqadu* and *muḫḫu*. The former designates the cutaneous layer around the skull, i.e., the outside of the head and its skin, whereas the latter designated the skull and brain, i.e., a bony structure with marrow (= the brain).[32]

Since the relevant passage in *BAM* 9 is duplicated by another Assur manuscript, *BAM* 3, which has the writing SAG.DU over UGU, *BAM* 9 does not seem to have been a varying tradition. Instead, it must be regarded as an idiosyncrasy on behalf of Kiṣir-Aššur, who either made the mistake when copying, or because he did not recall the difference between the terms anatomically (cf. Worthington 2012: 112). If Kiṣir-Aššur copied from a writing-board containing a version parallel to Nineveh Ugu, then *muḫḫu* would have been the subject until this prescription, in which the focus changed to *qaqqadu* (cf. Westenholz and Sigrist 2006: 4). A third possibility is that he consciously wrote this sign, as (*ṣētu*-)fevers may have been able to reside within the bones, i.e., the marrow or brain(?).[33]

29

BAM 9 obv. 23–24:	[DIŠ NA SAG].DU-*su* UD.DA TAB-*ma* SÍG UGU-*šú i-šaḫ-ḫu-ḫu*
	[x x x] [24] [TUKU]-*ši* *{x}* SAG.DU-*su* SAR-*ab* ...
BAM 480 col. iii 8–9:	DIŠ [NA] SAG.DU-*šú i-šaḫ-ḫu-uḫ*
	ZI SAG.KI TUKU.TUKU [9] *ana* x[...] SAG.DU-*su* SAR-*ab* ...
BAM 3 col. ii 27–28:	DIŠ NA UD.DA TAB-*ma* {TUKU} SÍG SAG.DU-*šú i-šaḫ-ḫu-uḫ* [28]
	ZI SAG.KI TUKU.TUKU SAG.DU-*su* SAR-*ab* ...
Jastrow 1913 obv. 18–19:	[ ]⸢TAB-*ma*?⸣ SÍG TA *raš* SAG.DU-*šú i-šaḫ-ḫu-uḫ* [19]
	[ ]

Edition in Worthington 2005: 11 line 141'–42' and p. 27 for comments on these lines.

30 Furthermore, this line contains an erasure and possibly only one TUKU sign to denote the Gtn stem. See Ch. 3 note 29.

31 In the edition of the 1st tablet (Worthington 2005) and the 2nd tablet (Attia and Buisson 2003) of the first subsection of Ugu the opening incipit has been translated as "If a man's head is feverish" or "Si le crâne d'un homme contient de la chaleur", although Geller at one point advocated a translation as "If a man's brain contains heat (fever)" (Geller 2001–02: 58, 68; cf. Westenholz and Sigrist 2006: 4).

32 The OB lexical list Ugumu lists body parts in Sumerian, in which we find a range of words related to the head in Sumerian (Couto Ferreira 2009; Westenholz and Sigrist 2008).

33 This is perhaps indicated in several diagnoses concerning (*ḫimiṭ*) *ṣētu*, e.g., *BAM* 145 obv. 11–12: "... the flesh above is cold (but) his bone below (feels) burning hot ..." (Scurlock and Andersen 2005: 53). See the NA royal letter *SAA* 10 no. 242: "... this fever has lingered inside the very bones" (obv. 10–12: *ina* ŠÀ *ša ḫu-un-ṭu* [11] *šu-ú ina* ŠÀ *eṣ-ma-a-ti* [12] *ú-kil-lu-u-ni*). See

BAM 9 is an extract (*nisḫu*), and all the entries are extracted according to uncertain principles from the first tablets of the 1st subseries of the therapeutic Ugu series, as shown in Table 20 in Section 9.3.4.[34] The entries duplicated in the Ugu tablets were chosen from sections concerning the *qaqqadu* and not the *muḫḫu*.[35] The choice of entries for *BAM* 9 may therefore have been based on their relation to physical symptoms occurring mainly on the outside of the head (i.e., not the internal brain-area). Perhaps the extracts were chosen according to instructions or maybe they were arranged as such on the writing-board from which Kiṣir-Aššur copied.

In two instances in *BAM* 9, Kiṣir-Aššur writes a dual of the cuneiform sign for eye (IGI^{II}) where the specification relates to the "right" or "left" eye.[36] Although this is not necessarily uncommon, it is not attested in the parallel Nineveh library copy *BAM* 482.[37] However, this was likely a scribal convention rather than anatomical unawareness (see, e.g., *BAM* 202 rev. 7', *KAR* 298 rev. 30).

The catch-line of *BAM* 9 is preserved in two Assur duplicates and states: "[If] *ṣētu*-fever burns [a man] so that the hair of his head continually stands on

also *BAM* 575 col. i 21 (2nd tablet of the *suālu* Ugu subseries): DIŠ NA ŠÀ-*šú* GIG-*ma* ŠÀ GÌR.PAD.DU-*šú* SIG$_7$ Š[À-*šú* G]IG.MEŠ SA$_5$ UD.DA SÁ.SÁ "If a man is ill in the 'abdomen', the inside of his bone(s) is yellow, his belly is covered with 'sores' (*simmu*), he is overcome by *ṣētu* (Cadelli 2000: 125). As a result, fevers such as *ṣētu* may occasionally have been related to the marrow and, by extension, the brain. Cf. Stol 2007a: 12, 22, 25, 27 with examples.

34 *BAM* 9 contain duplicate passages of lines 141'–146' and 148' from *BAM* 480 = 1st tablet (Worthington 2005 ms A) and lines 7–9, 67–67, 68–69, 84–89 and 169'–176' of *BAM* 482 = 2nd tablet (Attia and Buisson 2003 ms A).

35 Westenholz and Sigrist (2006: 4) noted that lines 1–140' and 190'–197' in *BAM* 480 (Worthington 2005) concerned the *muḫḫu*, whereas lines 141'–189' and 206'–end concerned the *qaqqadu*.

36 *BAM* 9 obv. 14: [x x x x ZA]G-*šú* DAB-*su-ma* IGI^{II} ZAG-*šú* ÉR *ú-kal* ⸢x⸣[...]
BAM 482 col. ii 20: DIŠ [NA SAG.KI ZAG]-*šú* DAB-*su-ma* IGI ZAG-*šú* ÉR *ú-kal* ...
BAM 9 obv. 16: [DIŠ N]A SAG.KI GÙB-*šú* DAB-*su-ma* IGI^{II} GÙB-*šú* ÉR *ú-kal* [...]
BAM 482 col. ii 22: DIŠ NA SAG.KI GÙB-*šú* DAB-*su-ma* IGI GÙB-*šú* ÉR *ú-kal* ...
See Attia and Buisson 2003: 6 line 84 and 86.

37 A few differences, however, suggest that *BAM* 9 was copied from a tradition varying from the Nineveh traditions. The diagnosis in *BAM* 9 obv. 35 is broken, but two duplicates have DIŠ KI.MIN and two have DIŠ NA SAG.KI.DAB.BA TUKU.TUKU-*ši* (Attia and Buisson 2003: 3 line 7). Neither line fits the *BAM* 9 entry. Furthermore, *BAM* 9 obv. 4 and another manuscript share an order of two drugs, [^{šim}GÚR].GÚR ... ^{šim}LI, which are reversed in three other duplicates, e.g., the Nineveh library copy *BAM* 482 (ibid.: 8 line 171'). *BAM* 9 also formulates the diagnosis in obv. 18 differently than in *BAM* 482 (ibid: 6 line 88).

end".[38] This diagnosis and its symptoms are known to have affected various bodily areas, and we must assume that Kiṣir-Aššur was supposed to move on to other illnesses or areas of the body after copying *BAM* 9.

3.3.1 *Treating Ghostly Afflictions*

The unpublished manuscript N4 no. 237 contains a prayer to Šamaš and two prescriptions for treating a man seized by a ghost.[39] The content is therefore directed against similar problems as some prescriptions in *BAM* 9. However, there are no symptom descriptions in N4 no. 237 and only a single preserved diagnosis (rev. 4: ⌜DIŠ NA GIDIM DAB⌝-*su*; cf. obv. 14–15). Presumably, all the treatments in N4 no. 237 were directed against this problem. The tablet mentions two ritual elements, which Kiṣir-Aššur could have learned in connection to this text. Obverse lines 20–21 mention: "You draw the line [... in the manner o]f a diviner" (*šiddu* [... *kīma š*]*a bārî tašaddad*), referring to an act of ritually marking an offering arrangement apart from the environment, and obverse line 22 states: "You distribute small heap(s) of flour" ([*zid*]*ubdubbâ tattanaddi*).[40]

The final prescription contains at least three notations of a "new break" in slightly smaller script, indicating that the original copied from contained a number of breaks (see Sections 3.4.1 and 7.4.3 for further discussion of such statements). This treatment is also preserved in Kiṣir-Aššur's *BAM* 9, Kiṣir-Nabû's *KAR* 56 from his *mašmaššu*-phase,[41] as well as a manuscript from contemporary Nineveh (*AMT* 93,1; see Scurlock 2006: 607 no. 290). The prescription is presented in partitur below with a composite translation:

---

38 *BAM* 9 rev. 69: [DIŠ NA] ⌜UD.DA TAB⌝.BA!-*ma* SÍG SA[G.DU]⌜-*šú*?⌝ GUB.MEŠ EG[IR?-*šú* ...]
BAM 145 obv. 1: [DIŠ NA U]D.DA TAB.B[A-*ma* ...]
BAM 146 obv. 29': [...]-*ma* SÍG SAG.DU-*šú* GUB.GUB-*az* IGI.ME[Š-*šú*]
For translations and the illness, see, e.g., Stol 2007a: 28–29; Scurlock and Andersen 2005: 53 no. 3.121. The colophon of *BAM* 145 is broken, but on the picture on CDLI (P285241) the middle of rev. 7 may read: ⌜*bà-rì*⌝. The end of rev. 9 may read: ⌜ŠÁMAN!?.LÁ⌝ [TUR(?)], but this requires further collation. See Ch. 5 note 57.

39 The partly damaged initial prescription (obv. 16–rev. 3) presumably described actions accompanying the prayer.

40 N4 no. 237 obv. 20–22: ... *šid*-⌜*du*⌝ [x x x] ^{21} [GIM *š*]*á* ^{lú}ḪAL GÍD-*ad* A SIKIL B[AL-*qí*] ^{22} [ZÌ.D]UB.DUB.BU ŠUB.ŠUB-*ma* ..., see Abusch and Schwemer 2011: 138, 145, 148 with further references. Note that N4 no. 237 is the only of Kiṣir-Aššur's *šamallû ṣeḫru* texts mentioning "flour heap(s)" *zidubdubbû*, whereas *BAM* 129 col. i 27 and 31 is the only of his text from this phase mentioning a "magical flour circle" *zisurrû*.

41 Edited, except for the colophon, in Scurlock 2006: 442 no. 177 (obv. 1–4), 448–449 no. 179 (obv. 12–rev. 10), 450 no. 180 (rev. 11–13), 607 no. 290 (obv. 5–11).

N4 no. 237 rev. 4:	⸢DIŠ NA GIDIM DAB⸣-*su*	*ú-ra-an-na*	
KAR 56 obv. 5a:	DIŠ NA GIDIM DAB-*su*	*ú-ra-an-na*	→
BAM 9 rev. 47a:	[DIŠ N]A ⸢GIDIM⸣ DAB-*su-ma*	*ú-ra-a-nu*	→
AMT 93,1 obv.$^{?}$ 2'a:	[	*ú-ra*]-⸢*a*⸣-*na*	→

N4 no. 237 rev. 5:	⸢^{ú}LAL KA⸣.A.AB.BA	ŠIM.^{d}MAŠ ⸢NITA *u* MUNUS⸣
KAR 56 obv. 5b–6:	^{ú}LAL ^{6} KA.A.AB.BA	ŠIM.^{d}MAŠ NITA *u* MUNUS
BAM 9 rev. 47b–48a:	⸢^{ú}⸣LAL ⸢KA⸣.A.AB.BA	⸢ŠIM.^{d}⸣[MAŠ] ^{48} [MUNU]S$^{!}$ →
AMT 93,1 obv.$^{?}$ 2'b:	^{ú}LAL KA.A.AB.BA	ŠIM.^{d}MAŠ NÍTA *u* MUNUS

N4 no. 237 rev. 6:	*ḫe-pí eš-šú*	GI.ŠUL.ḪI ⸢^{ú}⸣*a*[*k-tam*]	
KAR 56 obv. 7a:		GI.ŠUL.ḪI ^{ú}*ak-tam*	→
BAM 9 rev. 48b:		GI.[Š]UL.ḪI ^{ú}⸢*ak*⸣-*tam*	→
AMT 93,1 obv.$^{?}$ 3'a:	[	-*t*]*ám*	→

N4 no. 237 rev. 7:	*ḫe-pí eš-šú*	ÚḪ.⸢^{d}⸣[ÍD]	
KAR 56 obv. 7b:	*ḫe-pí eš-šú*	ÚḪ.^{d}ÍD	
BAM 9 rev. 48c:	^{na4}⸢*mu*⸣-*ṣa*	ÚḪ.^{d}ÍD	→
AMT 93,1 obv.$^{?}$ 3'b:	^{na4}*mu-ṣa*	ÚḪ.^{d}ÍD	

N4 no. 237 rev. 8:	⸢^{ú}LÚ.U$_{18}$⸣.LU	*ḫ*[*e-pí eš-šú*]	
KAR 56 obv. 8a:	^{ú}LÚ.U$_{18}$.LU	*ḫe-pí eš-šú*	→
BAM 9 rev. 48d–49a:	^{ú}NAM.L[Ú	] ^{49} [NUM]UN	→
AMT 93,1 obv.$^{?}$ 3'c:	^{ú}LÚ.U$_{18}$.LU	NUMUN	→

N4 no. 237 rev. 9:	⸢^{giš}ŠINIG⸣	SI GU$_4$ *tur-á*[*r*	ḪE.ḪE]	
KAR 56 obv. 8b–9a:	^{giš}ŠINIG ^{9}	SI GU$_4$ *tur-ár*	ḪE.ḪE	→
BAM 9 rev. 49b:	^{giš}*bi-ni*	SI GU$_4$ *t*[*u*]*r-ár*	ḪE.⸢ḪE⸣	→
AMT 93,1 obv.$^{?}$ 3'd–4'a:	^{giš}*bi-ni* ^{4}	[	] ḪE.ḪE	→

N4 no. 237 rev. 10:	⸢PIŠ$_{10}$.^{d}ÍD⸣	SUḪUŠ ⸢^{giš}MA⸣.NU [x x x (x)]	
KAR 56 obv. 9b–10a:	PIŠ$_{10}$.^{d}ÍD ^{10}	SUḪUŠ ^{giš}MA.NU *ḫe-pí eš-šú*	→
BAM 9 rev. 49c:	PIŠ$_{10}$.^{d}ÍD	SUḪUŠ ^{giš}MA.NU 1-*niš* ⸢SÚD⸣	
AMT 93,1 obv.$^{?}$ 4'b:	PIŠ$_{10}$.^{d}ÍD	SUḪUŠ ^{giš}MA.NU 1-*niš* SÚD	→

N4 no. 237 rev. 11:	*ina* ÚŠ ⸢^{giš}ERIN⸣ ḪE.⸢ḪE⸣ ŠÉŠ-*su*-⸢*ma*	TI⸣-[*uṭ*]
KAR 56 obv. 10b–11:	*ina* ÚŠ ^{giš}ERIN ḪE.ḪE ^{11} ŠÉŠ-*su-ma*	TI-*uṭ*
BAM 9 rev. 50:	[*ina*] ÚŠ ^{giš}ERIN ḪE.ḪE ŠÉŠ-*su-ma*	TI-*u*[*ṭ*]
AMT 93,1 obv.$^{?}$ 4'c:	*ina* ÚŠ ^{giš}ERIN ḪE.ḪE ŠEŠ.MEŠ-*su-ma*	TI

> If a ghost afflicts (lit.: seizes) a man, you char and mix (*list of ingredients*). Grind together *kibrītu*-sulphur (and) *ēru*-tree, (and) mix (there)in resin of *erēnu*-cedar. You anoint him (with it), and he will recover.

The edition above shows that *KAR* 56 also contained notations of a "new break" in smaller script in almost the exact same lines as N4 no. 237.[42] Furthermore, both these manuscripts contain identical spellings and writings of the prescriptions. The only difference is the addition of the comment "new break" in N4 no. 237 reverse line 6. Comparatively, the two additional duplicate passages in *BAM* 9 and *AMT* 93,1 contain different spellings and added ingredients in the passages where N4 no. 237 and *KAR* 56 noted breaks in the original.[43] Accordingly, these manuscripts differ, although they do not appear to represent a single divergent tradition.[44] N4 no. 237 contains passages also considered useful to Kiṣir-Nabû, and the knowledge was therefore employed in N4 at various career stages. Furthermore, the text was labelled as an *u'iltu*-tablet, which could indicate the purpose behind the text was different from other *šamallû ṣeḫru* manuscripts labelled as *ṭuppus* (see Section 5.3.2).

The prescription above is not the only duplicate passage in N4 no. 237 and *KAR* 57. The three opening lines of the initial prayer in N4 no. 237 are parallel to *KAR* 56 obverse lines 12–14, although the remaining spell and the following ritual instruction in *KAR* 56 differ from the prayer and the following prescription in N4 no. 237.[45] *KAR* 56 also contains two additional entries not incorporated into N4 no. 237 (*KAR* 56 obv. 1–4, rev. 11–13). The colophon of *KAR* 56 reads: "(*Catch-line*), a copy of an Assyrian writing-board, for undertaking a (ritual) procedure of Kiṣir-Nabû, the *mašmaššu*-exorcist, he [qu]ickly extracted (it)".[46] As discussed in Section 9.2.1, *KAR* 56 was presumably copied

42 N4 no. 237 rev. 7/*KAR* 56 obv. 7; N4 no. 237 rev. 8/*KAR* 56 obv. 8; N4 no. 237 rev. 10(?)/*KAR* 56 obv. 10.

43 E.g., N4 no. 237 rev. 7 vs. *BAM* 9 rev. 48; N4 no. 237 rev. 8 vs. *BAM* 9 rev. 48; N4 no. 237 rev. 8 vs. *BAM* 9 rev. 49; N4 no. 237 rev. 10 vs. *BAM* 9 rev. 49.

44 *BAM* 9 and *AMT* 93,1 do not agree on various spellings, see e.g., *BAM* 9 rev. 48 vs. *AMT* 93,1 obv.$^{?}$ 3' and *BAM* 9 rev. 50 vs. *AMT* 93,1 obv.$^{?}$ 4'. Other spellings in the two manuscripts are identical, although they differ from N4 no. 237 and *KAR* 56, see e.g., *BAM* 9 rev. 49 vs. *AMT* 93,1 obv.$^{?}$ 3'. *BAM* 9 and *AMT* 93,1 contain the same added ingredients in the "breaks", e.g., *BAM* 9 rev. 48/*AMT* 93,1 obv.$^{?}$ 3', *BAM* 9 rev. 49/*AMT* 93,1 obv.$^{?}$ 3'.

45 N4 no. 237 obv. 1–3: [ÉN ^{d}utu lu]gal ⸢an-ki-ke$_4$ ^{d}utu⸣ di-<ku$_5$>-kur-kur-ra-ke$_4$ ^{2} [^{d}utu] ⸢saĝ-kal⸣ diĝir-re-e-ne-ke$_4$ ^{3} [^{d}]⸢utu kala-ga⸣ pa.è.

46 *KAR* 56 rev. 14–17: DIŠ NA *lu* AN.TA.ŠUB.BA *lu-u* ^{d}*lugal-ùr-ra* ^{15} GABA.RI ^{giš}ZU *Aš-šur*^{ki}*-i* ^{16} *ana* DAB DÙ-*ši* ^{p}*Ki-ṣir-*^{d}PA MAŠ.MAŠ ^{17} [*ḫa*]-*an-ṭiš* ⸢ZI⸣-*ḫa*.

from a writing board with Assyrian sign forms.[47] Comparatively, N4 no. 237 is only "copied and checked according to its original".[48] Considering the numerous notes on breaks in identical places in N4 no. 237 and *KAR* 56, it is possible that the prescription was copied by Kiṣir-Aššur and later Kiṣir-Nabû from the same partly broken writing-board. The added note on a "new break" in N4 no. 237 rev. 6, which is not found in *KAR* 56, or filled out with an ingredient in the two additional duplicate manuscripts, indicates that Kiṣir-Aššur saw a broken space on the writing-board copied from, which had originally not listed an ingredient. Kiṣir-Nabû may have realized this when producing his copy since the note was not added to his manuscript. This indicates that Kiṣir-Aššur was an inexperienced copyist when he produced N4 no. 237, which is substantiated by a peculiar writing of his father's name as Nabû-bēssuni in the colophon (N4 no. 237 rev. 15: $^{\text{p.d}}$AG-*bi*-⸢*su*⸣-*ni*).

BAM 9 was a "first extract" and a "copy of a writing-board", which may have been further described in a broken passage (Section 9.2.1). Thus, it is possible to pose two hypotheses concerning this text in relation to N4 no. 237. Possibly, *BAM* 9 was copied from the same writing-board as N4 no. 237 and *KAR* 56, but the text served another purpose than the former.[49] Thus, broken spaces could have been filled and different spellings employed. Alternatively, *BAM* 9 was copied from another writing-board with a different text.

3.4 The "Strings" and "Inner" Body

Four of Kiṣir-Aššur's *šamallû ṣeḫru* texts attest to him learning about the mouth, lungs, abdomen, and "strings" (i.e., muscles, tendons, arteries, veins, etc.) of the body via the illnesses *sagallu-šaššaṭu* (*BAM* 129), *māmītu* and *kadabbedû* (*BAM* 201,), *maškadu* (N4 A 400), and *ašû, pašittu, lubāṭu*, as well as various lung illnesses (*RA* 40 pl. 116). *BAM* 129, *BAM* 201 and *RA* 40 pl. 116 are discussed individually here to provide a discussion of their content in relation to Kiṣir-Aššur's training. The manuscript N4 A 400 is still unpublished, and only a single general observation can be made. The text is likely the only tablet among Kiṣir-Aššur's *šamallû ṣeḫru*-phase manuscripts, which contain a single incantation and instructions for treating a concrete illness.

47 Whether or not the Assyrianism *i-bal-laṭ-ma*, instead of the expected Babylonian *iballuṭ* in *KAR* 56 rev. 9, can be attributed to the writing-board or Kiṣir-Nabû's idiosyncracies is uncertain.

48 N4 no. 237 rev. 12: [LIBIR.R]A.BI.GIM AB.SAR BA.AN.È.

49 Additionally, *BAM* 9 was labelled a *ṭuppu* and N4 no. 237 an *u'iltu*. The latter types may have served different purposes, see Section 5.3.2.

3.4.1 BAM *129*

BAM 129 has a preserved first and fourth column, only the beginning lines are preserved in column two, and none of column three survives. The two columns on the obverse consist of *abracadabra* incantations and ritual instructions against *sagallu*,[50] but without diagnoses, whereas column four contains diagnoses and elaborate prescriptions for treating *šaššaṭu*. Presumably, column three also contained cures for this illness. Unlike bilingual and monolingual Akkadian incantations, it is unclear if *abracadabra* incantations had any place in LB scribal education, and their appearance in the *šamallû ṣeḫru* manuscript *BAM* 129 is therefore peculiar.[51]

Kiṣir-Aššur included three annotations in spaces left blank in the first column of *BAM* 129, noting that the tablet copied from contained a "new break".[52] In two of these examples the presumed correct reading of the line is known:

BAM 129 col. i 8:	[DÙ.DÙ.B]I ú ta [x x x x GAR]-*an* A pa $^{ḫe\text{-}pí\ eš\text{-}šú}$ *ina* ^{dug}LA.ḪA.AN
CT 23 pl. 6 col. ii 9'–11':	[...] TI-*qé-šú-ma ana* IGI 20 ^{10} [... A].MEŠ *pa-ši-rì* ÍD ^{11} [...]
K. 2483+ obv. 4–5:	DÙ.DÙ.BI ú ta kil šá ti rat [...] ^{5} ^{dug}LA.ḪA.AN ...
BAM 129 col. i 10:	[x x x x x x x x x K]A$^{?}$ ^{giš}BAN$^{!}$ NU GAR-*nu šá* $^{ḫe\text{-}pí\ eš\text{-}šú}$
CT 23 pl. 6 col. ii 12'–13':	[...] ⸢*šá ana*⸣ K[A$^{?}$ ^{g}]^{iš}BAN NU GAR-*an* ^{13} [...]
K. 2483+ obv. 6–7:	*ana* ŠÀ ŠUB-*di* [...] ^{7} *šá ana* KA ^{giš}BAN *la* GAR-*nu šá* 7 K[A ...]
BAM 129 col. i 31:	[x x] ⸢x⸣ ŠUB-*di* ZÌ.SUR.RA-*a* NIGIN-*me* $^{ḫe\text{-}pí}$ [^{eš}]$^{\text{-}šú}$ DUG$_4$.GA
CT 23 pl. 7 col. ii 27':	[... .SU]R.R[A ...]

50 The *abracadabra* incantation beginning in *BAM* 129 obv. 12 is also attested as incipit against "roaring ears" in *AMT* 35,1 obv. 6': [...] ḫa gi ḫu ú-a na-an-ku-ud-ri KA.INIM.MA GEŠTUG^{II}-*šú i-šag-gu-ma*.

51 Cf. Gesche 2001: 50, 55, 173–77, 214–15. Finkel included one *abracadabra* incantation (Finkel 2000 no. 51). However, *sagallu*-illness may occasionally have been treated with *abracadabra* incantations, such as the ones found in *BAM* 129.

52 See *BAM* 129 col. i 8, 10, 31: *ḫe-pí eš-šú*. No breaks are noted in col. iv.

The ritual in *BAM* 129 col. i 8–11 is difficult to understand, even in the preserved Nineveh versions. The internal evidence suggests that Kiṣir-Aššur may have understood even less. In addition to the "new break" in col. i 8, the beginning of the line is broken and leaves room for no more than five reconstructed signs. This amount of space does not fit any of the duplicate versions. The break must therefore be reconstructed with another "new break" note, an unknown line from a different tradition, or represent a mistake in Kiṣir-Aššur's copy. Notably, Kiṣir-Aššur makes at least one mistake in this passage, copying ^{giš}GIM for ^{giš}BAN. Due to the similarity of the two signs, Kiṣir-Aššur possibly mistook BAN for GIM.[53]

Finkel has argued that the *ḫe-pí* glosses among his group of LB exercises may be an attempt by the writer to show his ability to faithfully preserve and transmit an older, fragmentary text (Finkel 2000: 180; cf. Worthington 2012: 26–27). Considering that the production of tablets to be integrated into the family's tablet collection seems to have been one of the goals of aspiring scholars,[54] *BAM* 129 may be an example of Kiṣir-Aššur showing his ability to copy a difficult and fragmentary tablet. Therefore, the copy here could be an exercise. Nevertheless, several passages in the treatments prescribe ritualistic acts, which Kiṣir-Aššur perhaps copied in order to aid his father. The same conclusions may hold true for N4 no. 237 above.

Peculiarly, Kiṣir-Aššur did not copy any of the numerous *maškadu-* or *araḫḫi-*themed incantations and rituals often prescribed against *sagallu*.[55] Unlike the entries chosen for *BAM* 9, the duplicate passages of *BAM* 129 run consecutively on the Nineveh (Ugu?) manuscript *CT* 23 pl. 5–14, which included all such incantations and ritual instructions (Section 9.3.4).

53 *BAM* 129 col. i 10. Worthington (2012: 93–98) classified such errors as "errors of sign identification" (see a similar example in Heeßel 2000: 306 note 30).

54 Memorization through repeated copying was an integral part of cuneiform training (Robson 2011a: 562–63). For apprentice manuscripts at Ḫuzirina, see ibid.: 564–65. Manuscripts from *šamallû ṣeḫrus*, such as K. 2016a+, were also excavated in Assurbanipal's tablet collection (Veldhuis 2014: 384–85; Lieberman 1990: 215–16). Many apprentices left behind few tablets in the N4 collection, perhaps to commemorate their time in the house (Maul 2010a: 215 and note 93; see Fadhil 2012: 34, 51). Comparatively, the LB text production was generally related to learning and teaching (Clancier 2014: 45–46, 50, 52; George 2003–04: 404). Several NB and LB examples exist of educational tablets donated to temple libraries, see Gesche 2001: 155, 158; Pearce 1993: 190; Cohen 1988: 25; Cavigneaux 1981.

55 See *CT* 23 pl. 4 rev. 9–11 and pl. 10–11 col. iii 26–28 (Arbøll 2018a; Abusch 2016: 169–70, 263, 350; Cavigneaux 1999b; Cooper 1996).

3.4.2 BAM *201*

The five preserved prescriptions on *BAM* 201 mainly concern *māmītu* and *kadabbedû* causing fever and swollen insides,[56] throwing up saliva with blood and pus,[57] and having yellow eyes.[58] None of the diagnoses or prescriptions has any direct duplicate, but all of the long prescriptions seem to contain one step in the treatment wherein the patient is bandaged with a cloth (TÚG).[59] The combination of clearly internal illnesses and mainly external applications suggests these were the factors behind the arrangement.

Of note, the tablet provides an alternative treatment method for the final application on the reverse, which is unusual in Kiṣir-Aššur's copies.[60] Additionally, almost all prescriptions on this tablet are quite long. The catch-line is also peculiar, as it does not spell out the following diagnosis, but simply

---

56 Obv. 23'–25': ⸢DIŠ⸣ NA KÚM *ṣar-ḫa* TUKU-*ma* ŠÀ^{II}-*šú* MÚ.MÚ-*ḫu i-te-*⸢*ne*⸣*-em-me-rù*$^{!}$ $^{24'}$ [...]-⸢*šú*$^{?}$⸣ MÚ.MÚ-{⸢*ḫu*$^{?}$ x⸣} ŠÀ-*šú* KA.<KEŠDA>-*tì* GÌR[^{II}]-⸢*šú*⸣ *t*[*e*]*-bu* $^{25'}$ [...]-⸢x⸣ NA BI ŠU.NAM.ÉRIM.MA KA.DAB.BÉ.DA, "If a man's insides continually becomes swollen and there is a hot fever, his(?) [...] is swollen (and) his inside (are) *constricted*, his fee[t] are raised [...]; that man (suffers from) 'Hand of Curse (or) *kadabbedû*" (cf. Maul 2019: 310–312).

57 Obv. 29': [DIŠ NA ...] GIG-*ma* KI ÚḪ-*šú* ÚŠ *u* LUGUD Š[UB$^{!}$.ŠUB$^{?}$], "[If a man] is ill with [...], and he [continually throws] up blood and pus with his saliva" (see Maul 2019: 310–312).

58 Rev. 31': [DIŠ NA (x)] ⸢IGI^{II}⸣-*šú* SIG$_7$ DIRI-*ut* NA BI ŠU.NAM.ÉRIM.[MA$^{?}$], "[If a man]'s eyes are full of yellow, that man (is ill from) 'Hand of Curse". Maul (2019: 310–312) reads [DIŠ NA ŠÀ(?)] IGI-*šú* SIG$_7$ SA$_5$ BABBAR NA BI ŠU NAM.ÉRIM, and states that the dual of IGI is not visible on the original tablet. However, there is at least one vertical wedge at the end of the partly visible IGI, which does not belong to this sign or -*šú*. Regarding the reading DIRI-*ut* over SA$_5$ BABBAR, see also BabMed onlines. Rev. 31' on Köcher's copy reads: ... ŠU NAM.ÉRIM. If we follow the Sa-gig principle, this could designate *māmītu* as "Krankheitsverursacher" and not only "Krankheitsname", which would be the only such example among Kiṣir-Aššur's texts (see Heeßel 2000: 50). However, the tablet may contain the remains of a damaged /MA/ on the side, which could negate this observation. It remains uncertain.

59 *BAM* 201 obv. 15': *ina* TÚG SUR-*ri* LÁ-*id*; 18': *ina* TÚG SUR-*ri ur-ra u* GE$_6$ LÁ; 22': *ina* TÚG SUR-*ri* LÁ-*id*; 28': [... UZ]U.MEŠ-*šú* LÁ-*id*; 30': [...] TAR ⸢sa/ru$^{?}$ al$^{?!}$⸣ LÁ [(x?)]; rev. 37'–38': *ina* TÚG SUR-*ri* $^{38'}$ *ina* KUŠ.EDIN *ur-ra u* GE$_6$ SAG ŠÀ-*šú* LÁL (see Maul 2019: 310–312). Note the new interpretation of *ṭerû* (SUR) in *CAD* (Ṭ: 103–4) as "to extract, squeeze or press out liquid (via a piece of leather, cloth)" over the previous translation "to rub into" (*CDA*: 414; *AHw*: 1388–89). Regardless, the patient must have been bandaged with the mentioned piece of leather or cloth.

60 *BAM* 201 rev. 40'–41': ... *saḫ-lé-e ina* KAŠ NAG-*ma ina-eš* $^{41'}$: ÚḪ ^{d}ÍD *ina* A NAG.

writes "If 'ditto' …".[61] Furthermore, in the colophon Kiṣir-Aššur writes *na-às-ḫa* with AŠ for ÀS, which is rare in Kiṣir-Aššur's colophons.[62]

The colophon specifies that the content was extracted from "a writing-board of prescriptions from the Gula temple".[63] The tablet is labelled as an *u'iltu*-tablet, which perhaps designates a commitment or an obligation inherent in the purpose for copying the text.[64] As this tablet was different from the others copied by Kiṣir-Aššur as *šamallû ṣeḫru,* I would argue that the *u'iltu* label here must designate some sort of exercise Kiṣir-Aššur was obligated to make. In this case, it is not inconceivable that Kiṣir-Aššur was tasked with finding *māmītu* treatments, which also included bandages.

3.4.3 RA *40 pl. 116*

RA 40 pl. 116 consists of six prescriptions on the obverse. As noted by its editors Labat and Tournay (1945–46: 113), the first diagnosis concerning *ašû, pašittu,* and *lubāṭu* illnesses is roughly duplicated in the 3rd tablet (*BAM* 578) of the *suālu* subsection of the Nineveh Ugu series that deals specifically with bile affecting the chest and epigastrium with or without fever (*ummu*) as well as jaundice (see Section 9.3.4).[65] The remaining five prescriptions and four diagnoses have no direct parallels, however, and appear to concern illnesses of the airways.[66] The opening diagnosis, mentioning the names of *ašû, pašittu,* and

---

61 *BAM* 201 rev. 42'–43': DIŠ KI.MIN ^{ú}ḪAB ^{ú}GÌR.NAGA.GA^{mušen} ^{ú}SIKIL $^{43'}$ EGIR-*šú iš-šaṭ-ṭar* (see Maul 2019: 310–312).

62 The only other instance is *BAM* 28 rev. 17': … *na-às-ḫa*. According to Borger (2003: 245), this reading was rare.

63 See Maul 2010: 213–214 and the discussion in Section 9.5.1; *BAM* 201 rev. 44'–45': TA ŠÀ ^{giš}ZU *šá bul-ṭi ša* É ^{d}ME.ME $^{45'}$ SAR È *ḫa-an-ṭiš*$^{!}$ *na-às-ḫa.*

64 *BAM* 201 rev. 46': ⌜*ú-ìl*⌝*-ti* ^{p}*Ki-ṣir*-AN.ŠÁR ŠÁMAN.LÁ TUR. See Section 5.3.2.

65 *RA* 40 pl. 116 obv. 1: [DIŠ] ⌜NA *a-šá-a pa-šit-tú*⌝ *u lu-*⌜*ba-ṭi* GIG⌝
BAM 578 col. ii 9a: DIŠ NA *a-šá-a pa-šit-tú u lu-*[*ba-ṭi* GIG …
Cf. *BAM* 578 col. ii 13a: *ana a-šá-a pa-šit-tú u lu-ba-ṭi* ZI-*ḫi* …
RA 40 pl. 116 obv. 2–3: ⌜Ú⌝.BABBAR ILLU LI.DUR ^{ú}*ak-tam kám-mu* 1-*niš* LÁL$^{!}$-*a*[*l*] ^{3} *ina* KAŠ NAG-*ma* TI-*u*[*ṭ*]
BAM 578 col. ii 9b–10: […] ^{10} ^{ú}KUR.RA URUDU.BAD 7 Ú.[ḪI.A …]
Cf. *BAM* 578 col. ii 13b: Ú.BABBAR ILLU LI.TAR […]
See Cadelli 2000: 195 lines 9–10 and 13. Labat and Tournay (1945–46: 114) read obv. 2: *tuballal*$^{a[l]}$ and Cadelli (2000: 195 note 25) notes this must be ḪE, albeit the reading is odd as obv. 17 has ḪE.ḪE. I would argue that the picture on CDLI looks more like LÁL$^{!}$ for *šaqālu* "to weigh out", which could also fit the context.

66 *RA* 40 pl. 116 obv. 8–9: "If a person is sick with wheezing *suālu* (barking-coughs) so that his windpipe (trachea and/or bronchi) is full of wind, he coughs (and) coughs (and) has phlegm …" (Scurlock and Andersen 2005: 48 no. 3.98).

lubāṭu, suggests that Kiṣir-Aššur previously may have copied material related to these illnesses with more thorough symptom descriptions.

Interestingly, Kiṣir-Aššur wrote the *ḫašû*-plant in obv. 19 as ᵘḪAR.MEŠ. Such a writing is unique, and Labat and Tournay (1945–46: 121) suggested that this was likely a graphic writing of *ḫašû*, the word for this plant and for "lungs". Since Kiṣir-Aššur had just copied two prescriptions concerning the "lungs", written MUR.MEŠ (MUR being identical to ḪAR) he likely made an "error of attraction" and wrote "plant (for) the lungs" (cf. Worthington 2012: 109).[67]

Certain illnesses could affect the stomach and induce vomit. One such affliction was *pašittu*, a dangerous bile-like fluid in the gastro-intestinal system.[68] Vomiting could be considered a symptom of imbalance within the body or be induced in order to expel the problem, which was the case in two instances in *RA* 40 pl. 116, for expelling *pašittu*-bile and phlegm.[69] As shown below in Chapter 4, this text and *RA* 15 pl. 76 likely enhanced Kiṣir-Aššur's knowledge about internal physiology, and also improved his skills for removing certain internal maladies by inducing vomit and using the nostrils to introduce medication.

3.5 Snakes, Scorpions and Horses: A Discussion of *RA* 15 pl. 76

The text published by Scheil in *RA* 15 on pl. 76 does not have a museum number. Consequently, the original cannot be consulted and one must rely on his problematic copy (see Appendix 2 with a new edition). The tablet consists of a number of one-line prescriptions against snakebites and scorpion stings on the obverse, and at least two longer prescriptions designed for horse ailments on the reverse (Stol 2011: 400–402).

3.5.1 *Snakes and Scorpions: The Obverse*

While incantations for stings and bites seem to be relatively well attested in the OB corpus,[70] Finkel stresses that "prescriptions for bites and stings by and

67 Note that the pharmacological text *BAM* 1 lists several plants with various names, which are listed as Ú MUR.MEŠ, i.e., "a plant for the lungs" (Attia and Buisson 2012: 27 lines ms B1 col. ii 21–26).

68 For this type of bile, see Section 4.1.3.

69 *RA* 40 pl. 116 obv. 4–7; obv. 8–12. Cf. *BAM* 201 obv. 16'–22'.

70 See SEAL section 5.1 (accessed 23/01/2017); George 2016: 98–118. The earliest incantations against scorpions and snakes were found in ED III Ebla and Fara (Krebernik 1984; Finkel 1999: 213 note 2 for further references).

large did not enter the traditional corpus of therapeutic medical texts".[71] The effects of snake and scorpion venom are, however, well attested in incantations in which venom became a metaphor for various illnesses.[72] The relatively few snake and scorpion treatments known from the first millennium primarily originate from the N4 collection and various works concerning plants.[73]

The prescriptions on the obverse of *RA* 15 pl. 76 consist mainly of so-called "simples", i.e., prescriptions comprising a single ingredient.[74] Presumably, the first diagnosis states: "If a snake bit a man",[75] and obverse line 14 changes the subject with the diagnosis: "If a scorpion stung a man".[76] *RA* 15 pl. 76 obv. 1'–6' is duplicated in the final section of *BAM* 42 (rev. 63–67). *BAM* 42 was written during an unknown stage by Aššur-šākin-šumi, likely a contemporary of Kiṣir-Aššur in the N4 collection (Maul 2010a: 216 note 101). According to Finkel (2000: 213 note 3), the snake treatments were added at the end in a smaller hand as an "afterthought". While this may be the case, it is noteworthy that the preceding treatments were directed against breathing illnesses (Köcher 1963a: XVII). The inclusion of snakebite treatments in *BAM* 42 could therefore be based on a symptomatic relationship between snake venom and such symptoms (see Section 4.1.2).

Peculiarly, several duplicate passages end with the present verbal form *ina-eš* in *RA* 15 pl. 76 and the stative form *né-eš* in *BAM* 42, both derived from the verb "to live, stay alive, recover" *nêšu*, suggesting that the two texts were not copied from the same original or that individual choice was involved (cf. *CAD* N/2: 197). Moreover, *RA* 15 pl. 76 obverse lines 8'–10' is found in parallel passages in the plant list *CT* 14 pl. 23. The parallel passages all make use of a "wad of reeds" (*ḫi-mu-ú*) applied to the bite, and they describe the "bandaging"

71 Finkel 1999: 213 and note 3. Finkel, however, noted that such treatments were considered as part of *āšipūtu*, cf. *KAR* 44 obv. 19: ZÚ M[U]Š TI.LA GÍR.TAB TI.LA …, "to cure a snake bite, to cure a scorpion (sting) …". For a discussion of prescriptions against snakebites in medical texts, see Steinert 2018d: 249–250.

72 E.g., Böck 2007: 290 line 155 (= ms j col. iv 14) in an incantation concerning *maškadu*: "It took half the venom of the snake; it took half the venom of the scorpion", *mi-šil im-ti ša* MUŠ *il-qí mi-šil im-ti šá* GÍR.TAB *il-qí*; see Arbøll 2018a: 269.

73 N4 tablets: *BAM* 42 rev. 63–67, *BAM* 176 obv. 11'–15' (Pedersén 1986, N4 no. 605 and no. 277), *RA* 15 pl. 76 obv. 1'–25'. Plant lists mentioning bites and stings include *šammu šikinšu* (Stadhouders 2012: 12–13). For *BAM* 42, see also Heeßel 2010c: 153–54. Note also *KAR* 181 (N4 no. 96), which contains incantations and rituals against scorpions, snakes, and dogs (Steinert 2018d: 250).

74 For the concept of "simples" in Babylonian medicine, see Geller 2005: 4.

75 *RA* 15 pl. 76 obv. 1' [x x x x x x x x x x x x x-*l*]*u*$^?$ ⸢GU$_7^{!?}$⸣-[*ma*$^?$ *ina*$^?$]-⸢*eš*⸣
BAM 42 rev. 63 DIŠ NA MUŠ ⸢*iš*⸣-*šuk-šú* ⸢x⸣ *ur-ba-*⸢*tì*⸣ *ta-qàl-lu* GU$_7$-*ma né-eš*

76 *RA* 15 pl. 76 obv. 14': [DIŠ NA G]ÍR$^!$.TAB SÌG$^!$-*su* …

in the infinitive (LÁ-*du*, NIGIN-*ú*).[77] Considering that *RA* 15 pl. 76 represents an extract from a writing-board (see Section 9.2.3), presumably with prescriptions, it is noteworthy that several entries in the plant list *CT* 14 pl. 23 largely correspond to those in the therapeutic text *RA* 15 pl. 76. Although these texts are not exact duplicates, they contain parallel entries with similar problems, plants, and how the drugs are to be administered. Such a correlation seems unexpected.[78]

3.5.2 *Horse Colic: The Reverse*

The reverse of *RA* 15 pl. 76 contains two prescriptions presumably intended for horses (Stol 2011: 400–402). Horses were important animals in the NA period (ibid.: 386). In addition to the corpus of Hippiatric texts from 13th century Ugarit,[79] treatments for horses are primarily known from the NA manuscripts *RA* 15 pl. 76, *BAM* 159, *BAM* 309, and some plant lists.[80] Such treatments were transmitted together with human treatments, although several of the prescriptions utilize plants and treatments exclusively attested in these contexts (ibid.: 392). Additionally, they typically are not considered part of the normal sphere of healing knowledge.[81] As a result, Scurlock suggested that the horse treatments in *BAM* 159 were inserted due to a thematic parallel in referring to the nostril (*naḫīru*).[82]

The reverse of *RA* 15 pl. 76 is fragmentary and poorly copied, but it refers to pouring liquid into the left "nostril" (*naḫīru*) in two instances (rev. 4', 7') and likely mentions "horse" in reverse line 8' (Stol 2011: 401). Administering ingredients into the irrational left nostril is only attested in veterinarian praxis, which indicates that both these prescriptions relate to horses (ibid.: 392). Unfortunately, the illness described in reverse line 8' remains unclear.[83] *RA* 15 pl. 76 also has a peculiar and previously unknown catch-line, which may read: "If a man's! stomach rises (to vomit) and *settles*!, (and) his stomach (after

77 The *ḫimû*-wad is mainly attested in these two texts (cf. *CAD* Ḫ: 193–94).

78 Some entries show slight changes; cf. *RA* 15 pl. 76 obv. 6 partly duplicated in *BAM* 42 rev. 68 and *CT* 14 pl. 23 obv. 9; *RA* 15 pl. 76 obv. 11' duplicated in *CT* 14 pl. 23 obv. 11.

79 Cohen and Sivan 1983; see Stol 2011: 386 note 171 for additional references.

80 *BAM* 159 was also excavated in N4, although it was written by one Bēl-apkal-ilāni from outside the Bāba-šuma-ibni family (Parys 2014: 8; cf. Stol 2011: 386–402).

81 However, such prescriptions were part of written knowledge early on. See the prescription for a calf from Ebla in Fronzaroli 2005.

82 Parys 2014: 4, 6; Scurlock 2014: 498; Stol 2011: 387; see the recent discussion and edition of *BAM* 159 in Parys 2014. The relevant sections can be found in *BAM* 159 col. v 33–36 (potion through the left nostril) and col. v 37–47 (enema). See also Cohen 1983.

83 Rev. 8': [*a*?]-*na* ANŠE!.KUR.RA *ša* bu ḫi DAB-*su* SIG_5-*iq*, "It is good [f]or a horse that is seized (by) *bu ḫi*". See the discussion of this sentence in Appendix 2 and Stol 2011: 401 and note 254.

having) settled *rises*(?) (again)".[84] Considering the two previous prescriptions dealt with horses, the catch-line likely reflects a continuation of symptoms that indicate a relationship with colic and the stomach. The content of the horse prescriptions are discussed in detail in relation to physiology in Section 4.4.3.

Comparatively, two prescriptions in *BAM* 159 deal with horse colic, of which the first was likely a prescription designed for horses, although the second may have been a human prescription applied to horses (Stol 2011: 387, 393–95). What is translated "horse colic" is written *kīs libbi* "binding of the 'heart'" or "abdomen, belly" in *BAM* 159. Colic is the most common horse illness, and it is also attested in the pastoral god Šakkan (ibid.: 397–98). In horses, colic can have many causes and it is defined as a digestive disease causing abdominal pain.[85] Due to the horse's animalistic nature, *kīs libbi* is a more complicated affair in humans, as there is slight evidence that it may also have had a psychological dimension that manifests as an emotional disturbance.[86]

The above evidence suggests that *RA* 15 pl. 76 may not be as extraordinary as has typically been assumed. In the so-called "Assur Medical Catalogue", hereafter referred to as the AMC (see Section 9.3.2), bites and stings as well as veterinarian knowledge are listed after works known to have been included in the Nineveh Ugu series. Their titles in the AMC could indicate that such knowledge was considered to be as important as human healing to the medical traditions in Assur.[87] However, it is unknown if application methods or other associative factors had created clusters of prescriptions that were transmitted in the medical tradition (cf. Geller 2010: 97–108).

---

84 *RA* 15 pl. 76 rev. 9': DIŠ NA! ŠÀ-*šú* E_{11}! *ù ú*!-*rad* ŠÀ-*ba-šú* E_{11} *a-lam*?. The verb *elû* with phonetic initial *a-* is attested in imperatives and second person singular forms, mainly from OB examples (*CAD* E: 116). The spelling cannot be explained here, but I fail to see other interpretations. For further discussion of this line, see Appendix 2 and Scheil 1918: 77, 79.

85 Gonçalves et al. 2002.

86 Cadelli (2000: 363 and note 457) quotes a dream omen wherein *kīs libbi* is given as an opposite to "joy" *ḫūd libbi* (see *CAD* K: 433b; possibly also *AbB* 1 no. 36 obv. 17). This probably stemmed from the fact that emotions were linked to the heart (ŠÀ) and by extension the entire abdomen (Parys 2014: 4–5; Chalendar 2013: 14–17; Steinert 2012: 232–33; Böck 2010a: 69; Cadelli 2000: 363–65, 372–73). However, the reference is not from a purely medical context. For *kīs libbi*, see also Steinert and Vacín 2018: 708–709, 713–715. Considering *kīs libbi*'s affect on the gastro-intestinal system, it may also have been related in some way to bile. Böck (2014a: 121–128) has suggested that bile regulated the intestinal fluids. Interestingly, "heart-break" *ḫīp libbi* was translated as "panic" by Stol (1993: 27–31) and he relates this to melancholy and bile. However, *kīs libbi* should probably be considered distinct from *ḫīp libbi*.

87 AMC lines 76–78: [... N]A! ⌜MUŠ⌝ *iš-šuk-š*[*u*] 77 ... Ú.ḪI.A *ša* BÚR *ša ni-šik* ⌜MUŠ⌝ 78 [UR.GI_7] ⌜*lu*?⌝ [... *zi-q*]*it* GÍR.TAB SÌG-*iṣ* ...; line 122: 1 DUB *ša*! ANŠE.KUR.RA.[MEŠ *u*] *ša* GU_4.M[EŠ]. See also Panayotov 2018b: 91.

The common theme of *RA* 15 pl. 76 seems to be animals influencing other individuals or being influenced. However, a tentative suggestion could be that the stings/bites and affected horses were connected, as animals in the fields were likely more susceptible to being stung or bitten.[88] Thematically, it therefore describes venomous animals as disease agents with either humans or domestic animals as victims or patients. Apart from being an introduction to these different genres of healing literature, *RA* 15 pl. 76 likely initiated Kiṣir-Aššur into the anatomical conceptions lying latent in the cuneiform medical literature. At least one OB incantation could be applied to humans and animals alike, and Stol argues that the second horse treatment in *BAM* 159 was originally designed for humans.[89] By extension, the veterinarian material could perhaps be utilized by students to understand some aspects of human anatomy.[90] This was also the case in several instances in the history of Greek and Roman medicine (see Mattern 2013: 145–55, 158–60, 163; Stol 2011: 395 note 224 with references; van der Eijk 2008: 398–99; Nutton 2004: 49, 77, 119–120, 128, 132, 214–15, 231–32).

3.6 Gaining an Understanding of Anatomy and Physiology

As previously discussed, Kiṣir-Aššur, and his teacher(s), likely drew on the healing texts copied as *šamallû ṣeḫru* to widen his diagnostic and anatomical understanding. But while anatomical conceptions in the ancient sources (e.g., Steinert 2016: 206; Couto Ferreira 2009; Westenholz and Sigrist 2008; Stol 2006; Landsberger 1967), as well as descriptions of anatomical terms in specific corpuses (e.g., Heeßel 2000: 25, 28–29; Böck 2001),[91] have been the

88 See Section 4.2.2. Scorpions are occasionally compared to angry bulls (see the Ur III incantation in Finkel 1999: 234, text 10; the OB incantation *RA* 88 pl. 161 obv. 1–2; see also George 2016: 102–4; SEAL text 5.1.19.4 ((accessed 23/01/2017)). This comparison could originate in the observation of a bull's reaction after being stung. Note that the first Ugaritic prescription for horses edited by Cohen and Sivan (1983: 9–10, 13 line 2) utilizes the ingredient *'qrbn* translated as a "scorpion-like plant".

89 Stol 2011: 395 and note 223; cf. Böck 2009a: 117–118. See the OB incantation *CT* 4 pl. 8a obv. 33f. (*lū awīlūtum lū alpu lū immeru*, Steinert and Vacín 2018: 720–722 line 217, 726). Horse sweat is also used in a prescription as a metaphoric ingredient in a prescription for use on humans (Scurlock 2014: 412), and bull saliva was used in *RA* 15 pl. 76 against a scorpion sting (see Appendix 2). For a livestock remedy amid human remedies, see George 2016: 132–34.

90 If Steinert's suggestion that the Mesopotamian healers visualized the human body as a container filled with fluids can be generalized, one could imagine animals were occasionally visualized similarly (Steinert 2016: 209–210).

91 See also Dhorme 1923 and Holma 1911.

subject of individual studies, it has also been pointed out on occasion that some Mesopotamian anatomical descriptions do not always appear coherent or specific.[92]

One particular problem seems to be the descriptions of internal areas and organs of the torso.[93] Autopsy was to the best of our knowledge not performed on the human body.[94] As a result, the internal processes were formulated in a tradition that combined observable external symptoms with anatomical features observed in animals and possibly human war casualties (see Section 4.4.1). Therefore, many blank holes had to be filled in order to produce even a rough understanding of how the insides functioned.[95]

As hypothesized in Section 3.1.1, the material copied in Kiṣir-Aššur's *šamallû ṣeḫru* tablets attests to a wide range of bodily areas and was possibly used to achieve an associated understanding of the bodily processes through the written diagnoses. Considering that *BAM* 9 was described as a "first extract" from either one or several writing-boards and *RA* 15 pl. 76 was the "32nd? extract", it is possible that *BAM* 129 and *RA* 40 pl. 116 also once contained a phrase that designated them as extracts.[96] Although this remains uncertain, Kiṣir-Aššur likely copied 31 extracts before *RA* 15 pl. 76, and, if so, it stands to reason that he copied these as *šamallû ṣeḫru*.[97] Additionally, *BAM* 9, *RA* 15 pl. 76, and *RA* 40 pl. 116 contain two general types of protective phrases, namely "you must not erase my written name" and "he who takes (the tablet) away, let Nabû order his disappearance" or "let [DN] take aw[ay] his eyesight".[98]

---

92 E.g., Steinert 2016: 205–9 and note 32–33; Stol 2006; Geller 2004; Attia 2000; Cadelli 2000: 290–292. This was perhaps occasionally the case among the ancient Greek sources as well (Nutton 2004: 77; see Steinert 2016: 203; Geller 2010: 116).

93 E.g., Steinert 2016: 205–6; Böck 2014b: 103–4, 106, 111–15; Geller 2010: 21–22; Westenholz 2010; Stol 2006.

94 E.g., Steinert 2016: 203; Geller 2010: 21; cf. Scurlock and Andersen 2005: 43, 117, 135, 416–17.

95 The enhanced focus on four organs in attributing illnesses to body parts in the LB *SpTU* I no. 43 may have been related to astral medicine (Steinert 2016: 230ff., 241–242; Geller 2014: 291–293; cf. Heeßel 2010b: 30–31; Köcher 1978: 24–25; for astral medicine in general, see Heeßel 2008a).

96 However, *BAM* 129 may have been intended to function as a library copy. This remains unclear.

97 As argued in Section 9.2.3, *RA* 15 pl. 76 likely represented one of the later extracts in this sequence. For a discussion of Kiṣir-Aššur's numbered extracts, see Section 9.2.

98 *BAM* 9 Rev. 74–76(?): [MU$^{?}$ ^{d}PA$^{?}$ *u*$^{?}$ ^{d}AM]AR.UTU *šu-mì šaṭ-rù la t*[*a-pa-šiṭ*] ^{75} [… ^{d}]AG ⌜*ù*⌝ ^{d}A[MAR.UTU] ^{76} […]⌜x x x x x-*šú*⌝-*m*[*a* …]

RA 15 pl. 76 Rev. 14'–15': [MU *šaṭ-r*]*u la ta-pa-šiṭ šá* NÍG.GIG ^{d}ŠE.NAGA $^{15'}$ […]⌜x x x⌝ *ni-ṭil* IGI^{II}-*šú li-i*[*t-bal*]

RA 40 pl. 116 Rev. 4–5: MU ^{d}AG *u* ^{d}AMAR.UTU *šu-mi šaṭ-rù la ta-pa-*[*šiṭ*] ^{5} *šà* IR ^{d}A[G] ZÀḪ-*šú liq-b*[*i*]

Beside these texts, similar statements are found at the end of colophons in *BAM* 131, Beckman and Foster 1988 no. 21, *KAL* 10 no. 4, *LKA* 77 and N4 no. 175. Possibly, Kiṣir-Aššur

BAM 9, *BAM* 201, and *RA* 15 pl. 76 also explain what originals Kiṣir-Aššur copied from, and in all three cases this was a writing-board. *BAM* 201 even adds that it was copied from "a writing-board of prescriptions from the Gula temple", which was likely located in Assur (see Section 9.5.2). This suggests that Kiṣir-Aššur drew his medical *šamallû ṣeḫru* material from one or several writing-boards, perhaps all of which were located in a library in the temple dedicated to the goddess of healing. Unfortunately, little is known about the Gula temple in Assur, its library, and whether or not Kiṣir-Aššur received any education there (cf. Wiggermann 2008). Additionally, the unpublished text N4 A 2191 was perhaps copied from a tablet by a certain [...]-Marduk, an *asû* from the land of [...].[99]

This evidence could tentatively be interpreted as an indication that Kiṣir-Aššur was made to copy out the pertinent parts of a writing-board, which contained a text relevant for education and practice, in order to learn (and discuss) the passages required to educate him in the subjects described. This education also included physiological conceptions. This is supported by the general evaluation of the Bāba-šuma-ibni family's numbered extracts investigated in Section 9.2. Preliminarily, Kiṣir-Aššur copied out an idiosyncratic handbook, which consisted of a number of relevant extracts (*nisḫu*), and these adhered to his family's school of thought and his own education.

3.6.1 *Kiṣir-Aššur's Diagnostic Training and Sa-gig*

Kiṣir-Aššur's *šamallû ṣeḫru* texts show relatively few complex diagnoses affecting several bodily areas, and they are probably extracted from one or more collections of therapeutic texts possibly arranged from head-to-toe according to specific bodily areas (*BAM* 9, *BAM* 129, *RA* 40 pl. 116). Additionally, Kiṣir-Aššur copied at least one exercise(?) according to a malady that affected several bodily areas (*māmītu* in *BAM* 201; ghost in N4 no. 237(?)). Therefore, Kiṣir-Aššur studied both select groups of chosen illnesses that affected certain bodily areas, as well as how one or more complex illnesses could manifest themselves in a multitude of areas (cf. Wee 2012: 239).

---

did not write a title in the final example; the remaining three are from Kiṣir-Aššur's *mašmaš bīt Aššur* phase.

99 N4 A 2191 colophon line 2: [x x x x]⸢x da?⸣-dAMAR.UTU lúA.ZU *šá* KUR [x]. The interpretation is uncertain. Kiṣir-Aššur may also have copied *LKA* 113 from an IM.GÍD.DA of someone else (see Ch. 8 note 86). Kiṣir-Nabû copied at least two tablets from *u'iltus* of a certain Aššur-šarrāni (*LKA* 96, *LKA* 100).

Complex diagnoses, as the ones discussed in Section 3.1, seem to require advanced medical understanding. Correlating symptoms with diagnoses and subsequently determining the cause behind the illness, is often described as a process illustrated by the Esagil-kīn-apli recension of the diagnostic prognostic handbook Sa-gig, especially its 2nd subseries "When you approach the patient" (Heeßel 2007b: 120–29; Heeßel 2000: 49–52; cf. Wee 2012: 183–84, 186).[100] The 2nd subseries was arranged head-to-toe according to the symptom that was mentioned first in the description (Wee 2012: 222, 240; Heeßel 2000: 19, 24–30). Therefore, this subseries prioritizes symptom over illness in its arrangement (Wee 2012: 156, 476, 479). However, Sa-gig's practical use as well as its function for education is less clear (Robson 2008: 474; Heeßel 2000: 90–94; cf. Wee 2012: 239). Contemporary exorcist at the royal court in Nineveh never quoted the series, perhaps relying on observation, experience and pragmatism for prognostic purposes (Robson 2019: 118). Other scholars at the royal court quoted omen series such as *Enūma Anu Enlil* extensively (Rochberg 2011: 627). A few of Kiṣir-Aššur's *šamallû ṣeḫru* diagnoses are comparable to concrete entries in Sa-gig.

The *šaššaṭu* diagnosis in *BAM* 129 col. iv 3' was partly duplicated in two sections of Sa-gig, namely tablets 10 and 33.[101] The line in *BAM* 129 states: "[If a man]'s [neck] (and) his hips are stiff: *šaššaṭu* is its name".[102] This line is almost duplicated in the two sections of Sa-gig, but with a variation between *šaššaṭu* in Sa-gig 33 and "Heavy Strings" (SA.DUGUD) – another name for *šaššaṭu* – in Sa-gig 10. Furthermore, all passages in Sa-gig add the symptoms stiff (*ašṭu*) hands and feet.[103]

---

100 In general, Sa-gig lists fewer illnesses as diagnoses than are known throughout the therapeutic corpus, and only around 40 actual reasons for why an illness was caused are listed (Koch 2015: 277; Heeßel 2000: 58–60). See Johnson (2018) for a discussion of illness names in prescriptions and the diagnostic-prognostic series Sa-gig.

101 Sa-gig 10 = *AMT* 106,2 and *TDP* pl. 19 (Labat 1951: 80ff.; Scurlock 2014: 74ff.); Sa-gig 33 = *SpTU* IV no. 152 (Heeßel 2000: 353ff.).

102
BAM 129 col. iv 3'	[DIŠ NA GÚ-*su*] MURUB$_4$II-*šú* *aš-ṭa šá-áš-šá-ṭa* MU.NI *ana* TI-*šú*
SpTU IV no. 152 rev. 95	[… MURU]B$_4$-*šú* ŠU^{II}-*šú u* GÌR^{II}-*šú* *aš-ṭa šá-aš-*[*šá-ṭa* x x]
TDP pl. 19 obv. 10	DIŠ GÚ-*su* MURUB$_4$-*šú* ŠU^{II}-*šú* GÌR^{II}-*šú* *aš-ṭa* SA.[DUGUD]
AMT 106,2 obv. 10	[DIŠ … ŠU^{II}]-*šú u* GÌR^{II}-*šú* *aš-ṭa* SA.DUGUD

SpTU IV 152 = Sa-gig 33; *AMT* 106,2 = Sa-gig 10.

103 Although hands and feet are not mentioned in *BAM* 129 col. iv 3', they are mentioned in the diagnosis following this entry:

Such correlations between Sa-gig and the therapeutic material seem to appear irregularly.[104] However, a connection in Kiṣir-Aššur's tablets to Sa-gig is evident. It is unknown at what stage an *āšipu* would have learned Sa-gig, although the N4 exercise *BAM* 310 suggests that such omens could have been introduced at an early stage.[105] Unlike Finkel's (2000: 142) hypothesis, adopted by Wee (2012: 87, 452) that Sa-gig and its commentaries would be the work of advanced students, the evidence from Kiṣir-Aššur does not show any traces of the Sa-gig series during his traceable educational phases. It should therefore be noted that no copies of Sa-gig were found in the N4 collection, and almost no evidence for the series exists in Assur.[106] In comparison, the N4 collection has not yielded a single regular manuscript of *Maqlû* (Schwemer 2017: 50). Yet, in a list of tablet incipits (VAT 13723+), presumably listing texts held in the N4 collection, the enumeration of the nine tablets of *Maqlû* (col. i 5'–13') ends with the summary: "Eight (tablets) of *Maqlû* (incantations) together with the ritual (instruction)s of *Maqlû*: 2 (copies?)" (ibid.: 51; Geller 2000: 227). The question remains how to interpret the last number, but Schwemer suggests that the collection held two complete copies of the whole series, perhaps on

---

BAM 129 col. iv 14': DIŠ NA GÚ-*su* ^{uzu}SA.SAL.MEŠ-*šú* ŠU^{II}-*šú* GÌR^{II}-*šú* […] NA BI *šá-šá-ṭ*[*a* …

AMT 31,2 rev. 5': […]⸢x x⸣-*ma* NA BI *šá-*⸢*áš*⸣*-šá-ṭa* GIG

104 Heeßel 2000: 87–89 and note 69; Stol 1991–92: 49–50; cf. Wee 2012: 156–57. Another parallel appears in Kiṣir-Aššur's *BAM* 131 obv. 9 duplicating Sa-gig 33 = *SpTU* IV no. 152 rev. 96 (Heeßel 2000: 353ff.), which Kiṣir-Aššur copied at an unknown stage of his career. In the first subseries of the Nineveh Ugu series, the 2nd tablet (*BAM* 482) contain 10 passages duplicating diagnoses from Sa-gig 4 (Attia and Buisson 2003, MS H = Sa-gig 4: line 60 (= H 124), 126' (= H 31), 130' (= H 32), 134' (= H 17), 136' (= H 13), 238' (= H 15), 240' (= H 12), 241' (= H 10), 242' (= H 11), 243' (= H 8)). In the *suālu* subseries of Ugu edited by Cadelli (2000), we find one passage in the 3rd tablet (*BAM* 587) col. iii 7 duplicated in Sa-gig 18 line 24 (*TDP*: 170 line 24) and Sa-gig 33 line 92 = *SpTU* IV no. 152: 92, and one passage in col. iv 26 duplicated in Sa-gig 9 line 13 (*TDP*: 72 line 13) and Sa-gig 33 line 93 = *SpTU* IV no. 152: 93 (Heeßel 2000: 353ff.). SAG.KI.DAB.BA is not attested in Sa-gig, but it does occur several times in the first tablets of Ugu. However, several entries in Sa-gig begin with "his temple is seized" (SAG.KI-*šú* DAB-*su*), which could indicate that the relationship between the two was self-evident (Wee 2012: 238 and note 90 for references). Wee's discussion of the diagnosis in *BAM* 129 col. iv 6' in relation to Sa-gig 33 rev. 96 is not relevant, as the entry in Sa-gig 33 likely relates to the *šaššaṭu* diagnosis in *BAM* 131 obv. 9–10 (cf. Wee 2012: 473).

105 N4 no. 57 (= *BAM* 310) consists of nine lines and is designated as "questions of Sa-gig" on obv. 3–4: *maš-al-a-te* ⁴ *ša* SA.GIG. The tablet is certainly an early school tablet.

106 Pedersén 1986: 50–51 and note 31; Heeßel 2010a: 158. As noted by Pedersén (1986: 51) *BAM* 114 (N4 no. 354) opens with 10 single-line diagnoses concerning renal and rectal maladies (Geller 2005: 70–71), and *KADP* 22 (= N4 no. 487 = 3rd tablet of Uruanna) col. i–ii comments on the nature of certain diagnoses.

clay tablets or writing-boards. Noticeably, if the N4 collection held complete texts on writing-boards not represented in the surviving clay tablets, this has the implication that Sa-gig may have existed in the collection as well.[107] This remains uncertain.

The pre-Esagil-kīn-apli recension(s) of Sa-gig appears to have been grouped according to particular maladies, prognoses, or divine agents with disconnected symptom descriptions, and they mirror tendencies in groupings found in therapeutic texts (Wee 2012: 272, 279; *CMAwR* 1: 434–43; Heeßel 2000: 105–11; Stol 1993: 91–98). This tradition was still copied around 700 BCE in Ḫuzirina (cf. *STT* 89).[108] Considering that Assur and Ḫuzirina may have shared intellectual traditions to some extent,[109] coupled with the fact that Assur has provided almost no examples of Sa-gig (Heeßel 2010a: 160–61), Kiṣir-Aššur may well have been taught according to different principles than the established Sa-gig series. Furthermore, these observations tentatively imply that the 2nd subseries of Esagil-kīn-apli's Sa-gig was not required when learning about physiology or acquiring the ability to perform differential diagnosis.

Although most therapeutic texts contain a lower density of symptom descriptions compared to Sa-gig, Wee (2012: 312) observed that therapeutic tablets frequently include several similar maladies, facilitating a degree of differential diagnosis (distinguishing similar illnesses) by juxtaposing noteworthy symptoms that were used to distinguish the maladies (e.g., *BAM* 129). In the absence of Sa-gig, I believe acquiring the skill to perform differential diagnosis was among the purposes of Kiṣir-Aššur's *šamallû ṣeḫru* texts. In addition to providing him with the relevant prescriptions for such maladies, the diagnoses coupled with oral teachings received from his father in professional situations would have enabled him to diagnose illnesses.[110] Only circumstantial

107 Cf. Pedersén 1986: 50–51 and note 31; Heeßel 2000: 94, 109 and note 55. Maul (2010a: 207) proposes that the largely missing Sa-gig recensions in N4 may be related to the existence of separate collections. Presumably, the brother of Nabû-bēssunu and of Kiṣir-Aššur made their own collections elsewhere, and perhaps they subdivided their work into areas of responsibilities. Although the existence of more libraries is plausible, it remains uncertain if Esagil-kīn-apli's Sa-gig was accepted in Assur (Heeßel 2010a: 161). For an example of a writing-board from N4, see Klengel-Brandt 1975. See also Section 9.2.1 on the use of writing-boards in N4.

108 *STT* 403, however, is a commentary on the Esagil-kīn-apli recension of Sa-gig tablet 1–3. This version was therefore also known in Ḫuzirina (Wee 2012: 543ff.; Stol 1993: 91–98).

109 The evidence is tentative, and only overlaps have been pointed out (Reiner and Civil 1967: 209; Lambert 1959: 122, 124, 127–28). Furthermore, at least one son was sent to the Ḫuzirina school from Assur, albeit none from Nineveh, Kalḫu, or Dūr-Šarrukēn (Robson 2014: 154; Robson 2013: 50). See Heeßel 2010a: 161.

110 For therapeutic texts in relation to illness identification, see Johnson 2015.

evidence describe how aspiring *āšipu*s were taught the material they copied, but it is likely that the content copied became subject to dissemination within a scholarly context.[111] Thus, these combined factors would have filled the gap left by the missing (written) Sa-gig tradition. Additionally, the following chapter argues that Kiṣir-Aššur also acquired his physiological understanding of the human body from the therapeutic texts in combination with tangible experience gained from aiding his father.

3.7 Preparation for Other Duties as *šamallû ṣeḫru*

As *šamallû ṣeḫru*, Kiṣir-Aššur copied *KAL* 4 no. 19, a fragmentary ritual text perhaps similar to a *namburbi*-ritual, *LKA* 43, a *šuʾilla*-prayer (lit.: "hand-lifting") to Madānu, a divine personification of judgement related to Marduk (Krebernik 2007: 356–57),[112] N4 A 2191, a ritual against a ghost duplicating an uncertain part of *BAM* 323 (cf. Scurlock 2006: 712–713), and N4 no. 289, a ritual intended to provide a patient with a substitute for the goddess Ereškigal of the netherworld (Verderame 2013: 315ff.; Tuskimoto 1985: 125ff.). All three genres are among the categories for practicing *āšipūtu*.[113] Generally, *namburbi*-rituals were used apotropaically against worrying terrestrial, astrological, and birth omens, as well as to safeguard the diviner (Koch 2010: 46, 53; Maul 1994: 12–13). The *šuʾilla*s were adaptable prayers used by individuals to address particular concerns by petitioning (greeting) a specific deity.[114]

KAL 4 no. 19 is very poorly preserved, and considering that the first healing instruction for *garābu* in *KAL* 4 no. 41 ended similarly to one of three relatively badly preserved lines in *KAL* 4 no. 19: "you throw (it) into the river",[115] *KAL* 4 no. 19 was perhaps not a *namburbi*-ritual. Section 6.4 evaluates Kiṣir-Aššur's other *namburbi*-ritual texts, which are all from his later phases. This adds to the suspicion that *KAL* 4 no. 19 was likely not a *namburbi*-ritual. Possibly, both

---

111 Zamazalová 2011: 318; van der Toorn 2007: 58; Gesche 2001: 5, 198; Sjöberg 1972.

112 *LKA* 43 contains a few mistakes in sign forms underlining that Kiṣir-Aššur was a young apprentice when he copied this text. See obv. 7: *ga*-; obv. 11: … -*li*-.

113 Jean 2006: 83–86, 99. Three types of *šuʾilla*-prayers can be distinguished: Emesal Sumerian prayers of the *kalû*, Sumerian prayers for the *mīs pî* ritual, and (largely) Akkadian prayers as part of *āšipūtu* (Frechette 2012: 3–4). A few more are also known from other professions via incipits (ibid.: 4–5). It is unclear if the ritual "A substitute for Ereškigal" was included in the EM (see Geller 2018b: 299 line 20, 306).

114 Frechette 2012: 4, 7–8, 165–66. These prayers were included in, e.g., *bīt rimki* and some *namburbi*-rituals.

115 *KAL* 4 no. 19 rev. 4′: [… N]U? *a-na* ÍD ⸢ŠUB⸣-[*di*].
KAL 4 no. 41 obv. 8: […]⸢x⸣ *a-na* ÍD ŠUB-*di*.

KAL 4 no. 19 and *LKA* 43 functioned as part of rituals that were intended to cure the divine cause behind some illnesses, and they attest to Kiṣir-Aššur's training in these areas of practice (see Koch unpublished: 11 note 63; Heeßel 2000: 81–86; see Ch. 6 note 72). N4 no. 289 transfers illness through the use of ritual substitution.

3.7.1 *Kiṣir-Aššur's* šu'illa-*prayers*

Šu'illa-prayers usually consist of an invocation of a deity, presentation of the worshipper and his/her need, petition for what is wished for, and a thanksgiving (Hrůša 2015: 120; Frechette 2012: 130–31; Zgoll 2004).[116] Therefore, *šu'illa*s were used to gain the aid of a deity by creating (= restoring) a favourable relationship between supplicant and the divine sphere (Frechette 2012: 9).

LKA 43 is addressed to Madānu and the text is largely similar to a *šu'illa*-prayer to Nusku.[117] The text is known in multiple duplicates from the N4 library and Assur in general, and must have been broadly circulated among these specialists.[118] The prayer is listed as part of *bīt salā' mê*, performed during Tašrītu in connection to the New Year celebrations, as well as the *bīt rimki* ritual, which was associated with the substitute king ritual (Ambos 2013a: 42, 262ff.; Frechette 2012: 166, 169, 178; Læssøe 1955: 25 col. iii 61).

The various copies show slight individual differences in terms of content, division of lines as well as number of lines, in addition to variants in writings.[119] Consequently, at least *LKA* 43 appears not to have been written according to poetic principles that divide lines into evenly distributed verse units. Unfortunately, *LKA* 43 is the only duplicate of this prayer with a copying statement, which specifies that it was "written and checked according to its original".[120] We can therefore hypothesize that *LKA* 43 was either not copied

116 *KAR* 44 obv. 4: ŠU.ÍL.LA.KAM.

117 Madānu 1; Frechette 2012: 170 note 10, 178 note 6, 259; Mayer 1976: 394, 406. Nusku was also important in relation to the lamp present during healing ceremonies (Panayotov 2016).

118 *KAL* 4 no. 58, *KAL* 4 no. 59(=*LKA* 46 and 47a+b), *LKA* 44, *LKA* 45 (Frechette 2012: 259; *KAL* 4: 112–14). It appears as though all five examples of this prayer, including *LKA* 43, were written without instructions (Frechette 2012: 144 note 3). At least one *šu'illa*-prayer to Nabû was part of Gesche's 2nd school phase and is also found on prisms (Gesche 2001: 177, 193ff.).

119 Lines divided differently: *LKA* 43 obv. 1–2 vs. *LKA* 44 obv. 1, *KAL* 4 no. 58 obv. 1; *LKA* 43 obv. 7–8 vs. *LKA* 44 obv. 4, *KAL* 4 no. 59 obv. 1'–2', *KAL* 4 no. 58 obv. 4. Couplets divided onto two lines: *LKA* 43 obv. 2–3 vs. *LKA* 44 obv. 2, *KAL* 4 no. 58 obv. 2; *LKA* 43 obv. 5–6 vs. *LKA* 44 obv. 3, *KAL* 4 no. 58 obv. 3. Differing text in the various manuscripts: *LKA* 43 obv. 13–14/*LKA* 44 obv. 8/*KAL* 4 no. 59 obv. 6'; *KAL* 4 no. 59 obv. 14'–15'. Editions in Mayer 1976: 459ff.; *KAL* 4: 112–14.

120 Rev. 15: *ki-ma* SUMUN-*šú šá-ṭir ba-ri.*

from the same tablet as the other examples, or that individual choice in lines and divisions was an active component when copying this text.

Incidentally, only one additional *šuʾilla*-prayer can be identified among Kiṣir-Aššur's tablets with colophons, namely *LKA* 40 for Tašmētu.[121] As argued in Section 7.2.1, this tablet likely derived from his *mašmaššu*-phase. Despite these two being the only explicit examples of *šuʾilla*s copied by Kiṣir-Aššur, the N4 collection contained many "Hand-lifting"-prayers (Pedersén 1986: 50).

Although such texts could function in a variety of "official" state or temple contexts, they could also be used to heal the cause behind an illness (see Ch. 6 note 72). Several lines of petitioning in *LKA* 43 focus on health and healing, which supports this proposal.[122] Certain "Curses" *māmītu* are frequently observed as Kiṣir-Aššur's opponents, and perhaps Madānu (justice) could dispatch as well as remove such an affliction. As such, this prayer may be considered an *ad hoc* item in Kiṣir-Aššur's ritualistic inventory.

3.7.2 *N4 no. 289: A Substitute for Ereškigal*

The ritual known as "A man's substitute for Ereškigal" (*ana pūḫi amēli Ereškigal*) was copied by Kiṣir-Aššur during his *šamallû ṣeḫru*-phase. This unpublished manuscript was listed by Pedersén (1986) as N4 no. 289. Only the upper half of the obverse and the colophon on the reverse are extant. The text duplicates Kiṣir-Nabû's *LKA* 79, written during an uncertain stage of his career "for undertaking a (ritual) procedure" and copied according to some unknown original,[123] as well as the damaged text *KAR* 245 from an uncertain place in Assur.[124] Furthermore, the N4 manuscript *LKA* 80 (N4 no. 324) partly duplicates some passages of N4 no. 289 and *LKA* 79 (see Tsukimoto 1985: 128–129). These texts have hitherto been the only known copies of this ritual, intended to substitute a patient with a female goat kid. The text may have been circulated particularly in Assur,[125] although the ceremony must have been known in Nineveh since the rite was mentioned in two letters from the royal court: one inquiring why the ceremony had not been not performed for the king (*SAA* 10 no. 89),

121 *LKA* 40 rev. 12′: KA.INIM.MA ŠU.ÍL.LÁ ^{d}*Taš-me-t*[u_4?].

122 E.g., obv. 20: [*m*]*u-bal-liṭ* ^{lú}⸢ÚŠ⸣ "the reviver of the dead"; obv. 21: … *šá bul-lu-ṭu i-ram-m*[*u*] "who loves keeping (people) alive"; rev. 8: *u*[*k*]*-kiš* GIG.MU *qí-bi* TI.LA "remove my illness, command life!".

123 *LKA* 79 rev. 23–24: *ana* DAB AG! ^{p}*Ki-ṣir-*^{d}PA ⸢x⸣[…] ^{24} *ina pi-i* ⸢x⸣[…].

124 Verderame 2013: 315–316; Nasrabadi 1999: 41–43; Tsukimoto 1985: 125–130; Ebeling 1931a: 65–69 no. 15, 69–70 no. 16. Individual spellings in N4 no. 289 and *LKA* 79 only show small variations.

125 All currently known copies of the ritual are from Assur.

and another stating that the ritual had been performed for Assurbanipal when he was crown prince (*SAA* 10 no. 193).[126]

The actions described in the preserved section of N4 no. 289 are described as follows: the ritual begins before sunset and takes place in the patient's house (obv. 2–5). The exorcist digs a hole in the earth, intended to function as a grave, and he makes the patient and the goat lie on the ground (obv. 6). He touches the patient's throat with a dagger made of tamarisk wood, and he cuts the throat of the goat with a dagger made of bronze (obv. 7–8). The insides of the "dead" (*mītu*, ÚŠ-*ti*), i.e., the goat, are washed, anointed and filled with aromatic plants (obv. 8–9). It is dressed in a garment, its feet supplied with sandals, its eyes smeared with kohl, oil is poured on its head, and it is wrapped in the patient's turban (obv. 9–12). The goat is thereafter arranged and disposed of "as a dead man" (obv. 12–13: … ⸢GIM ^{lú}ÚŠ *te-pu-si*⸣ ^{13} ⸢*tu-kan-na-ši*⸣). The patient leaves, and various incantations and a lamentation are performed (obv. 13–15). N4 no 289 breaks off after this passage. In the duplicate *LKA* 79, the ritual concluded with funerary offerings (*kispu*) for Ereškigal, the family's collective ghost, as well as the substitute animal itself, in order to keep the substitute in the netherworld and to ensure that it was accepted as a deceased family member. Finally, the goat is buried and the patient returns into the chamber (Verderame 2013: 315–317; Tsukimoto 1985: 134–135).

The purpose of the ritual was to remove illness through substitution, i.e., by transferring the patient's persona to a female goat kid, and letting the prognosticated outcome of the ailment come to fruition. As such, the ceremony did not appease the cause of illness or eliminate the actual malady, but it moved the sufferer's identity to a substitute animal.[127]

Although Kiṣir-Nabû's copy was likely from a later phase of his career,[128] Kiṣir-Aššur may have copied the ritual in N4 no. 289 during an early stage of his *šamallû ṣeḫru*-phase. In the colophon, Kiṣir-Aššur supplies his father Nabû-bēssunu with the title *mašmaššu aššurû*(?).[129] This title for Nabû-bēssunu is

126 Verderame 2013: 315 note 54; see *SAA* 10 no. 89 rev. 5–6: "… and (the ritual) 'A substitute for Ereškigal' should be performed …", *ù* ⸢*pu-u-ḫi* LÚ$^{!}$⸣ *ana* ^{d}*Ereš-ki-gal* ^{6} *na-da-a-nu lu-u e-piš-ma*; *SAA* 10 no. 193 obv. 14-rev. 1: "We shall perform (the ritual) 'A substitute for Ereškigal' for the crown prince", *pu-u-ḫi* LÚ *a-na* ^{d}*Ereš-ki-gal* $^{\text{rev. 1}}$ *a-na* DUMU.MAN *né-pa-áš*. *SAA* 10 no. 89 was sent by the Aššur temple scholar Akkullānu (Section 2.3.5).

127 In some cases, it is possible that Ereškigal's messenger "Death", *mūtu*, hid underneath the patient's bed and was ready to take a patient to the netherworld (Plantholt in press; Wiggermann 2011: 313–14; Wiggermann 2007b: 106–109; see also Arbøll 2019: 10).

128 I suggest this on the basis of the purpose statement in the colophon of *LKA* 79, see Section 7.4.

129 N4 no. 289 rev. 3': DUMU $^{\text{p.d}}$AG-*bi-su-nu* ^{lú}MAŠ.MAŠ BAL.TIL^{ki}-*u*. If *BAM* 9 was copied around Kiṣir-Aššur's *šamallû ṣeḫru*-phase, as argued in Section 5.4.1, then Nabû-bēssunu may have been *mašmaššu aššurû* in the broken colophon of this text as well.

otherwise only preserved among his own texts (see Ch. 2 note 44). Unless Nabû-bēssunu held various titles at the same time, or was able to employ different titles according to duties, N4 no. 289 would have been one of the earliest texts with colophons copied by Kiṣir-Aššur (see also Section 5.4.1). This observation is substantiated by a mistake in obverse line 13.[130]

In general, the rite was presumably employed in cases where a patient was considered severely ill, and if the household could afford the prescribed materials (see Tsukimoto 1985: 130). Considering the copies from various career phases of the Bāba-šuma-ibni family members, it is plausible that the ritual was employed in this family as an *ad hoc* cure used in cases of severe illness. Kiṣir-Aššur may have acquired knowledge about this ritual so he could aid his father in preparing and conducting the ceremony or for educational reasons without immediate practical application.

3.7.3 *Activities Unrelated to Healing*

The unpublished manuscript N4 no. 241 contains brief words and phrases in Sumerian and Akkadian. The individual lines are ruled off from one another, clearly denoting individual entries. The outline suggests the text held incipits of individual compositions. However, the entries are not incipits, and individual words are awkward and cannot be properly contextualized.[131] Following 18 lines with individual entries, the text states: "including 18? *explanatory comments*" (rev. 3: EN ⌜18? *ṣa-a-ti*⌝).[132] The problematic term *ṣâtu* can refer to lexical lists, commentaries, explanatory word lists, or generalized "lemmata" (see, e.g., Gabbay 2016: 51–52, 82–83, 101–103, 297; Rochberg 2015: 229 note 88; Frahm 2011a: 48ff.). However, the exact nuances of the term can be difficult to evaluate in individual contexts, and my translation above is a tentative suggestion. The inclusion of the term in N4 no. 241 indicates that the manuscript was meant

130

N4 no. 289 obv. 13:	⌜*tu-kan-na-ši* ^{lú}GIG⌝ {aš}	*i*-⌜*teb-bi*	*ina*? *bi-rit*⌝ KÁ	<UD>.DU-*ma*
LKA 79 obv. 15–16:	*tu-kan-na-ši* ^{lú}GIG	*i-teb*-⌜*bi*⌝ ^{16}	*ina bi-rit* KÁ	È-*ma*
KAR 245 obv.? 245:	[	*i*]-⌜*teb*⌝-*bi*	*ina bi-rit* LÚ	È-*ma*

Kiṣir-Aššur seems to have misread the passage on the original, perhaps intending to write *ina* KUN_4(I.DIB) "by the threshold/doorsill" instead of *i-teb-bi*. Thus, the line was misunderstood and several mistakes occur, among these the superfluous *ina* and a lacking UD near the end.

131 E.g. obv. 2: "For [N]inurta", [^{d}N]in-urta-ra, obv. 9: "My *big*? brother", šeš-ḪAL$^{(\textit{mistake for GAL?})}$-ĝu$_{10}$, obv. 11: "he goes", ⌜*il*⌝-*lak*. If Kiṣir-Aššur acted as a teaching assistant, as suggested below, the content could originate in a specific teaching context, although the colophon specifies the text was "copied and checked according to its original" (Appendix 1).

132 The use of *adi*/EN in the meaning "including" is frequently attested in lists of various works (see Geller 2018b: 301 and note 29; Steinert 2018d: 204).

to function as a commentary on various entries. However, this interpretation does not seem suitable based on the content. If the text functioned as a commentary, the explanatory element must have been supplied orally. Before the colophon, N4 no. 241 contains seven lines of uncertain content, which is located in a badly damaged section of the reverse of the tablet. If this peculiar text contains an inherent organizing principle, it cannot be understood from the preliminary reading.

The colophon informs us that N4 no. 241 was copied and checked according to an original, that the text was an *u'iltu* of Kiṣir-Aššur, and finally that the tablet was copied on behalf of Kiṣir-Aššur.[133] As shown in Section 7.4.2, the three additional examples of tablets copied on Kiṣir-Aššur's behalf all originate among his *mašmaššu* and *mašmaš bīt Aššur* tablets. N4 no. 241 is therefore the only text copied on Kiṣir-Aššur's behalf from any apprentice phase, and the text must be considered peculiar.[134] Texts with similar content from early education phases are not widely attested in N4. The tablet N4 no. 241 therefore appears, to the best of my knowledge, to be unique in the N4 text collection.

Judging from the content and colophon of N4 no. 241, the text seems to have been copied by a young pupil, who was presumably in the process of developing his writing skills and literacy.[135] N4 no. 241 therefore suggests that the junior apprentice Kiṣir-Aššur acted as a teaching assistant to at least one younger student. However, this remains conjecture. We can only speculate on who this young student might have been. Yet, it is noteworthy that Nabû-bēssunu's title "exorcist of the Aššur temple" was written with a Babylonian form of the sign É. The sign suggests that the writer of the colophon had been exposed to Babylonian in addition to NA sign forms during his initial schooling.[136]

133 See Appendix 1. Sadly, the context of the final statement is damaged and the line contains an erasure, rev. 13: [*ḫa*$^{?}$-*a*]*n*$^{?}$-⸢*ṭiš*$^{?}$⸣ *ú-šá-áš*-⸢*ṭir*⸣ *{*ma*}*.

134 Although the sign SAR in colophons, here and in other publications, tends to be read as a G-stem of the verb *šaṭāru* "to write, copy", it cannot be excluded that some of these generic statements could have been causative Š-stems. E.g., *LKA* 119 from Kiṣir-Aššur's *mašmaš bīt Aššur*-phase was "copied and checked" (SAR-*ma ba-rì*), but it appears to have two mistakes in the colophon, which Kiṣir-Aššur cannot have made at this stage of his career: a missing <*aš*> in Kiṣir-Aššur's name rev. 16 and Bāba-šuma-ibni's name spelled in an otherwise unattested manner in the family's colophons as $^{p.d}$*Ba*-⸢*ba*$^{?}$⸣. Still, one would have expected the writing SAR.SAR or SAR.MEŠ for a Š-stem of *šaṭāru*.

135 This observation confirms the interpretation of the title *šamallû* as "apprentice", as a person striving towards becoming skilled at a trade. In the case of *āšipu*s, the title implies that the person had acquired basic literacy.

136 Kiṣir-Nabû explicitly notes that several manuscripts from which he copied were in Babylonian writing (Section 9.2.1).

3.8 Summary

Kiṣir-Aššur's *šamallû ṣeḫru*-phase tablets mainly focus on treatments of bodily symptoms, although he also copied material related to soothing the cause of an illness. The diagnoses attested in the texts can generally be considered complex. It is therefore peculiar that the diagnostic-prognostic series Sa-gig is completely missing from the written remains of Kiṣir-Aššur's education, and it remains uncertain when Kiṣir-Aššur was educated in Sa-gig and if the family made use of this series at all. The material indicates that the diagnoses in the therapeutic texts were intended to function as the basis for Kiṣir-Aššur's education in how to diagnose and treat illnesses.

Tablets appear to have been copied according to assignments focusing on, for example, a physiological area, a section of a collection of therapeutic prescriptions, or according to a specific malady. Furthermore, in at least Kiṣir-Aššur's case, snakebites, scorpion stings, and horse treatments were studied on equal footing with the other treatment texts. Kiṣir-Aššur presumably extracted an idiosyncratic sourcebook from one or more writing-boards related to a recension of Ugu, throughout his *šamallû ṣeḫru*-phase. This is discussed further in Sections 9.2 and 9.3. Additionally, this chapter showed that Kiṣir-Aššur copied tablets concerning *šu'illa*-prayers and ritual instructions, possibly to familiarize himself with methods for treating a cause of illness. Kiṣir-Aššur also copied a ritual to provide a substitute for a patient. They were therefore part of the relevant tools for Kiṣir-Aššur's education as a healer. Finally, a tablet copied on behalf of Kiṣir-Aššur suggests he may have functioned as a teaching assistant for novice students.

Venom treatments and veterinary prescriptions may have been used to conceptualize several physiological processes of the human body and perhaps human prescriptions could be applied to animals in some instances. These suggestions form the basis for a broader discussion of Kiṣir-Aššur's education in physiology as *šamallû ṣeḫru* in the following chapter.

CHAPTER 4

Training in Anatomy and Physiology as *šamallû ṣeḫru*

Kiṣir-Aššur copied treatments for snakebites, scorpion stings, and horse maladies on *RA* 15 pl. 76, and these cures only occur during Kiṣir-Aššur's *šamallû ṣeḫru*-phase. They are found on a tablet that was labelled as the 32nd(?) extract. This tablet likely played a role in Kiṣir-Aššur's education as *šamallû ṣeḫru*, although it is difficult to evaluate what impact this knowledge had on his overall education. This chapter discusses the possible benefit in practical, physiological, and educational knowledge that Kiṣir-Aššur may have gained from *RA* 15 pl. 76.

The first section investigates the snakebite and scorpion sting treatments on the obverse of *RA* 15 pl. 76 in the context of envenomation. By analysing the cultural and physical role of snakes and scorpions in Mesopotamia, the section argues that the physical effects of venom produced remarkable effects. These outcomes were observed as an awe-inspiring force, which also illustrated vividly how various physiological processes functioned in actual patients. Whether or not Kiṣir-Aššur was involved in these treatments himself, the section argues that this knowledge introduced him to powerful fluids which were associated with bile and saliva in humans. By extension, venom may have been used to illustrate awe-inspiring fluids inherent in various species.

By discussing the role of veterinarian knowledge among exorcists in the NA period, Section 4.2 evaluates Kiṣir-Aššur's use of such knowledge for understanding human physiology based on the reverse of *RA* 15 pl. 76. Additionally, it discusses Kiṣir-Aššur's possible practical use of such treatments. The following section discusses animal variants of human illnesses to contextualize veterinarian medicine within the therapeutic corpus. Finally, Section 4.4 evaluates the use of animal anatomical terms in medical texts to argue that animal physiology and anatomy were occasionally used to explain human physiology and anatomy. Thereupon, certain physiological overlaps related to breathing, with a focus on the nose, are investigated to argue that Kiṣir-Aššur may have acquired anatomical knowledge about the nose, throat, lungs, and breath from certain treatments applied via a tube into the nose.

DOI:10.1163/9789004436084_005

4.1 The Role of Venom in Kiṣir-Aššur's Anatomical Understanding

This section argues that Kiṣir-Aššur was introduced to cures related to snake and scorpion venom on the obverse of *RA* 15 pl. 76. By applying these treatments to envenomed patients, Kiṣir-Aššur gained experience with the effects of venom. Thus, he was exposed to the power of venom as a concept, which helped him gain an improved understanding of physiological processes. Snake and scorpion venom (*imtu*) have pronounced physical effects on the victims (see below). What follows demonstrates that venom was considered an important cultural concept for illustrating the physiological processes of the body and for metaphorically expressing the function of illnesses. By extension, knowledge of venom and its effects was probably more important than has previously been recognized (cf. Finkel 1999: 213).

4.1.1 *Snakes and Scorpions in Mesopotamia*

Snakes (*ṣēru*) and scorpions (*zuqaqīpu*)[1] were common in Mesopotamia and both must have been observed frequently in people's houses,[2] and their sightings were integrated into the 1st subchapter of Sa-gig.[3] Evidence suggests that scorpions could be found under the bed or in storerooms,[4] and snakes could

1 The word "scorpion" was frequently written with the Sumerogram GÍR.TAB, which could be translated as "the burning dagger" (*patru ḫamāṭu*), describing the painful sensation of being stung.

2 Several tablets in *Šumma ālu* were devoted to occurrences involving snakes (tablet 22–26) and scorpions (tablet 30–31) (Freedman 2006a; see Freedman 2006b for a commentary on the snake omens). Only fragments of *Šumma ālu* exist from N4 (*KAL* 1 no. 19, 35, 45, and 55; cf. the *namburbi*-rituals against snakes in Maul 1994: 270ff.). For a discussion of this series in Assur, see Heeßel 2007a: 2–10; cf. Freedman 1998: 322–23. *Šumma ālu* concerns everyday phenomena in the immediate environment of a man and his house (Koch 2015: 233ff. with a comprehensive overview; see also Guinan 2014: 117–18; Guinan 1996). However, a purely empirical basis for *Šumma ālu* seems unlikely (Rochberg 2011: 623–24).

3 See Labat 1951: 8–11. Snakes and scorpions were not the only creatures whose appearance was assessed during the diagnostic process.

4 Scorpions are observed in a number of "bed-scenes" under the marriage bed (Stol 2000: 118 and note 46 with references). A number of omens in *Šumma ālu* concern observing a scorpion on, e.g., a man's bed (Freedman 2006a: 136–37 tablet 30 line 35'–36'). Scorpion incantations indicate the places in which scorpions were found (Foster 1996: 861): "It is green in the thornbush(?), it is silent in the sand, it is venomous in the brickmold", *wa-ru-uq i-na ba-aš-tim* [8] *ša-ḫur i-na ba-ṣí* [9] *im-ta i-šu i-na na-al-ba-ni* (Pientka 2004: 389 and note 1; Nougayrol 1972: 141–42 obv. 7–9); *CT* 38 pl. 38 obv. 59 refers to a scorpion as the "wolf of the storeroom, lion of the larder" (Pientka 2004: 394; Foster 1996: 861; see also George 2016: 111ff.; Maul 1994: 344ff.; Caplice 1965: 121–23).

easily make their way into one's house through, e.g., a drain or sewer.[5] Furthermore, both were part of the magical sphere and were used metaphorically in various cultic contexts.[6] Both creatures also appear frequently on amulets against the demon Lamaštu (Wiggermann 2000: 239, 341).

The use of these creatures in Mesopotamian metaphorical and associative thought is well attested. Snakes were for example used to describe an infant child coiled up within the mother and coming out slithering like a snake.[7] Scorpions were the symbol for motherhood and were related to fertility and the image of the married woman through the goddess Išḫara.[8] By extension, the scorpion and snake illustrate domestic life and combine the concepts of life (renewal, birth), family (motherhood, womanhood), and death (venom).

---

5 *Šumma ālu* (Freedman 2006a: 46) tablet 23 line 102–4 states: "If a snake gives birth in the *asurrû* of a man's house: … (negative apodosis), [103] If a snake nests in the *asurrû* of a man's house: … (negative apodosis), [104] If a woman catches a snake unaware in the *asurrû* and lets it go: … (positive apodosis)"; DIŠ MUŠ *ina a-sur-re-e* É NA *ú-lid* … [103] DIŠ MUŠ *ina a-sur-re-e* É NA NÁ-*iṣ* … [104] DIŠ MUŠ MUNUS *ina a-sur-re-e ina la mu-de-e* DAB-*su-ma* BAR-*šú* … (George 2015: 93 with further references; cf. George 2009: 156 no. 19 obv. 2–3: "The drain bore it" *ú-ul-da-šu-ma*[!] [3] *a-sú-ru-um* …). The *asurrû* can refer to either a "sewer" or the "wall footing" (George 2015: 99–102). Although the first millennium meaning seems to favour the latter, omen literature retains the original meaning (ibid.). Snakes were also associated with water and the underworld (Pientka-Hinz 2009: 217).

6 Snake charmers (*mušlaḫḫu*) were known at the NA court and are mentioned in *Maqlû* (Abusch 2015: 72–73 line 42, 132–33 line 94; Radner 2009: 223–24; Pientka-Hinz 2009: 214; *CAD* M/2: 276–77.). Foundation deposits with clay snakes are also known from 8th and 7th century Assur, (Pientka-Hinz 2009: 221 with references; Ismail 1982: 199 and fig. 3; Klengel-Brandt 1968 pl. 8). Various gods, such as Ereškigal and Ningišzida, are associated with mythological beings, which are part snake or viper (e.g., *mušḫuššu*, *bašmu*) (Pientka-Hinz 2009: 215). Furthermore, both the constellations "scorpion" (MUL GÍR.TAB) and "snake" (MUL [d]MUŠ) are mentioned in the astrological compendium Mul-apin (see "scorpion" and "snake" in Watson and Horowitz 2011; Hunger and Pingree 1999; Koch 1995; Hunger and Pingree 1989; see also Hallo 2008: 238).

7 Böck 2009c: 270–72; Stol 2000: 10 and note 59. Snakes may have been related to fertility or youth on the basis of their "renewal" when shedding their skin (Pientka-Hinz 2009: 216; see George 2003: 722–23 lines 305–6). It is noteworthy that the snake who steals Gilgameš' plant of life smells the plant. Concerning smell and life, see Ch. 4 note 88.

8 Zernecke 2008; Stol 2000: 118; Prechel 1996; van der Toorn 1996: 173; van Buren 1937–39. A number of bed scenes also display a scorpion underneath the bed, probably referring to the couple's married aspect (Winter 2012: 355). The scorpion was also the symbol of the palace women in the NA palaces, and it can be found on various objects excavated in these (Melville 2004: 50–51; Ornan 2002: 470–71). Their relationship to motherhood is clear from the fact that they carry their young around on their back after birth (Pientka 2004: 396–97). The NA queen Ḫamâ's seal likely features Gula and her dog, with a scorpion behind the goddess (Hussein 2016 pl. 133a; see also the articles in Curtis et al. 2008 concerning the royal queens' tombs in Nimrud). Occasionally, the false mother Lamaštu is depicted with a scorpion beneath her legs (Wiggermann 2000: 234).

Snakes and scorpions were therefore important for the metaphoric expression of the Mesopotamian understanding of the world, and, as we shall see below, their venom was important in the Mesopotamian understanding of how illnesses affected the body. Therefore, encountering patients suffering from these bites and stings also taught the student about both the body's physiological processes, on the basis of observable features, and the metaphoric relationships between medical knowledge and the cause of symptoms.[9]

4.1.2 *Venom and Physiology*

Many types of scorpions and snakes were differentiated in ancient Mesopotamia, as listed, for example, in Ur$_5$-ra tablet 14.[10] While it is difficult to correlate the historical evidence with modern taxonomy, we know at least eight species of venomous snakes and three species of venomous scorpions native to Iraq (Habeeb and Rastegar-Pouyani 2016: 67; Chippaux and Goyffon 2008: 72). Among the widely distributed venomous snakes are the Desert Horned Viper (*Cerastes cerastes gasperetti*), the Levantine Viper (*Macrovipera lebetina obtusa/euphratica*), and Field's or Persian Sand Viper (*Pseudocerastes persicus persicus/fieldi*).[11] Among the venomous scorpions are the Deathstalker Scorpion (*Leiurus quinquestriatus*) and the Fattail Scorpion (*Androctonus crassicauda*).[12] Venomous snakes and scorpions can inject venom through bites and stings, which have a variety of physical effects, as shown in Table 5.

Due to the effects of venom, the Akkadian concept *imtu* was generally considered to be awe-inspiring and was used as a metaphor in incantations to establish the effects of an illness or demon.[13] Furthermore, symptoms such as "paralysis" (*šimmatu*) that were commonly experienced with bites or stings

9 See the tablet published by Nougayrol (1972: 141) with a drawing of a scorpion. It is unclear if the writer had observed a scorpion up close.

10 Pientka 2004: 395; Landsberger 1962: 7–9, 39–40. See also Landsberger 1934: 45–46, 54ff.

11 Habeeb and Rastegar-Pouyani 2016: 72–73; Harkins 2012; Warrell 1995: 435–38, 450, 454–55. During an excavation in the 1950s in northeastern Iraq, a group collected several venomous snakes, e.g., Eastern Montpellier Snake (*Malpolon monspessulana insignitus*) and Desert Cobra (*Walterinnesia aegyptia*) (Reed and Marx 1959: 114).

12 See Chippaux and Goyffon 2008: 72; Shalita and Wells 2007; Fet et al. 2000: 72–73, 155–57; Lucas and Meier 1995: 212–13; see also Gilbert 2002: 41–42. In the Al-Anbar province in 2009, various snakes and scorpions, including both the Deathstalker and Fattail Scorpion, were observed (Fadhil et al. 2009: 38).

13 E.g., in relation to the illness *maškadu*: "It took half the venom of the snake (and) it took half the venom of the scorpion", *BAM* 124 col. iv 14: *mi-šil im-ti šá* MUŠ *il-qé mi-šil im-ti šá* GÍR.TAB *il-qé*. Other examples include Lamaštu's venom, which is occasionally described in a similar manner (Farber 2014: 156–57 line 127; Pientka 2004: 399).

TABLE 5 Attested effects of snake and scorpion venom[a]

Attested and reported effects of venom	Snake	Scorpion
Local Symptoms		
Pains	+	+
Swelling	+	+
Redness	+	+
Numbness	+	
Burning sensations	+	+
Haemorrhaging	+	
Tissue necrosis	+	
Systemic Symptoms		
Abnormal coagulation[b]	+	
Sluggishness, paralysis, muscle rigidity	+	+
Nausea, Vomiting	+	+
Renal and general organ failure	+	+
Dark urine	+	
Low blood pressure (Hypotension)	+	+
Sweating	+	
Weakness of one entire side of the body (Hemiparesis)	+	
Brain stroke (Ischemia)	+	
Respiratory failure	+	+
Convulsions		+
Abdominal pain		+
Diarrhoea		+

a For snakes, see Rebahi et al. 2014: 169–70; Alirol et al. 2010: 3; Cesaretli and Ozkan 2010: 579; Göçmen et al. 2006: 160; Lifshitz et al. 2002: 1227–28; Warrell 1995: 456–57, 471, 474–75. Note that several of the acute systemic symptoms are attested infrequently (cf. Rebahi et al. 2014; Cesaretli and Ozkan 2010: 583). For scorpions, see Bawaskar and Bawaskar 2012: 48–50; Chippaux and Goyffon 2008: 76; Dehesa-Davila et al. 1995: 228–30; Sofer 1995; Sofer et al. 1994: 973–74. Note that "irrespective of different species of scorpions, clinical manifestations are similar with varying degrees of severity" (Angsanakul and Stiprija 2013: 81; cf. critique in Boyer et al. 2009: 632). Only few patients experience a majority of symptoms, although children are especially susceptible to die from the venom (Chippaux and Goyffon 2008: 76–77; Sofer et al. 1994: 973). Generally, children are more affected by venom.

b Coagulopathy and disseminated intravascular coagulopathy. This can lead to, e.g., bleeding gums (Alirol et al. 2010: 3).

TABLE 5 Attested effects of snake and scorpion venom (*cont.*)

Attested and reported effects of venom	Snake	Scorpion
Involuntary eye movement (Nystagmus)		+
Dilation of pupils (mydriasis)		+
Involuntary and painful erection (priapism)		+
Excessive salivation		+
Low body temperature (Hypothermia)		+
Heart attack		+

became identified as an illness category.[14] Some of the very visible effects of envenomation may have been used to establish relationships between illnesses associated with snakes and scorpion venom.

One example is the so-called *araḫḫi*-incantations, which were used in connection to love magic, fertility, scorpion stings, "string" illnesses, and witchcraft.[15] By combining these incantations' themes with one noticeable symptom of scorpion envenomation, priapism, one cannot help but associate the scorpion stings with potency, as well as the various metaphoric relationships inherent in scorpions, such as motherhood and the (marriage) bed (see above).[16] Furthermore, the name for scorpion in Akkadian, *zuqaqīpu*, may derive from the verbal root *zaqāpu* "to erect, to point upward". The Akkadian scorpion, *zuqaqīpu*, has therefore been translated as the "erector", because its venomous stinger stands erect when confronted with danger (Pientka 2004: 391). Scorpion venom could cause priapism and this symptom may provide an additional reason for this name.[17]

Notably, the symptoms from a lethal envenomation would have affected most bodily functions, thereby demonstrating the venom's effect on breathing,

14 E.g., Böck 2007: 266–67, 299.

15 Arbøll 2018b: 269–70; Abusch 2016: 169–70, 263, 350; Cavigneaux 1999b: 258–59; Cooper 1996.

16 This relationship between venom and its connection to potency may have influenced the reasoning behind the following medication: "If a man is ill at his testicle(s), you crush a dried scorpion, you drink it in beer and he will live"; *BAM* 396 col. iv 13–14: DIŠ NA ŠIR-*šú* GIG GÍR.TAB ḪÁD.DU *ta-sàk* [14] *ina* KAŠ NAG-*ma i-ne-eš*; or "If a man [is ill] at his testicle(s), you soak a living scorpion <in> a hardened vessel with oil …"; *BAM* 396 col. iv 15: DIŠ ⸢NA *ina* ŠIR x?⸣ GÍR.TAB TI.LA <*ina*> DUG.KAL Ì.GIŠ DIR (Scurlock 2014: 544–46; Pientka 2004: 400 and note 85–86).

17 Although this symptom mainly occurs in "older" children (Sofer et al. 1994: 976), it is also attested in adults in relation to scorpion stings from, e.g., the Fattail Scorpion (Bawaskar and Bawaskar 2012: 49).

the "strings", the abdomen (renal and rectal symptoms), mouth, the impaired function of the motoric system (via pains, paralysis and convulsions), and perhaps even death. Furthermore, the symptoms affecting the mouth and anus would have been particularly obvious through vomiting and defecation. I therefore propose that Kiṣir-Aššur did not only learn treatments related to snakebites and scorpion stings in order to heal them, but he also used his observations of the effects of venom to visualize how the human body functioned when engaged with its awesome power.

As will be shown in the next section, venom (*imtu*), bile (*martu*) and spittle (*ruʾtu, rupuštu, illātu*) were to some extent conceptually interconnected. Despite being different fluids, they were equated in lexical lists and were possibly believed to possess some of the same qualities.[18] The physiological functions of bites and stings may therefore have been part of a larger theoretical illustration of how interspecies physiology and such fluids in particular were believed to function. Thus, Kiṣir-Aššur may have been exposed to the framework of a "universal" venomous substance inherent in all animals and humans when learning about venom treatments. Interestingly, the majority of symptoms encountered in all the therapeutic diagnoses that Kiṣir-Aššur copied as *šamallû ṣeḫru* could be caused by an especially venomous bite or sting. Therefore, being exposed to victims of bites or stings would have demonstrated a majority of bodily functions for a student, on the basis of which it would have been possible to conceptualize how some aspects of human physiology functioned.

4.1.3 *The Physiological Conception of Venom, Bile, and Saliva*

The term "venom" (*imtu*), attested in connection to a variety of animals such as scorpions and snakes, was linked in lexical lists to other fluids believed to possess some of the same awe-inspiring qualities that affected various bodily processes.[19] In a recension of the lexical list Diri, known from both NA Nineveh and Assur,[20] lines 117–123 of the the first tablet provide readings of the Sumerogram ÚḪ as "spittle, saliva, phlegm" *ruʾtu*, "spittle, saliva, phlegm, froth"

18 Wee (2012: 253–55) and Scurlock and Andersen (2005: 696 note 261, 728 note 29) have criticized the use of lexical lists as sources for establishing connections between illnesses, as they mainly group illnesses together based on "logographic rather than pragmatic affinities" (Wee 2012: 254–55). However, Wee (ibid.: 329) himself saw a use of certain lexical material in commentaries, and Scurlock and Andersen (2005: 693, note 195, 728 note 29) stated that some illnesses associated in writing also shared symptoms. Regardless, interpretation was likely a central undertaking in understanding the scholarly written traditions, and, e.g., lexical lists and commentaries could be used to interpret omens (Frahm 2010a: 97–99; see also Veldhuis 2014: 19–23).

19 *CMAwR* 1: 195; Geller 2010: 152; references can be found in *CAD* I–J: 139.

20 The examples from Assur are exercise tablets with extracts, Civil 2004: 104–5. For Diri, see Veldhuis 2014: 182–87.

rupuštu, "saliva" *illātu*, "venom, poison" *imtu*, "phlegm, slime" *uḫḫu*, "spittle, slime, (chough as illness)" *ḫaḫḫu*, and "foam" *ḫurḫummatu* (MSL 15: 108–9). Venom and bile were lexically equated in Uruanna[21] and in *Malku* tablet 8.[22]

The question of what motivated these conceptual overlaps is discussed in what follows, beginning with bile in the human body followed by a discussion of saliva in relation to witchcraft.[23] Bile (*martu*) was known, then as now, as a yellow-green fluid derived from the gallbladder that had a significant colour and smell.[24] Due to its significant colour and smell, bile was related to a variety of human problems and illnesses, such as jaundice (*aḫḫāzu*, *amurriqānu*).[25] Furthermore, it may have been believed to govern certain physiological processes. Böck has recently argued: "The association of 'bile' with the accumulation of water … points to two Ancient Mesopotamian ideas of the body: one is that bile was believed to cause, regulate or distribute abundant water in the body; and the other is that abundant water in the intestines was believed to cause severe troubles" (Böck 2014a: 127–28).[26] In

21 Köcher cites the fourth tablet of Uruanna line 25: "Wenn jemand durch Geifer/Gift (von Dämonen/Schlangen etc.) (*imtu*) krank wird, so leidet er an der Galle (*martu*)" (Köcher 1978: 35–36 note 59).

22 *Malku* tablet VIII line 124: *imtu* : *martu* (Hrůša 2010: 144).

23 Although lexical evidence is regularly criticized as a source for conception rather than groupings according to similarities in Sumerograms, the fact that all the terms quoted above could be read from the same Sumerogram indicates that these terms were related concepts (see Ch. 4 note 18).

24 In addition to butchers noticing bile during the removal of the liver and the gallbladder from butchered animals, inspections connected to extispicy noted whether or not the gallbladder was intact and if bile flowed from it (Koch 2000: 514 with textual references; Meyer 1987: 143–44).

25 This overlap occurs particularly because of the shared yellow-green colour, which in Akkadian is the same word ((*w*)*arqu*, SIG_7). Jaundice can cause yellow discolouration of the eyes, base of the tongue, and skin, and bile is naturally yellow-green. Furthermore, gall-bladder disorder can result in miscoloured stools and urine. The two common terms for jaundice are *aḫḫāzu* "catcher-(demon)" from *aḫāzu* "to seize, hold a person" and *amurriqānu* from *warāqu* "to be yellow-green". For these illnesses and associations in cuneiform medicine and incantations, see Böck 2014a: 74, 122–28, 138–39; Scurlock 2014: 522–23; Scurlock and Andersen 2005: 32–34, 136–38; Cadelli 2000: 66, 196–98, 373; Velduis 1999: 37–38; Michalowski 1981; Alster and van Dijk 1972.

26 See also Arbøll forthcoming; Böck 2014a: 107–110. Water was related to the process of creation and birth (Stol 2000: 4–6, 62, 125–26; cf. the beginning of *Enūma eliš* in Lambert 2013: 50ff.), and the connection between jaundice and bile – the latter as a regulator of water – may have been linked to the fact that infants, i.e., the product of creation and birth, regularly suffered from jaundice. For the connection between bile and stomach pains, see Steinert and Vacín 2018; George 2016: 132ff. as well as Lambert and Millard 1969: 92–93 line 47: "For his heart was broken and he was vomiting gall", *ḫe-pí-i-ma li-ib-ba-šu i-ma-a' ma-ar-ta-am*. Bile was also related to "burning" *ḫamāṭu*, as evidenced by *Malku*

one reference, divine saliva is also associated with jaundice, and by extension with bile.[27]

In addition to *martu*, another type of bile is also recognized, namely *pašittu*.[28] *Pašittu* was related to the abdomen and the epigastrium through an association with vomiting.[29] Furthermore, *pašittu* was connected to Lamaštu.[30] Importantly for the present discussion, it could be written with the Sumerogram ZÚ.MUŠ.Ì.GU$_7$.E.[31] One translation of this Sumerogram could be "the snakebite's hurtful 'oil'", as a reference to the venom emanating from the snake's

---

tablet 4 line 54: *ḫa-mi-ṭa-at lìb-bi* = *mar-tú* "that which burns in the inside of the body = bile" (Hrůša 2010: 94–95; CAD Ḫ: 65).

27 The OB incantation *UET* 5 no. 85 obv. 1–10: *i-za-an-na-an* ^{2} *ki-ma ša-me-e* ^{3} *el-li-at* ^{4} ^{d}PIRIG-AB-GAL ^{5} *el-li-tu-šu* ^{6} *ki-ma še-li-pí-im* ^{7} *li-i-r*[*i-iq*] ^{8} *i-na a*$^{!}$*-wu-ri-*[*qá-nim*] ^{9} *ši-pa-a-a*[*t*] ^{10} *a-wu-ri-qá-n*[*i*]*m*, "Nergal's saliva pours down like rain, may his spittle become yellow as a turtle because of jaundice. Incantation against *awurriqānu*-jaundice" (Veldhuis 1999: 37–38; Landsberger and Jacobsen 1955: 14 note 7; CAD I–J: 85).

28 See Böck 2014a: 123; Scurlock and Andersen 2005: 137; Köcher 1978: 36; Labat and Tournay 1945–46: 117. *Pašittu* etymologically means "the destroyer, eraser" (CAD P: 249; Böck 2014a: 123–24 and note 99; Scurlock 2014: 522). Böck (2014a: 123) translates the malady as "bile liquid" (cf. CAD P: 256–57). Scurlock and Andersen (2005: 137) identified *pašittu* as "cholecystitis". Köcher (1978: 36) translated *pašittu* as "Gallenblasenkolik". Labat and Tournay (1945–46: 115) translate "de regurgitations bilieuses" (see Scurlock and Andersen 2005: 704 note 119). Meier (1939: 302) translated *pašittu* as "Gallenflüssigkeit". See also Cadelli 2000: 343, 379; Wiggermann 2000: 225 note 44.

29 See examples in Böck 2014a: 123–24; Scurlock and Andersen 2005: 137. The illness is featured several times in the second column of the 3rd tablet of the *suālu* subsection of the therapeutic series Ugu (Cadelli 2000: 62–63). *Pašittu* is observed in the LB *SpTU* I no. 43 obv. 11, read by Geller as: KI.MIN MIN *pa-šit-t*[*u*$_4$] ^{mí}*mar-tu*$_4$ "ditto, ditto ('from the mouth of the *karšu*' (pylorus?)) : *pašittu*, the daughter" (Geller 2014: 3 with references). Neither Köcher (1978: 24), Heeßel (2010b: 30), Böck (2014a: 124) nor Steinert (2016: 231) read the MÍ and therefore read "Gallensaft, Gallenblase(nkrankheit)". However, at least the copy indicates that the MÍ was present, and the question is how to interpret it. If we follow Geller's transliteration, ^{mí}*mar-tu*$_4$, it could be a reference to "daughter", indicating *pašittu* was "the daughter", i.e., like Lamaštu (see Wiggermann 2000: 225–26). Or perhaps the illness was considered the daughter of Lamaštu, i.e., an associative symptom/demon? Notably, Lamaštu is mentioned directly above in the text in obv. 10 (Geller 2014: 3).

30 In Atra-ḫasīs *pašittu* is described as follows: "Let there be among the peoples the *Pāšittu*-demon, to snatch the baby from the lap of her who bore it" (Lambert and Millard 1969: 102–3), vii 3'–5': *li-ib-ši-ma i-na ni-ši pa-ši-it-tu* $^{4'}$ *li-iṣ-ba-at še-er-ra* $^{5'}$ *i-na bi-ir-ku a-li-it-ti*. This role was traditionally Lamaštu's (Farber 2014: 1–7; Wiggermann 2000: 236ff.). Wiggermann (2000: 238) provides an explanation for Lamaštu's mythological and pathogenic roles wherein she is a (frustrated) mother (*ummu*) and rejected daughter (*martu*) of Anu who causes fever (*ummu*) and bile (*martu*).

31 Scurlock and Andersen 2005: 137; CAD P: 256. Note also "*pašittu* of blood" *pašittu ša dāmu* in Böck 2007: 224 ms A (pl. 28–29) col. i 17'–18', which is the Akkadian translation of the Sumerian ZÚ.MUŠ.Ì.GU$_7$.E.ÚŠ.

tooth.[32] This Sumerogram therefore seems to equate the problem with a venomous fluid ("oil"), which hurts, and is associated with the mouth (or literally "tooth" in the snake analogy). A first millennium Babylonian commentary on Sa-gig tablets 13 and 12 or 14 states: "*Pašittu* venom means *pašittu* that holds bile".[33] Kiṣir-Aššur also encountered *pašittu* once, namely in his *šamallû ṣeḫru* manuscript *RA* 40 pl. 116.[34] As such, both fluids were associated with venom and bodily processes, possibly indicating that bile may have been considered a "venom" inherent in mammals.

Phlegm, spittle, and saliva (*ru'tu, rupuštu*) were connected to witchcraft (*kišpu*).[35] An incantation could therefore be expressed simply as "spittle", i.e., something thrown (*nadû*) from the mouth (*CMAwR* 1: 4; Schwemer 2007a: 16–21). Spittle was an ambivalent substance, much like bile, and could grant life and recovery as well as contamination and illness.[36] Furthermore, witchcraft could produce a number of characteristic symptoms. One group of symptoms comprised various abnormal states in the mouth involving phlegm and the overproduction of saliva (Schwemer 2007a: 169–70 and notes 23, 25). Excessive saliva could also be caused by scorpion envenomation and be observed as venom in the mouth of snakes about to bite. Therefore, such fluids may have been compared to spittle in the mouth of ill-wishers who were magically manipulating a victim through witchcraft or as phlegm in the lungs and throat of people under attack from witchcraft. This requires further investigation

32 I read the Sumerogram as ZÚ.MUŠ "snakebite" (for ZÚ as "bite", see Appendix 2), Ì "oil", and GU_7.E "hurtful" (cf. SA.GU_7.E = *ekketu* "scratching", Böck 2014a: 29; *CAD* E: 69). Labat and Tournay (1945–46: 117) analyzed the Sumerogram differently, and saw it as a reference to an attack on the dental nerves (Cf. Köcher 1978: 36). Scurlock and Andersen (2005: 704 note 119) agree with "snake bite" for ZÚ.MUŠ, and see the Sumerogram as "a reference to the quality of the pain". Cf. Böck's discussions of the image of the snake spitting venom in relation to bile to express fury and anger (Böck 2014a: 126 and note 108 with references).

33 GCBC 766 obv. 4: *pa-šit-tú im-tú* : *pa-šit-tú šá mar-tú ú-kul-lu*, see Jiménez 2015 with further references and discussions concerning this tablet. Jiménez reads the entry differently as: "The 'poisonous *pāšittu*-demon' means 'the *pāšittu*-demon that holds bile'".

34 Obv. 1: [DIŠ] ⸢NA *a-šá-a pa-šit-tú*⸣ *u lu-*⸢*ba-ṭi* GIG⸣.

35 *CMAwR* 1: 4. However, note that such references were more frequently written $UŠ_7$ or $UŠ_{11}$. The sign $UŠ_{11}$ was also equated with *imtu* "venom" in bilingual incantations and the phrase *imat marti* "venomous bile" could therefore be understood as "spittle mixed with bile" (ibid.: 195).

36 *CMAwR* 1: 4. Note the 1st tablet of Atra-ḫasīs lines 231–34 in connection to the creation of man: "After she had mixed that clay, she summoned the Anunnaki, the great gods. The Igigi, the great gods, spat upon the clay …", *iš-tu-ma ib-lu-la ṭi-ṭa ša-*⸢*ti*⸣ 232 *is-si* ᵈ*a-nun-na i-li ra-bu-*⸢*ti*⸣ 233 ᵈ*i-gi-gu i-lu ra-bu-tum* 234 *ru-u'-tam id-du-ú e-lu ṭi-iṭ-ṭi* (Lambert and Millard 1969: 58–59). However, saliva's use in healing rituals appears to be limited (Schwemer 2007a: 18 note 60).

elsewhere. Although Kiṣir-Aššur may not have encountered witchcraft (*kišpu*) as *šamallû ṣeḫru*, several symptom descriptions mention phlegm.[37]

Regarding saliva, it is interesting to note that the Mesopotamians do not seem to have described rabies metaphorically as connected to spittle. We know from incantations that the ancient Mesopotamians were aware that rabies infected new hosts through saliva (Finkel 1999: 213–223). However, references are largely to the dog's semen (*nīlu*) being in the mouth (*pû*) or on its teeth (*šinnu*) and infecting through a bite (*nišku*).[38]

Thus, several relationships between venom and other bodily fluids can be explained through analogies inherent in the symptoms of, e.g., scorpion envenomation. As such, the overarching conceptions investigated here could have been taught to Kiṣir-Aššur in connection with his encounter with scorpion and snake venom and possibly with envenomed patients.

4.2 Veterinarian Knowledge in Kiṣir-Aššur's Education

Veterinarian prescriptions only appear during Kiṣir-Aššur's *šamallû ṣeḫru*-phase, i.e., his first (traceable) stage of education, and they therefore played a role in the education that he received during this period. Kiṣir-Aššur acquired the requisite knowledge for his education from a therapeutic tradition that may have been specific to Assur (see Section 9.5.3). Within this tradition, there existed various veterinarian remedies. Although veterinarian *asû*s had existed in the OB period, there is, to the best of my knowledge, no evidence in the written documentation for *asû*s or *āšipu*s specialized in any type of animal medicine during the NA period.[39] As a result, who administered animal healing in the NA period remains uncertain.

37 *BAM* 201 obv. 29': … KI ÚḪ-*šú* ÚŠ *u* LUGUD Š[UB!.ŠUB?]; *RA* 40 pl. 116 obv. 9: … ÚḪ TUKU-*ši*. Note the alternative ingredient in *BAM* 201 rev. 41: ÚḪ dÍD *ina* A NAG.

38 Wu 2001: 34. However, note the description of the *asakku*-demon in Lugal-e, which also references a scorpion attack, in line 172: "he drips the (venomous) water (or saliva?) over his side", a da-bi-a mu-un-sur-sur-re (ibid.: 42; van Dijk 1983: 73). For *nīlu*, see Stol 2000: 4–5.

39 See Stol 2011: 379–80 with references; *CAD* A/2: 347e. *CAD* attests to specialized *asû*s in the 3rd millennium BCE, as well as in the OB and NB periods. The only NA example stems from the annals of Esarhaddon. A broken list of deportees mentions the word *muna''išu*, "veterinarian" (*CAD* M/2: 199) or "animal surgeon" (*CDA*: 216); a participle derived from the otherwise unattested D-stem of the root *nêšu* "to live" (cf. Stol 2011: 379; Borger 1967: 114 section 80 col. i 10'). The word is attested in the lexical series Lu I as: A.ZU ANŠE = *mu-na-'i-i-šú* (see *CAD* M/2: 199 for further references). Maul (2013: 18) considered the knowledge of the unknown "Pferdedoktoren" to be so important that it was

Some anatomical terms were derived from animal anatomy (see Section 4.4.1). Human and animalistic physiology therefore likely coalesced to an indeterminable extent.[40] Thus, knowledge of animalistic anatomy may have been useful for understanding human anatomy and physiology. Comparably, veterinary medicine appears as a separate discipline in the later *Hippiatrica* (5th–6th century CE), although some healing for horses is reported to have been borrowed from the realm of human healing and some cures are said to be effective for humans.[41] Labat even saw a thematic relationship between the Akkadian medical texts and Greek and Latin hippiatric texts, suggesting that veterinarians in Anatolia drew upon Akkadian human medicine in their works (Labat 1951: XLIII–XLV).[42]

The inclusion of these cures in human medicine, such as the references to horse treatments in *šammu šikinšu*,[43] could suggest that these genres were not considered separate in Mesopotamian thought. It is therefore plausible that (Assur) healers drew both on human and veterinarian prescriptions to apply treatments to humans in the NA period, even though there are only a few indications for this. Additionally, there is evidence that healers in theory also used treatments designed for humans to treat animals (see Section 3.5.2).

4.2.1 *Horses and Specialists*

Horses were very valuable in the NA period (Radner 1997: 305–6) and were historically part of a specialist sphere of written knowledge in Assur. Horses were important for the Assyrian army from the MA period onwards (Maul 2013: 17–18 and note 9), for which role they needed to be trained. A specialist called the *susānu*, "horse trainer", was responsible for training horses for chariots (see *CAD* Š/3: 378–80). A number of MA texts written by a *susānu* instruct the reader in the "Trainierung von Wagenpferden",[44] and one such text is even stated to

---

included in the written human healing texts. In general, there may occasionally be an overlap in terminology. The *asû* Ur-Lugaledena from Lagaš (ca. 2100) was described as *asû* even though he was dedicated to Šakkan and his seal features equipment for the birth of cattle (Stol 2011: 379). In OB Mari, references to *asûtu*, the craft of the *asû*, may describe veterinarian praxis (ibid.: 379 and note 120 with references).

40 Animals were occasionally used for comparison in the physiognomic omens (Böck 2000: 40 with references).

41 McCabe 2007: 4, 6, 15, 42–43, 144–145, 276, 278.

42 A study of the Akkadian loanwords in the Ugaritic hippiatric texts suggests that these drew on Akkadian material as well (Watson 2004).

43 E.g., Stadhouders 2012: 3 §15'; Stadhouders 2011: 8 §15'.

44 Pedersén 1985 M1 and M2; Ebeling 1951. These MA texts were perhaps associated with similar Hittite texts (cf. Ebeling 1951: 58–60; Cohen and Sivan 1983: 2 note 6; Stol 2011: 373–74 and notes 78–80 for references; Maul 2013: 17).

be the "2nd [tablet/writing-board]" of some unknown collection.[45] Although this knowledge was not transmitted in writing into the NA period, the tradition exemplified by these texts may have been kept alive through oral transmission into the NA Period.[46]

Texts connected to the wellbeing of animals were also included in the AMC[47] and the EM, of which the latter example was probably intended to prevent the spread of illness in horse stables and cattle pens, as well as camp areas.[48] Perhaps included under these headings is a *namburbi*-ritual from Nineveh, which was performed so "that *di'u*-illness, plague and pestilence may not approach the king's ho[rses and] troops".[49] This ritual even included the participation of the king himself, was performed in camp (lines 27 and 65),[50] and included the exorcist making amulets for the horses (line 60).[51]

Maul (2013) recently edited a group of texts attested from the MA period to the 7th century in Nineveh that are connected to the purification of the stables.[52] The MA tablet VAT 10035 (= ms A) contained an initial incantation only in Sumerian, to which the later copies added interchanging lines of Akkadian (Maul 2013: 20–21). Although ms A states that it was copied from an "Akkadian tablet", probably referring to Babylonia, this tradition was surely sustained, translated, and transmitted through the first millennium in an Assyrian tradition.[53] The texts mention that horses were subject to an elaborate ritual performed by an exorcist. Therefore, these MA and NA texts,

45 Ebeling 1951: 11, ms A rev. 4'–6': [x (x) x] 2-*ú* ⌜x x 30?⌝ x? šu-[…] 5' [ŠU Px-(x)-x]-*ki-ni su-sa-ni* DUMU […] 6' *ša pi-i li*-[…]; cf. Stol 2011: 373–74 and note 76.

46 The commentary VAT 9426 is perhaps younger than the MA texts (Ebeling 1951: 6).

47 AMC line 121: "If horses in the stable [… are] reduced (and) there [is] an epidemic", *šúm-mu* ANŠE.KUR.RA.MEŠ *ina tar*-[*ba-ṣi* … T]UR? BAD-*a-nu* G[ÁL.MEŠ]; see Steinert 2018c: 181; Steinert 2018d: 276–277.

48 Maul 2013: 19 and note 25; *KAR* 44 rev. 24, see Ch. 4 note 60.

49 Maul 2013: 18–19 and notes 19 and 26 with references ; Caplice 1970: 118–23. Lines 1–2: *a-na di-i'-ḫu šib-ṭi* NAM.ÚŠ.MEŠ *a-na* AN[ŠE.KUR.RA *u*] 2 ERÉN.ḪI.A LUGAL NU TE-*e* …

50 Caplice 1970: 119, 121 line 27: "You have the king recite 'Lord, the strong one of all the great gods'", UMUN.E GÌR.RA DÌM.ME.ER.GAL.GAL.E.NE ANA LUGAL *tu-šad-ba-ab*. Caplice 1970: 120, 123 line 65: "(and) anger (of the gods) will not approach the king's horses (and) camp, and …", *ug-ga-tu*4 *a-na* ANŠE.KUR.RA.MEŠ KARAŠ LUGAL NU TE-*ḫi-ma* …

51 Caplice 1970: 120, 123 line 60: "… You [place] (the pouch) on the necks of the horses", … *ina* GÚ ANŠE.KUR.RA *ta*-[*šak-kan*]. Amulet stones for the king's and royalty's chariots are also mentioned in other exorcistic texts (Schuster-Brandis 2008: 354–56; cf. Maul 2013: 18–19 and note 21–23 with references). Such stones were also included in a newly built trough area in connection to Sennacherib's new *ekal māšarti* in Nineveh, as listed on an inscription from an inscribed trough (MacGinnis 1989: 189). See also Nadali and Verderame 2014.

52 The MA copy VAT 10035 (= ms A) was copied by an *āšipu* (Maul 2013: 19).

53 Maul (2013: 20–21) also noted several Assyrianisms in the later copies.

combined with the examples of veterinarian medicine found in the N4 collection, point to the existence of various traditions concerning knowledge of horses in Assur.

However, only in an unpublished and undated Assur document regarding a number of equids to be delivered to the city Ubasê do we encounter an exorcist, called Nabû-gamil(?), in connection to an actual equid.[54] Although the text does not seem to describe a regular levying of horses, known from the so-called Horse Lists from Assur and Nimrud,[55] it is unclear if the equid was a "donation".[56] Furthermore, at least one *tamītu* divinatory question (*KAR* 218 = N4 no. 108) excavated in N4 concerns a white horse's suitability to pull Marduk's chariot, and even makes use of a tube (^{giš}SAG.KUD) to whisper the prayer into the ear of the horse (Lambert 2007: 80–83). This document could therefore point to a relationship between horses, the Aššur temple, and exorcists.[57]

Nonetheless, we must imagine that ill animals were in need of care. Although a veterinarian professional not attested in the written documents could have administered such treatments, the Assur horse traditions together with the horse prescriptions inherent in the N4 collection and their place in Kiṣir-Aššur's training suggest that some *āšipu*s could have performed certain functions as veterinarians in 7th century Assur (see also Steinert 2018d: 276; Panayotov 2015: 486–488).

4.2.2 *Kiṣir-Aššur and Veterinarian Knowledge*

Kiṣir-Aššur's copying of texts during his *šamallû ṣeḫru* education suggests that veterinarian knowledge was as important as treatments designed for humans, even though it represents a smaller part of his textual production.[58] As written

---

54 Jean 2006: 176, Ass. 10804 = VAT 20401 rev. 8–10: ANŠE NÍTAḪ *ša* ^{giš}BAN ^{9} $^{\text{p.d}}$PA-*ga*$^{?}$-*mil* ^{lú}MAŠ.MAŠ ^{10} x x TI x [x].

55 Found in Assur (Schroeder 1920 no. 31–38, 131–132; Pedersén 1985: 30 note 7) and Nimrud (Dalley and Postgate 1984: texts nos. 85, 98–118; Maul 2013: 17), perhaps to be dated to Sargon's reign (Dalley and Postgate 1984: 18–20).

56 High-ranking members of society occasionally made deliveries of equines to the army (Jean 2006: 176, 183).

57 Kiṣir-Aššur may later have been connected to the Aššur temple, as attested by his title *mašmaš bīt Aššur* (see Section 8.1). For exorcists in connection to horses, see also a prescription utilizing horse sweat in Básckay 2018: 99, 106; Scurlock 2014: 413, 416. The text *SAA* 16 no. 70 concerns a horse that is possibly ill. A sales document of a field from 742 BCE excavated in the N24 archive in Assur demands that should any of the selling party's family members file a lawsuit, they shall make various payments and "tie two white horses at the feet of (the statue of) Aššur" (Deller et al. 1995: 126–28 no. 136; see May 2018: 73–74 and note 91).

58 See Section 3.5.2.

veterinarian knowledge only seems to be found in Assur during the NA period, the fact that such knowledge was copied by Kiṣir-Aššur attests to its importance among his medical texts. The question is what purpose these prescriptions served. *RA* 15 pl. 76 improved Kiṣir-Aššur's repertoire of cures, yet, from the arguments put forth in Sections 3.5 and 4.2, three possible hypotheses can be established as to why Kiṣir-Aššur acquired this knowledge related to horses, snakebites, and scorpion stings:

1) To practice veterinarian medicine. Animals in the fields were prone to be bitten or stung, and *RA* 15 pl. 76 was designed to heal various types of animal illnesses (bites, stings, colic).[59]
2) As part of a training curriculum. *RA* 15 pl. 76 was the 32nd(?) extract in a hypothesized row of copies and could be part of a syllabus Kiṣir-Aššur needed to learn, regardless of its applicability.[60]
3) To improve Kiṣir-Aššur's physiological understanding of the human body, and perhaps also his knowledge of animal physiology.

Kiṣir-Aššur's training possibly depended on a combination of these three hypotheses, although it is difficult to evaluate which focus was the most important. As suggested in Section 5.2.3, Kiṣir-Aššur may have been in charge of treating children (prophylactically) as *šamallû mašmaššu ṣeḫru* before becoming a responsible ritual supervisor, healing adults as *mašmaššu*. If Kiṣir-Aššur aided his father in healing animals during his *šamallû ṣeḫru*-phase, I cautiously suggest that he initially may have been allowed more autonomy when administering treatments (perhaps under supervision) to horses and other animals before moving onto human babies. Further reasons for this suggestion are explored in Section 5.2.3.

4.3 Excursus: Animal Variants of Human Illnesses

In ancient Mesopotamia, certain illness names were used to describe what were considered animal variants of human afflictions.[61] Several of these names

59 However, note that animal symptoms resulting from envenomation may differ from human reactions (Al-Asmari and Al-Saif 2003: 65).

60 Bites, stings, and veterinary prescriptions appear late in the AMC lines 76–78: [... N]A! ⌜MUŠ⌝ *iš-šuk-š*[*u*] 77 ... Ú.ḪI.A *ša* BÚR *ša ni-šik* ⌜MUŠ⌝ 78 [UR.GI$_7$] ⌜*lu*?⌝ [... *zi-q*]*it* GÍR.TAB SÌG-*iṣ* ...; and lines 121–22: *šúm-mu* ANŠE.KUR.RA.MEŠ *ina tar-*[*ba-ṣi* ... T]UR? BAD-*a-nu* G[ÁL.MEŠ] 120 1 DUB *ša*! ANŠE.KUR.RA.[MEŠ *u*] *ša* GU$_4$.M[EŠ]. The EM refers to symptoms and cleansing of the domesticated animal abodes, *KAR* 44 rev. 24: "To purify the pen of cows, bulls and sheep (and) horses", TÙR ÁB.GU$_4$ḪI.A *u* U$_8$.UDU.ḪI.A ANŠE.KUR.RA SIKIL.E.DÈ.

61 Stol (2011: 380–81) defines an ill animal by its inability to perform its duties, but he also discusses defects described in the omen series *Šumma izbu*, liver omens, injuries inflicted

designate illnesses that resemble the symptoms observed in humans, albeit mainly in relation to externally observable symptoms.

In the NA period, sheep variants of a number of human illnesses are known via Ur$_5$-ra tablet 13, including sheep-*sikkatu*, sheep-*samānu*, sheep-*rapādu*, and sheep-*šaššaṭu*.[62] Additionally, a "Hip illness" is known in cattle and sheep variants,[63] and we also know sheep with "Sick inside(s)", *garābu*, and ill lungs.[64] Another illness called *rāšānu* could afflict cattle and sheep and likely caused hair loss,[65] and we also know a type of mange.[66] Several of these maladies seem to manifest themselves as skin disorders.

Gods or demons could inflict illness upon animals as well as humans.[67] Similarly, an evil afflicting an animal could likely be transferred to the owner.[68] This probably gave rise to a contagion model similar to our concept

---

on animals by their owner or others, as well as various defects inflicted on animals by humans.

62 Ur$_5$-ra tablet 13 (*MSL* 8/1: 10, 12) line 44: UDU.GAG.ŠUB.BA = *šá sik-*[*ka-ti*]; lines 57–60: UDU.[SA].AD.NIM = ditto *sa-ma-nu* ^{58} UDU.[S]A.AD.NIM = ditto *ra-pa-du* ^{59} UDU.[S]A.AD.GAL = ditto *šá-áš-šá-ṭu* ^{60} UDU.[SA].AD.GAL = ditto *ra-pa-du*. *Utukku*-demons and *samānu* were considered deadly for livestock (Geller 2016: 43, 234–35; Stol 2011: 382 and note 138). Sheep-*sikkatu* was treated with incantations in the OB period (*YOS* 11 no. 7 obv. 17: KA.INIM.MA UDU.GAG.ŠUB.BA; Stol 2011: 385 and notes 159, 161 and 163–64; see also *YOS* 11: 45 and no. 69). Perhaps related to sheep-*šaššaṭu* is a type of vertigo and paralysis (Stol 2011: 384 and note 158; Sjöberg 1973: 114, 119 lines 166–67: udu sag-nigin lú-al-dib-ba ^{167} é-gar$_8$ šu-ur$_4$-a …).

63 Ur$_5$-ra tablet 13 line 42 and 339b refers to UDU.ÍB.GIG "Sheep ill hip(s)" and ÁB.ÍB.GIG "Cow ill hip(s)" (*MSL* 8/1: 10, 48; Stol 2011: 385–86 notes 165–166).

64 Oppenheim and Hartman 1945: 158–59 lines 42–46: UDU.<ÍB>.GIG : *šá qab-lu maḫ-ḫa* ^{43} UDU.<ŠÀ>.SUR : *šá nis-*[*ḫu*] ^{44} [UDU.GA]G.ŠUB.BA : *šá sik-*[x-x] ^{45} UDU.GA$^{(!)}$].ŠUB.BA : *šá ga-ra-bi* ^{46} [UDU.UR$_5$].ŠUB.BA : *šá ḫa-še*$^{!}$*-e*. Sheep *garābu* was perhaps called *girriṣānu* (see *CAD* G: 90a; Scurlock and Andersen 2005: 232, 722 note 127).

65 Stol 2011: 384; *CAD* R: 191a. It was perhaps related to the human skin illness *ra'šānu*, which typically afflicted the head (Scurlock and Andersen 2005: 244–45).

66 Possibly a variant of "itching" (SA.GU$_7$.E) named SU.GU$_7$ MÁŠ.ANŠE (Kinnier Wilson 1962: 59).

67 Gods could "touch" (*lapātu*), "hit" (*maḫāṣu*), and "devour" (*akālu*), see Salin 2015; Stol 2011: 382 and note 136; van der Toorn 1985: 71.

68 An example of this from OB Mari is perhaps quoted by Stol (2011: 382 note 134). Omens could designate the outbreak (*miqittu*) of an epidemic among the owner's animals (e.g., Böck 2000: 300–301 line 57), adding misfortune to the man. *CAD* (M/2: 100) lists *miqittu* as "downfall, misfortune, epidemic, death". Therefore, the misfortune of a man is an epidemic among his animals.

of "zoonosis", i.e., diseases spreading from animals to humans.[69] Evidence suggests that domesticated animals were often afflicted in herds or flocks due to their proximity.[70] Therefore, we find references to epidemics and stalls,[71] as well as purification rites for the pens of cattle, sheep, and horses in the healers' corpora.[72]

As we have already seen, horse colic (*kīs libbi*) was also an identifiable illness. In addition to the known prescriptions, we also find plants that are described as useful against horse colic in two copies of *šammu šikinšu* and a fragment of a "therapeutic vademecum".[73] Why this horse disorder was one of the only animal illnesses found in the therapeutic material is uncertain, although we know that cattle and horses were considered especially important to individual households. It is therefore conceivable that the owners would go to great lengths to ensure their survival.[74]

Only veterinarian medicine concerning horses seems to exist in the NA therapeutic corpus. However, the lexical traditions in particular points towards an overlap between human illnesses and their animal counterparts. As argued in Section 4.2, the relationship between veterinary and human healing in Mesopotamia seems to have been fluid. Animals were for many reasons useful to both men and gods combined, and animal metaphors as well as physiological concepts were used to describe how humans functioned.[75] That animal ailments overlapped with predefined human illnesses could explain why there are so few veterinarian texts because human medicine may have been applicable to animals.

---

69 Some zoonotic diseases must have existed (e.g., rabies, see Wu 2001; perhaps *maškadu*, see Wasserman 2012; cf. Arbøll 2018a).

70 Codex Ḫammurabi paragraph 266: "If, in the enclosure (*tarbaṣim*), an epidemic (*lipit ilim*) should break out …" (see also paragraph 267; Roth 1995: 130; cf. Stol 2011: 381–82, 385–86 note 165; Maul 1994: 193 lines 14–17). Note a *namburbi*-ritual for protecting the king's horses and troops (Caplice 1970: 118f.; cf. Stol 2011: 383 and note 141). See also the so-called "heart-grass" incantation (George 2016: 129–32; Veldhuis 1990).

71 AMC line 121–22; see Ch. 4 note 60.

72 *KAR* 44 rev. 24; see Ch. 4 note 60. One incantation related to these purifications is INIM.INIM.MA TÙR.ANŠE.KUR.RA SIKIL.E.DA.KAM (Tsukimoto 1985: 178–83; see Stol 2011: 377 and note 104 with further references). For magic against field pests, see George 1999.

73 E.g., Stadhouders 2012: 3 §15', 12 §10'; Stadhouders 2011: 8 ms A §15', 26–27 ms C §10'; Stol 2011: 393, discussion of *CT* 14 pl. 41 (= Rm. 362).

74 Cattle were part of the family in the OB period and were given names (Postgate 1992: 164 and note 254 with further rerences). Horses were also valuable in the NA period (Radner 1997: 305–6).

75 E.g., Stol 2006; Foster 2002; Scurlock 2002a; Watanabe 2002.

4.4 Animal and Human Physiology: The Reverse of *RA* 15 pl. 76

The Mesopotamians often used vague or unclear terminology regarding the organs contained in the torso and other areas of the body.[76] The term *libbu* (ŠÀ), for example, designates the heart, entrails, womb, and abdomen (belly).[77] As it was probably not easy to gain knowledge of human insides, animal anatomical terms as well as common concepts were used to describe and metaphorically illustrate the human innards. This section discusses some of these aspects in order to argue why a conceptual overlap between animal and human anatomy may have existed concerning how the stomach and nose were understood in diagnostic descriptions and treatments. Thus, this section evaluates the purpose of the reverse of *RA* 15 pl. 76 and provides an interpretation regarding Kiṣir-Aššur's educational use of this text.

4.4.1 *Animal Anatomical Terminology*

As previously mentioned, animal dissection for various purposes (extispicy, butchers) or human battle wounds must have been sources for gaining knowledge of the insides.[78] A common anatomical description, *rapaštu* (*CAD* R:

76 Steinert 2016: 205–9 and note 32–33 with references; Westenholz 2010; Stol 2006; Geller 2004; Attia 2000.

77 *CAD* L: 164; Böck 2014a: 103–4, 106, 111–19; Böck 2014b: 101–105, 111–19; Geller 2007a: 189; Stol 2006: 103.

78 Geller 2010: 21–22; Westenholz 2010: 9–14; Stol 2006: 103; Cadelli 2000: 290; Attia 2000: 49. As shown in the following section, incantations and treatments used by exorcists referred to specific anatomical parts of animals. Whether such knowledge was derived visually and orally from butchers, from lexical lists (e.g., Steinert 2016: 199 and notes 13–14 with references; Couto Ferreira 2009; Westenholz and Sigrist 2008; Stol 2006; Landsberger 1967), or the knowledge of the *bārû* is unknown. A connection between *āšipu* and *bārû* in which such knowledge could have been shared is only rarely visible, but for example an exorcist named Banūnu from Nimrud owned texts consisting of *tamītu*-prayers, which typically are considered part of the *bārû*'s work (Koch unpublished: 10 and note 57; Koch 2015: 125–27; Lambert 2007 no. 1 and 2). For extispicy in relation to anatomy, see, e.g., Wyplosz 2006; Glassner 2005; Koch 2000: 43ff.; Starr 1990: XXXIX–LV; see also Cohen 2016. While campaigning, many wounds were probably treated ad hoc, see Esarhaddon's succession treaty line 643–45 (*SAA* 2 no. 6). Several reliefs and NA royal annals illustrate that the soldiers of conquered cities in the 7th century were occasionally flayed (e.g., Grayson and Novotny 2012: 15–16) and hung on stakes surrounding the city (e.g., Leichty 2011: 83). Anyone interested in anatomy would have had a chance to inspect the human body in these cases. For a discussion of experts accompanying the Assyrian army on campaigns, see Nadali and Verderame 2014. Wee (2012: 5) makes a strong case that little could be learned from repeated human dissection that could not be learned from animal dissection (see also Geller 2010: 3–4, 22).

152–53), was derived from a cut of meat, thereby rendering it difficult to understand as a demarcated description for a bodily area.

Ruminant gastrointestinal physiology seems to have been relatively well known, and an incantation describes two stomachs: "The ewe eats and it *regurgitates*?, a[nd] the mouth gives (the food) to the first stomach (*karšu*), the first stomach to the omasum (*riqītu*), the omasum to the rear (*arkatu*). The dung falls down, and the grass receives (it)".[79] The extispicy corpus with its thorough knowledge of the insides of sheep includes even more terms: *karšu* (rumen), *pî karši* (reticulum), *riqītu* (omasum), and *kukkudru* (abomasum).[80] Humans only have one stomach, and it is therefore peculiar that several of these terms are also attested in human medicine.[81]

The human *karšu* can be translated as "belly, stomach" or even "womb", depending on the context.[82] In relation to animal anatomy, *karšu*, as the rumen, and *pî karši*, as the closely connected reticulum, became associated with the human stomach and perhaps the opening to the stomach from the oesophagus (lower oesophageal sphincter) or the opening from the stomach to the intestines (pylorus).[83] Ur$_5$-ra tablet 15 lists various readings of UZU.ŠÀ

79 Cf. Stol 2006: 105–6; Starr 1983: 91–93; Cadelli 2000: 297 note 57–58. *KAR* 165 obv. 9–12 (partial duplicate BM 76986): *ik-kal im-mer-tú-ma i-ʾa-ra-m*[*a*(?)] [10] *pu-u a-na kar-ši kar-ši a-na ri-q*[*í-ti*] [11] *ri-qí-tu a-na ár-kàt i-nam-*[*din*] [12] *i-ma-qut* A.GAR.GAR-*ma* Ú.KI.KAL *i-*⸢*ma-ḫar*⸣; see *CAD* A/2: 275; *CAD* R: 367. Stol (2006: 105) reads *i-ʾa-ra* as a verbal form from the root *âru* translating "it advances to". I understand it as a form of *arû* "to vomit", as this makes sense in the context of ruminants "regurgitating" (cf. Cadelli 2000: 335–37). It was also translated as "vomit" by Scurlock and Andersen (2005: 117 no. 6.3). However, *arû* verbal forms usually end in *u* and rarely note the first weak root in writing (cf. *CAD* A/2: 316).

80 Although the *bārû*'s knowledge of the insides of sheep is typically not part of the *āšipu*'s knowledge, there may be indications of an overlap of some anatomical knowledge. In particular, *karšu* is also mentioned as cuts of meat for consumption (see Stol 2006: 106 note 13, 107; Bottéro 1995: 31, 205). The *karšu*– perhaps designating the entire stomach of ruminants – was offered to the Aššur temple (*SAA* 7 no. 188–90, 192–94, 197–98, 200–201, 203, 206–213, 216, 219). Thus, these cuts were not known exclusively to divinatory experts. That, e.g., the *karšu* was also known outside of specialist spheres is evident from the reference of a kitchen technique called "contorting (*zâru*) the rumen (*karšu*)" (Stol 2006: 107 note 25; Bottéro 1995: 46, edition of *YOS* 11 no. 25 line 41: *ši-i-tum ka-ar-šu tu-li-mu-ú ta-za-ar-ma*). For the relationship between medicine and cooking, see Worthington 2003: 10–11.

81 The *kukudrum* is attested once in a medical context (Stol 2006: 107 and note 23). Several hemerologies prohibit eating dates on certain days or "he will be sick of the *riqītu*" (Stol 2006: 106 and note 15; see *AMT* 6,6 line 6 and *CT* 51 pl. 161 rev. 20).

82 *CAD* K: 223–25; Stol 2006: 106; Cadelli 2000: 297; Köcher 1978: 23–24). The term is attested in *Šumma izbu*, but here it is an organ or part thereof (Cadelli 2000: 298 and note 62; Leichty 1970: 163 tablet 16 line 49').

83 See Steinert 2016: 231–32, 235–36; Geller 2014: 3; Heeßel 2010b: 30–31; Cadelli 2000: 298 note 65; Köcher 1978: 23–24.

as *libbu*, *karšu*, *qerbu*, and *irru*, perhaps indicating a descending anatomical order in the gastrointestinal system (Cadelli 2000: 298; *MSL* 9: 9 lines 98–101; see also Böck 2014b: 111–19). The *karšu* is, however, rarely attested in the diagnostic statements (Cadelli 2000: 298 and note 65).

The *pî karši*, "mouth of the *karšu*", is better attested in human medicine. It is known especially in relation to *dugānu*-illness and illnesses of the epigastrium (Stol 2006: 107, 111; Cadelli 2000: 243–44 and notes 257–58). A LB medical text groups several illnesses according to four internal organs or anatomical areas, and here *pî karši* occurs as an anatomically discernable "organ".[84] Stol (2006: 107) emphasized that this anatomical idea must have originated in animal physiology, and it is therefore peculiar that it was adopted in human physiological descriptions.[85] As a result, animal anatomical terminology was employed on various occasions in both metaphor and practice to describe the human insides. This conceptual overlap between animal and human physiology may therefore have been useful for explaining various physiological aspects of humans.

4.4.2 *Human and Equine Physiological Aspects of the Nose*

The mouth and nostrils are the orifices opening to the lungs and the stomach. The nose was associated with breath and life.[86] The throat and neck area was called *napištu*, a word that can also be read as "life, opening, air hole"

84 *SpTU* I no. 43; Steinert 2016: 230–32; Geller 2014: 3–9; Heeßel 2010b: 30–31.

85 Several aspects of animals and humans were compared, such as physiology, sexuality, reproduction, family, children, and death (Steinert 2012: 22–25). Animals, however, did not have ghosts (*eṭemmu*) (Cooper 2009: 25–26), or intellectual abilities (Steinert 2012: 25 and notes 19–21). The ancient Mesopotamians were therefore aware of differences between humans and animals, although the anatomical and physiological similarities seem to have enabled an overlap. Note a mystical text in which various animals are described as the ghosts of various gods (Livingstone 1986: 83).

86 Although a major problem in these analyses concern the Sumerogram for nose (KIR_4) and mouth (KA), which are written with the same cuneiform sign and are therefore identical (see for example a discussion of how to transliterate the sign in Wee 2012: 174 note 120 and 176 note 125 with references). Nonetheless, e.g., *SAA* 10 no. 322 states that placing tampons in the openings of the nostrils (*naḫīru*) "will cut off the breath" (rev. 15–16: *šá-a-ru* [17] *i-ka-si-ir*). Furthermore, several diagnoses refer specifically to the nostrils (*naḫīru*) or write "nose" phonetically (*ap-pa-šú*), making the examples less ambiguous (Wee 2012: 459–60 and note 66). A LB commentary also clarifies in one example that the reading is KIR_4 and not KA (ibid.: 710). Therefore, it seems that nostrils were associated with breath in general, at least in a relaxed state. The phrase *napīš* KIR_4-*šú* DUGUD "breathing of his nose is difficult" (ibid.: 711 note 3') indirectly demonstrates this as well. Stol (2000: 198) noted a distinction in relation to fluids from KA (*nadû* "thrown, ejected") or KIR_4 (*alāku* "flow"). In the OB recension of the Gilgameš Epic, Enkidu's wake lasts seven days and nights "until a maggot dropped from his nostril" (George 2003: 278–79 col. ii 9': *a-di tu-ul-tum im-qú-tam i-na ap-pi-šu*, 680–81, 686–87, 692–93).

and is related to *napīšu* "breath, breathing" (CAD N/1: 296–305; Steinert 2012: 271 and note 1).[87]

In Sa-gig we find the formulation *šār appi* "wind of the nose" associated with breath.[88] Therefore, the diagnostic literature associated breath with the nose, although this may be more of an idiom than actual conceptualization.[89] Perhaps because of the nose's relationship to life, nosebleed treatment was considered a particular skill.[90] Unfortunately, it is difficult to evaluate if the Mesopotamians were aware of the epiglottis' function of directing food into the oesophagus.[91] In general, breathing through the nose seems to have reflected a healthy state.[92] It is therefore interesting that "wind" (*šāru*) was also perceived as an agent that could inflict illness.[93]

---

87 Etymologically, *napištu* is derived from *napāšu* "to breathe freely, to rest, to expand, to become abundant" (CAD N/1: 288).

88 See Steinert 2012: 275 and note 19. Sa-gig tablet 6 was concerned with the nose and nostrils, and herein we find that a blocked nose with breath coming out the mouth or breath violently drawn from the nose leads to death (Scurlock 2014: 53; Scurlock and Andersen 2005: 590–92; TDP: 56 lines 33–36'). See TDP: 84 lines 30–31: DIŠ ZI-*šú* GU_4.UD.ME *u* ŠÀ.MEŠ-*šú it-te-nen-bi-ṭu* GAM [31] DIŠ ZI-*šú* GU_4.UD.ME *u* SA.MEŠ-*šú šap-ku* GAM DIŠ ZI-*šú i-tar-rak-ma qit-ru-bat* [G]AM, "If his breath becomes rapid (lit.: jumps) and his insides are continually cramped, he will die. If his breath becomes rapid (lit.: jumps) and his 'strings' are tense, he will die. If his breath throbs and comes closely spaced, he will [d]ie" (Scurlock and Andersen 2005: 340). TDP: 54 line 4b: DIŠ KIR_4-*šú* BAD.BAD-*ir* GAM "if his nose is completely blocked off, he will die" and TDP: 82 line 24: DIŠ … PA.AN. BI *ina* KIR_4-*šú* DAB.DAB GIG BI NU DIN "if … his breath is 'seized' in his nose, that patient will not get well" (Scurlock and Andersen 2005: 537). TDP: 56 line 32 may read: DIŠ IM KIR_4-*šú ina* KA-*šú* È-*a* … "If his breath (*šār appi*) is 'seized' in his mouth …".

89 In prescriptions, "heavy" (*kabātu*/DUGUD) could describe both the nose and mouth due to the reading of the Sumerogram, see Scurlock and Andersen 2005: 206 no. 9.118 with references. Note Sa-gig tablet 3 line 63: "his breath is seized in his nose so that he makes his breath go out through his mouth, it will make death mount to this throat […], *na-pi-is-su ina* KIR_4-*šú* DIB-*ma ina* KA-*šú* GARZA *uš-ti-ṣi mu-tim ana* ZI-*šú ú-šel-la-a* x x […] (Scurlock 2014: 15, 21; Labat 1951: 24 line 54).

90 KAR 44 obv. 18: ÚŠ.KIR_4.KU_5.DA $BURU_8$.KU_5.RU.DA *du-ga-nu* GIG *u* ŠÀ.SUR.KU_5.RU.DA ⌈*qa*⌉*-na ši-ta-šú*. For such treatments, see Scurlock and Andersen 2005: 207, 539.

91 The epiglottis is located around the uppermost part of the larynx. Note Sa-gig tablet 9 line 62: "If … his breaths have become short (and) his breath constantly enters his throat as if he were thirsting for water …", DIŠ … ZI.ME-*šú* LÚGUD.MEŠ ZI-*šú* GIM *šá* A *ṣa-mu-ú i-te-ner-ru-ub* … (Scurlock 2014: 68, 71; Labat 1951: 76). Here breath and water goes down the throat. In RA 40 pl. 116 obv. 8, we find the description "windpipe" (GI.GÍD MUR. MEŠ-*šú*; CAD E: 137–38), which may attest to the knowledge that the trachea differed from the oesophagus in the throat, although this description of the "windpipe" is mainly attested in connection to coughs (CAD E: 138).

92 Wee 2012: 468–69 note 76. Note the NA letter ABL 771 obv. 6–7 in which the king places a "Plant of Life" at the nostrils (Selz 2014: 658).

93 Böck 2014a: 36–37 and notes 148 and 150, p. 152; Geller 2010: 94–95; Cadelli 2000: 345–46. Winds could also be indicative of good or bad fortune in relation to astrological omens,

Only one clearly defined illness attacked both the nostrils and mouth together, namely *bu'šānu*.[94] The illnesses treated through the nostrils, however, include *bu'šānu*,[95] "Ill lungs",[96] *suālu*,[97] and *ašû*.[98] In general, the nostrils are rarely used during healing, but aside from some examples related to human illness, one good example is for horses with colic to ensure ingestion (*CAD* N/1: 137 with references; see Section 4.4.3). Horses are obligate nasal breathers, i.e., they breathe through their noses (Holcombe et al. 2007: 454–455). Notably, horses display symptoms such as pain through a variety of facial expressions, which importantly include dilated nostrils (Gleerup et al. 2015: 103, 109, 113; Ashley et al. 2005: 566). As a result, a horse's state of illness could in several instances be evaluated via the nostrils, with the metaphoric relationship between breath and life. This is discussed further below.

The lungs were associated with wind and the connecting windpipe.[99] Peculiarly, lungs may have been considered related to the digestion of food in connection to eating and drinking bewitched foodstuffs.[100] While it is difficult to envision how the Mesopotamians conceptualized something other than air going into the lungs and moving into the gastrointestinal system, it should be

---

see Rochberg 1988: 57–60. The female south wind had an evil aspect, and was associated with, e.g., the *alû*-demon, Lamaštu, and *lilû* spirits (Wiggermann 2007a: 134–35; Wiggermann 2000: 227–28, 242; see Jacobsen 1989: 271–73). Incidentally, Pazuzu was linked with a positive aspect of wind and became an apotropaic protector against such forces (Wiggermann 2007a: 134ff.; Heeßel 2002a: 1–3, 66–69, 84–85, 88–89). See also Wiggermann 2007a: 130; Izre'el 2001: 38 lines 15'–16', 69 note 18, 145–46. I have not had access to Jiménez' unpublished PhD on *The Winds in Cuneiform Literature*.

94 *CAD* B: 350–51; Böck 2014a: 157–58; Scurlock 2014: 389ff.; Scurlock and Andersen 2005: 40–42, 413–14; Collins 1999: 90, 185–99; Kämmerer 1995: 157; Kinnier Wilson 1966: 51–55. The incantations against *bu'šānu* differentiate one additional area of the throat, occasionally defined as "soft", called the *nurzu* (see *CAD* N/2: 351). It is unclear if "cutting-of-the-throat" *zikurudû* (ZÍ.KU$_5$.RU.DA) magic could affect a victim's ability to breathe or use the throat (*CMAwR* 1: 3, 199; Abusch 2008: 64–65; Schwemer 2007a: 63–64, 100–101; cf. Geller 2007a: 197–99).

95 *BAM* 543 col. i 61': DIŠ NA KA-*šú u na-ḫi-ri-šú bu-'-šá-nu* DAB …; col. i 66': DIŠ KI.MIN …

96 *AMT* 54,1 obv. 8: DIŠ NA MUR.MEŠ GIG …

97 *RA* 40 pl. 116 obv. 8–9: DIŠ NA *su-alu ši-ḫi* GIG-*ma* GI.GÍD MUR.MEŠ-*šú* ^{9} IM SA$_5^!$ *ú-sa-al ú-gan-na-aḫ* ÚḪ TUKU-*ši*.

98 *BAM* 3 col. i 37: DIŠ NA *a-šu-ú* DAB-*su* …; col. i 40: DIŠ NA *a-šu-ú* DAB-*su* … (cf. *BAM* 497 col. ii 14; *BAM* 500 col. i 1). See Fincke 2000: 102 and note 804. Cf. *BAM* 35 col. i 20: KI.MIN relating to the illness in col. i 15'.

99 *Suālu* has its seat "between the lungs", *birīt ḫašê*, whereas *bu'šānu* has its seat in the "windpipe" *ebbūb ḫašê* (Cadelli 2000: 386; Collins 1999: 185–88, 260–61).

100 Stol 2006: 104–5 with examples. This was perhaps connected to the presence of "phlegm, foam" *rupuštu* (ÚḪ) in relation to certain lung and epigastric illnesses, which were associated with witchcraft (*CMAwR* 1: 4; see also Geller 2010: 149–50; Geller 2007a: 196 note 36).

noted that the kidneys are also anatomically disconnected from the digestive tract, but were still recognized as linked to urine (see Geller 2005: 1–2; Scurlock and Andersen 2005: 104; Geller and Cohen 1995). Perhaps a magical component of bewitched food could be explained through the manner in which the gods receive the offering in Atra-ḫasīs, namely via smell.[101]

Thus, the nose appears to have been the principal breathing orifice that was considered a marker for a healthy (perhaps relaxed) state for both humans and horses. Breath was associated with wind and the throat, as well as with the lungs. Furthermore, bewitched foodstuff was related to both the lungs and areas of the epigastrium.

4.4.3 *Discussion of the Veterinarian Prescriptions on* RA *15 pl. 76*

Kiṣir-Aššur dealt with veterinarian knowledge in his *šamallû ṣeḫru* manuscript *RA* 15 pl. 76. In the two horse treatments, a particular tube (DUG *ziriqi*), comparable to a "feeding tube", was used for reaching down the oesophagus to administer solutions to a horse, presumably with colic, through its nose.[102] A similar method of administering a medicament was encountered in

101 However, only divine beings received offerings like this. Lambert and Millard 1969: 98–99, 3rd tablet col. iv 34–36: "[The gods sniffed] the smell, they gathered [like flies] over the offering. [After] they had eaten the offering …", *[i-ṣi-nu i-l]u e-re-ša* 35 *[ki-ma zu-ub-b]i e-lu ni-qí-i pa-aḫ-ru* 36 *[iš-tu-m]a i-ku-lu ni-qí-a-am* (see Foster 1996: 183). See also, e.g., the end of Ištar's Descent to the Netherworld (Lapinkivi 2010: 22, 28, 33) line 138: "Let the dead come up and smell the incense", BA.ÚŠ.MEŠ *li-lu-nim-ma qut-ri-in li-iṣ-ṣi-nu* (see Foster 1996: 408), and the 5th tablet of the Erra Epic (Cagni 1969: 126–29) lines 49–50: "In the sanctuary of the god who honours this poem may abundance accumulate, but let the one who neglects it never smell incense", DINGIR *šá za-ma-ru šá-a-šú i-na-du ina a-šìr-ti-šú lik-tam-me-ra ḫé-gál-lum* 50 *ù šá ú-šam-sa-ku a-a iṣ-ṣi-na qut-rin-na* (see Foster 1996: 788; Bottéro 1985: 249). Food offerings could also be equated with "insence (offering)" (*qutrīnu*), see *CAD* Z: 106. Maybe this is why some of the treatments for the nostrils mentioned above also utilized fumigation, as this would be directed towards the lungs (see *CAD* N/1: 137 for examples). However, witchcraft texts generally mention that a patient has ingested or imbibed bewitched food or drink, and not as such smelled it. Yet, the two aspects of consuming foodstuff may not be mutually exclusive, as most people will smell as well as eat/drink their food. The relationship between foodstuff, fumigation, and the divine world requires further investigation in relation to medicine.

102 *RA* 15 pl. 76 rev. 1'–4', 5'–8'; Stol 2011: 401–2 and note 257–58 with references. *CAD* (Z: 134) interprets it as a sort of pipette, von Soden as "Ton-pipette" (*AHw*: 1532), and Stol (ibid.) translates it as "…-Röhre". The DUG designates it as a clay object comparable to various fluid containers (ibid.: 401 and note 256). Stol stresses the uniqueness of the instrument, as this is the only example (cf. *BAM* 159 discussed in Parys 2014: 23 and Böck 2009a: 117 and notes 56–57). This method for treating horses and especially colic is also attested in the Ugaritic hippiatric texts (Cohen and Sivan 1983: 9–10, 16–17 with references) and the method is still applied today (e.g., Lopes et al. 2004: 696, 702).

Kiṣir-Aššur's *šamallû ṣeḫru*-phase copy *RA* 40 pl. 116. In this text, Kiṣir-Aššur treats various cough afflictions (*suālu*) associated with the "windpipe" (GI. GÍD MUR.MEŠ) by trickling a fluid onto the tongue and pouring it into the nostrils with a *takkussu*-pipette, in addition to drinking a potion to induce vomiting.[103] Thus, Kiṣir-Aššur acquired knowledge about administering medicaments through the nose and possibly also anatomical insight into the functions of the throat, lungs, and stomach.

As previously stated, only four NA prescriptions are known for treating horses, all from N4 (*BAM* 159, *RA* 15 pl. 76), of which three specify pouring the fluid into the "left nostril".[104] Stol noted that flushing ingredients through the left nostril over the right nostril must be considered an irrational practice only attested in veterinary treatments (Stol 2011: 392).[105] However, the mention of right and left nostrils also occurs in *Šumma izbu* in relation to the features of human foetuses: "If a woman gives birth, and (the child) has no left nostril; (the child) is endowed with happiness".[106] A similar nostril distinction occurs among symptoms observed in babies in Sa-gig: "If the air of an infant's right 'nostril' gets cold and that of the left gets hot, 'Hand' of Lamaštu".[107]

In general, the various omen series tend to focus on positive and negative omens, where the interpretation depended on different schemata such as right/left as favourable/unfavourable, and they frequently incorporate impossible phenomena.[108] As such, they function as artificial constructs and can-

103 *RA* 40 pl. 116 ovb. 8–12: DIŠ NA *su-alu šá ši-ḫi* GIG-*ma* GI.GÍD MUR.MEŠ-*šú* ^{9} IM SA$_{5}$! *ú-sa-al ú-gan-na-aḫ* ÚḪ TUKU-*ši* ^{10} [GA]ZI^{sar} ^{ú}ḪAR.ḪAR 1-*niš* SÚD *ina* Ì *ḫal-ṣi* ÚŠ KIR$_{4}$ EME-*šú* ^{11} [*t*]*u-qar-ra-ár u* ^{giš}SAG.KUD! DIR-*ma ana na-ḫi-ri-šú* DUB [x?] ^{12} EGIR-*šú* KAŠ SAG NAG.MEŠ-*ma i-àr-rù* (Labat and Tournay 1945–46: 114–15; see *CAD* T: 79). For pipettes on humans, see Stol 2011: 401 and note 255–56. For *appi lišāni* see *CAD* L: 212.

104 *BAM* 159 col. v 36: … *ina na-ḫir* GÙB-*šú* DUB-*ak-ma* TI; *RA* 15 pl. 76 rev. 4': [… *ina*] *na-ḫir* 2,30-*šú* DUB-[*ak* …]; rev. 7': [*ina*] ⸢DUG?⸣ *zi-ri-qí ana n*[*a*]-*ḫir* 2,30-*šú* DUB-*ak*.

105 This is echoed in the descriptions of plants for horse *kīs libbi* in *šammu šikinšu* poured into the horse's left nostril (see Stadhouders 2012: 3 §15', 12 §10'; Stadhouders 2011: 8 ms A §15', 26–27 ms C §10').

106 Leichty 1970: 57 tablet 3 lines 29–32 (the line quoted is 31): BE MUNUS Ù.TU-*ma* KIR$_{4}$ *u na-ḫi-ri* NU GÁL … ^{30} BE MUNUS Ù.TU-*ma na-ḫi-ir* 15 NU GÁL … ^{31} 150-*šú* NU GÁL … ^{32} BE MUNUS Ù.TU-*ma na-ḫi-ra-šú* NU GÁL.MEŠ … (cf. Scurlock and Andersen 2005: 396–97). See most recently De Zorzi (2011: 59), who emphasized obstructions of orifices as a general negative omen in *Šumma izbu*.

107 Scurlock 2014: 260, 266 line 54; Labat 1951: 224 line 54: DIŠ LÚ.TUR IM KIR$_{4}$-*šú šá* 15 ŠED$_{7}$-*ma šá* 2,30 KÚM-*im* ŠU ^{d}DÌM.ME.

108 Koch 2015: 12–14; De Zorzi 2011: 46–47; Rochberg 2010; Guinan 1996. In *Šumma izbu*, the normal right/left opposition as favourable/unfavourable is reversed, as the observations concern malformation. A malformation on the right side makes it an unfavourable omen and vice versa (De Zorzi 2011: 52–53; Guinan 1996: 6–7; Leichty 1970: 7).

not always be taken as representative of actual occurrences or their frequency. However, the focus on nostrils is noteworthy in connection to the discussion of infants and horses. Furthermore, infants appear generally to be nasal breathers like horses (Bergeson and Shaw 2001; see Section 5.2.2).

As discussed above, horses externalize their pain, such as that experienced by colic,[109] especially through the facial features. Infants can also suffer from infantile colic (Hyman et al. 2006; Wessel et al. 1954), and among the symptoms are irritability, compulsive crying, shortness of breath, and abdominal pain.[110] Interestingly, both horses and infants would have been unable to communicate their symptoms properly, and therefore other indicators were needed to diagnose the problems. Thus, breathing through the nose by horses and infants, or the lack of breathing (e.g., children screaming), was indicative of possible problematic physiological states.

Digestive problems, such as *kīs libbi* in horses, could be treated through their noses. In addition to the advantage of administering a potion to an animal that would otherwise not have imbibed it, there may be a metaphoric relationship between *kīs libbi* and the nose. As breath (or life) seems to be linked to the nose, this could explain why one could treat the physical and (in humans) emotional effects of *kīs libbi* via the flaring nostrils of a hose. The horse would look emotionally disturbed, which would add to the diagnosis of *kīs libbi*.

Regardless, it seems that knowledge about the function of the oesophagus and trachea was difficult to gain, and, by exposing Kiṣir-Aššur to these veterinarian as well as human treatments with pipettes, he would have learned about these physiological areas. An overlap may have existed between human and animal physiology in terms of the nose and breath. Kiṣir-Aššur could therefore have been introduced to the underlying physiological conceptions and the possible focus on the nose as a health indicator in animals and at least babies when he was *šamallû ṣeḫru*.

4.5 Summary

The manuscript *RA* 15 pl. 76 was examined due to its unexpected content, following the microhistoric approach seeking to solve such mysteries. The tablet illustrates that the treatments of snakebites and scorpion stings and veterinarian knowledge played a role in Kiṣir-Aššur's education. Snake and scorpion

109 For one definition of horse colic, see Gonçalves et al. 2002: 650.

110 Such problems were also mentioned in the 40th tablet of Sa-gig (Volk 1999: 13; Cadelli 1997: 12–13, 26, 29). See Section 5.2.2.

venom were probably used for illustrating many bodily processes. The effects of potent venom would demonstrate most bodily functions to a student, and, as such, the concept was terrifying as well as an exemplar in relation to the human body. In general, snake and scorpion venom was used metaphorically to explain the power of various illnesses. As a result, various analogies and lexical overlaps existed between venom, bile in mammals, and saliva in relation to witchcraft. These overlaps drew on the power of venom to explain how these other fluids functioned to regulate and problematize various bodily processes.

Although veterinarian prescriptions appear infrequently, the city of Assur had several written traditions linked to knowledge about horses. Kiṣir-Aššur may have made use of these to treat animals. This chapter suggests that Kiṣir-Aššur used methods of treatment via the nose to acquire knowledge about human physiology from horses, as well as perhaps to treat ill animals himself. The overlap of some treatments and illnesses between animals and humans supports this proposal.

Human internal organs and processes were not properly understood in the ancient world, due to a lack of knowledge about the insides and a partial inability to use this knowledge in medical practice. It is therefore likely that animal physiology was occasionally used to explain human bodily processes. One aspect of basic bodily experience used was the relationship between the nose and breath in horses and children, who were unable to verbally communicate their symptoms. Furthermore, breathing through the nose indicated a healthy state for adults as well (see Ch. 4 notes 86–88). Kiṣir-Aššur's treatments related to the nose would also have improved his understanding of the throat, lungs, and stomach during examination and healing, thereby improving his physiological understanding.

CHAPTER 5

Further Apprenticeship: *šamallû* to *mašmaššu ṣeḫru*

This chapter discusses the limited material that exists from Kiṣir-Aššur's "apprentice" *šamallû*, "junior apprentice exorcist" *šamallû mašmaššu ṣeḫru* and "junior exorcist" *mašmaššu ṣehru* phases to provide an overview of what is currently known about these intermediate phases of his training. Furthermore, a text related to calming an infant or a child from Kiṣir-Aššur's *šamallû mašmaššu ṣeḫru*-phase is used to suggest that he acquired healing competences related to children. This chapter therefore discusses Kiṣir-Aššur's possible involvement in healing infants and considers the general theories on infant and child healing in relation to Kiṣir-Aššur's previous tablets. Texts from Kiṣir-Aššur's nephew, Kiṣir-Nabû, are used to contextualize and discuss Kiṣir-Aššur's manuscripts from his *šamallû mašmaššu ṣeḫru*- and *mašmaššu ṣeḫru*-phases. Furthermore, Kiṣir-Aššur's tablets labelled as *u'iltu*s are also discussed in general.

Additionally, this chapter examines Kiṣir-Aššur's use of the phrase "(he) whose trust is Nabû" (*ša Nabû tuklasssu*) in colophons from his *šamallû ṣeḫru* and *šamallû mašmaššu ṣeḫru* phases, as well as on tablets without titles. This facilitates the distribution of a few tablets without titles onto Kiṣir-Aššur's apprentice career phases.

5.1 The *šamallû*-phase

After Kiṣir-Aššur's relatively well-attested *šamallû ṣeḫru*-phase, Kiṣir-Aššur became a *šamallû* "apprentice" (Maul 2010: 208 and note 67). The phase is unfortunately only attested by two texts, of which one is unpublished. What follows presents the relevant tablets and their content in order to facilitate a cautious discussion of the manuscripts in relation to Kiṣir-Aššur's career. The texts are listed in the table below.

KAL 10 no. 4 is a large tablet with an introductory diagnostic statement as well as a multitude of incantations and brief instructions directed at releasing a "Curse" (rev. 46: [KA.INI]M.MA ⸢NAM⸣.É[RIM.BÚR]. ⸢RU⸣.DA.KÁM).

TABLE 6 Texts assigned to Kiṣir-Aššur's *šamallû*-phase

Text	Content	Format and designation
KAL 10 no. 4	Obverse and reverse: a diagnostic statement and ritual instruction (obv. 1–11), nine incantations (obv. 12–13, 14–33, 36–49, 50–55, obv. 57–rev. 5, rev. 6–20, 22–30, 32–37, 39–44) and six brief instructions (obv. 34–35, 56, rev. 21, 31, 38, 45) all against a "Curse" (*māmītu*) (rev. 46)	Portrait; *ṭuppu*
N4 no. 175[a]	Obverse and reverse: instructions for performing sections of the *bīt mēseri* ritual (obv. 1–rev. 7, rev. 8–17) with at least 15 incantation incipits preserved and associated brief ritual instructions (obv. 15, 17, 19, 26, 37(?), 39, 41, 43, 45, 52, rev. 3, 9, 14, 15, 16)	Portrait; *u'iltu*

a Kiṣir-Aššur's title is preserved in rev. 19 as [lú]ŠAB.T[UR]. Seeing as the line is not tightly written, there is no reason to assume further signs should be reconstructed, although the side of the tablet is broken and it could technically have held [lú]ŠAB.T[UR TUR].

The colophon provides the writing [lú]*šam-lu-*⸢*ú*⸣ for the title *šamallû* (rev. 48).[1] The text ends with a curse: "[He who] carries off th[is tablet], may the gods of heaven and earth ta[ke away] his eye(sight)".[2]

The unpublished text N4 no. 175 outlines parts of the ritual known as *bīt mēseri* "the house of confinement" (Borger 1974; see also ibid. 1994). As shown in the detailed discussion of this ritual in Section 6.3.2, *bīt mēseri* made use of a number of figurines and drawings alongside incantations and ritual actions, in order to rid a patient and his house of demons (Seidl and Sallaberger 2005–06: 67; Wiggermann 1992: 106–13; Meier 1941–44: 140). A line in N4 no. 175 indicates that the ritual was somehow connected to the ritual action of "rubbing" (*muššu'u*, rev. 6; see also Böck 2007; ibid. 2003). In the colophon, an erased line

1 Such a spelling is not attested in Kiṣir-Aššur's other tablets with titles composed of the word *šamallû* (*ṣeḫru*/*mašmaššu ṣeḫru*). However, the abbreviated form is attested elsewhere in Assur and Ḫuzirina (e.g., Fadhil 2012: 55; Hunger 1968: 10).

2 *KAL* 10 no. 4 rev. 51: [*ša ṭuppa šu*]-⸢*a*⸣-*tú* TÙM DINGIR ⸢*ša-me-e*⸣ *qaq-qa-ri* IGI[II]-*šú lit-*[*ba-lu*]. Note also the writing IGI.KÁR in rev. 48 for *bari* "checked", which is otherwise only attested in Kiṣir-Aššur's N4 no. 224 from an uncertain phase of his career.

between rev. 18 and 19 still has ŠID-*nu* legible, and the line may once have held additional instructions.

In N4 no. 175 Kiṣir-Aššur's name is written ᵖZÚ.KEŠDA-ᵈ*aš-šur*, which is otherwise only attested in *BAM* 121 from an uncertain phase (see Sections 5.4 and 7.2.1). Furthermore, he copied his father Nabû-bēssunu's title *mašmaš bīt Aššur* with a Babylonian form of the sign É, possibly indicating that Kiṣir-Aššur was trained in Babylonian sign forms.[3] The tablet was also described as "quickly extracted for his (own) 'reading'".[4] In this context, the word *tāmartu* can be translated "viewing, reading" (*CAD* T: 111–114; *AHw*: 1313), and it must be considered a technical term related to knowledge acquisition, although the exact nuances are not clear (see Robson 2019: 124 and note 117; ibid. 2014: 152; Geller 2010: 134, 136–138). However, N4 no. 175 is the only tablet among Kiṣir-Aššur's manuscripts with this phrase (cf. *ACh Supp.* 2 24 in Section 7.6). By comparison, Kiṣir-Nabû copied at least three tablets "for his (own) 'reading'", and these are all commentaries.[5] The colophon of N4 no. 175 ends with a warning to the reader: "He who carries (the tablet) off, wherever he lifts his hands to (praise) Nabû, let him (i.e. Nabû) not hear his prayer, [he who fea]rs Nabû and Marduk shall not erase my written name!".[6]

Both Kiṣir-Aššur's *šamallû*-phase tablets contain portions of two types of rituals, which were integral to the *āšipu*'s profession according to the EM (Geller 2018b; ibid. 2000). The manuscripts indicate that Kiṣir-Aššur as a *šamallû* focused on acquiring further ritual means to treat a so-called "Curse", possibly as a cause of illness, as well as gaining an insight into how the important demarcation ritual *bīt mēseri* was performed. The latter observation is supported by the addition of the phrase "for his 'reading'" in the colophon. Overviews of rituals slightly similar in form to N4 no. 175, although with different aims, are otherwise found during Kiṣir-Aššur's *mašmaššu*-phase (*KAR* 298) and on a tablet without a title (*KAL* 10 no. 1). Presumably, Kiṣir-Aššur's two *šamallû* tablets enabled Kiṣir-Aššur to apply ritual treatments towards "Curse" as a cause of illness and aid in preparing or performing the *bīt mēseri* ritual.

---

3 The É in Nabû-bēssunu's title *mašmaš bīt Aššur* was also written with a Babylonian form of the sign in N4 no. 241, copied on behalf of Kiṣir-Aššur as a *šamallû ṣeḫru* (Section 3.7.3). Note also the Babylonian form of the sign LÚ in the colophon of *BAM* 28 (see Ch. 8 note 18).

4 Rev. 22: *ana* IGI.DU₈.A-*šú ḫa-an-ṭiš is-su-ḫa*.

5 *AfO* 12 pl. 13–14 (*ana* IGI.DU₈.A-*šú*), a commentary on *Tummu bītu* and *Šurpu* tablet 2 (CCP 2.1.C); N4 no. 163 (*ana* IGI.LÁ-*šú*), a commentary on Marduk's Address to the Demons (CCP 2.2.1.A.a); N4 no. 220 (*ana a-ma-ri-šú*), a commentary on *Tummu bītu* and *Maqlû* tablets 1–2 (CCP 2.1.A). Kiṣir-Nabû also copied three texts with related terminology: *BAM* 52 (*malsūtu*), *BAM* 106 (*malsūtu*) and *Iraq* 62 no. 35 (*maš'altu*, see Frahm 2011a: 268–270; CCP 2.2.1.A.b).

6 Rev. 23–25: [*š*]*á* IR *e-ma a-na* ᵈAG ŠU^II^-*su* ÍL-*ú* ²⁴ [*s*]*u-up-pi-šu a-a i-šam-mé* ²⁵ [MU]D ᵈAG *u* ᵈAMAR.UTU MU SAR *la ta-pa-šiṭ*.

5.2 The *šamallû mašmaššu ṣeḫru*-phase

After the "apprentice"-phase, Kiṣir-Aššur became a "junior apprentice exorcist". Previous research has not been able to differentiate these phases beyond the change in titles.[7] Due to the meagre *šamallû* evidence presented above, doing so remains difficult. Regardless, it is still possible to present some observations in relation to the available evidence. Kiṣir-Aššur only copied three preserved texts during his *šamallû mašmaššu ṣeḫru*-phase, and these are presented in the table below:

TABLE 7 Texts assigned to Kiṣir-Aššur's *šamallû mašmaššu ṣeḫru*-phase

Text	Content	Format and designation
LKA 89+*LKA* 90	Obverse and reverse (col. i–iv): diagnostic statement(?) (col. i 1'), instruction with embedded incantation (col. i 2'–26'+ col. i 1"–9"), prayers and incantations (col. i 10"27"+col. ii 1–12, col. ii 14–22+col. ii 1'–30'+col. iii 1–9, col. iii 12–30, col. iii 32–47, col. iii 49–68+col. iv 1–4, col. iv 5–18+col. iv 1'–3'), and brief instructions (col. ii 13, col. iii 10–11, col. iii 31, col. iii 48) all directed against ghostly afflictions	Two-columned; *ṭuppu*(?)
LKA 141	Obverse and reverse: prayers (obv. 1–3, 17–20+[...]), an incantation (rev. 1'), and ritual instructions (obv. 4–15, rev. 3'–8') for reconciling a man with his god.	Portrait(?); *ṭuppu*
N4 no. 24[a]	Obverse and reverse: incantation revolving around Lamaštu (obv. 1–rev. 15) with a rubric stating it was designed to "calm a child" (rev. 16: LÚ.TUR.ḪUN.GÁ)	Landscape; IM.GÍD.DA

a According to the most recent copy by Farber (1989: pl. 13), Kiṣir-Aššur was *mašmaššu ṣeḫru* (MAŠ.MAŠ TUR) when he copied this text. However, recent collations by Daniel Schwemer (personal communication) revealed the writing ŠÁMAN.LÁ in a smaller script underneath his title. This addition indicates Kiṣir-Aššur was *šamallû mašmaššu ṣeḫru* when the tablet was copied.

7 E.g., Robson 2014, 2011a; Maul 2010a; Gesche 2001: 213; Pearce 1993; Hunger 1968: 9–10.

LKA 89+ is a two-columned tablet with incantations and ritual instructions against ghostly afflictions.[8] These instructions aimed to free the patient of a ghost and to banish it to the netherworld, taking the generic "Any Evil" (*mimma lemnu*) with it.[9] Ghosts were regularly treated in Kiṣir-Aššur's texts, and he had previously treated the effects of these to some degree in the *šamallû ṣeḫru* manuscript N4 no. 237 and the presumed *šamallû ṣeḫru* tablet *BAM* 9. Interestingly, *LKA* 89+ is described as an extract, although it is a library copy (multi-columned).[10] The reason for this discrepancy could stem from the text having been copied from a writing-board and originally having been part of an even bigger text. It is therefore possible that the *nisḫu* label could describe both multi-columned tablets as well as brief extracts in N4.[11] As a result, it can be difficult to establish what purpose a text served after its immediate use in the N4 collection. The multi-columned format could perhaps indicate a wish to keep the text for reference in the library afterwards,[12] although in the case

8 For the most recent edition and copy, see *CMAwR* 2: 189ff. text 8.25 ms B; see also Scurlock 1988a no. 85, 87; Ebeling 1931a: 122ff.; cf. Abusch 2002: 76–78; Bottéro 1983. The join between *LKA* 89+ and *LKA* 90 was previously noted by Pedersén 1986: 72 no. 523; see also Verderame 2008: 56.

9 Abusch 2002: 76–77. The removal of *mimma lemnu* is also frequently stressed in the Ištar-Dumuzi incantation rituals (Farber 1977: 9). Ghost rituals were also used in, e.g., *bīt rimki* and the New Year festival, and were therefore not exclusively related to healing, but also stately or royal rituals (see Ambos 2013a: 52, 57ff., 201ff.; Scurlock 1988a: 127). Large parts of the row of entries and content are duplicated in the multi-columned *KAR* 227 (= N4 no. 88) written without a colophon. However, the end of *LKA* 89+ col. iv cannot be found on *KAR* 227. Although large parts of *LKA* 89+ are broken and cannot be assessed, the differences observed are on the reverse in col. iii of both examples, where the incantation in *KAR* 227 col. iii 8'–24' is duplicated in *LKA* 89+ col. iii 2'–17'. The *LKA* 89+ entry opens with ÉN, which is not written in *KAR* 227. Furthermore, *LKA* 89+ col. iii 17' and the small instruction in 18' were divided onto two lines each in *KAR* 227 col. iii 13'–14' and 15'–16'.

10 *LKA* 89+ col. iv 9': [(x) x x x x x x]⸢x⸣ *na-as-ḫa*. Presumably, the line read *ḫanṭiš* or *zamar* before, but the line ends with *nasḫa* written very tightly, and likely more than three signs were originally on the line. It is therefore difficult to account for so many broken signs without considering that the line originally contained another statement, such as a purpose statement (*ana ṣabāt epēši*; see *KAR* 374 rev. 21; *LKA* 157 col. iv 12'). Such statements are argued in Section 7.4 to occur around the *mašmaššu*-phase. However, other texts only contain the *ḫanṭiš nasāḫu* statement on the last line, although the lines could easily hold more signs (*BAM* 81 rev. 18'; *BAM* 186 rev. 34; *BAM* 188 rev. 13; *BAM* 351 rev. 15; cf. *BAM* 333 rev. 4'). *LKA* 89+ is said to be "written and checked according to its original", *LKA* 89+ col. iv 5': LIBIR.RA.BI.GIM AB.SAR.ÀM *bà-rì*.

11 It is unclear if *nasāḫu* always designates extracts in N4, or if the verb could be used to designate a copy (cf. Black 1985).

12 This suggestion is built on the assumption that such formats normally served such purposes. However, this cannot be substantiated, although this was likely the case at Nineveh. Robson (2014: 146–47) has shown that this collection was in fact atypical in

of *LKA* 89+, the format may simply imply that Kiṣir-Aššur needed to copy out more text than what could be copied onto a single columned format tablet.

LKA 141 contains at least two prayers and accompanying ritual instructions (Pedersén 1986: 73 no. 543), which concern one(?) ritual for reconciling a man with the god (or goddess) of his house (Ebeling 1953a: XIII).[13]

N4 no. 24 was designated as a "recitation to calm a child" (KA.INIM.MA LÚ.TUR ḪUN.GÁ.KE_4).[14] The term translated as "child" here, *ṣeḫru* or *šerru*, can also designate a baby or an infant (see Farber 1989: 132–36). The incantation revolves around the demoness Lamaštu and therefore does not contain typical lullaby-like child calming motifs (e.g., Farber 1990a). Instead, it describes how Lamaštu stalks around a house and among the domesticated animals, luring the children to her venomous teats (Farber 2014: 301; Wiggermann 2000: 231 and note 93). The unsettling fear established by the crying of an infant heralded the presence of Lamaštu (ibid.: 237; Cadelli 1997: 26), and the family's ancestors and domestic cult could be severely disturbed by children crying (Stol 2000: 212–13; van der Toorn 1996: 18–19, 121, 125).

Lamaštu was the daughter of Anu, she killed babies by posing as a midwife and was formally installed by the gods to keep population growth in check (Wiggermann 2000: 224–25). She preferably attacked babies and pregnant women by causing a number of symptoms (e.g., fever, intestinal problems, red rash) related to other illnesses (e.g., jaundice, *pašittu*) potentially leading to death (Wiggermann 2000: 236–39; Stol 2000: 210). Problems during pregnancy and birth as well as protecting and curing ill babies were all part of *āšipūtu*, and these areas are therefore expected to appear during the training of exorcists.[15]

The themes encountered during this particular level of education appear to revolve around the cult of the house, i.e., the family cult, the personal deities attached to a house as well as calming infants crying, and how to appease and

---

several ways. In general, good copies could have been kept as library copies to replace older tablets in worse condition, although this would not necessarily depend on format (Clancier 2014: 46).

13 *LKA* 141 rev. 2': KA.INI[M.M]A DINGIR LÚ KI LÚ ⸢x⸣[x x x (x)]. The first prayer mentions in obv. 1: … *lu-u* DINGIR É *lu-u* ^{d}15 É *lu-u* DING[IR LÚ$^{?}$ …]. Furthermore, this colophon is the only instance where Kiṣir-Aššur writes the divine element of his father, Nabû-bēssunu's name phonetically: *na-bi-um*. However, the spelling is peculiar. The tablet remains unedited.

14 Farber 1989: 102–107 ms L, pl. 13; Farber specifies that such incantations could serve to calm a crying child, to heal an ill child or to protect a child from dangers prophylactically (ibid.: 3; George 1993b; cf. van der Toorn 1996: 120).

15 Jean 2006: 66; Geller 2000: 245, 256–58; Stol 2000: 59ff.; *KAR* 44 obv. 15: $^{\text{MUNUS NU}}$ ⸢*el-lu*⸣ ^{mí}PEŠ$_4$.KÉŠ.DA ^{mí}LA.RA.AḪ ^{d}DIM$_8$.ME.KÁM *u* LÚ.TUR.ḪUN.GÁ, "(When) a woman is unclean Woman not able to give birth, travailing woman in difficulty because of Lamaštu, (incantations) to calm a child".

remove the evils induced by the divinities' dissatisfaction with the inhabitants. Apart from the possible uses to treat the cause behind an illness,[16] reconciling a man with his god and treating ghosts as causes of domestic troubles implies that something could upset a household's various deities. In the first half of the second millennium, crying children were notorious for disturbing the peace of the family, as well as the domestic cult (van der Toorn 1996: 120–21, 125–28; cf. Farber 1989: 1–4; Farber 1990a), and sleeping or resting gods evidently considered noise a disturbance.[17] With N4 no. 24, Kiṣir-Aššur became able to calm a child and prophylactically keep Lamaštu at bay while ensuring that domestic cultic aggravation, which he also learned to handle as *šamallû mašmaššu ṣeḫru*, was less prone to happen.

Although one can only consider this evidence tentative, Kiṣir-Aššur appears to have learned these genres in order to remove domestic misfortune and possible sources of illness. Exorcistic healing of illness appears to have involved a dual approach by ritually soothing the anger of the divine cause and providing a physical treatment (Heeßel 2000: 94–96; cf. Stol 1991–92: 44ff.; van der Toorn 1985: 67ff.). Kiṣir-Aššur may therefore have focused his attention on the latter during his *šamallû ṣeḫru*-phase in particular, whereas especially the *šamallû mašmaššu ṣeḫru*-phase could have focused on soothing (possible) causes of illness. As stated above, it is unknown if the rituals were learned in order to treat possible estranged divinities before illness, or as a dual approach while healing illness. Furthermore, as argued in the following sections, N4 no. 24 may inidicate that Kiṣir-Aššur also had pediatric duties during his *šamallû mašmaššu ṣeḫru*-phase.

5.2.1 *The Child Calming Incantation N4 no. 24 and Duplicates*

Kiṣir-Aššur's nephew, Kiṣir-Nabû, copied roughly the same Lamaštu incantation as Kiṣir-Aššur's N4 no. 24, although Kiṣir-Nabû produced his copy as *mašmaššu* and included a ritual.[18] N4 no. 24 contains no ritual instruction and deals explicitly with Lamaštu and is intended to calm a child, whereas the

16 Koch unpublished: 11 and note 63; Heeßel 2007b: 127–28 and notes 28–29; Heeßel 2000: 81–86; cf. van der Toorn 1985: 123; Lambert 1974: 267–322.

17 Heffron 2014: 88–93; Stol 2000: 211–213; van der Toorn 1996: 18–19, 121, 125; Farber 1990a: 146–47. A frequently cited example is the motif of noise in Atra-ḫasīs causing Enlil to become so angry it results in the flood (Lambert and Millard 1969). Michalowski (1990: 385–89) argues that the metaphor of noise in mythological narratives "establishes a privileged position for the concept of creation, activity, independence", which in Atram-ḫasīs asserts humanity as "an independent, creative being" (ibid.: 389). Therefore, he does not regard noise as a literal mark of overpopulation. See also Machinist 1983 for noise as a motif in the Erra Epic.

18 N4 no. 247; see Farber 2014: 300–301; Farber 1989: 102–107 ms K, pl. 12; cf. Köcher 1949: 22–27.

ritual instruction in Kiṣir-Nabû's N4 no. 247 indicates that the purpose was to keep the child safe by applying ingredients to the child to keep Lamaštu, as well as "Any Evil" (*mimma lemnu*), at bay.[19]

The colophon of Kiṣir-Aššur's N4 no. 24 contains a tablet designation, his name, and a title. The tablet is labelled as an IM.GÍD.DA (lit.: "Long tablet"), a label interpreted in other studies as an exercise (see Ch. 6 notes 4–5). In comparison, Kiṣir-Nabû's N4 no. 247 was categorized as an *u'iltu*, perhaps indicating an obligation of some sort (see Section 5.3.2). N4 no. 247 was copied when Kiṣir-Nabû was *mašmaššu*, and it was copied according to a Nineveh(?) writing-board copied from Nippur.[20] Kiṣir-Aššur provided no copying statement for his content in N4 no. 24. Kiṣir-Nabû's N4 no. 247 contains several Assyrianisms not present in Kiṣir-Aššur's duplicate, despite N4 no. 247 being copied from an alleged Babylonian original (Farber 1989: 103, 105; cf. Farber 2014: 210). Other minor differences in choice of spellings and line division are present in N4 no. 24 and N4 no. 247, although it is currently unclear if the alterations stem from differing recensions (Farber 1989: 103–7). One example of such differences between the texts is:

N4 no. 247	obv. 2	*ap-re-e-šá*	*up-pu-rat*	AGA-*š*[*á* ...]
N4 no. 24	obv. 2–3	*up-ru-šá*	*up-pu-rat* 3	*a-ga-šá ap-rat*
LKU 32	obv. 12	*up-ri-šá*	*up-pu-ra*[*t* ...	]

The later Babylonian duplicate *LKU* 32 also shares features with both N4 no. 24,[21] as well as N4 no. 247.[22] Thus, it is unclear how many recensions these three texts represent. Notably, the IM.GÍD.DA *BAM* 102 copied by Kiṣir-Aššur

19 Cf. Farber 2014: 35, 301; N4 no. 247 rev. 19, 22–23: [DÙ.D]Ù.[B]I(?) ... [22] ÉN *an-n*[*i*]-*t*[*ú*] 3-[*šú*] ŠID-*nu* LÚ.TUR [ŠÉŠ] [23] *mim-ma* ḪU[L *u*] ^{d}DÌM.ME [NU TE-*šú*] (Farber 1989: 104–105). Incantations against *mimma lemnu* also appear on Lamaštu amulets (Wiggermann 2000: 220). The incantation is stated to be for "fumigation and stones" (rev. 18: *a*[*n*]-*n*[*a*]*m* 3$^{?}$-[*š*]*u ina* UG[U x$^{?}$ *q*]*u-ta-ri u*$^{?}$ NA_4.ME[Š ŠID-*nu*(?)], Farber 1989: 104–5).

20 N4 no. 247 rev. 24–26: *ina* ZAG$^{!}$ ^{giš}⸢ZU⸣ [NI]NA$^{!ki}$ GA[B]A.RI EN.LÍL^{k}[^{i} ...] [25] *ú-ìl-ti* ^{p}*Ki-ṣir*-^{d}PA MAŠ.MAŠ *ša* [...] [26] DUMU $^{p.d}$UTU-Ù.TU MAŠ.MAŠ DUMU $^{p.d}$PA-*b*[*e*-...].

21 Mainly choice of words and writings, for example:

N4 no. 24 obv. 5	*du-ra-niš* ⸢*uš*⸣-*ta-na-ár*
N4 no. 247 obv. 4	*ṣe-ra-niš ut-ta-*[*na-šak*(?)]
LKU 32 obv. 13	*du-ra-niš uš-ta-na-ár* ...

Farber (2014: 35) noted that *LKU* 32 contains "several Assyrianisms not present in the Assur 'version'", which is presumably represented by Kiṣir-Aššur's N4 no. 24. However, Kiṣir-Nabû's N4 no. 247 also contains Assyrianisms (Farber 1989: 103).

22 Especially the ritual instruction. *LKU* 32 also contains at least three other associated incantations and ritual instructions.

as *mašmaššu* is largely similar in structure to N4 no. 24, i.e., only an incantation and an explicit statement about not having written a ritual, which could indicate that Kiṣir-Aššur was practicing certain shorter incantations for a specific purpose during these phases (see also the *šamallû ṣeḫru* manuscript N4 A 400). Comparably, his father Nabû-bēssunu copied KAL 4 no. 6 as *mašmaššu ṣeḫru*, and this tablet likely only contained a single prayer related to a *namburbi*-ritual.

5.2.2 *Excursus: Paediatricians and Treatments*

Unlike veterinarians, no titles are known for ancient paediatricians, but only for midwives.[23] Nevertheless, the exorcist was involved in assessing the physiognomy of humans in general, as well as providing prophylactic or therapeutic treatment of children.[24] The 40th tablet of Sa-gig attests to 112 diagnoses of child symptoms (Volk 1999: 13; Cadelli 1997: 12–13).[25] The most dominant among the problems diagnosed are behavioural problems, such as the ones presumably treated by N4 no. 24, and digestive disorders such as colic (Cadelli 1997: 26, 29).[26] Although age is rarely specified, the entries may often concern newborns as well as babies (Cadelli 1997: 13).

Already during pregnancy, Lamaštu and witchcraft could pose a threat to the unborn child (Cadelli 1997: 15). Some demonic beings could even be born with the child, such as Lugal-urra or Šulpaea (Cadelli 1997: 15; Stol 1993: 89). This portended a scattered house (Volk 1999: 18 note 108). Cramps associated with epilepsy were particularly ominous (ibid.: 16–17; Cadelli 1997: 23–24). These symptoms could foreshadow a fatal end for mother, father or the entire household (Volk 1999: 17 and note 102; Stol 1993: 89).[27] Jaundice (*aḫḫāzu* in

23 OB Mari was probably famous as a centre for healing child illnesses (Volk 1999: 29–30 and notes 179–80 with references). For midwives, see Stol 2000: 171–76.

24 Steinert 2018c: 181; Böck 2000: 32, 313, 315; Stol 2000: 59–72. However, the exorcist is advised not to see the mother for a duration of one month after birth (Stol 2000: 206). Note that at least one incipit related to birth is only attested in the N4 text collection (Steinert 2018d: 272; N4 no. 167).

25 The general writing is LÚ.TUR for "baby, newborn, infant, child", which can be read *šerru*, the more literary *la'û/lakû*, or the common designation for a child *ṣeḫru* (Stol 2000: 176; cf. Volk 1999: 12 note 73 with references to discussion).

26 Infant colic can present itself as a regular occurring emotional response involving crying, screaming and occasional difficulty in breathing because of the "fussing", combined with physical manifestations such as stomach pains, regurgitation and diarrhoea (Hyman et al. 2006: 1522–1523; Wessel et al. 1954).

27 See also Sa-gig tablet 29, in which various ominous portents are specified if a child is born with Antašubba or Šulpaea or if these demons fall on a child during various periods of the child's life (Scurlock 2014: 219–220; Heeßel 2000: 318–338).

tablet 40), which could signal the presence of Lamaštu in children,[28] was also considered ominous, and the birth of a yellow child heralded the death of the owner of the house.[29]

Some physical symptoms could therefore herald the destruction of a household. Treatments safeguarding the household and keeping it in balance were essential, and such purposes seem to correspond to Kiṣir-Aššur's *šamallû mašmaššu ṣeḫru* texts and large parts of his *mašmaššu* texts concerning, e.g., *namburbi*-rituals (see Sections 5.2 and 6.4).

Little is known about what therapeutic treatments for diseases were applied to babies.[30] The best information stems from the NA royal correspondence,[31] although we often find only brief remarks that a child is doing well.[32] Nontheless, some exorcists practicing at the contemporary NA royal court at Nineveh, may been involved in observing and healing infants or children in addition to adults (e.g., Parpola 1993 nos. 213–215, 218, 302, 305). Volk (1999: 11) regarded it as a chance of discovery that child treatments are so poorly documented in medical literature. However, child healing is not listed as an identifiable category in the AMC.[33]

Nonetheless, many illness diagnoses for children are attested in "adult" versions (Cadelli 1997: 32). It is therefore plausible, although impossible to prove, that at least older children received the same (modified) treatments as adults

28 Lamaštu was known as "the goddess who (makes) his face yellow" *ul-tú* ⌜*ša*⌝ IGI-*šú* SIG_7 (Volk 1999: 24 note 137 with reference).

29 De Zorzi 2014: 441; Cadelli 1997: 31; Leichty 1970: 66; tablet 4 line 5: [BE SAL Ù.TU]-*ma* MIN-*ma* (= *ul-la-nu-um-ma*) SIG_7 *ma*-[*li*] EN É ÚŠ, "If a woman gives birth, and at the birth (the child) is already fully yellow (Leichty: flecked with green (spots)) – the owner of the house will die."

30 For boy's problems, see George 2016: 167–68. Note *BAM* 248 col. iv 39–43 with prophylactic treatments for keeping "hands" of various deities from approaching infants (Scurlock 2014: 626ff.). Scurlock (ibid.: 621) furthermore states: "Treatments specifically and exclusively designed for infants or toddlers are relatively rare and usually scattered among prescriptions for adults with similar problems." For additional examples of treatments for adults or children, as well as cures exclusively for children, see Steinert 2018d: 228.

31 Volk 1999: 8. Letters mentioning children's health, regardless of age and description: *SAA* 10 no. 187, 193, 194, 196, 197, 202, 213, 214, 215(?), 217, 218, 219, 222, 223, 231, 238, 239, 244, 245, 247, 293, 296, 298, 299, 300(?), 301, 302, 304(?), 305, 306(?), 309, 319, 320, 321, 322, 323.

32 The evidence from the antechamber to the third NA tomb at Nimrud showed several individuals ranging 6–12 years of age, a fully grown foetus (8th–9th lunar month), and a baby (3–9 months) (Macgregor 2012: 81; Müller-Karpe et al. 2008: 144). Although these individuals must date to the 8th century, it is uncertain whether or not these were royal children.

33 Apart from pregnancy and birth which occur near the end of the AMC, the best candidate is an earlier entry in line 98: [...] ⌜*ana* ᵈDIM_9⌝.M[E] Z[I-*ḫi*? x x x], "for era[dicating(?)] Lamaštu [...]".

(ibid.: 33 note 159).[34] A human adult treatment was perhaps also modified into at least one horse prescription in *BAM* 159 (Stol 2011: 395 and note 223; cf. Böck 2009a: 117–18). I would also like to emphasize the recent findings by Heeßel (2006: 19–20) concerning the possible lack of differences between the treatment of men and women in major parts of the first 35 tablets of Sa-gig. This could indicate that the diagnostic and therapeutic corpora may not always have been applied exclusively to the identified gender, even species, and perhaps also age group.

In relation to horses in particular, it is noteworthy that they and children are prone to nasal breathing and regurgitation (Section 4.4.2).[35] Furthermore, gastro-intestinal disorders are regularly observed in both horses and infants (Hyman et al. 2006: 1519; Gonçalves et al. 2002: 643). This may indicate an overlap in physiological conception, and due to the possible physiological knowledge taught to Kiṣir-Aššur as *šamallû ṣeḫru* concerning horses, we can perhaps hypothesize an overlap between some child and horse illnesses, and maybe adult treatments for similar problems.[36]

34 The AMC may indicate that conditions occurring in both children and adults were integrated into the adult sections of such medical texts, e.g., AMC line 23 adds *šá* LÚ.TUR and AMC line 28 adds *ù* LÚ.TUR *su-alu* GIG (Steinert 2018d: 227–228, 230). However, such cures are not found in the majority of therapeutic manuscripts, and the phrases above could therefore indicate that the prescriptions for adults referenced in AMC line 23 and 28 could be modified and applied to children.

35 It is unclear if Sa-gig tablet 40 lists any cases of "regurgitation", although it may be described by the verb *šurruḫu* (Cadelli 1997: 17, 20, 30; cf. Scurlock and Andersen 2005: 749 note 120). It therefore remains uncertain if "regurgitation" was differentiated from "vomiting" in terminology (cf. Volk 1999: 20–21; see translation by Scurlock 2014: 263–269).

36 This would require an understanding of how little medication a baby or an infant would need. Today, presumably as in ancient times, children are usually treated for issues connected to nutrition, common and infectious diseases, as well as injuries or trauma (see, e.g., Scurlock and Andersen 2005: 410ff.; Cadelli 1997: 20–21, 27–29). It is noteworthy that such issues are often treated similarly regardless of age. However, symptoms of diseases can be subtler in babies, and the physician must diagnose beyond specialization. Yet, there is generally little doubt when a child is in pain. Paediatricians today assess pain in infants and young children via a variety of pain scales in order to determine their levels of discomfort (e.g., Beltramini et al. 2017). Infants are prone to non-epileptic motor phenomena, such as tremors, jitters, forms of myoclonus, and brainstem release phenomena (Huntsman et al. 2008). The ancient medical texts seem to focus on such experiences in relation to the infant's motor system because they could foreshadow severe afflictions, which in turn could affect the entire household (Volk 1999: 16–17; Cadelli 1997: 23–24). These problems would therefore have been a matter of concern for a healer regardless of the medical knowledge gained from treating children. Practicing on infants and children would have allowed a healer to study failures to thrive in a non-verbal environment, how the body communicates problems and levels of pain under such conditions, as well as sharpening their diagnostic abilities, regardless whether or not this could be transferred

5.2.3 *An Interpretation: Kiṣir-Aššur as Paediatrician?*

In Section 4.2.2, I suggested that Kiṣir-Aššur might have worked (alongside his father) with animals, perhaps only horses, in addition to humans after having acquired veterinarian knowledge as *šamallû ṣeḫru*. Following this line of reasoning, the evidence presented here tentatively suggests that he may have moved on to (aid his father when) treating infants, babies or children at least as *šamallû mašmaššu ṣeḫru*. In addition to the obvious dangers of doing more harm than good when practicing medicine, there may have been an economic and ethical value system explaining why practicing on ill animals and babies provided more professional security than on human adults.[37]

In comparison, the OB laws of Ḫammurabi contain several clauses for both physician (*asû*) and veterinarian (*asî alpim ulu imērim*) accidents or malpractice, which are instructive for understanding what was at risk. Although law collections such as the laws of Ḫammurabi may not reflect actual practice, and instead relate to "cultural assumptions and values of their drafters and copyists" (Roth 1995: 4–7 with references),[38] they certainly reflect a concern for justice when wronged, which can be used to emphasize tendencies towards punishment:

LḪ paragraph 218: "If a physician (*asûm*) performs major surgery with a bronze lancet upon an *awīlum*-man and thus causes the *awīlum*'s death, or opens an *awīlum*'s temple with a bronze lancet and thus blinds the *awīlum*'s eye, they shall cut off his hand" (Roth 1995: 123).[39]

---

directly to adults. These observations were formulated following a personal communication with Elisabeth Lund, chief paediatrician at Kolding Hospital, Denmark. However, it is also possible that Kiṣir-Aššur copied the incantation N4 no. 24 because he himself became a father around this time (JoAnn Scurlock, personal communication). It cannot be excluded that some texts were copied by Kiṣir-Aššur for reasons unrelated to his profession, similar to one of Nabû-zuqup-kēnu's manuscripts containing the 12th tablet of the Gilgameš Epic (Frahm 1999).

37 One example is the area of surgery, although it is unclear who practiced this in most periods outside of the OB period where the *asû* is mentioned in this role in the laws of Ḫammurabi (Böck 2014a: 19–20; Geller 2010: 53, 56, 58, 60–61). Even today, there are potential problems related to infections during surgery, and the occasional threat in incantations concerned with "the obsidian blades of Gula" (*ṣurrū naglabū Gula*) emphasizes that this was likely considered an equal threat to illness and patient alike as a last resort (Böck 2014a: 19; Geller 2010: 3, 54; Collins 1999: 94, 217–18, 233).

38 Johnson 2015: 295–300 and Charpin 2010b: 77–82 and note 43 with further references; see also Westbrook 2003: 17–21. See Guinan 2014: 117 on laws in relation to omens.

39 However, other rules applied if the man was a slave of a commoner (*muškēnum*), see paragraph 219–20.

LḪ paragraph 225: "If he (i.e., a veterinarian, *asî alpim ulu imērim*) performs major surgery upon an ox or a donkey and thus causes its death, he shall give one quarter(?) of its value to the owner of the ox or donkey" (ibid.: 124).[40]

Causing the death of an ox or donkey while performing surgery on it resulted in a fine of one-fourth(?) of the animal's value. However, if a physician caused a man's (*awīlum*) death or blinded his eye during surgery, he would have his hand cut off, effectively ending his practice. Therefore, less may have been at stake when treating an animal compared to an adult. Although the laws of Ḫammurabi stem from the OB period, they were actually copied, probably for their historic value, in the N4 collection.[41] Still, we do not know if regulations for malpractice stipulated in the laws of Ḫammurabi are applicable to the *āšipu*'s trade.

Children are not mentioned in the extant law collections in relation to healing, but it must be considered certain that infants were vulnerable during pregnancy and in the time following birth, and that they were occasionally in need of medical assistance (Stol 2000: 27–48, 129–34, 209–14).[42] It is therefore plausible that the failed healing (or assisted delivery?) of a prominent family member's baby could damage your reputation, although you may have been allowed to continue your practice elsewhere.[43] If this analysis is correct, it is possible to identify three hypothetical and generalized steps with increased professional consequences as a result of a failed healing:

1) Animals → Economic penalty
2) Infants, babies → Damaged social reputation/social exclusion
3) Adults → Physical penalty/termination of practice

This could imply that some apprentice healers, if trained in all such treatments, may have had greater autonomy when healing animals and babies, as the cost of failure would have been more manageable in terms of continuing

40 One fourth or one fifth of the price is unclear (Roth 1995: 142 note 41).

41 Ismail 1982: 199. It is currently unknown if the content related to the laws or the prologue.

42 For birth at the NA court, see Melville 2004: 37 note 1, 42–43, 47. For birth incantations, see Couto-Ferreira 2017: 58, 60, 64; Böck 2009c: 272–74; Stol 2000: 59–71. Concerning birth, see Steinert 2018d: 272–76 with further references. It seems the death of a child could be associated with misfortune (ibid.: 269–270 with further references).

43 This appears to have been the case for Urad-Gula, the son of Esarhaddon's chief exorcist Adad-šumu-uṣur. One tenuous suggestion is he was dismissed from the royal court in disgrace because he had failed to oversee the successful delivery of a child, perhaps Assurbanipal's (*SAA* 10 no. 293; see Parpola 1983a: 354–56). Perhaps this was the reason for his petition to Assurbanipal in the famed "Forlorn Scholar" letter (*SAA* 10 no. 294; cf. Geller 2010: 77–79; Parpola 1987: 268–69)?

his career.[44] In these cases, it is likely that the apprentice gained autonomy in treating animals such as horses before babies, which in turn were treated with greater autonomy by the apprentice before adults. However, this remains hypothetical. It should be kept in mind that medical healing often had a religious aspect. In relation to rituals, the success of such performances may have depended on the gods (see Ambos 2010: 17–18). Although healers were likely to be held responsible to some extent for failed healings, it is possible that failure could be interpreted as the will of the gods.[45] Yet, no available sources describe the consequences of an unsuccesful treatment by an *āšipu*.

The hypothesis above may, however, be tentatively substantiated in relation to Kiṣir-Aššur's career. As shown in Section 3.5, Kiṣir-Aššur's *šamallû ṣeḫru* tablet *RA* 15 pl. 76 relates to venomous stings and bites as well as horse treatments (colic?). This tablet may therefore relate to knowledge acquisition or perhaps even practice in these areas of treatment. Kiṣir-Aššur's *šamallû mašmaššu ṣeḫru* tablet N4 no. 24, discussed above, relates to prophylactically treating a child. The evidence is therefore vague and limited. A number of texts copied by Kiṣir-Nabû and related to children and pregnancy are copied during his *mašmaššu ṣeḫru*- and *mašmaššu*-phases, thus indicating such material belonged to later phases.

The surviving evidence indicates that Kiṣir-Aššur may have worked with treatments related to horses before children, although he also copied adult treatments as *šamallû ṣeḫru*. Though it is possible that Kiṣir-Aššur aided in practicing on adults alongside animals and children throughout his apprenticeship, I draw on the value system outlined above to suggest that he may have experienced greater autonomy when treating on animals and children before becoming an autonomous healer of adults as well. I therefore hypothesize that Kiṣir-Aššur, in addition to periodically aiding his father with a range of healing activities, may have had greater autonomy when treating horses (and other animals?) and babies before moving on to practice healing on human adults without supervision as *mašmaššu*.

44 Adults were probably also the most valuable members of a household to keep healthy. Furthermore, adults would also have been able to complain verbally, whereas animals and babies can mainly communicate their distress non-verbally if crying and screams are disregarded.

45 For a survey of ritual failures and mistakes, see Ambos 2007. Some texts stress illnesses that the healer should not attempt to heal (Schwemer 2011: 434).

5.3 The *mašmaššu ṣeḫru*-phase

Kiṣir-Aššur's "junior exorcist" *mašmaššu ṣeḫru*-phase is poorly attested, with only one text preserved. Sadly, the manuscript is unpublished and little is known about the content. Nonetheless, a few observations can still be made.

Although the exact content of N4 A 2727 is currently unknown, the text contains two incantations with instructions for application, of which the first incantation duplicates *BAM* 105 obv. 1–6 and presumably also *STT* 97 col. iv 25–29 (Daniel Schwemer, personal communication). This brief incantation mentions various (gynaecological?) problems concerning a young woman,[46] although the brief ritual instruction in *BAM* 105 obv. 7 explains that the incantation was widely used, as it could be recited over any suppository, ointment and enema against "Anus illness" (DÚR.GIG) (Section 8.4.1; see also Kiṣir-Aššur's *BAM* 102 in Section 6.1). Therefore, it is unclear against what problem N4 A 2727 was directed. However, considering the widely applicable use of the incantation and instruction in *BAM* 105, it does not seem accidental that N4 A 2727 contains the label "tested prescriptions, which are *suitable for use*(?)" (*bulṭī latkūti ša ina qāti šūṣû*). These are presumably the earliest prescriptions labelled as "tested" (*latku*) copied by Kiṣir-Aššur (see Section 8.3). The phrase *ša ina qāti šūṣû* seems to indicate the treatment in question was considered especially useful, although the exact nuances are uncertain (see Ch. 6 note 25).

TABLE 8 Texts assigned to Kiṣir-Aššur's *mašmaššu ṣeḫru*-phase

Text	Content	Format and designation
N4 A 2727	Obverse and reverse: two incantations with instructions, of which one may have been against "Anus illness"	Landscape; *u'iltu*

46 *BAM* 105 obv. 2–3: *nab-ni-sa da-mu u šar-*⌜*ku*⌝ *iṣ-bat* KAL *ina* $MURUB_4$-⌜*šá*!?⌝ ³ *iṣ-bat* KI.SIKIL *ina pag-ri-šá*. Perhaps the incantation concerned menstruation or a severe gynaecological problem. It was certainly employed for "Anus illness" on account of the associated bleeding. The association between menstruation and bleeding from male pelvic orifices were also used in diagnoses concerning "if a man passes blood from his anus" or "if a man's penis drips blood", see Stol 2016: 438; Geller 2005: 40–41, 68–69, 94–95, 104–105, 140–141, 188–189, 212–215, 218–219.

Noticeably, only around five tablets represent the various Bāba-šuma-ibni family members' *mašmaššu ṣeḫru*-phases.[47] This observation could tentatively indicate that this family did not keep tablets, did not inscribe their names or titles, or kept their tablets elsewhere during the *mašmaššu ṣeḫru*-phase. Kiṣir-Nabû probably copied three tablets related to pregnancy and babies during his *mašmaššu ṣeḫru*- and *mašmaššu*-phases. In combination with Kiṣir-Aššur's child-calming incantation N4 no. 24, the evidence indicates that such material belonged to the *šamallû mašmaššu ṣeḫru*, *mašmaššu ṣeḫru* and *mašmaššu* phases.[48] However, he also copied a tablet with prescriptions for skin illnesses of the head (*BAM* 33) and a commentary to the incantation *tummu bītu* and *Šurpu* tablet 2 (*AfO* 12 pl. 13–14) as *mašmaššu ṣeḫru*. At least the first incantation in Kiṣir-Aššur's N4 A 2727 was a tested remedy used elsewhere against "Anus illness".

5.3.1 *Discussion of the* mašmašsu ṣeḫru-*phase*

Little is known about the concrete competences demanded during the "junior" (*ṣeḫru*) phases of various professions. For the MA period, Wagensonner has elucidated various aspects concerning the training of three *ṭupšarru ṣeḫru*s who were sons of the MA royal scribe Ninurta-uballissu (Wagensonner 2014a; Wagensonner 2014b; Wagensonner 2011: 647–49). At least two of the brothers wrote tablets or controlled each other's work.[49] Although we cannot determine if they were still engaged in a learning process at this stage, Wagensonner (2011: 649) considered it likely they were already at the peak of their education (cf. ibid. 2014b: 459).

---

47 See Kiṣir-Nabû's *mašmaššu ṣeḫru* tablets *AfO* 12 pl. 13–14, *BAM* 33 and perhaps *KAR* 114(?), as well as Nabû-bēssunu's *KAL* 4 no. 6; cf. Maul 2010a: 208–10. *KAR* 114 contains another child calming incantation and ritual (Farber 1989: 98–101 no. 32 ms h).

48 Kiṣir-Nabû copied *KAR* 114 as *mašmaššu* (*ṣeḫru*?), rev. 11: … MAŠ.[MAŠ (TUR?)], (almost no space), and *LKA* 143 and N4 no. 247 as *mašmaššu* (cf. Fadhil 2012: 37 note 2). See also *KAR* 223 for postponing a birth from happening in the first month of the year, which was copied by Kiṣir-Nabû without a title, but including the *ša Nabû tuklassu*-phrase (Stol 2000: 93 and note 19 with references). Furthermore, knowledge related to children is also found in Late Babylonian scholarly texts from Uruk. Stevens suggested a correlation existed within this material between knowledge related to the professional specialism of a tablet owner and the occurrence of so-called protective formulae in the colophons (Stevens 2013: 211–12; see the discussion of such phrases in Section 6.2.3). If we accept this division, it would seem that diagnoses, treatments, and omens for women, birth, and babies were part of their specialization and this knowledge likely belonged to the *mašmaššu ṣeḫru*- and *mašmaššu*-phases of the Urukean scholars examined by Stevens (e.g., *SpTU* I no. 38, no. 48, no. 59, *SpTU* III no. 90, *SpTU* V no. 248; Stevens 2013: 234–36).

49 Wagensonner 2014b: 462; Wagensonner 2011: 649.

In the LB scribal education, incantations against Lamaštu, as well as incantations from, e.g., *Maqlû* and *Šurpu*, were copied in the second phase (Gesche 2001: 176). A brief catalogue of five related incantation incipits from the Lamaštu series, as well as a number of prescriptions for treating "Anus illness", are also among the medical school tablets published by Finkel (2000: 144, 195–96). Stevens (2013) also found some shared features in the LB Uruk Šangû-Ninurta family's tablet collection, which might mark certain tablets as part of specialist training or as advanced pedagogical texts. These features included the tablets written by *ṣeḫru*s, designated as commentaries, being *malsûtu*s or IM.GÍD.DAs (i.e., exercises; cf. Gesche 2001: 50), and containing errors, notes, or brief colophons without ownership or copying statements.[50] Stevens suggests the "junior" status may have lasted "many months or even years" (Stevens 2013: 220–21).

Interestingly, in *SAA* 10 no. 290 Urad-Gula writes to the king concerning the exorcist Nabû-leʾutu and his son who was performing rituals with him: "Even I have noticed that this son of his is (still) in the unsteadiness of youth (*ṣaḫḫurānūtu*)" (Parpola 1993: 277).[51] Therefore, the participating son in this case was clearly considered immature. The question is if he was a (*mašmaššu*) *ṣeḫru* at this time.[52]

Considering that Kiṣir-Aššur also wrote at least two IM.GÍD.DAs as *šamallû mašmaššu ṣeḫru* and *mašmaššu*, we might consider it likely he was still in training as a *mašmaššu ṣeḫru*. In terms of content, Kiṣir-Aššur and his nephew tentatively appears to have been closer to the educational principles of the LB healers than the MA *ṭupšarru*s during his *mašmaššu ṣeḫru*-phase.

5.3.2 *Excursus: Kiṣir-Aššur's* u'iltu-*tablets*

Kiṣir-Aššur copied numerous tablets labelled as *u'iltu*s throughout his career. Seeing as the label may in some contexts have had a pedagogical nuance (see below), I have included an excursus on the term in this chapter before examining Kiṣir-Aššur's *mašmaššu*- and *mašmaš bīt Aššur*-phase in the following chapters. However, the exact nuances of the term *u'iltu* in the N4 text collection are poorly understood. Kiṣir-Aššur likely copied four such texts as *šamallû ṣeḫru*, one as *šamallû*, one as *mašmaššu ṣeḫru*, possibly four as *mašmaššu*,

---

50 Stevens 2013: 219–20 and notes 49–54 and 56; Frahm 2011a: 313 note 1492, 314 note 1495. Kiṣir-Nabû's commentary *AfO* 12 pl. 13–14 was written as *mašmaššu ṣeḫru*. See also Pearce and Doty 2000: 337–41.

51 *SAA* 10 no. 290 rev. 15-s. 1: … *u a-na-ku* [16] *a-ta-mar* DUMU-*šú an-ni-i* [s. 1] [*ina*] ŠÀ *ba-ra-ar ṣa-ḫu-ra-nu-tú šú-u*.

52 For NA apprentices, see Robson 2014: 152–53; Robson 2013: 50; Robson 2011a: 564–65.

five as *mašmaš bīt Aššur*, and at least three during an uncertain phase.[53] The *u'iltu* label was written systematically with the signs *ú-ìl-tì/ti* by Kiṣir-Aššur and Kiṣir-Nabû.

In the *CAD* (U-W: 51), the word is translated as "a type of tablet about twice as wide as long, inscribed parallel to the longer axis containing a scholar's report, obligation, debt, promissory note, debt note" (see also *AHw*: 1405; Gesche 2001: 147), and it is further specified at Nineveh as containing astrological reports and generally having a ratio between its sides of 1:2 with a landscape format (Radner 1995: 72; Radner 1997: 60–61; Parpola 1983a: 65; Parpola 1983b: 2 note 5; Hunger 1992: XV). The word originates etymologically from "to bind (by an agreement)" *e'ēlu* (*CAD* E: 40; *AHw*: 189), and it is therefore related to something owed to someone.[54] As mentioned in the *CAD*, *u'iltu*-reports were often written to the NA kings concerning celestial omens (Hunger 1992: XV). Scholars "kept the king's watch" (*maṣṣartu ša šarri naṣāru*), which involved watching, guarding and protecting the king by ensuring he knew what course the gods had decreed for him (Parpola 1993: XXI–XXII). The inherent responsibility between observation and report may have been reflected in the label *u'iltu*. As discussed in Section 5.3.2, the *u'iltu* label in N4 may tentatively designate the content as an exercise, obligation or commitment on behalf of the copyist. The word *u'iltu* can therefore cautiously be proposed in some instances to indicate a duty or exercise administered by, or made in relation to, a senior teacher, practitioner or colleague. There is currently no evidence to suggest that the label could also designate a healer's obligation in relation to a patient. None of Kiṣir-Aššur's *mašmaš bīt Aššur*-phase *u'iltu*s are copied on his behalf, which suggests that Kiṣir-Aššur copied them himself. However, it cannot be excluded that the anonymous "written and checked" statement, spelled SAR-*ma* È, could hide a Š-stem of *šaṭāru* in some cases (see Section 7.4.2 as well as Ch. 3 note 134). This remains uncertain.

Noticeably, Kiṣir-Aššur's *u'iltu*s all seem to be one-columned tablets in portrait format, which is unexpected (see also Maul 2019: 312). The only

53 *Šamallû ṣeḫru*: *BAM* 201; N4 A 400; N4 no. 237; N4 no 241(?); *šamallû*: N4 no. 175; *mašmaššu ṣeḫru*: N4 A 2727; *mašmaššu*: *BAM* 81; *BAM* 122; *KAL* 4 no. 7(?); *KAR* 230; *mašmaš bīt Aššur*: *BAM* 300; *KAR* 62; *KAR* 63; *LKA* 83; N4 no. 110; broken title: *KAL* 7 no. 24(?); *KAL* 10 no. 13; *LKA* 137. Kiṣir-Aššur or Kiṣir-Nabû: *BAM* 260; *LKA* 146.

54 By comparison, the OB *galamāḫu* Ur-Utu from Sippar owned 46 letters referring to an etymologically similar "binding" (*e'iltu*) that was to be released (*paṭāru*) by the gods, probably through a ritual (Tanret 2011: 283–284). The word is translated "obligation, liability, sin" in *CAD* (E: 51–52), and in the case of Ur-Utu, it could lead to illness and the eventual loss of life (Tanret 2011: 283–284).

exceptions appear to be Kiṣir-Aššur's three *u'iltus* LKA 83, N4 A 400 and N4 A 2727 in single-column, landscape format. Peculiarly, the majority of Kiṣir-Nabû's *u'iltus* seem to be in the landscape format. Why Kiṣir-Aššur's *u'iltus* largely differ from the expected landscape format is unclear. Perhaps it was no different from choosing paper with lines over paper with squares (Ulla Koch, personal communication). There does not seem to be any distribution of such texts according to specific career phases or content (cf. Finkel 2000: 146). The meaning of the term and the shape of *u'iltus* in general require further investigation.

5.4 Excursus: The *ša Nabû tuklassu*-phrase

At least five of Kiṣir-Aššur's texts contain the phrase "whose trust is Nabû" (*ša Nabû tuklassu*) or a variant thereof, usually written *ša*/*šá* ^{d}AG/PA NIR-*su*/GISKIM-*su*/*tuk-lat-su*.[55] Of these texts, three can be attributed to the *šamallû ṣeḫru*-phase (RA 15 pl. 76) and *šamallû mašmaššu ṣeḫru*-phase (LKA 89+, LKA 141). This leaves two texts, BAM 9 and BAM 121, which do not contain a title related to a career phase. Although Section 7.1 argues that Kiṣir-Aššur's tablets without titles belong to later career phases, the presence of this phrase in earlier phases could indicate that BAM 9 and BAM 121 belong somewhere before the *mašmaššu*-phase (see below).[56] These two colophons read:

55 BAM 9 rev. 72: [... ^{d}A]G *tuk-lat-su* ⸢^{d}⸣[*T*]*aš-me-tu*$_4$ ⸢x⸣[...]; BAM 121 rev. 25: ... *ša* ^{d}PA NIR-*su*; LKA 89+ col. iv 6': ... *šá* ^{d}AG GISKIM-*su*; LKA 141 rev. 10': ... ⸢*šá*⸣ [...]; RA 15 pl. 76 rev. 11': ... *ša* ^{d}PA *tuk-lat-su*; cf. KAL 4 no. 37 rev. 8': [... NI]R-*su*. The last text was likely copied by Kiṣir-Aššur or Kiṣir-Nabû (see Section 7.3). Kiṣir-Nabû has at least nine tablets with this or similar phrases: *CMAwR* 1 pl. 25–26 rev. 27: *šá a-na* ^{d}[A]G *u* ^{d}KURNUN [*t*]*a-ak-lum*; BAM 52 rev. 103: ... *šá* ^{d}PA NIR$^{?}$-*su*; BAM 106 rev. 9': ... *ša* ^{d}AG *tuk*-[*lat-su*]; BAM 147 rev. 28': ... *šá* PA NIR-*su*; KAR 223 rev. 14: ... *šá* DAG NIR-*su*; LKA 100 rev. 8: ... *šá* ^{d}PA *tuk-l*[*at*]-*s*[*u*]; LKA 118 rev. 4': [...]⸢x⸣ *u* ^{d}*Taš-me-tu*$_4$ *ta-a*[*k-lu*$^{?}$]; N4 no. 163 (= Geller 2016: 394–96; Geller 2014: 64ff.) rev. 26: ... *šá* ^{d}⸢NÀ⸣ NIR-*su*; N4 no. 247 rev. 25: ... *ša* [...]; cf. CT 15 pl. 43f. rev. 11': ... ⸢*ša* ^{d}AG⸣ *tuk-lat-s*[*u*]; KAL 4 no. 37 (see above); KAV 182 col. iv 9': [...] ^{d}AG *tuk-lat-su*. Notably, Kiṣir-Nabû regularly seems to choose the same Sumerogram for Nabû (PA/AG) as the theophoric element of his name.

56 Generally, the phrase *ša Nabû tuklassu* is included directly after the personal name of the copyist or owner of the tablet. However, Kiṣir-Aššur's BAM 9 and Kiṣir-Nabû's LKA 118 differ, and in BAM 9, Kiṣir-Aššur writes an altered version of the phrase after his father Nabû-bēssunu's name (see below). Kiṣir-Nabû's texts published in *CMAwR* 1 pl. 25–26 and LKA 118 also show alternative formulations over this thematic sentence.

BAM 9 rev. 69: [DIŠ NA] ⸢UD.DA TAB⸣.BA$^{!}$-*ma* SÍG SA[G.DU]-⸢*šú*$^{?}$⸣ GUB.MEŠ EG[IR$^{?}$-*šú iš-šaṭ-ṭar*]
BAM 9 rev. 70: [(*nis-ḫu*)] IGI-*ú* GABA.RI ^{giš}ZU [x x x x x x x x x(?)]
BAM 9 rev. 71: [D]U[B (*blank*)] ^{p}*Ki-ṣir*-AN.ŠÁR DUMU $^{p.}$⸢^{d}⸣AG-*bé*-[*sun* ^{lú}MAŠ.MAŠ BAL.TIL^{ki}/É AN.ŠÁR(?)]
BAM 9 rev. 72: [(x x?) *šá* ^{d}A]G *tuk-lat-su* ⸢^{d}⸣[*T*]*aš-me-tu*$_{4}$ ⸢x⸣[(x x x x x?)]
BAM 9 rev. 73: [DUMU $^{p.d}$*B*]*a-ba*$_{6}$-MU-DÙ ^{lú}ZABAR.DAB.BA *É*-[*šár-ra*]
BAM 9 rev. 74: [(*niš* ^{d}PA$^{?}$ *u*$^{?}$) ^{d}AM]AR.UTU *šu-mì šaṭ-rù la t*[*a-pa-šiṭ*]
BAM 9 rev. 75: [(x x x?) ^{d}]AG ⸢*ù*⸣ ^{d}A[MAR.UTU]
BAM 9 rev. 76: [(x x x x?)]⸢x x x x x-*šú*⸣-*m*[*a* (x x x?)]

(*Catch-line*); ^{70} First [extract], a copy of a writing-board [*from*$^{?}$ ...], ^{71} [ta]bl[et] (of) Kiṣir-Aššur, son of Nabû-bē[ssunu the Assur exorcist/ exorcist of the Aššur temple], ^{72} [...] whose trust is [Na]bû, [T]ašmētu [...], ^{73} [son of B]aba-šuma-ibni, the *zabardabbû*-priest of *Ešarra*; ^{74} [on oath of Nabû and Ma]rduk, do not [erase] my written name! ^{75} [...] Nabû and M[arduk ... (*curse*?), ^{76} ...] him, and [...].

BAK 200 ms A

BAM 121 rev. 24: *a-na ṣa-bat e-pe-še* ZI-[*ḫ*]*a*$^{!}$
BAM 121 rev. 25: DUB-*pi* ^{p}ZÚ.KEŠDA-AN.ŠÁR *ša* ^{d}PA NIR-*su*
BAM 121 rev. 26: DUMU $^{p.d}$AG-*be-sun* ^{lú}MAŠ.MAŠ É AN.ŠÁR

Extracted for undertaking a (ritual) procedure, ^{25} tablet of Kiṣir-Aššur, whose trust is Nabû, ^{26} the son of Nabû-bēssunu, the exorcist of the Aššur temple.

BAK 198 ms B

BAM 9 is a "first [extract], a copy of a writing-board [from$^{?}$ ...]" and is designated as a *ṭuppu* of Kiṣir-Aššur. We should note that Kiṣir-Aššur's *RA* 15 pl. 76 and *RA* 40 pl. 116, both copied as *šamallû ṣeḫru* and the former with the *ša Nabû tuklassu* addendum and described as "the 32nd$^{?}$ extract" copying a writing-board, were also designated as *ṭuppu*s. This is not the case for Kiṣir-Aššur's later numbered extracts.[57]

57 The catch-line of *BAM* 9 is repeated as the opening of the single prescription found on *BAM* 145. This tablet's colophon is unfortunately too broken to determine who wrote it and for what purpose, although Scurlock remarks that "it is of the 'excerpted for specific performance' type" (Scurlock 2014: 423). Therefore, it is uncertain if we can regard this

However, the *ša Nabû tuklassu*-phrase in *BAM* 9 does not resemble the way Kiṣir-Aššur ordinarily writes this phrase, as it also includes an uncertain passage concerning Tašmētu.[58] Although this may be a variation, it is also noteworthy that the phrase occurs after Kiṣir-Aššur's father's name and in the middle of his geneology. No comparable examples can be identified among Kiṣir-Aššur's colophons. As such, it may be an elaborate praise of his father's devotion to the god of writing and his consort. Furthermore, the text contains a protective statement, and such statements only appear in the surviving evidence on tablets from Kiṣir-Aššur's *šamallû ṣeḫru-*, *šamallû-* and *mašmaš bīt Aššur*-phases, as well as an uncertain phase (Section 6.2.3).

BAM 121 consists of one-line "ditto" (KI.MIN) prescriptions,[59] it may have covered several physiological areas with changes marked with a double horizontal ruling,[60] and it ends with a longer prescription on the reverse. Due to the *ana ṣabāt epēši*-phrase, however, the tablet was likely copied for the specific treatment of an afflicted patient, perhaps overseen by Kiṣir-Aššur himself (see Section 7.4). Furthermore, Kiṣir-Aššur used a logographic writing of his name in the colophon (Arbøll 2018b). This is one of only two surviving tablets from Kiṣir-Aššur in which this writing occurs (see also N4 no. 175). As such, it is unusual, although the content is not particularly unique.

5.4.1 *Kiṣir-Aššur's Use of the* ša Nabû tuklassu*-phrase*

In general, the *ša Nabû tuklassu*-phrase in this form seems to occur mainly in connection with individuals connected to the N4 collection, such as the Bāba-šuma-ibni and Bēl-kundi-ilāya families (Borger 1970b: 167; cf. Hunger 1968: 12–15).[61] A somewhat comparable phrase occurs in several of the colophons

---

tablet as the one Kiṣir-Aššur wrote following *BAM* 9, although *BAM* 145 contains a number of erasures marked in Köcher's copy. See Ch. 3 note 38.

58 Cf. the following phrase in an Assurbanipal colophon on K. 9404 (Maul 1994: 540) rev. 3'–4': *ša a-na* A[N.Š]Á[R *u Mullissu taklu*] [4'] *ša* [d]AG *ù* [d]*T*[*aš-me-tu*$_4$ *uznu rapaštu išrukūš*], "He who trusts in Aššur and Mullissu, onto whom Nabû and Tašmētu bestowed broad understanding" (Maul 1994: 280, 282 ms C). See also Hunger 1968 no. 217, 237, 255, 319, 322–23, 326, 329–32, 336, 338, 460.

59 Obv. 4, 5, 6, 7, 13. See Section 3.2.

60 Obv. 1: DIS NA SAG […], repeated in obv. 4, 5, 6, 7 and 8(?). Whether the initial diagnosis concerns the head (SAG.[DU]), headache (SAG.KI.DAB.BA), or the epigastrium (SAG ŠÀ) remains uncertain, but the focus was probably different to when it changes in obv. 9: DIŠ NA GÌ[R[II]-*šú*(?) …], repeated in obv. 10, 12, 13 and rev. 14.

61 The Bēl-kundi-ilāya family's colophons can be found in *BAK* 252–54, 504, 508–10, 518 and 519 (Borger 1970b: 166; cf. Fadhil 2012: 41). Borger writes: "Die Floskel 'dessen Zuversicht Nabû ist' wird anscheinend nur in den Familien von Bel-Kundi-ilāya and vor Bāba-šuma-ibni … gebraucht; Nr. 248 läßt sich freilich noch nicht auf diese Weise einordnen." (Borger 1970b: 167). *BAK* no. 248 (= *BAM* 87 lines 25–26) reads: [25] LIBIR.RA.BI.[GI]M AB.SAR

from Assurbanipal's libraries.[62] Maul interprets the *ša Nabû tuklassu*-phrase mainly as a pious and praising supplement, signalling that the copyist was a faithful trainee of Nabû, but without an exact function in N4 (Maul 2010a: 215 and note 96). Although he did not pursue his analysis further, the subordinate relationship to Nabû seems to occur most frequently diachronically within texts related to training (Gesche 2001: 159–61; Maul 1998: XII–XIV, XVI; Cavigneaux 1996: 24–27; Cavigneaux 1981: 37–38).

As shown by the *šamallû ṣeḫru* and *šamallû mašmaššu ṣeḫru* tablets on which this phrase occurs, it seems to be connected to a number of Kiṣir-Aššur's student tablets. This is corroborated comparatively by at least one commentary from Kiṣir-Nabû with this phrase (N4 no. 163 = Geller 2014: 64ff.), albeit this text is from an unknown phase. A number of Kiṣir-Nabû's numbered extracts (*BAM* 52, *BAM* 106, *BAM* 147), of which two are instructional (*BAM* 52, *BAM* 106), also contain this phrase without a title.[63] However, Kiṣir-Nabû's *mašmaššu*-phase tablet N4 no. 247 likely also included the phrase, which argues against the above observations.[64] The phrase may in Kiṣir-Aššur's case have been used primarily on apprentice phase tablets, although the evidence is far from conclusive.

Where does this place *BAM* 9 and *BAM* 121? As argued in Section 7.1, titles were probably not omitted on tablets with names before Kiṣir-Aššur's later phases. The use of the *ša Nabû tuklassu*-phrase on these two tablets indicates they may have been part of Kiṣir-Aššur's apprentice phases. However, the phrase in *BAM* 9 may relate to Kiṣir-Aššur's father, Nabû-bēssunu, which would make this text the only example of such a use of the expression by Kiṣir-Aššur. This could indicate the text was earlier than other preserved texts with the *ša Nabû tuklassu*-phrase. This observation, together with the fact that *BAM* 9 was a first extract related to the head, could support the text being from around Kiṣir-Aššur's *šamallû ṣeḫru*-phase. *BAM* 9 was also labelled a *ṭuppu*, much like the other numbered extract from his *šamallû ṣeḫru*-phase, *RA* 15 pl. 76. Kiṣir-Aššur's later extracts were not labelled as *ṭuppu*s. However, the evidence is

BA.AN.È ^{26} *šà-ṭír* $^{p.d}$30-[x x] *šá* ^{d}PA NIR-*s*[*u*], but since the name is broken and a genealogy is not mentioned, this text cannot be placed. However, it does originate from the N4 library (Pedersén 1986: 64 no. 188 = Ass. 13955/gz). The text *CT* 15 pl. 43f. published as *SAA* 3 no. 37 is reconstructed by Livingstone (1989: 95) as Kiṣir-Nabû's on the basis of a partially visible [^{d}]⸢PA *ša* ^{d}AG⸣ *tuk-lat-s*[*u*]. However, the text was excavated in Nineveh and the relationship to Kiṣir-Nabû remains uncertain.

62 E.g., Hunger 1968: 98 lines 2–6.

63 Kiṣir-Aššur's texts also include numbered extracts from the *mašmaš bīt Aššur*-phase, thus these texts cannot be generalized according to training (Section 9.2.3).

64 N4 no. 247 rev. 25: *ú-ìl-ti* ^{p}*Ki-ṣir-*^{d}PA MAŠ.MAŠ *ša* [x x x (x)].

tenuous at best. Perhaps the lack of a title should be explained with this text being from before Kiṣir-Aššur officially became *šamallû ṣeḫru*.

BAM 9 contains a catch-line that opens the fragmentary tablet *BAM* 145 with a broken colophon (see Ch. 3 note 38). This text appears to be an exercise of some sort (Köcher 1963a: XII). If *BAM* 145 was copied by Kiṣir-Aššur after *BAM* 9, this would further support *BAM* 9 as an earlier phase tablet. Considering the indications, although none are conclusive, I regard *BAM* 9 as a *šamallû ṣeḫru* tablet in this study.

BAM 121 contains a purpose statement, which indicates that this text is from a later phase of Kiṣir-Aššur's career (see Section 7.4). The combined use of the *ša Nabû tuklassu*-phrase together with a purpose statement may very tentatively indicate this was one of the first tablets Kiṣir-Aššur copied for a healing treatment. I suggest that the text may have been written slightly before or during the *mašmaššu ṣeḫru*-phase, in order to account for the *ša Nabû tuklassu*-phrase combined with a purpose statement.

5.5 Summary

The evidence for Kiṣir-Aššur's *šamallû*-, *šamallû mašmaššu ṣeḫru*- and *mašmaššu ṣeḫru*-phases is problematic as there are few texts, and the manuscripts in general probably cover several years of Kiṣir-Aššur's career. During his *šamallû*-phase, Kiṣir-Aššur copied incantations and brief ritual instructions for treating a "Curse" (*māmītu*), as well as guidelines for performing sections of the ritual *bīt mēseri*. The latter text was copied "for his (own) 'reading'", which suggests an instructive purpose. As a *šamallû mašmaššu ṣeḫru*, Kiṣir-Aššur copied texts connected to the domestic cult and infants. One ritual was aimed at reconciling a man with his god and another at treating ghosts, possibly related to the ancestral cult. Albeit very uncertain, Kiṣir-Aššur may have focused on such rituals to be able to treat possible causes of illness. Another of his *šamallû mašmaššu ṣeḫru* texts, an IM.GÍD.DA, attests to him copying a peculiar tradition of an incantation to calm an infant, baby or child. This focus on infants could be seen in relation to his other texts from this phase, as crying infants were known causes of disturbance for the family cult.

The incantation to calm an infant focused on Lamaštu, a known killer of infants and children. If Kiṣir-Aššur treated infants or children medically is uncertain. In general, such treatments are difficult to identify, and it is possible that adult treatments could be administered in revised versions to infants, babies or children. If so, Kiṣir-Aššur could have treated children, but this remains hypothetical. Nevertheless, there existed an overlap in physiological conceptualisation between infants and horses, which Kiṣir-Aššur had previously encountered as *šamallû ṣeḫru*. As a result, it is possible that he used this overlap to gain deeper insight into human physiology in order to provide better treatments. Due to the increasing economic and cultural worth of horses, children and adults, this chapter hypothesized that Kiṣir-Aššur may have experienced greater autonomy when aiding his father, first when treating horses, thereafter infants or children, and finally adults. If so, Kiṣir-Aššur would have been able to build upon previous insights into animal-human physiology. The argumentation follows the microhistoric approach seeking to illuminate the subject's world via comparative evidence to fill gaps in the documentation.

Kiṣir-Aššur was probably still training to become an exorcist during his *mašmaššu ṣeḫru*-phase, although the evidence is unclear (see Sections 5.3.1 and 6). His sole text from this phase consists of an *u'iltu* with two incantations and instructions. At least one of the incantations duplicates a relative simple spell used elsewhere for treating "Anus illness" (DÚR.GIG), which is ordinarily considered a relatively simple ailment (see Sections 3.1 and 3.1.1). The content of Kiṣir-Aššur's manuscript was described as "tested prescriptions, which are *suitable for use*(?)". In the surviving material, such statements were mainly employed after Kiṣir-Aššur became *mašmaššu* (see Sections 6.2.2 and 8.3; cf. Section 5.3). The text suggests that Kiṣir-Aššur acquired certain treatments considered useful for practice during his *mašmaššu ṣeḫru*-phase. Comparative material from Kiṣir-Aššur's nephew, Kiṣir-Nabû, indicates that initiation into advanced knowledge may have begun during the *mašmaššu ṣeḫru*. The fact that the material copied in Kiṣir-Aššur's sole text from this phase may have been used for treating "Anus illness", implies it may not have been considered advanced knowledge. Furthermore, his *šamallû* manuscript N4 no. 175 suggests that he began copying texts for gaining a deeper understanding of the content earlier during his training.

Concerning the differences in skill and responsibility that may be implied in the sequence of titles borne by Kiṣir-Aššur before he became *mašmaššu*, a number of relevant observations have been presented throughout Chapters 3–5. However, the publication of further texts assigned to Kiṣir-Aššur may alter individual observations as well as the importance of identified focuses. We may therefore not yet be in a position to fully understand all aspects of Kiṣir-Aššur's training. Nonetheless, I have argued extensively for my ideas, which are supported by comparative evidence. Thus, I consider the hypothesised progression in patient groups, defined by a social hierarchy and autonomous practice, a likely scenario. Although he copied numerous medical texts with treatments for adults, I have on the basis of thorough discussions proposed that some material could perhaps be modified and applied to animals and children as well (Section 5.2.2). Furthermore, I have argued that he likely aided his father simultaneously in treating adults and preparing healing ceremonies during his training.

Alternative hypotheses may be suggested, although a progression from simple to complex material is not reflected in the material. Almost all of Kiṣir-Aššur's *šamallû ṣeḫru* manuscripts concern healing or rituals instructions for a single individual. During his *šamallû*-phase, he copied two rituals related to the individual and his house. As a *šamallû mašmaššu ṣeḫru*, Kiṣir-Aššur copied texts connected to the domestic cult and infants. When he became *mašmaššu ṣeḫru*, he learned tested healing procedures. As a *mašmaššu*, he copied an increasing number of different text types relevant to practice (Chapter 6), and a wide variety of rituals were copied during this and his *mašmaš bīt Aššur*-phase (Chapter 8). Thus, a tentative progress from individual to household in terms of illness, and finally a change in focus towards social problems, evil omens and official cult can be proposed.

CHAPTER 6

Kiṣir-Aššur's *mašmaššu*-phase

In this and the following chapter, I examine the *mašmaššu*-phase of Kiṣir-Aššur's training, alongside associated material from the *mašmaššu*- and *mašmaš bīt Aššur*-phases. Chapter 6 consists of a close examination of the texts that can be securely assigned to this phase by means of the colophons, in which Kiṣir-Aššur is identified as a *mašmaššu*, and it provides an in-depth discussion of the significance of some of these texts for Kiṣir-Aššur's career. In chapter 7, the tablets that can be assigned to the *mašmaššu*-phase on the basis of text-internal criteria are discussed, even though they do not explicitly identify Kiṣir-Aššur as *mašmaššu*. The medical texts from Kiṣir-Aššur's *mašmaššu*-phase are discussed in relation to his entire production of magico-medical texts in Section 9.1.

The texts written during the *mašmaššu*-phase indicate that Kiṣir-Aššur's education was not completed until sometime during this phase, yet the precise date on which he would have "graduated" is unclear. It is possible that we have to assume an on-the-job transition from student or trainee to independent practitioner, but this has to remain hypothetical. If my reconstruction is correct, it is possible that some time after he was qualified as an exorcist he was able to begin treating patients on his own, i.e., without supervision, and he was also allowed to conduct house calls.

6.1 Texts with Colophons including the Title *mašmaššu*

Table 9 shows that only eight tablets can be securely assigned to Kiṣir-Aššur's *mašmaššu*-phase of training, as well as one text that may have been copied by either Kiṣir-Aššur or Kiṣir-Nabû. As in the previous phases, none of the tablets are dated. Consequently, the tablets are discussed according to their contents, because no chronological order or sequencing can be established at this point.

I have tentatively grouped the tablets in groups of medical texts, ritual texts, and other technical literature perhaps connected to scholarship. The tablets indicate that Kiṣir-Aššur focused on more diverse areas, in contrast with the earlier phases of his education. According to the available evidence, it is also the first time since the *šamallû ṣeḫru*-phase that he copied symptom descriptions with medical diagnoses. During this phase he also copied out treatments

© TROELS PANK ARBØLL, 2021 | DOI:10.1163/9789004436084_007

TABLE 9 Texts assigned to Kiṣir-Aššur's *mašmaššu*-phase[a]

Group	Text	Content	Format and designation
Medical texts	*BAM* 81	Obverse: (broken) Reverse: three prescriptions for a bandage against *maškadu*-illness (rev. 1'–7'), a potion to be drunk (rev. 8'–9') and an enema (rev. 10'–16')	Portrait; *u'iltu*
	BAM 102	Obverse (broken) and reverse: one broken incantation (rev. 1') against "Anus illness" (DÚR.GIG) (rev. 2'), where the ritual is explicitly "not written" (rev. 3')	Landscape; IM.GÍD.DA
	BAM 122	Obverse: three prescriptions for a bandage (obv. 1–7) and a wash (obv. 8–15) against a shin repeatedly slackening (obv. 1), hurting feet that change place with one another with paralysis and stiff "strings" (obv. 8–10) and paralyzed feet where the patient has difficulty walking (obv. 16–17) Reverse: one broken entry (rev. 1') and four prescriptions for a bandage (rev. 2'–10'), ointment (rev. 11'–17') and a potion to be drunk (18'–19') against stiff "strings" of the feet where the patient is unable to walk (rev. 2'–4', cf. rev. 11'–13')	Portrait; *u'iltu*
Ritual texts	*KAL* 4 no. 7	Obverse and reverse: one prayer (obv. 11'–15') and three instructions (obv. 7'–10', rev. 1'–3', 4'–6') for a *namburbi*-ritual against witchcraft (obv. 1'–6')	(Fragmentary, portrait?); *u'iltu*(?)

a Bibliography for individual tablets can be found in Appendix 1. The colophon of *BAM* 81 is partly reconstructed and could also have referred to Kiṣir-Aššur as *mašmaššu* (*ṣeḫru*): MAŠ.[MAŠ (TUR?)].

TABLE 9 Texts assigned to Kiṣir-Aššur's *mašmaššu*-phase (*cont.*)

Group	Text	Content	Format and designation
	KAR 230	Obverse and reverse: incantation (obv. 1–14) for the exorcist going to the patient's house and a ritual instruction (obv. 16–rev. 8) involving figures of Marduk and Ninurta, followed by a secrecy formula (rev. 9–11)	Portrait; *u'iltu*
	KAR 298	Obverse and reverse: 25 entries providing instructions with incantation incipits (obv. 2–11, 12–14, 15–16, 17–18, 19–20, 21–25, 26–28, 29–32, 33–37, 38–40, 41–42, 43–44, 45–46, 47–48, rev. 1–2, 3, 4–5, 6–7, 8, 9–10, 11–12, 13, 14, 15–17, 17–22) for producing figurines for the ritual "To block (the entry of) 'the foot of evil' into a man's house" (obv. 1) and eight entries providing instructions (rev. 23–25, 26–29, 30–35, 36–37, 38–40, 41–42, 43–44, 45–46) for rituals connected with "To avert *di'u*-illness, plague and epidemic"	Portrait; [...]
	LKA 115	Obverse and reverse: *namburbi*-ritual against any observation in a man's house (obv. 1–2), ritual instruction (obv. 3–8), incantation with instructions(?) (obv. 9–rev. 6') and final instruction (rev. 7'–9')	Portrait; N/A
Other texts	*CT* 37 pl. 24f.	Obverse and reverse (col. i–iv): bilingual Lú lexical list providing entries with Sumerian titles for professions with Akkadian translations	Two-columned; [...]

TABLE 9 Texts assigned to Kiṣir-Aššur's *mašmaššu*-phase (*cont.*)

Group	Text	Content	Format and designation
		Kiṣir-[Aššur/Nabû?]	
Ritual texts	*LKA* 146	Obverse and reverse: mythological incantation (obv. 1–21) related to 21 *mêlu*-poultices from Ea (obv. 22–23) and instructions (obv. 24–rev. 15, 16–24(?)) for making these	Portrait; *u'iltu*

of illnesses related to the lower body and the "strings" (*BAM* 81 and 122),[1] on which he may have focused later as well, and it is likely also the first time that he copied *namburbi*-rituals. Among the limited medical texts from Kiṣir-Aššur's *mašmaššu*-phase, *BAM* 81 contains a prescription possibly against *maškadu*, which partly duplicates another treatment in *BAM* 122 likely designed for ill feet.[2]

Other text genres copied during this phase were rituals connected to ill patients (a ritual for going to a patient's house, *KAR* 230) and preventing evil and illness from entering a house (a ritual intended to safeguard a house from evil demons, *KAR* 298). The only non-related text is *CT* 37 pl. 24f., which is a fragmentary copy of a Lú lexical list (Veldhuis 2014: 252–53; Civil 1969: 223ff.).[3]

1 The *maškadu*-illness treated in *BAM* 81 is compared to modern vertebral arthritis and muscle strains (see Scurlock and Andersen 2005: 257–58, 488, 505, 720 with further references), but can also affect the *qablu*, groin/thigh area, maybe the renal and rectal functions, and the "strings" of the lower body producing stiffness (see Arbøll 2018a; Wasserman 2012; Geller 2005: 3).

2 *BAM* 81 rev. 8'–9', *BAM* 122 rev. 18'–19', and N4 no. 210 = *BAM* 257 rev.$^{?}$ 11–16:

BAM 122 rev. 18': ^{ú}TE.GÍL$^{!}$.LA ^{ú}*pu-qut-tú*

BAM 81 rev. 8'a: KI.MIN ^{ú}*ti-gi-la-a* ^{ú}*pu-qut-tú* →

BAM 257 rev.$^{?}$ 11–12: ^{ú}*ti-gi-la* ^{12} ^{ú}*pu-qut-tú*

BAM 122 rev. 19': ^{ú}K[A.Z]A[L.L]Á$^{?}$ *{x}* *ina* KAŠ NAG

BAM 81 rev. 8b–9: ^{ú}KA.ZAL.LÁ ^{9} UR.BI SÚD *ina* KAŠ NAG-*šú-ma* TI

BAM 257 rev.$^{?}$ 13–16: ^{ú}KA.ZAL.LA ^{14} ^{ú}*kur-ka-nu-u* ^{15} 4 Ú sa-[x x (x)] ^{16} *ina* KAŠ NAG

It is uncertain if Kiṣir-Aššur intended to produce a phonetic writing of *tigilû*/*tegilû* in *BAM* 81 and *BAM* 122, or if the Sumerogram was written in a peculiar manner. I follow the *CAD* (T: 397) in my transliteration. *BAM* 257 rev.$^{?}$ 15 may have held an illness name, e.g., SA.[GAL(?)].

3 See Pedersén 1985: 20. *CT* 37 pl. 24f. is edited alongside a number of other tablets generally labelled with the title "Miscellaneous LU-lists" 6.212 ms B (Civil 1969: 225ff.).

LKA 146, copied by either Kiṣir-Aššur or Kiṣir-Nabû, contains a mythological incantation that describes how Ea endowed humanity with 21 poultices and provides the associated prescriptions for these (*LKA* 146; Lambert 1980; Lambert 1956: 144; cf. Lawson 1994: 47–48).

Several of the tablets contain specific features that either are observed for the first time (see below) or appear during the *mašmaššu*-phase, although one would expect such types of texts earlier. An example of the latter is the IM.GÍD.DA (lit.: "long tablet") label found in *BAM* 102. The NA reading of the label remains uncertain,[4] but it is typically interpreted as having had an education or pedagogical function throughout most periods.[5] The label therefore either indicates that Kiṣir-Aššur was not fully trained as a *mašmaššu* or that the label was used differently in N4. Kiṣir-Aššur also copied another IM.GÍD.DA, N4 no. 24, during his *šamallû mašmaššu ṣeḫru*-phase and he or Kiṣir-Nabû copied the single-columned tablet *BAM* 206 in portrait format during an uncertain phase (Section 5.2). Although the term IM.GÍD.DA may not necessarily refer to format during the NA period, both *BAM* 102 and N4 no. 24 were copied as single-column tablets in landscape orientation.

LKA 115 is not only one of the first *namburbi*-rituals from Kiṣir-Aššur, which can be assigned to a career phase, but it is also the first tablet containing a "purpose statement", i.e., a statement declaring that the content was copied "for undertaking a (ritual) procedure" (*ana ṣabāt epēši*). Such statements are investigated in Section 7.4. *LKA* 115 also states that Kiṣir-Aššur had someone copy the text on his behalf (*ú-šaš-ṭir-ma íb-ri*). Such authority indicates Kiṣir-Aššur was in a position to supervise junior exorcists, and this evidence will be further examined in Section 7.4.2.

The following sections evaluate the specific content and use of Kiṣir-Aššur's *mašmaššu*-phase tablet *KAR* 230 for making house calls, *KAR* 298 for providing rituals securing houses, *LKA* 115 and *KAL* 4 no. 7 in relation to a general discussion on his use of *namburbi*-rituals, and finally *CT* 37 pl. 24f. and its connection to scholarship.

---

4 Possibilities include *imgiddû* (*CAD* I-J: 115), *giṭṭu* (*CAD* G: 112), *liginnu* (*CAD* L: 183), *u'iltu* (ibid.: 184), and *nibzu* (*CAD* G: 113; cf. *CAD* N/2: 206). See also Stevens 2013: 220 note 52; Frahm 2011a: 29 and note 96; Beaulieu 1992: 103 and note 16.

5 For possible uses of IM.GÍD.DA tablets in NB and LB second phase school tablets, see Gesche 2001: 49–50. In NA royal letters, the IM.GÍD.DA tablet perhaps designates a text recited for educational purposes (see Zamazalová 2011: 324; Livingstone 2007: 104–5; *SAA* 10 no. 39 rev. 8–9 *SAA* 16 no. 28 obv. 3–4). The term was used in the advanced pedagogical tablets from the later phases of education in the LB Urukean libraries (Stevens 2013: 219–20). Note that "extraneous" (*aḫû*) scholarly knowledge is occasionally written on IM.GÍD.DA tablets (e.g., Fincke 2001: 23–25).

6.2 Making House Calls: Discussion of *KAR* 230

It is possible that making house calls could be interpreted as marking the transition from trainee to practitioner. We know that exorcists made house calls to diagnose illnesses and cure them. The opening phrase of the 1st subseries of Sa-gig was also the name of the series: "When the exorcist goes to the house of the sick man" *enūma ana bīt marṣi āšipu illaku* (Heeßel 2000: 19, 20–21).[6] Furthermore, several healing ceremonies explicitly refer to the house and especially the bed of the patient.[7] Although it has been suggested that patients were treated in their homes because of impurity (Avalos 1995: 177–82), Stol has stressed that phrases such as "his bed has seized him" must be considered as evidence that one was also bedridden in a physical sense (Stol 1997: 408; Arbøll 2019; see *CAD* E: 318a for examples).

There is no indication before Kiṣir-Aššur's *mašmaššu*-phase that he was in charge of patients and made house calls to diagnose and treat people's maladies on his own. The unedited text *KAR* 230, written during Kiṣir-Aššur's *mašmaššu*-phase, may designate the critical point at which Kiṣir-Aššur was considered qualified to be responsible for a patient's healing.[8] The text consists of a Babylonian ritual for making house calls and contains an incantation and ritual designated as: "Recitation: the exorcist goes to the house of the sick man".[9] Heeßel (2000: 70 and note 7) originally saw this incantation as a means for the exorcist to determine the cause of an illness en route to the patient's house, although this was not necessarily the only purpose. The text remains unedited and without known duplicates. In what follows, I discuss some aspects of the incantation and ritual instruction in *KAR* 230 in order to contextualize this text in relation to Kiṣir-Aššur's use during his *mašmaššu*-phase.

6 A. 3739a+b (Geers 1926) obv. 1: DIŠ *e-nu-ma ana* É GIG KA.PIRIG GIN-*ku* (Labat 1951: 2). For the reading KA.PIRIG as *mašmaššu*/*āšipu*, see Geller 2010: 45–50; Geller 2007c: 5–6; Jean 2006: 26–31; Heeßel 2001–02: 28. Note *KAR* 26 obv. 25 in a prayer to Marduk that mentions that the exorcist does not walk along the streets without Marduk (Mayer 1999: 150, 157; see Schwemer 2007b: 57–58; Jean 2006: 184). Whether or not the N4 exorcists practiced healing in their own home remains uncertain (cf. Robson 2019: 130, 259; May 2014: 64, 78).

7 The bed is also mentioned in several symptom descriptions. For examples concerning a bed, see Farber 2014: 171, 187, 193; *CMAwR* 1: 35, 91–92, 119, 144, 240, 329, 343–44, 359, 397–98, 440; Schramm 2001: 8–9; Stol 1993: 25, 38–41, 49–50, 72; Wiggermann 1992: 108–110, 116, 121. See also Kiṣir-Aššur's reference to the patient's bed in *BAM* 129 (Farber 2004: 127 note 54).

8 Nils Heeßel is currently preparing new copies and editions of *KAR* 230 and *KAR* 31. For the latter text, see below. I would like to thank him for discussing *KAR* 230 and sharing his personal notes with me.

9 *KAR* 230 obv. 15: KA.INIM.MA ^{lú}MAŠ.MAŠ *ana* É ^{lú}GIG DU-*ma*.

6.2.1 *The Incantation of* KAR *230*

The first line of the incantation in *KAR* 230 states: "Incantation: Who attacked him (i.e., the patient) and changed his mind? His heels [*are swollen*(?), and] he is unable to [wa]lk about".[10] The line refers to two commonplace evils encountered in Mesopotamian diagnostics, namely the "attack" (*maqātu*) of a god or demon (Salin 2015; Heeßel 2000: 1–6; van der Toorn 1985: 68–69), indicating the physical symptoms, and the "changed mind" (*ṭēmu šanû*), indicating a mental illness (*CAD* Ṭ: 95–96; Arbøll 2019 with references; Stol 2009; Kinnier Wilson 1965).

The word *ṭēmu* combined with the verb *šanû* "to be changed, become different" indicates an alteration of the mind, which is often translated as "insane" (*CAD* Ṭ: 95–96d ; Stol 2009; Farber 1977: 74–75). However, an affected *ṭēmu* is also occasionally hinted at during severe illness or imbalance.[11] In *SAA* 10 no. 196, for example, an advice reads: "not eating and not drinking confuse (D-stem *ašāšu*) the mind (*ṭēmu*) and *adds to* illness" (Parpola 1993: 159; *CAD* Ṭ: 95b).[12] Likewise, a variant in a diagnosis in Sa-gig illustrates a concrete affliction's diagnostic traditions, ranging from physical to psychological: "[If …] his affliction keeps changing: (*var.*) his mentality keeps changing, 'Hand' of Sîn […]".[13] Although *ṭēmu šanû* refers specifically to a state of insanity, and not a generic symptom of illness,[14] it is not impossible that the phrase in *KAR* 230 intends to cover other alterations of the mind as well.

Several lines of the incantation are too broken to be completely restored, although the recitation seems to relate to whether or not a divine power can hurt the patient.[15] The more legible ending reads:

---

10 See Heeßel 2000: 70 note 7. Obv. 1–2: ÉN *man-nu im-qut* UGU-*šú-ma ú-*⸢*šá*⸣*-an-ni ṭè-en-šú* [2] *eq-ba-*⸢*šú*?⸣ [MÚ?.MÚ?-*ma i-tál*]*-lu-ku ul i-le-*ʾ*i*. For the provisional readings of line two, see similar examples in *CAD* E: 248; *BAM* 122 rev. 2′–3′, 11′–12′ (Nils Heeßel, personal communication). Obv. 1 literally opens "who fell on his 'top' (*muḫḫu*)", and in combination with the reference to "heel" (*eqbu*) in obv. 2, it is possible the text intended to hint at the head-to-toe arrangement found in, e.g., Sa-gig, Ugu, and the AMC.

11 Perhaps this is why *imḫur-ešrā*, "it cures twenty (maladies)", was also considered good against *ši-ni-it ṭè-me* (Stadhouders 2012: 16; Stadhouders 2011: 35 line 53′). Note also an OB letter stating: "… I was almost insane for three days. I did not touch food or even water" (Oppenheim 1967: 87).

12 *SAA* 10 no. 196 rev. 16–18: *la a-*[*ka*]*-lu la šá-tu-u* [17] *ṭè-e-mu ú-šá-šá* [18] *mur-ṣu ú-rad*.

13 Sa-gig tablet 19/20 line 13′: [DIŠ …] DAB-*su* KÚR.KÚR-*ir* : UMUŠ-*šú* KÚR.KÚR-*ir* ŠU ^{d}30 […] (Scurlock 2014: 177, 179; Wee 2015: 273; Heeßel 2000: 227; cf. Wee 2012: 608, 679). The reference may refer to changes in behaviour in connection to either physical or psychological symptoms.

14 Although it is unclear if a delirium could be included in this state.

15 E.g., obv. 8 … *ana ka-me* ZÚ.KU[D? …], "in order to bind the bit[e]".

Obv. 10 *a-na* KUR.NU.GI.A
Obv. 11 GIM ^{lú}ÚŠ NU *rud-u* TI.LA[16]
Obv. 12 *ù* ^{d}*Kù-bu la in-ni-qu* GA AMA-*šú*
Obv. 13 *a-pa-qid-ka* {⸢*ki*⸣} *ana* 7 ^{d}Ì.DU$_8$.GAL *šá* ^{d}*ereš-ki-gal*[17]
Obv. 14 *mim-ma lem-nu* NU TE-*a-šú šá* ^{d}MAŠ EN INIM *šu-ú* ÉN

To *kurnugia* (the Netherworld), like a dead man cannot 'add (to) life' and Kūbu (the divine stillborn baby) cannot suckle the milk of its mother, I entrust you to the seven gatekeepers (*idugallu*) of Ereškigal; *mimma lemnu* shall not approach him! It is (an incantation) of Ninurta, lord of the command.[18]

These lines imply that the malady was sent to the netherworld.[19] The text symbolically cuts off the devouring malady by referring to the dead's inability to become well and the divine unborn fetus *Kūbu*'s inability to suck at its mother's breast (Stol 2000: 26–32). The demonic force is then handed over (*paqādu*) to the gatekeepers of Ereškigal and thereafter kept in the netherworld.[20] Finally, the incantation specifies that the generic *mimma lemnu* "Any Evil" should not approach the patient, and that this command – i.e., the entire incantation – is a spell of Ninurta.

16 It is unclear how to interpret the signs after NU. I have chosen to read *rud-u* for D-stem *ruddû* "to add" (*CAD* R: 239–243), although the writing is ackward. In at least one NA letter, a verbal form of *ruddû* and *balāṭu* are used in hendiadys to designate "to feel better" (ibid.: 243). Alternatively, the sign *rud* could be emended to TUK$^{!}$-*u* for *rašû* ""to acquire, obtain", although the writing seems to be unattested (cf. *CAD* R: 193ff.). An unlikely alternative would be ŠÌTA-*u* for *rāṭu* "sustenance tube", though it would be unclear why it should have a long –*u*. For *rāṭu* in general, see *CAD* R: 220c; van der Toorn 1996: 60–61; Tsukimoto 1985: 23–26. Another solution is to interpret the reading as corrupt.

17 Ebeling writes "rasur" on the copy *KAR* 230 in relation to the *ki* in obv. 13, although this is not entirely clear on the original. This requires further collation. The use of *paqādu* "to entrust" is also used of patients in relation to protective deities or sections of the royal palace in which case it may indicate confinement or protection (see Parpola 1983a: 109–10). See also the negative use of *paqādu* in relation to pregnancy and children (Steinert 2018d: 269).

18 Obv. 9 likely contains the verbal form *a-ṭa-rad-ka* "I will send you away".

19 This seems to resemble the purpose of the Ištar-Dumuzi rituals published by Farber (1977), wherein the generic evil *mimma lemnu* is also mentioned several times (ibid.: 9). Note that Kiṣir-Aššur's only dated text, *KAR* 267, contained a ritual associated with these Ištar-Dumuzi rituals (see Section 7.5). However, Kiṣir-Aššur is not supplied with a title in the text's colophon.

20 These gatekeepers are referenced in the myth of Nergal and Ereškigal, see Ponchia and Luukko 2013: 13, 23. Only one gatekeeper (^{lú}Ì.DU$_8$) is specified in Ištar's Descent, see Lapinkivi 2010: 9, 29.

Several largely unedited Ḫulbazizi incantations also revolve around themes of identifying *mimma lemnu* (*at-ta man-nu mim-ma lemnu*), and at least one example explicitly hands the evil over (*paqādu*) to the doorkeepers of the underworld (*SpTU* III no. 82 col. ii 27–33). The incantation therefore addresses any malady that may have come upon a patient and attempts a dismissal of a generic and unidentified evil, perhaps before the healer has provided a diagnosis or as a broadly applicable means against any cause of illness.[21]

6.2.2 *The Ritual and Purpose of* KAR *230*

The ritual instruction largely adds to the above section. The instruction contains four relevant points. First, two figurines of Marduk and Ninurta are made out of wax, the exorcist performs mouth-washing to enable them to receive a number of offerings placed before them on *paṭiru*-tables, and the incantation is recited three times.[22] Thereafter, the incantation is recited three times over the sick patient before performing a *takpirtu* purification rite.[23] Then, the Marduk figurine is placed at the head of the patient's bed and the Ninurta figurine is placed at the lower end, and for one day the incantation is recited three times before them while a brazier is supplied with *burāšu*-juniper.[24] Finally,

21 Another possible example of a universal ritual against many different maladies and various portends is *KAR* 26 (= N2 no. 8), see Schwemer 2007b: 57–58; Mayer 1999; Pedersén 1986: 32.

22 *KAR* 230 obv. 16: NU ^{d}AMAR.UTU *u* ^{d}MAŠ *ša* GAB.LÀL DÙ-*uš*; the end of obv. 17: … MAŠ.MAŠ KA.LUḪ.U.DA DÙ-*uš*, written onto the edge, contains a third person description of what occurs in relation to the presumed second person in obv. 18; obv. 18–19: KA-*šú-nu* LUḪ-*si* GI.DU$_{8}$.MEŠ ^{19} *ina* IGI.MEŠ-*šú-nu* KÉŠ-*as*; offerings in obv. 20–23; obv. 24: ÉN 3-*šú ina* IGI.MEŠ-*šú-nu* ŠID-*nu*, "you recite the incantation 3 times in front of them".

23 *KAR* 230 rev. 1–2: [ÉN] 3-*šú ina* UGU ^{lú}GIG ŠID-*nu* ⸢x$^{?}$⸣ ^{2} EGIR-*šú tak-pir-tu* DÙ-*uš* …

24 *KAR* 230 rev. 3–5: NU ^{d}AMAR.UTU *ina* SAG GIŠ.NÁ NU ^{d}MAŠ *ina* ⸢*še-pit*⸣ [GIŠ.NÁ] ^{4} *ina* UD.1.KAM$^{?}$ ÉN *an-ni-tú* 3-*šú ana* IGI-*šú-nu* ŠID-*nu* $^{5\ (on\ side)}$GIM *ka-a-a-an* NÍG.NA ^{šim}LI GAR-*an* ⸢x (x?)⸣. Both the *ina* (rev. 4) and GIM (rev. 5) are written on the left side, almost as a note, although not in smaller handwriting. This is not entirely clear on Ebeling's copy, but has been collated. The OB adverbial expression *kīma kayyantim*(*ma*) "as normal, customary" is the only example with these two words (*CAD* K: 41; *CDA* 154). Perhaps the GIM was a note to designate to Kiṣir-Aššur that "when(ever you recite the incantation), constantly you …"? The term *kayyān*(*u*) was also used from the 7th century BCE onwards to designate the literal or regular sense of a word in a context in commentaries (Gabbay 2016: 182–194). Although *KAR* 230 likely stems from an older tradition, the GIM is placed conspicuously on the left side of the tablet, which could indicate there was something to notice here for the copyist/reader of the text. However, any interpretative function *kayyān* could possible have in *KAR* 230 is uncertain at this point. For the understanding of supplying a brazier with juniper, see Mayer 1994: 114; Mayer and van Soldt 1991: 112. It is unclear if the sign SAR in the colophon (rev. 12) could indicate an unexpected Š-stem, and

the last two lines of the ritual instruction likely relate to the efficacy of the ritual and how it was obtained:

Rev. 7 *ne-pi*$_5$*-šam lat-ku šu-*⸢*ú*?⸣ [x (x)]
Rev. 8 *ina* KA IM.GÍD.DA *šá ana* <ŠU> È-⸢*u*?⸣[x?]-⸢x x x x⸣-*ḫa*[25]

This is a tested ritual procedure [x?]; [*extra*]*cted*? 'according to' an *imgiddû*-tablet, which (is) *suitable for use* [...].[26]

The ritual itself does not focus on determining the cause of illness. Instead, it produces two figurines of deities that are intended to combat the non-specific evil,[27] provides a purification ritual for the idols and the patient, and provides an attempt at a scholarly reasoning why this ritual was applied and how it was conceived. As such, the ritual intends to protect the patient and provide a "universal" protection ritual, which could presumably be performed at the start of a healing ceremony.

The last section of the ritual instruction cited above describes the ritual as a "tested ritual procedure" (Section 8.3). Furthermore, this section likely states that the text was extracted from an unspecified IM.GÍD.DA, maybe for checking something (e.g., the effect of the ritual?) or possibly considered suitable for use. As a result, the ritual instruction contained a statement similar to those

---

therefore designate that the tablet was copied on Kiṣir-Aššur's behalf by someone else (cf. Ch. 3 note 134).

25 I have interpreted a corrupt reading of the phrase *ša ana qāti šūṣû*, although only *šá ana* and È (*barû, waṣû*) are visible. As such, it is possible that the line referred to "checking" the effect(?) of the ritual procedure. However, if my restoration is correct, the understanding of *ša ana qāti šūṣû* is a problem. Meanings range between "what is at hand, available" or "which is suitable for use(?)" (for references, see *CMAwR* 2: 416; *CMAwR* 1: 64, 121). Abusch and Schwemer (*CMAwR* 1: 235) in one instance cautiously propose: "that *is well proven*" as an alternative translation. The end of the line remains uncertain and needs further collation. However, it seems reasonable to assume the final *ḫa* relates to a verbal form of *nasāḫu*. Perhaps the ending read ⸢ZI!?⸣-*ḫa*, although this reading does not account for the remaining signs. Another possible suggestion could be: [*ḫa-a*]*n-ṭiš* ⸢*as*!*-su*!?⸣*-ḫa* (Nils Heeßel, personal communication).

26 Such tested ritual procedures are also mentioned in, e.g., BAM 322 rev. 89, see Ch. 9 note 147; Steinert 2015: 129 and note 84. See also AMT 105,1 col. iv 21'–24': [*na*]*p-šá-la-tú tak-ṣi-ra-nu lat-ku-tu*$_4$ *ba-ru-ti šá ana* [Š]U? *šu-ṣú-ú* 22' *šá* KA NUN.ME.MEŠ*-e la-bi-ru-ti šá la-am* A.MÀ.URÙ, "Tested (and) proven salves (and) strings of amulet stones, *suitable for use*, from the mouth of ancient sages from before the flood" (Geller 2010: 17 and notes 15–16; Rochberg 2004: 215; Elman 1975: 31; Hunger 1968: 142 no. 533; Reiner 1961: 10 and note 1; Lambert 1957: 8).

27 Marduk and Ninurta were associated with war metaphors, which were regularly invoked by the exorcist, see Böck 2014a: 183–85.

found in colophon describing how the text itself was conceived. However, this was not the colophon, and the statement therefore served another purpose than the copying statements found in colophons. It may have been a description of a scholarly method for obtaining the cure found within the text or simply intended to underline the usefulness of the ritual.

6.2.3 *The Secrecy Statement of* KAR 230

KAR 230 contains a section between the ritual instructions and the final colophon, separated from them by horizontal lines, stating: "A secret of exorcism (*āšipūtu*). An expert may show an expert; a non [exper]t may not see (it). (As) for your son whom you love, make him swear by Asalluḫi and Ninurta and (only) then show (it to) him!" (see Lenzi 2008a: 166–78).[28]

The statement focuses on keeping knowledge within a professional sphere. But how these phrases should be understood is still unclear. Such so-called "secrecy labels" and the associated "*Geheimwissen* colophons"[29] have had a problematic research history due to the recurring problem of their inconsistent and low distribution over time and space (Stevens 2013: 211–13; Lenzi 2008a: 204; Beaulieu 1992: 107).[30] Earlier studies, such as Borger 1957–71, listed the examples and provided a typology. Later, Beaulieu (1992: 109–10), for example, suggested secrecy statements in LB Uruk could work to restrict dissemination of certain learning within a social setting. In the past decade, Lenzi (2008a: 204, 214, 380) conceded that texts with such statements cannot be distinguished from others based on content. However, he suggested that texts with such secrecy statements were "restricted to authorized individuals" (Lenzi 2008a: 160; cf. Stevens 2013: 211 note 3).

Others have argued that the phrases merely attest to professional pride (Koch 1995: 95–96; Livingstone 1986: 1; Neugebauer 1969: 144).[31] Recently, Stevens (2013: 211, 214–15) has reasoned for both secrecy and protective phrases[32] working together towards protecting knowledge and categorising texts linked

---

28 Rev. 9–11: *ni-ṣir-te* MAS.MAŠ.MEŠ ⸢ZU⸣-*a* ⸢ZU⸣-*a* IGI.LÁ ⸢NU⸣ [ZU]-*a* NU IGI.LÁ ^{10} *ana* DUMU-*ka šá ta-*⸢*ram*!⸣-*mu* MU ^{d}*Asal-lú-ḫi* ^{11} *ù* ⸢^{d}MAŠ? *šu*⸣-*úz-kir-šú-ma kul-lim-šú*. See also Rochberg 2004: 212–13. The writing MAŠ.MAŠ.MEŠ may stand for *āšipūtu*, as it does not have a ^{lú} determinative. MEŠ can also be found in writings such as LÚ.MEŠ for *amēlūtu* (see *CMAwR* 1: 310 line 105", 431 line 9).

29 These statements also focus on secrecy, but they are part of the actual colophons.

30 For the most recent overviews, see Stevens 2013: 211 note 3 and Lenzi 2008a: 2–15 with further references.

31 Rochberg (2004: 213) agrees with Neugebauer and takes the term "esoteric" as a reference to exclusivity and therefore not incomprehensibility.

32 These phrases, occurring in colophons, are intended to protect the knowledge, and they include the so-called "*Geheimwissen* colophons" and statements such as: "Whoever

to professional and individual intellectual identity in LB Uruk. As a result, Stevens stated that the marked texts express "a network of clearly articulated relationships between the professional specialism(s) of the individual scholar and the text he sought to protect" (ibid.: 231). Regardless, these results cannot be compared directly to the NA evidence.

Among Kiṣir-Aššur's texts with colophons, two "*Geheimwissen* colophons" are attested: *KAR* 230, copied when Kiṣir-Aššur was *mašmaššu*, and the cultic explanatory text *KAR* 307, copied when he was *mašmaš bīt Aššur*.[33] Considering Kiṣir-Aššur's wider use of protective phrases, such as curses, these are found on seven of Kiṣir-Aššur's texts.[34] Among these texts, four are from his *šamallû ṣeḫru*-phase,[35] two are from his *šamallû*-phase, and one is from his *mašmaš bīt Aššur*-phase. These texts include both numbered extracts (*RA* 15 pl. 76) and text copied according to known rows of entries from standardized therapeutic Nineveh tablets (*BAM* 129, see Section 9.3.4).

No truly recognizable features can be deducted from the texts with secrecy and protective phrases. Although they may have been particularly important to Kiṣir-Aššur, one can easily find groups of texts comparable to these, but without such phrases. The texts relate to all areas of importance for Kiṣir-Aššur's career, i.e., healing (*BAM* 129, *BAM* 131, *RA* 15 pl. 76, *RA* 40 pl. 116), making house calls (*KAR* 230), ritually demarcating houses (N4 no. 175), performing exorcistic rituals (*KAL* 10 no. 4, *LKA* 77), and possibly participating in rituals connected to the Aššur temple (*KAR* 307).

6.2.4 *Interpretation of* KAR *230*

In relation to *KAR* 230, Lenzi (2008a: 167) argued that this secrecy phrase may have represented an actual formalized procedure wherein a father or master may have passed on the knowledge contained on a "secret" tablet to a son or apprentice, and therefore this procedure would have provided "an objective

---

reveres Anu, Ellil and Ea shall not take it (i.e., the tablet) away by theft" (Stevens 2013: 213–14; cf. Lenzi 2008a: 204).

33 The fact that the statement in *KAR* 230 occurs in a separated section could indicate that it was originally part of the text copied. It is therefore not strictly speaking a colophon. Several of the examples listed by Lenzi (2008a: 171–86, 216–19) are from Kiṣir-Aššur and Kiṣir-Nabû's texts, as well as texts excavated within N4. Among Kiṣir-Nabû's texts focusing on secrecy in statements or colophons include *BAM* 199 and N4 no. 80.

34 *BAM* 9, *BAM* 131, *RA* 15 pl. 76, *RA* 40 pl. 116, *KAL* 10 no. 4, *LKA* 77, N4 no. 175. Several of these also contain statements prohibiting the erasure of the copyist's name. See also Beckman and Foster 1988 no. 21, which contains a broken colophon with a prohibition against erasing the copyist's name.

35 Including *BAM* 9, which lacks a title but is placed in this category due to text-internal features. See Section 5.4.

marker in the subordinate's experience to indicate that he passed from normal activity into one that was marked as in some way special". Although this interpretation entails a literal understanding of the statement and a synthesis of ancient practices based on conjecture, it is appealing to accept such an understanding in relation to how *KAR* 230 functioned in Kiṣir-Aššur's training.

Regardless of how the secrecy statement is interpreted, *KAR* 230 may have represented Kiṣir-Aššur's initiation into a special ritual procedure, perhaps particularly appreciated and transmitted within this family.[36] The text is without known duplicates, which underlines its significance among the N4 tablets. Furthermore, the tablet was designated as a "copy from Babylon" and labelled as an *u'iltu*.[37] Such *u'iltu*s can perhaps be considered a commitment of some sort (see Section 5.3.2). Maybe Kiṣir-Aššur was expected to know this or similar rituals as part of his specialized training in order to become a practicing exorcist, and the *u'iltu*-label, if understood as a commitment, may have been the task of acquiring the final pieces necessary to practice.

Presumably, when Kiṣir-Aššur copied *KAR* 230 he acquired the knowledge this text represents (Section 1.4). If this was the case, *KAR* 230 may have been a ritual Kiṣir-Aššur copied before being able to make house calls on his own, although he was already *mašmaššu* at the time and dabbled in scholarly matters (see Section 6.5). Maul (2010a: 216) has suggested that approbation probably took place when one was awarded the title *mašmaššu*, but in this case we may assume the authorization for making house calls may have occurred when Kiṣir-Aššur gained the necessary ritual. I suggest that *KAR* 230 represents the dividing line between Kiṣir-Aššur acting as an assistant and taking charge of a patient's healing. Perhaps Kiṣir-Aššur's family used the secrecy phrase in the particular case of *KAR* 230 to emphasize the meaning of this text. Though this may have been the case, secrecy labels must have varied over time and place and cannot generally be explained in relation to exorcistic training.

6.2.5 *Nabû-bēssunu's Ritual for Approaching a Patient:* KAR *31*

Another ritual from Kiṣir-Aššur's father, Nabû-bēssunu, relates directly to attending patients as a healer. Nabû-bēssunu copied the bilingual incantation *KAR* 31 at an unclear stage of his career (edited in Maul 2018; Geller 2016: 38–39).

36 Lenzi's comment that the content of *KAR* 230 is "nothing special" has been disproven by the analysis above (cf. Lenzi 2008a: 167).

37 *KAR* 230 rev. 12–13: GABA.RI KA.DINGIR.RA[ki] SAR È [13] *ú-ìl-ti* ...

The incantation was a recitation to keep various demons from approaching the exorcist when he approaches a patient.[38] The ritual states:

> Its ritual: grind up male and female *nikiptu*-plant, mix it in honey and ghee, when you will approach the patient, you first anoint yourself, (so that) in order to approach the patient, 'Any evil' (*mimma lemnu*) will not approach you.
>
> GELLER 2016: 40[39]

The incantation and ritual are therefore designed to make the exorcist apply a cream to his skin to protect himself from the potential danger inherent in being in close proximity to illness (Maul 2018: 181; Geller 2016: 40).[40] Such protection for the healer is also prescribed in the third tablet of Udug-ḫul, which in all respects resembles the colophon of the second tablet of Sa-gig: "If you approach a patient; until you cast an incantation onto yourself, you should not approach the patient".[41]

The two incantations and rituals *KAR* 31 and *KAR* 230 therefore cover two crucial areas connected to healing, which are also attested as two vital points in Sa-gig, namely: going to the patient's house and approaching the patient. Whereas *KAR* 230 covers the first part, *KAR* 31 covers the protection of the exorcist when approaching the patient. At least Kiṣir-Aššur and his father

---

38 *KAR* 31 rev. 19–20: KA.INIM.MA GAL$_5$.LÁ MÁŠKIM ^{d}*lugal-ùr-ra* SAG.ḪUL.ḪA.ZA A.LÁ ḪUL ^{20} AN.TA.ŠUB.BA *mim-ma šum-šú ana* MAŠ.MAŠ NU TE-*e*, "Incantation: that the *Gallû*-demon, *Rābiṣu*-demon, Lugal-urra (epilepsy demon), *Sagḫulḫaza*-demon, evil *Alû*-demon, Antašubba-epilepsy, and whatever else should not approach the exorcist" (see Maul 2018: 186, 188; Geller 2016: 39–40). *HKL* (vol. II: 55) lists the Nineveh parallels K. 9836+K. 10338+K. 20638, and K. 10565.

39 *KAR* 31 rev. 21–23: DÙ.DÙ.BI ŠIM.^{d}MAŠ NITA *u* MUNUS SÚD *ina* LÀL *u* Ì.NUN.NA ḪE.ḪE ^{22} *e-nu-ma ana* ^{lú}GIG *te-ṭè-eḫ-ḫu-ú ra-man-ka* 1-*niš* ŠÉŠ-*ma* ^{23} *ana* ^{lú}GIG TE-*ḫe mim-ma lem-nu* NU TE-*ka* (see the pictures in Maul 2018: 178–79).

40 In an OB medical text edited by Wasserman (1996) concerning carbuncles (*kurāru*), the final passage may encourage the healer(?) to protect himself as follows: "[As] soon as he finishes you should *rub* (lit.: anoint) your face so that [the illness will not] return to you"; ibid.: 4–5. Israel Museum 87.56.847 rev. 20–22: [*ki*]-⸢*ma*⸣ *i-ga-am-ma-ru* ^{21} [*i*/*a*]-*na pa-ni-ka ta-pa-aš-ša-/aš-ma* ^{22} [GIG? *ul*?] ⸢*i*⸣-*tu-ur-ra-ku-ma*. See also Gurney's original restoration and interpretation of lines 117–122 in the Poor Man of Nippur (Gurney 1956: 156–57; cf. Stol 1997: 410; Foster 1996: 934).

41 Geller 2016: 40–41; Heeßel 2001–02: 37, 40; Labat 1951: 18–19 and note 27: DIŠ *ana* GIG *ina* TE-*ka* EN ÉN *ana* NÍ-*ka* ŠUB-*ú ana* GIG NU TE-*ḫi*. Note the warning to cast an incantation onto a patient with particular symptoms before approaching him (Wee 2012: 71 note 114; Tsukimoto 1999: 193 lines 41–42).

Nabû-bēssunu seem to have focused on and transmitted this knowledge as part of the family trade.

6.3 Ritually Protecting the Houses of Clients: Discussion of *KAR* 298

Kiṣir-Aššur also copied *KAR* 298 as *mašmaššu*. The text contains several rituals intended to protect households from illness and epidemics. Kiṣir-Aššur had previously worked with prophylactic measures as *šamallû mašmaššu ṣeḫru* in relation to calming a crying child in order to revoke the evils heralded by its cries. However, the rituals in *KAR* 298 provide the performer(s) with the power to keep out various demons and plagues. This is another relatively new area of ritual performance learned by Kiṣir-Aššur during his *mašmaššu*-phase, and the following sections investigate *KAR* 298 and discuss it in relation to Kiṣir-Aššur and his family's use of certain quarantine measures in connection to illness treatments.

6.3.1 *The Purpose and Content of* KAR *298*

KAR 298 contains extracts of two texts listed in the EM as 1) "to block (the entry of) 'the foot of evil' into a man's house" and 2) "to avert *di'u*-illness, plague and epidemic …" (Wiggermann 1992: 41ff., 91).[42] The text likely had a broken label in the colophon and it was "quickly [extracted]".[43]

In order "to block (the entry of) 'the foot of evil' into a man's house", the ritual used protective figurines buried in various places underneath a house. This ensured that *šēp lemutti* "the foot of evil" would not enter a man's house.[44]

42 *KAR* 44 obv. 20: GÌR ḪUL-*tim ina* É LÚ KUD-*is di-ḫu* : *šib-ṭa* NAM.ÚŠ.MEŠ *šu-tu-qí u* SÍSKUR GABA.RI. Wiggermann (1992: 90, 92–93, 219) translates *šibṭu* as "stroke, blow" and relates it to an epidemical illness. Comparatively, *CAD* (Š/2: 387) translates "plague, epidemic" and *AHw* (1228) "Schlag, stoß" from *šabāṭu* "to strike, hit, blow, sweep". *KAR* 298 opens in obv. 1: ⌜*ana* ᵈ⌝A[LAD? NU TE-*ḫ*]*i ù* ⌜GÌR^II x ḪUL⌝ *ina* É NA ⌜KUD-*si*⌝ "to [keep] a *š*[*ēdu*-deity(?) from approachi]ng and to block (the entry of) 'evil …? feet' into a man's house" (cf. Wiggermann 1992: 42).

43 *KAR* 298 rev. 47: […] ᵖ*Ki-ṣir-Aš-šur* MAŠ.MAŠ *za-mar* [(ZI-x?)]. Wiggermann (1992: 41) follows Hunger (1968: 70 = *BAK* 201 ms I line 1) in reconstructing [*ana ṣabāt epēši*] before Kiṣir-Aššur's name. Although this is possible, as something was likely broken before Kiṣir-Aššur's name, it is more plausible that the text contained a copying statement. However, the copy does not show clearly how many signs were broken.

44 The ritual was also performed for Esarhaddon's sister Šadditu in *SAA* 10 no. 273 (cf. Parpola 1983a: 206–7; Maul 1994: 36). Here, the performer Šumaya was deemed "not able" (rev. 16: *la*!-*a le-'e-e*) by the writer Nabû-nadin-šumi, who states that instead of protecting her he "[has *exp*]*osed her*" (rev. 13: [*ú-se*]-*ṣi-a-ši*).

Households experiencing ominous happenings could be diagnosed with *šēp lemutti* "foot of evil", which forewarned about other maladies, such as *mūtānu* "plague" (Wiggermann 1992: 96). Comparable rituals such as "to keep *di'u*-illness (and) plague, pestilence from nearing the horses and the army of the king" (Maul 2013: 18 and note 19) and for purifying the stables (ibid.: 19ff., 22 note 43) suggest (zoonotic) epidemics must have been regularly attested.

Wiggermann (1992) edited both *KAR* 298 (text II) and the standard Nineveh recension of "to block (the entry of) ..." (text I), and he noted several differences between the two texts. The Nineveh recension, for example, describes figurines made of *ēru*, tamarisk, and clay consecutively, whereas *KAR* 298 breaks this sequence to describe groups of related figurines (ibid.: 87). Additionally, *KAR* 298 differs by specifying the place of interment of each statue in the relevant entry, providing more complete descriptions of figures, and quoting incipits of incantations in the relevant instructions (ibid.: 89–90). These discrepancies may stem from an unidentified Assur recension (ibid.: 88), but could also attest to a manageable reference layout for eased use.

Furthermore, *KAR* 298 has double rulings between obverse lines 40–41 and reverse lines 10–11. The first ruling seems to mark a shift from a related group of gods and sages to a group of monsters, whereas the purpose of the second ruling is unclear (Wiggermann 1992: 45). At reverse line 23, the text changes to another group of rituals known as "to make *di'u*-illness, stroke, and plague pass by" (ibid.: 90). This second group of rituals may have had a similar purpose to the first group in *KAR* 298, although they use different means of accomplishing this (ibid.: 91–92). In addition to using wooden ships to carry the illness away (rev. 23–25), the third and penultimate sections prescribe smearing certain substances on the doorpost of the house in question (rev. 41–42), as well as burying substances at the outer gate (rev. 43–44) in order to ensure that witchcraft does not approach a man's house (*CMAwR* 1: 215 ms U, 233, 426 ms B, 428).[45] The third to last entry also specifies the duration of the prophylactic effect: "illness, *di'u*-illness, distress, and pestilence will not come near the man or his house for one year" (*CAD* M/2: 297c).[46]

As mentioned in Section 2.3, many figurines were excavated underneath the floor of the N4 house.[47] However, Wiggermann (1992: 99–100, cf. 102–3)

45 The instructions describe a "creaking gate" to express that witchcraft was approaching (*KAR* 298 rev. 43: DIŠ NA KÁ É-*šú* <*ḫu*>-*ub-bu-ub kiš-pi ana* É NA.B[I] {*ina*} NU TE-*e* ...). Kiṣir-Aššur likely forgot a /*ḫu*/ and wrote an /*ina*/ too much in *KAR* 298 rev. 41. This may be compared to the episode described in Exodus 12.7 regarding marking one's house with sacrificial blood so that the angel of death will pass by one's house.

46 *KAR* 298 rev. 40: ... GIG *di-ḫu di-lip-tú u* ÚŠ.MEŠ *ana* NA *u* É-*šú* MU.1.KAM NU TE-*šú*.

47 See Klengel-Brandt 1968. For protective figures in the Aššur temple, see Huxley 2000.

concluded that the figurines found in N4, albeit the house is incompletely excavated, "show differences with the figurines of the ritual" in details and "their positions do not conform strictly to the prescriptions of the ritual but rather to the general ideas underlying these prescriptions". He conceded, however, that we do not know for what ritual these figurines were installed. Perhaps the rituals in *KAR* 298 were ideal models, which could be modified according to need and context.

Kiṣir-Aššur's hypothesized position as head of ceremonies, possibly foreshadowed by *KAR* 230 as argued above, was likely cemented before or after *KAR* 230 through his acquisition of the relevant rituals for protecting clients' houses in *KAR* 298. *KAR* 298 may represent a convenient *aide mémoire*, which Kiṣir-Aššur could consult easily upon having to perform the necessary part of the rituals. The text is therefore similar to other of his manuscripts concerning the information it provides (e.g., *KAL* 10 no. 1 and N4 no. 175). The inherent responsibility in providing ritual protection for an entire house and its household also indicate that Kiṣir-Aššur was in a capacity to supervise rituals.

6.3.2 KAR *298 in the Context of Associated Rituals*

The focus on keeping out various evils in *KAR* 298 illustrates that Kiṣir-Aššur as *mašmaššu* utilized certain procedures to protect houses. Considering Kiṣir-Aššur's function as a healer, it is not surprising that the rituals in *KAR* 298 contain elements comparable to *bīt mēseri* "the house of confinement", which was a ritual intended to confine a patient already afflicted with a malady (Wiggermann 1992: 105–6).[48] As such, evidence suggests part of the production of figurines in *KAR* 298 could be adapted to serve as a "quarantine procedure" in cases of illness. This is substantiated through associated texts within Kiṣir-Nabû's material discussed in this section.

The ritual *bīt mēseri* was also known in N4. Kiṣir-Aššur copied an overview of the ritual with incantation incipits as *šamallû* (N4 no. 175) as well as part of this ritual(?) during an uncertain phase of training.[49] Furthermore, an extract of the second tablet was excavated in the N4 collection (no. 572, VAT 13666+; Meier 1941–44, ms C). Unfortunately, both Kiṣir-Aššur's texts and the

48 The ritual appears as "to confine the patient", *marṣa ana esēri* in the "almanac of the exorcist" (Wiggermann 1992: 105–6 with references to texts). Udug-ḫul tablet 12 was largely duplicated in *bīt mēseri* (Geller 2016: 16; Wiggermann 1992: 113–14; Gurney 1935: 76ff.). Geller (2016: 16) also notes a relationship between Udug-ḫul tablet 12 and *KAR* 298.

49 The tablet is N4 no. 254, which remains unpublished. Reportedly, the colophon is broken. The first incantations(?) from the four tablets of *bīt mēseri* may be listed in an incantation catalogue from N4 no. 291 (= VAT 13723+) published as text A in Geller 2000, see fragment A_2 lines 4'–6' (ibid.: 232; cf. Meier 1941–44: 139).

ritual series *bīt mēseri* in general remain largely unpublished and unedited.[50] Generally, *bīt mēseri* used a number of figurines and drawings, which through incantations and rituals rid the patient and his house of demons, as well as ensuring that additional evils were kept out of the house (Seidl and Sallaberger 2005–06: 67; Wiggermann 1992: 106–13; Meier 1941–44: 140). A certain type of figurine produced in both *KAR* 298 and *bīt mēseri* includes depictions of "sages" (*apkallus*).[51] However, ritual loci,[52] actions performed during and after the ritual,[53] as well as the use of some depictions[54] differed in several instances between *KAR* 298 and *bīt mēseri*.

Nonetheless, there is further evidence for the use of rituals demarcating houses to exclude or expel evil among the Bāba-šuma-ibni family members, through their association with an incantation known as: "The house is put under a spell" (*tummu bītu*). The so-called "Curse, curse" rituals (Sag-ba sag-ba; Schramm 2001: 12) were used for producing flour circles to create ritual enclosures, and these also made use of this incantation. The incantation was also associated with *bīt mēseri* (Wiggermann 1992: 105, 111–12, 117). The incantation is mentioned on the fifth tablet of *bīt mēseri* (*AMT* 34,2) where a goat (*urīṣu*/ MÁŠ) was tied to the head of the patient.[55] A similar "scapegoat" ritual was

50 Sections of the ritual have been published in various locations: Wiggermann 1992: 105–17 collected a majority of references; see also Lenzi 2008b; Borger 1994; Borger 1974; Reiner 1961; Meier 1941–44: 139ff. See also *SpTU* II no. 8 and *SpTU* III no. 69.

51 Wiggermann 1992: 108–9; Borger 1974: 186; Reiner 1961: 6; see also Lenzi 2008b: 145; Borger 1994; Parpola 1993: XVII–XXI. Furthermore, Udug-ḫul tablet 12 was largely duplicated in *bīt mēseri* (Geller 2016: 16; Wiggermann 1992: 113–14; Gurney 1935: 76ff.). Both *KAR* 298 and *bīt mēseri* use figurines of Lulal (LÚ.LÀL, "Honey man") and Lātarāk, which were both related to Dumuzi in an apotropaic function (Wiggermann 2010: 344–345; Wiggermann 1992: 52, 64, 100, 111). Kiṣir-Aššur copied a ritual related to the Ištar-Dumuzi rituals (Farber 1977) as *mašmaš bīt Aššur* (Section 8.5).

52 The initial focus in *bīt mēseri* was the bedroom from which the ritual radiates out (Seidl and Sallaberger 2005–06: 67).

53 *Bīt mēseri* ended with the removal of figurines and drawings, and throwing the figurines in the river (Seidl and Sallaberger 2005–06: 67 and note 38).

54 See Wiggermann 1992: 102–3, 116.

55 Wiggermann 1992: 111–12; *AMT* 34,2 obv. 1 and 5: [... MÁŠ] *ina* SAG [lú]GIG KÉŠ ... [5] [...] ŠID-*nu* ⌜DA?⌝ ÉN *tu-mu* É ŠID-*ú*. Cf. Udug-ḫul tablet 12 line 159–60: *ana mi-iḫ-ri-it er-ši-šú ú-ri-ṣa ina re-eš mar-ṣu ir-ku-us* [160] [giš]ÙRI.GAL *ina re-ši-šú ú-zaq-qip*, "he tied a goat to the patient's head at the front of his bed, he set up an *urigallu*-standard at the (patient's) head" (Geller 2016: 430). Such *urigallu*-standards were also featured individually or in groups in *bīt rimki*, *mīs pî*, *šēp lemutti ina bīt amēli parāsu* and *bīt mēseri* (Seidl and Sallaberger 2005–06: 61–71). For a relationship between *bīt mēseri* and *mīs pî*, see Walker and Dick 2001: 9, 15. The Assyrian sacred tree possibly was also named *urigallu* (Selz 2014: 662 with references; Seidl and Sallaberger 2005–06: 54–61.

known as "a substitute for Ereškigal" (Tsukimoto 1985: 125ff. with references),[56] and it was copied by both Kiṣir-Aššur as *šamallû ṣehru* (N4 no. 289) and Kiṣir-Nabû at an uncertain stage of his career (*LKA* 79).

Tummu bītu was featured in two of Kiṣir-Nabû's commentaries,[57] perhaps indicative of its likely use as part of advanced education (Gesche 2001: 176; Finkel 1991: 102). Unfortunately, only individual lines of *tummu bītu* are known, e.g., via Kiṣir-Nabû's commentaries.[58] The commentaries are fortunately illustrative and show that the incantation focused on ritually demarcating a house:[59]

> The house is put under a spell, the floor has been prepared,
> (*Meaning*) GIŠ.ḪUR *is esēqu* (*which*) *is* 'to incise, make a drawing' (*which*) *is* a drawing,[60]
> Do not enter to him through the window of the side (of the house),
> (*Meaning*) the window of the bathroom (*bīt ramāki*),
> … (*Variety of windows follows with explanations*) …
> Ditto (i.e., do not enter to him) hidden in the shadow of a man,
> (*Meaning*) in secret,
> … (*Variety of entrance-related materials follows with explanations*).[61]

The incantation therefore emphasizes shutting out evil and denying it a place to hide within a house. This mirrors the purpose of the rituals in the prophylactic

56 *LKA* 79 obv. 1: *ana pu-u-ḫi* LÚ *a-na* ᵈ*Ereš-k*[*i-gal* …]. For some examples of rituals employing scapegoats, see Geller 2016: 430; Maul 2013: 28; Maul 1994: 98.

57 *AfO* 12 pl. 13–14, N4 no. 220. See Frahm 2011a: 121–23.

58 See for example Frahm 2018b and Frahm et al. 2013a; Wiggermann 1992: 117. For this incantation, see Farber 2014: 257; *CMAwR* 1: 397; Schramm 2008: 22–23; Böck 2003: 6; Schramm 2001: 8–9; Wiggermann 1992: 111–12; Finkel 1991: 102 no. 30; Borger 1969: 10–12 and Borger 1970a: 172; Abusch 1974: 254 note 10.

59 Cf. Schramm 2001: 8, 12. In *muššu'u*, *tummu bītu* is recited at the end of the ritual alongside the Sag-ba sag-ba incantation, see Böck 2003: 6–8, rev. 38–42: "The incantation 'Oath, oath' (Sag-ba sag-ba) – you draw a circle of flour [around the sickbed]. 39 The incantation 'Be conjured, house' (*tummu bītu*) – you pile up roasted flour and 40 you draw a circle of flour around the gate. You close the gate, but your hand does not have to touch the door!". The incantation is also used in a ritual intended to secure "brisk trade" of the innkeeper where various types of dust and fluids are smeared onto a man's door (Panayotov 2013; Caplice 1974: 23–24).

60 "Has been prepared" is written *šu-ta-as-suq* and must stem from the verbal root *nasāqu* and therefore not *esēqu* as stated in the text itself (Frahm 2018b: note 1).

61 See Frahm 2018b with commentary; Meier 1937–39: 241–43. *AfO* 12 pl. 13–14 obv. 1–4, 11–12: ÉN *tùm-me* É *qaq-qa-ru šu-ta-as-*⌜*suq*⌝ 2 GIŠ.ḪUR: *e-se-qu* : *e-se-qu* : *iṣ-ṣur-tú* 3 [*ina*] ⌜*ap*⌝*-ti ṣe-li la te-rab-šú* 4 *ap-tu šá* É *ra-ma-ki* … 11 *ina* GISSU *pu-uz-ri* ⌜LÚ⌝ KI.MIN 12 *ina pi-i-ši-ri* …; the obverse of the commentary N4 no. 220 seems to comment on the same lines. Cf. the related text Wiggermann 1992: 117 and fig. 8.

KAR 298 and the curative *bīt mēseri*. Several elements in this and associated rituals therefore appear to have functioned as a sort of "quarantine", admittedly more ritually than medically.[62] KAR 298 and its associated rituals include procedures for marking the gate of a patient's house.[63] Although such actions were ritualistic, these markings could also have indicated that the home of the patient was that of an afflicted patient under treatment.

6.4 *Namburbi*-rituals and House Calls: KAL 4 no. 7 and LKA 115

Rituals designed to remove the future effects of an evil omen were called *namburbi*-rituals (lit.: "its release").[64] Kiṣir-Aššur copied the *namburbi*-rituals KAL 4 no. 7 and LKA 115 as *mašmaššu*, the former to release the evil portended and caused by witchcraft[65] and the latter to avert the evil portended by any observation made within a man's house (*CMAwR* 2: 427–30 no. 11.5 ms A; Maul 1994: 446–52, 502ff.). KAL 4 no. 7 may be a copy by Aššur-šākin-šumi from one of Kiṣir-Aššur's tablets (see below), whereas LKA 115 was copied on the request of Kiṣir-Aššur (*ú-šaš-ṭir-ma íb-ri*), presumably by an apprentice, and thereafter checked by Kiṣir-Aššur.

These are the first *namburbi*-rituals attributed to any career phase with certainty.[66] The attestation of *namburbi*-rituals, whereof LKA 115 was copied

62 Geller (2010: 144) points to the LB commentary *SpTU* I no. 27 and the omen: "If a pig enters into the bedroom, a female captive will enter [into] her master's house", obv. 14': [ŠÀ-*bu-u*] DIŠ ŠÁḪ *ana qé-reb ur-ši* KU$_4$-*ub e-si-ir-ti* [*ana*] É EN-*šú* ⌜KU$_4$⌝-*ub* (see also George 1991: 155). Here, the "female captive" suggests "the sick man's confinement", obv. 15': … *a-si-ir-ti šá* E-*ú e-sér* ^{lú}GIG (Wee 2012: 515, 518).

63 E.g., Udug-ḫul, wherein bitumen and gypsum are smeared on the threshold of a house (Geller 2016: 314 and note for line 75'). Livingstone (1986: 172–73) edited a commentary in which these substances were identified as Ninurta (gypsum) and the *Asakku*-demon (bitumen) pursuing each other. SAA 10 no. 238 obv. 12–13 mentions an exorcist combatting an *alû lemnu* or Antašubba by hanging "a mouse and a shoot of a thornbush on the vault of the (patient's) door", PÉŠ.QA.GAZ$^{!}$ NUNUZ ^{giš}DÌḪ ^{13} *ina šib-še-ti ša* KÁ *e'-i-la* (Parpola 1993: 189). Smearing substances on the doorposts is also attested in *bīt rimki* (Seidl and Sallaberger 2005–06: 62). Furthermore, drawing figurines on the outer gate in *bīt mēseri* would be a visual marker of problems inside the house (Wiggermann 1992: 116).

64 Maul 1999b; Maul 1994: 12–13 and note 100; Caplice 1974: 7–13. See also the discussion of other uses of such rituals in Koch 2010: 45–47, 53.

65 Witchcraft could involve the witch sending unfavourable signs (*CMAwR* 1: 3, 199; Abusch 2008; Schwemer 2007a: 63, 100–101).

66 Kiṣir-Aššur's KAL 4 no. 19, written as *šamallû ṣeḫru*, was perhaps not a *namburbi*-ritual, despite its classification by Maul (cf. Maul and Strauß 2011: 13, 48–49). Only very little remains on the obverse and it likely included a passage mentioning "[…] for a man […]" (obv. 1) and something recited before Šamaš (obv. 5). The reverse mentions a vessel

on behalf of Kiṣir-Aššur, could also indicate that Kiṣir-Aššur became a fully-fledged practitioner sometime during his *mašmaššu*-phase. This is underlined by the inclusion in *LKA* 115 of a purpose statement (Section 7.4), likely indicating that the tablet was copied for a particular ceremony.

KAL 4 no. 7 and *LKA* 115, alongside all Kiṣir-Aššur's and his family's other manuscripts containing *namburbi*-rituals, are analysed in the following two subsections to provide a broader understanding of when such rituals were generally employed and for what purposes.

6.4.1 Namburbi-*rituals and Ceremonial Supervisors*

The *namburbi*-rituals were mentioned at least once in the EM and must be considered an integral part of the exorcist's duties in official and private contexts.[67] Most such rituals are generally well attested and they are directed against many different signs (Koch 2010: 45–47, 53; Maul 1994). Furthermore, the *namburbi*-rituals were incorporated into a variety of works such as *Šumma ālu* (Freedman 1998: 12–13). *Namburbi*-rituals were also written on amulets and used prophylactically.[68] Almost all *namburbi*-rituals from Assur stem from the N4 collection, although none of the amulets with such related rituals from Assur were found in this collection.[69] It is currently unknown if *namburbi*-rituals were considered advanced knowledge,[70] but *namburbi*-rituals were not among the school tablets treated by Gesche.

Kiṣir-Aššur does not seem to have practiced *namburbi*-rituals until he had *LKA* 115 copied for a performance as *mašmaššu* and Aššur-šākin-šumi copied *KAL* 4 no. 7 from a tablet written by Kiṣir-Aššur as *mašmaššu*. In total, Kiṣir-Aššur is attested in the colophons of at least six *namburbi*-rituals during his *mašmaššu*- and *mašmaš bīt Aššur*-phases. In comparison, his nephew Kiṣir-Nabû copied five *namburbi*-rituals and his father Nabû-bēssunu at least three. What appears to be the common denominator for all the examples with

(rev. 3') and later a figurine thrown into a river (rev. 4') (see ibid.: 49). It may have been another type of ritual, such as *KAL* 4 no. 41 written by Kiṣir-Aššur as *šamallû ṣeḫru*. See also Sections 3.7 and 7.4.1.

67 Maul 1994: 13, 159, 169. *KAR* 44 obv. 14: ḪUL *ka-la*, "All evil" (perhaps related to the *namburbi* genre, Jean 2006: 66, 69; Geller 2000: 257; Bottéro 1985: 71–72) and rev. 29: NÍG.AK.A.MEŠ NAM.BÚR.BI Á.MEŠ AN *u* KI-*tim ma-la ba-šá-a*, "the rites, *namburbi*-ritual(s) (for) the signs of heaven and earth, as many as there are".

68 Maul 1994: 13. One amulet with a *namburbi*-ritual is published in Panayotov 2013; see also Panayotov 2018a. For amulets, see Heeßel 2014.

69 Maul 1994: 159 and note 13, 176. The lack of amulets in N4 is likely because they were produced for and kept by the client, unlike the texts kept by the performer.

70 In relation to the EM, this depends on whether or not the second section is analysed as representative of advanced knowledge. See Section 9.4.

TABLE 10 *Namburbi*-rituals assigned to career phases[a]

Phase	Nabû-bēssunu	Kiṣir-Aššur	Kiṣir-Nabû
mašmaššu ṣeḫru	*KAL* 4 no. 6	–	–
mašmaššu	–	*KAL* 4 no. 7, *LKA* 115	*LKA* 112, N4 no. 404
mašmaššu aššurû(?)	*LKA* 109	–	–
mašmaš bīt Aššur	–	*KAR* 38, *LKA* 113, *LKA* 119	–
No Title	*RA* 18 pl. 28(?)	–	*KAR* 72
Broken Title	–	N4 no. 224	*LKA* 110, *LKA* 118

a *KAL* 4 no. 6 (Maul 1994: 409ff. ms A), *KAL* 4 no. 7, *KAR* 38 and *RA* 18 pl. 28 (Maul 1994: 421ff. ms A and B), *KAR* 72 (Maul 1994: 446–52 and C), *LKA* 109 (Maul 1994: 465ff. ms A), *LKA* 110 (Maul 1994: 49 note 19, 50 note 36, 51 note 49–50, 52 note 88, 107 note 3, 202f., 216 note 434, 218), *LKA* 112 (Maul 1994: 332 ms A; cf. Caplice 1967: 14–16 no. 15A), *LKA* 113 (Maul 1994: 207f.), *LKA* 115 (Maul 1994: 502ff.), *LKA* 118 (Maul 1994: 55 note 129), *LKA* 119 (Maul 1994: 8 note 67, 52 note 86, 90 note 64), N4 no. 224 (Maul 1994: 445 note 15), N4 no. 404 (Maul 1994: 378ff. ms B, 546–47 with copy; see also Butler 1998: 46ff.).

colophons is that all *namburbi*-rituals attested within the Bāba-šuma-ibni family seem to stem from their later career phases. Table 10 contains an overview of the attested phases.

Keeping in mind that tablets without titles may stem from the *mašmaššu ṣeḫru* phase and onwards (Sections 7.2 and 7.4), the evidence here tentatively suggests that *namburbi*-rituals were not copied, kept or written with colophons until the *mašmaššu ṣeḫru*-phase within the Bāba-šuma-ibni family. Why such rituals do not appear in the Bāba-šuma-ibni family's earlier material may be due to chance survival, and unfortunately the sample size is too small to generalize. Still, a suggestion could be that Kiṣir-Aššur learned the structure of such rituals before his *mašmaššu*-phase, although he was perhaps not expected to copy *namburbi*-rituals until he needed them.

6.4.2 Namburbi-*rituals and House Calls*

LKA 115 was written with a purpose statement, which Section 7.4 argues may indicate that the purpose of the text was pragmatic in relation to a ritual performance. The ritual within *LKA* 115 was designed to annul any type of evil omen observed within a man's house. This ritual was therefore broadly applicable, and it is difficult to pin the use of such rituals to specific duties. However,

Kiṣir-Aššur and his family's *namburbi*-rituals in general may provide an indication regarding their use within this family's responsibilities as healers.

Due to ominous sightings often occurring in the city or a house, *namburbi*-rituals were generally closely connected to the terrestrial omen series *Šumma ālu* (Koch 2015: 261–62; Heeßel 2007a: 4; Freedman 1998: 12–13; Maul 1994: 29, 163–65). Therefore, several of the specific evils to be averted in *namburbi*-rituals were related to *Šumma ālu*.[71]

There exists an overlap between sightings in *Šumma ālu* and the 1st subseries of Sa-gig, which is concerned with omens observed en route to and within the patient's house (Freedman 1998: 11–12). Such observations were ominous in combination with the patient's symptoms for establishing a diagnosis and prognosis (Heeßel 2001–02: 24). The omens in Sa-gig's 1st subseries have not previously been considered in the context of *namburbi*-rituals, perhaps because the main bulk of Sa-gig has occasionally been considered as different from other areas of Mesopotamian divination (Geller 2010: 90–91; Heeßel 2007b: 105–110; Heeßel 2000: 4–5; Stol 1991–92: 42–43; cf. Koch unpublished: 12–14; Koch 2015: 274).[72]

Reiner stressed that omen collections are expected to have had parallel apotropaic rituals, although the surviving evidence indicates to her that omens regarding future events could be treated via *namburbi*-rituals, whereas diagnostic and physiognomic omens could not.[73] However, this relates to the idea

71 Some examples include sightings of (wild) cats (Freedman 2017: 41ff.) where the *namburbi*-ritual *LKA* 112 could be used, or sightings of frogs (Freedman 2017: 156ff.) where the *namburbi*-ritual *LKA* 118 could be used.

72 Heeßel (2000: 81–86; see also Heeßel 2007b: 127–28 and notes 28–29) suggested that *šu'illa*-prayers, DINGIR.ŠÀ.DIB.BAs and other such prayers and rituals could be used to appease an angry god causing the illness (see Maul 1988: 25–32; van der Toorn 1985: 123; Lambert 1974). However, as noted by Koch (unpublished: 11 and note 63) Heeßel does not list *namburbi*-rituals, and he has actually argued against their use in relation to appeasing divine anger and reconciling a patient with a god (cf. Heeßel 2007b: 127). Maul (1994: 12–13) mentions *namburbi*-rituals against, e.g., human illness, but states they are not against physiognomic omens. Koch (unpublished: 11 note 63) suggests the universal *namburbi*s, such as Nabû-bēssunu's *LKA* 109, could perhaps be used in relation to illness (see Avalos 1995: 136; Caplice 1974: 9 note 4; cf. Maul 1994: 465–506). Stol (1991–92: 53–54 and notes 68–69) provided a reference to a *namburbi*-like ritual, which was used to avoid a prognosis stating that the patient will die. See also Lenzi 2011: 24–46.

73 Reiner 1995: 82–85. There were, for example, no apotropaic rituals for *Alamdimmû*, see Koch 2015: 289; Koch 2010: 45–47; cf. Böck 2002: 244; Maul 1994: 12 and note 100; Caplice 1974: 7–9. However, Koch (2015: 274–75) has stressed that divination such as extispicy can be used in relation to both past and future. Guinan regarded divination and magic as having an inverse relationship in the sense that magic can dissolve what divination reveals (Guinan 2002: 18). For some of the various uses of *namburbi*-rituals in connection to divination, see Koch 2011: 465.

that the *namburbi*s influence the diagnosis. Most recently, Koch (unpublished: 11 note 63) has suggested certain *namburbi*s may have played a role in treating the cause of illness. Perhaps they could even affect the illness' prognosis, i.e., the patient's future (Maul 1994: 12), if we assume that the omens from Sa-gig's 1st subseries were sent by divine causers of illness to herald their presence or provide indications concerning the prognosis of the illness. I therefore hypothesize that the terrestrial omens in at least Sa-gig's 1st subseries could

TABLE 11 The Bāba-šuma-ibni family's *namburbi*-rituals

Name	*Namburbi*-rituals		(Partial) Duplicate	
	KAL 4 no. 7	Evil portended by witchcraft	*KAR* 72	Kiṣir-Nabu
Kiṣir-Aššur	*KAR* 38	Divine anger from poorly executed ritual	*RA* 18 pl. 28	Nabû-bēssunu
	LKA 113	Evil portended by a bow	–	
	LKA 115	Evil portended by any observation in a man's house	–	
	LKA 119	Contagion by dust from an evil place	–	
	N4 no. 224 (unpublished)	Evil portended by a "curse" (*arratu*)	–	
Kiṣir-Nabû	*LKA* 110	Evil portended by a lost, broken or missing cylinder seal	–	
	LKA 112	Evil portended by certain behaviour of a wildcat	–	
	LKA 118	Evil portended by a frog	–	
	N4 no. 404	Evil emanating from a man's bed(room?)	–	
Nabû-bēssunu	*KAL* 4 no. 6	Remove alienation between two long separated persons	–	
	LKA 109	Universal *namburbi*	–	

perhaps be averted or manipulated apotropaically to treat the cause of illness via *namburbi*-rituals.[74]

Some of the Bāba-šuma-ibni family members' *namburbi*-rituals overlap terrestrial omens found in *Šumma ālu* and the 1st subseries of Sa-gig (cf. Veldhuis 1995–96: 152). Table 11 presents the content of the *namburbi*-rituals with colophons naming Bāba-šuma-ibni family members in order to discuss the possible use of such rituals. At least two of the *namburbi*-rituals above cover specific instances, which are recorded in the 1st subseries of Sa-gig:

Sa-gig tablet 2 line 37:	"If a cat or a mou[se? fill] the floor in the house of a patient: that [pati]ent will die."
Sa-gig tablet 2 line 38:	"If a cat or a [(type-of)]-m[ouse?] fi[ll] the floor in the house of a patient: that patient will live."
	…
Sa-gig tablet 2 line 43:	"If the seal of a patient is lost: that patient will die."[75]

The example from the 2nd tablet line 43 was not cited in *Šumma ālu* and refers to the loss of the seal of the administrator of a household (Maul 1994: 12, 205, 208). This omen could be removed by Kiṣir-Nabû's *namburbi*-ritual *LKA* 110. Furthermore, Kiṣir-Nabû's *LKA* 112 concerns the bad omen derived from a wildcat (*muraššû*) wailing (*bakû*), howling (*damāmu*) and continually crossing (a path) (Ntn-stem of *egēru*) (Maul 1994: 329–35, esp. 332 and note 32; cf. *CAD* B: 38). Despite the fact that the omens from Sa-gig concern an ordinary cat (*šurānu*) "filling the floor", almost all *namburbi*-rituals directed specifically against cats concern omens connected to *muraššû*-cats, and Maul (1994: 329) only provides one example (VAT 13988) mentioning a *šurānu*-cat.[76] As such, these rituals could relate to such omens as the ones quoted above from Sa-gig.

74 However, Sa-gig, and especially Sa-gig's 1st subseries, is largely unattested in Assur (Heeßel 2010a: 158; Heeßel 2001–02: 27–28; Labat 1951: 2 note 1; see Section 3.6.1).

75 Heeßel 2001–02: 32, 38–39. The following quotes consist of a collective reading of the best preserved parts of the various manuscripts in order to provide an overview of the content rather than aim at exact citation:
Line 37: DIŠ *ina* É [lú]GIG *lu* SA.A *lu* PÉ[Š] *qaq-qa-r*[*a umallû* GI]G.BI BA.ÚŠ.
Line 38: DIŠ *ina* É [lú]GIG *lu* SA.A *lu* P[ÉŠ] *qaq-qa-ra ú-ma-a*[*l-lu*]-⸢*ú* GIG.BI⸣ AL.TI.
Line 43: DIŠ [na4]KIŠIB [lú]TU.RA *iḫ-liq* GIG.BI BA.Ú[Š].

76 Note that the 45th tablet of *Šumma ālu* was devoted to omens concerning *šurānu*- and *muraššû*-cats (Freedman 2017: 41ff.; Maul 1994: 329 and note 1–3). Maul (1994: 329, 494ff.) only quotes Ass. 13988 (= N4 no. 561) as an example of a *namburbi* mentioning a *šurānu*-cat, although the ritual is directed against all sorts of bad omens and is a so-called "universal *namburbi*-ritual".

In connection to house calls, it is possible that at least two of Kiṣir-Aššur's *namburbi*-rituals were broadly applicable for rituals performed in a client's house. *LKA* 115 could serve to dispel problematic omens experienced in the patient's house, and *KAR* 38 could serve to protect Kiṣir-Aššur from any wrongdoing on behalf of himself and his assistant(s) while performing a ritual. His father apparently used this ritual as well. Kiṣir-Nabû also copied a *namburbi*-ritual for a bad omen concerning a frog (*muṣa''irānu*) (*LKA* 118),[77] and evil emanating from a man's bed (*mayyālu*) in case of nocturnal enuresis (N4 no. 404).[78] Especially the last ritual could have been useful in connection to a majority of healing ceremonies taking place around the patient's bed. Nabû-bēssunu, in addition to the duplicate above, also copied a ritual to remove alienation between two long separated persons (*KAL* 4 no. 6) and a so-called universal *namburbi*-ritual (*LKA* 109).[79]

Although several of the *namburbi*-rituals above do not directly reflect the elimination of bad omens listed in relation to house calls in Sa-gig, it is plausible that some of the more general types would have been employed to negate the effect of omens counteractive to the purpose of the visit, i.e., to heal an ill patient, or intended to soothe some of the divine anger behind an illness. If at least some of Kiṣir-Aššur's *namburbi*-rituals were connected to making house calls, such as *LKA* 115, this may fit the hypothesis from Section 6.2, that an exorcist would not lead healing ceremonies connected to house calls until he was *mašmaššu*. Following this hypothesis, *LKA* 115 would have been copied on behalf of Kiṣir-Aššur for his ceremony.

77 *LKA* 118 obv. 1: [... NAM.BÚR.B]I ḪUL BIL.ZA.ZA [...]; cf. Maul 1994: 55 note 129. The text is listed in *BAK* as no. 217, although Hunger simply transliterated ᵖ*Ki-ṣir*-dingir.[x], even though the text copied by Ebeling shows ᵈA[G]. Furthermore, the text in rev. 5' reads: [...] ᵈUTU-DÙ, and the name must have been Kiṣir-Nabû.

78 *LKA* 110, see Maul 1994: 202f.; *LKA* 112, see Maul 1994: 332f. text A and Caplice 1967: 14–17 no. 15A; N4 no. 404 (VAT 13682), see Butler 1998: 46–47; Maul 1994: 379ff., 546–47 (copy). The catch-line of *LKA* 112 refers to a *namburbi*-ritual against an *izbu* born in a man's house, such as the one preserved on *LKA* 114 (= N4 no. 507) with a broken colophon (Maul 1994: 334–337). The tablet could therefore have been written by a member of the Bāba-šuma-ibni family for a specific purpose (*ana ṣabāt epēši*; Maul 1994: 341). Furthermore, the catch-line of *LKA* 111 (= N4 no. 511; Maul 1994: 330ff.), a modified universal *namburbi*-ritual against *muraššû*-cat omens, is the first line of *LKA* 112, and *LKA* 111 could therefore have been written by, e.g., Kiṣir-Nabû. For rituals against enuresis, see also Verderame 2018.

79 *KAL* 4 no. 6, see also Maul 1994: 409ff.; *LKA* 109, see Maul 1994: 465ff.

6.5 Other Technical Literature: *CT* 37 pl. 24f.

Practice and pragmatic use of the exorcistic knowledge were not the only important aspects of becoming a *mašmaššu*. In addition to the practical capabilities, exorcists trained to become versed in interpretation of their text corpus. Therefore, contemporary texts focus on the competences needed to become an "expert" (*ummânu*), which included understanding the intellectual heritage learned and practiced up until becoming a *mašmaššu* (Section 9.4). Perhaps, therefore, Kiṣir-Aššur's *mašmaššu*-phase is the first part of his career wherein he copied a text relating to scholarship. The text *CT* 37 pl. 24f. is a fragmentary copy of a Lú lexical list (Civil 1969: 87ff., 223ff.).[80] Generally, lexical extracts are regarded as educational texts at some level in the first millennium, and the Lú lists may have been employed during the first school phase among the NB and LB tablets.[81] However, *CT* 37 pl. 24f. is not an extract and stems from Kiṣir-Aššur's *mašmaššu*-phase.[82]

The content of *CT* 37 pl. 24f. is probably similar or even related to the 25th tablet of Ur$_5$-ra (Civil 1969: 225 ms B).[83] The text contains two columns on each side. Each column consists of Sumerian words for a profession and the Akkadian equivalent of that word, with entries divided by a vertical line. The first column of the obverse likely provided Sumerian titles equivalent to *bārû* and *āšipu*, although it is now broken (ibid.: 227).[84] *CT* 37 pl. 24f. may therefore have been used in some way to emphasize a scholarly identity or read unusual Sumerograms as exorcistic titles via the broken beginning with Sumerian equivalents to the *āšipu* title (see Robson 2011a: 564; Gesche 2001: 130–31).

The text includes very elementary glosses and notes to individual words, e.g., spelling out the phonetic reading of a Sumerogram, and these are written in a smaller script.[85] Such notes are not commonly found in the N4 texts, but

80 See also Meier 1937–39: 246 note 38. For NA lexical lists, see Veldhuis 2014: 354ff.

81 Gesche 2001: 63, 124–29, 183. See the two lexical exercises *KADP* 46 and *KADP* 47 excavated in N4 (Veldhuis 2014: 369–70). Note also that some of the exercises copied on the Graeco-Babylonica tablets were derived from Ur$_5$-ra (Westenholz 2007: 276–77).

82 Gesche (2001: 63) listed *CT* 37 pl. 24f. as an example of a Lú list from Assur in connection to a discussion of school texts.

83 The content of texts such as CT 37 pl. 24f. may have become a separate list in the NB period called UM.ME.A = *ummânu* (Robson 2011a: 564; Gesche 2001: 125–32).

84 The title AZU (A-ZU) is listed as *bārû* in this and other lists. See *MSL* 12: 119 lines 14'–15', 227 lines 5'–6'. See also Landsberger's comment on this manuscript: it "gives the impression of a late secondary compilation of rather low quality" (*MSL* 12: 230).

85 Col. iii 13': ^{lú}AMA-A-TU$^{\textit{e-me-du}}$: *i-lit-ti bi-i-t*[*i*], col. iv 9': [^{lú}T]IBIRA$^{\textit{te-bi-ru}}$: <MIN>, col. iv 25': [^{l}]^{ú}MURUB$_4$.DUBUR$^{\textit{mu-ru-ub-du-bur}}$: *mu-ḫar-ri-*[*šu*] (Civil 1969: 228–29). For glosses in

are also seen on, e.g., Kiṣir-Nabû's copy of the EM, *KAR* 44.[86] At Nineveh, such glosses and notes occasionally appear in the royal correspondence in letters and astrological reports, and they have generally been interpreted as educational glosses for the king reading the text.[87] However, Talon (2003: 649, 653–54) has shown that the glosses in the royal letters cannot be regarded as proof of the king's schooling and must relate to idiosyncratic habits of a few courtly scholars. Several of the glosses in *CT* 37 pl. 24f. are simplistic readings of common signs and represent knowledge Kiṣir-Aššur must have known as *mašmaššu*.[88] Furthermore, similar glosses are also preserved in other Lú lexical lists from contemporary Nineveh (Civil 1969: 115ff.).[89] As a result, it may be that Kiṣir-Aššur used *CT* 37 pl. 24f. for scholarly activities during his *mašmaššu*-phase.[90]

6.6 Summary

According to the available evidence, Kiṣir-Aššur did not copy any medical prescriptions during his *šamallû* and *šamallû mašmaššu ṣeḫru*-phase. However, his *mašmaššu* texts attest to treatments of a variety of areas connected to the lower body. The medical texts are directed towards the treatment of "Anus illness", *maškadu*-illness, and the "strings" and muscles of the legs and feet. These texts are discussed further in Section 9.1.

---

general, see Krecher 1957–71.

86 *KAR* 44 obv. 2, 7, 8, 9, 10, 11, 12, 15, 18, 19, 21, rev. 32(?). What is noted on Geller's copy and is confirmed via collations is that the initial note to obv. 9 is written on obv. 8, and the final note for obv. 12 is written on obv. 11 (Geller 2000: 245). This cannot presently be explained by problems related to space on the tablet.

87 Veldhuis 2014: 382–84; Zamazalová 2011: 319; Villard 1997: 145 note 72, 147–48. Concerning some of the scholars at court who wrote such glosses and notes, see Verderame 2014: 725–27.

88 For glosses in a text copied by a *šamallû agašgû*, see Geller 2010: 130–32; see also Geller 2015.

89 Glosses reading the names of signs in lexical lists appear to be regularly attested in the first millennium (see Krecher 1957–71: 438; see Frahm 2011a: 16–17). At least one gloss listed in a Lú list from Nineveh is also preserved in *KAR* 44:
KAR 44 obv. 10: [*gu-ru-uš*]GURUŠ.LÍL.LÁ.MEŠ …
K. 2051+: [*gu-ru-uš*]GURUŠ : *eṭ-lum* (*MSL* 12: 126 line 79; Langdon 1917: 86 col. iii 13').

90 Whether or not such glosses were used explanatory remains uncertain, although Geller (2015: 37) has suggested this was the case for the N4 manuscript *KADP* 4. This text also listed certain Sumerograms apparently intended to be pronounced in Sumerian (ibid.: 35). The use of notes and glosses in relation to copyists' competence levels requires further investigation.

Although the *mašmaššu* title indicates that the holder of the title was an exorcist, Kiṣir-Aššur does not seem to have been an independent and fully trained practitioner when he gained this title. This chapter has argued that Kiṣir-Aššur did not make house calls on his own until he had copied and acquired a special ritual for going to the patient's house (*KAR* 230). The purpose of this ritual was to remove the cause of illness, possibly at the beginning of any treatment at a patient's house. The text was labelled as secret and, although it cannot be determined what this meant, it is not impossible that the phrase illustrated the Bāba-šuma-ibni family's view that this text was special to them. Kiṣir-Aššur's father, Nabû-bēssunu, also copied a related text, *KAR* 31, designed to protect the exorcist when approaching a patient. These texts combined therefore attest to a professional environment in relation to making house calls.

Kiṣir-Aššur's *KAR* 298 from his *mašmaššu*-phase was designed for prophylactically protecting a person's home via figures of magical beings. The text was likely aimed at practical adaption, and could have served as an *aide mémoire* for such rituals. The text was associated with *bīt mēseri* and other rituals for demarcating spaces and protecting them either for apotropaic or treatment purposes. Kiṣir-Nabû's associated texts related to the *tummu bītu* incantation attest to an environment dealing with demarcating rituals. These rituals therefore were adaptable and likely point to another side of Kiṣir-Aššur's practice, namely providing ritual quarantine for patients when healing them.

This chapter also evaluates Kiṣir-Aššur's production of *namburbi*-rituals, which appear to have begun around his *mašmaššu*-phase. As a result, these texts seem to be linked to the ritual performance. Kiṣir-Aššur was perhaps not a ceremonial supervisor before he copied *KAR* 230, and by extension, he did not copy *namburbi*-rituals previously. In addition, this chapter argues that the *namburbi*-rituals copied by the Bāba-šuma-ibni family in general may have been used to treat certain omens, such as those preserved in the 1st subseries of Sa-gig. Whether or not such rituals could be used in connection to such omens remains hypothetical, but, if they were indeed used, they would have been part of the appeasement of the divine cause behind an illness. However, further evidence is needed to corroborate this suggestion.

The final section discusses Kiṣir-Aššur's sole lexical text *CT* 37 pl. 24., which may have played a role in relation to his scholarly work at the time or for strengthening his professional identity.

CHAPTER 7

Additional Texts that May Belong to the *mašmaššu*-phase

This chapter contains a discussion of tablets that based on text-internal criteria, may be assigned to the *mašmaššu*- or *mašmaš bīt Aššur*-phases of Kiṣir-Aššur's career.[1] At least 14 of Kiṣir-Aššur's tablets do not provide his professional title and as many as 16 texts contain breaks in the colophons where a potential title would have been. As such, these tablets cannot be distributed properly to Kiṣir-Aššur's various career phases at present. However, certain features in the colophons can be used to propose a tentative assignment of some of these texts to certain career phases proximal to the *mašmaššu*-phase. Furthermore, the only dated tablet by Kiṣir-Aššur, and the Bāba-šuma-ibni family in general, *KAR* 267, is found among the tablets without titles, and this text will be discussed in order to assign this text to a section of Kiṣir-Aššur's career.

Kiṣir-Aššur's *mašmaššu*-phase tablet *LKA* 115 is the first text from any career phase that employs what will be referred to here as a "purpose statement". I use this term to refer to statements, which designate that the tablet was produced "for undertaking a (ritual) procedure" (*ana ṣabāṭ epēši*). By extension, such phrases are indicative of the texts' pragmatic purpose (e.g., Maul 2010a: 212–13; Hunger 1968: 12, 19–20). Outside of career phases, such statements are also found in nine of Kiṣir-Aššur's tablets without titles and in seven tablets with broken colophons. The present chapter argues that such statements are useful as a distributive criterion. Several manuscripts, including Kiṣir-Aššur's only commentary-like text without a title, *BAM* 307, also indicate they were copied at the request of Kiṣir-Aššur ([*ú-š*]*aš-ṭir-ma*). Therefore, this chapter also discusses Kiṣir-Aššur's use of assistants to copy relevant material.

7.1 Omission and Inclusion of Titles

The written name serves the purpose of remembrance, claiming ownership over the text as an object, or providing authority (Maul 2010a: 215 and note 94; Radner 2005: 70, 169). Perhaps for this reason, several of Kiṣir-Aššur's colophons

1 The title *mašmaš bīt Aššur* "Exorcist of the Aššur temple" designates the last traceable phase of Kiṣir-Aššur's career, which appears after his *mašmaššu*-phase. It is treated in Chapter 8.

include the phrase: “Do not erase my written name”.[2] Titles are additional elements that reference the level of competence within the professional group of which a copyist or writer was part.[3] All this information was stored in the colophons. The purposes of colophons differ over time, place and within individual careers, as discussed in Section 1.1 (cf. Gesche 2001: 153–54; Hunger 1968: 1, 15ff.; Leichty 1964: 147). However, while a copy frequently presents itself as the transmission of an ideally static textual tradition, Stevens (2013: 212) stated that the colophons must have served as the textual area for individual scholarly touch wherein scribes could practice “free choice over form and content”.[4] Still, Stevens (2013: 220 note 54) argued that colophons from advanced levels of scholarship tend to be more elaborate than earlier colophons, but in general this is not true of Kiṣir-Aššur’s colophons with titles.

Although the reasons for the addition or omission of titles in colophons is uncertain, a fair assumption may be that it depended on the audience, i.e., who was supposed to read the product in the present and future. Titles were included for both the scribe and his ancestors, although many works – some of which were integrated and preserved in tablet collections – were not supplied with a colophon at all (Hunger 1968: 9–11; Leichty 1964: 153). Comparative NB and LB material suggests that student or apprenticeship titles were not used during education before the professional specialization (Gesche 2001: 153ff., 213).[5] The question is therefore whether or not Kiṣir-Aššur could or would omit his apprenticeship title during his earlier attested phases. During his later career stages the purposes of the text may be indicative of who was supposed

2 *Šamallû ṣeḫru* title: *BAM* 9, *RA* 15 pl. 76, *RA* 40 pl. 116; *mašmaš bīt Aššur* title: Beckman and Foster 1988 no. 21, *LKA* 77. For quotations, see Appendix 1. It is unclear if names could actually be removed from tablets by applying, e.g., water to the colophon (see Taylor 2011: 19, 22; van de Mieroop 2006: 274, concerning erasing names from inscriptions). Maul (1994: 221) discusses the possibility that adding a name and stating that the person with this name wrote the tablet could bestow a benign divine effect on the copyist.

3 By extension, a title communicates professional credentials and identity to the reader. However, the recipient of a text, i.e., its reader(s), may have changed from text to text.

4 See also Rochberg 2004: 211. Yet, Stevens (2013: 212 note 6) argues the LB Uruk colophons show order in variation of elements, wording and sign choices in the colophon (see Robson 2011a: 566–69; cf. Lenzi 2008a: 206).

5 Gesche (2001: 153) seems to differentiate between school and library tablets’ colophons in the sense that the former were often dedicatory and the latter contained “Bibliotheksvermerken”. As such, especially the NB school texts donated to the *Nabû-ša-ḫarê* temple in Babylon were dedicated to this temple and by extension Nabû (Charpin 2010a: 47; Cavigneaux 1999a: 385–86; Cavigneaux 1981: 9–10, 37ff., 79–80, 101–2, 117–18, 125–26, 135ff.). Thus, such tablets with colophons likely functioned as votive objects in the temple (George 2003–04: 404; Gesche 2001: 153, 155, 158–60). Copying traditional texts may occasionally have been considered a service to the gods.

to read it, and consequently, whether or not a title was necessary. Perhaps certain "quickly extracted" tablets with purpose statements were produced rapidly (Maul 2010a: 213–14, 216). One possible result of the time constraints and the pragmatic purpose of such texts may have been that the copyist wrote minimalistic colophons.

Generally, texts copied during various training phases probably served the dual purpose of posing as an exercise in copying as well as providing a basis for practical training.[6] Nonetheless, the standard of *šamallû ṣeḫru* manuscripts must occasionally have been high, since there are several examples of such manuscripts being integrated into contemporary text collections (see Robson 2014: 152–53).[7] This is one possible reason why several of Kiṣir-Aššur's elaborate colophons appear during his *šamallû ṣeḫru*-phase. If so, the colophon likely served the purpose of creating an image of Kiṣir-Aššur as a skilled apprentice. Still, Kiṣir-Aššur may also have produced manuscripts without colophons, and the purpose of the colophon is therefore not always clear.

The recipient(s) of many of Kiṣir-Aššur's texts with colophons is uncertain. Nevertheless, even tablets with purpose statements were likely integrated into the tablet collection (Maul 1994: 169), although it is unknown if they were used after the specific ritual for which they were copied. Maul (2010a: 215) suggests the accumulation of tablets into a collection could be regarded as a means of identification of personal qualifications for individuals such as Kiṣir-Aššur. It may be that tablets without titles stem from later career phases in which the tablets would only be used by Kiṣir-Aššur, e.g., with purpose statements in relation to a ritual, or that Kiṣir-Aššur did not need a title to boost his image in particular texts. However, this remains speculative. The fact remains that Kiṣir-Aššur included a title in the majority of his colophons for reasons that are often unclear. I therefore find it unlikely that Kiṣir-Aššur would have copied, e.g., *šamallû ṣeḫru* tablets with colophons that omit both his title and the *ša Nabû tuklassu*-phrase (Section 5.4).

6 Robson 2013: 40; Schwemer 2011: 422; Maul 2010: 216–17; Geller 2010: 130–31; Beaulieu 2007a: 475–76; cf. Gesche 2001: 197, 212–13.

7 Whether these new copies were dedicated to the library as part of the training, they replaced older manuscripts, or were dedicated to, e.g., Nabû in connection with being placed in the library typically cannot be determined (cf. Clancier 2014: 46; Robson 2014: 150, 152–53; Cavigneaux 1981: 5). Although the NB school tablets from Babylon were often schoolwork, they were still kept in the temple as part of the floor filling, likely because they were dedicated to Nabû on behalf of the future scribe (Cavigneaux 1999a: 388). Maul (2010: 217), however, stressed that some N4 tablets without colophons contain poor spellings and a bad script (see Robson 2014: 154).

7.2 Tablets without Kiṣir-Aššur's Professional Title

There are in total 15 tablets without titles that may have belonged to Kiṣir-Aššur's *mašmaššu*-phase or later. It is unclear why these colophons do not mention his title explicitly, especially because some of the colophons do mention the titles of his forefathers. In addition to an overview of Kiṣir-Aššur's tablets without titles, this section includes a summary of textual features that are useful for suggesting possible phases wherein these tablets were copied. Table 12 contains an overview of the texts, divided into three groups according to the content of the texts, namely: medical texts, ritual texts, and texts relating to other areas of technical literature.

The diagnosis and prescription texts were directed against head maladies (*BAM* 9), a specific eye illness (*BAM* 351),[8] internal problems connected to the spleen(?) (*BAM* 78),[9] the lower body illness *šaššaṭu* and associated stiffness (*BAM* 131), and finally feet maladies (*BAM* 121).[10] Several tablets only contain incantations or prayers,[11] whereas others contain both incantations and rituals to combat ghosts (*KAR* 21, *KAR* 267), a diagnosis and an incantation ritual against an "Adversary" (*bēl dabābi*, *KAR* 171), incantations and ritual actions against a "Curse" (*māmītu*, *KAL* 10 no. 5), and a long and unpublished *namburbi*-ritual against another type of curse (*arratu*, N4 no. 224, see Section 6.4.2).[12] *KAL* 10 no. 1 provides incantation incipits and ritual instructions as guidelines for performing a long ritual against a "Curse". The text therefore appears similar in scope to the *šamallû* manuscript N4 no. 175 and the *mašmaššu* manuscript *KAR* 298. Note that the text contains a number of erasures (rev. 3', 4', 5', 7', 27'). N4 no. 228 is a unique text with a previously unattested Sumerian-Akkadian bilingual incantation for washing the mouth (KA LUḪ) on a statue of the king made from various materials. Finally, *BAM* 307 was likely a scholastic manuscript containing the right side of a commentary-like text, as discussed below.

---

8 *Birrat īnī*, see Fincke 2000: 90–91.

9 The *tulīmu*/*ṭulīmu* (*CAD* Ṭ: 124–25) designates the "spleen" or perhaps "pancreas"(?). See Westenholz 2010 for a discussion. Regarding the initial diagnosis in *BAM* 78, see also a commentary related to the Ugu series, 11N–T4, in Civil 1974: 336–37 line 6.

10 *BAM* 121 may have opened with prescriptions for the head, temples or the epigastrium, obv. 1: DIŠ NA SAG […]/SAG.[KI …]/SAG [ŠÀ …] etc.

11 *BAM* 333, *LKA* 40 and N4 no. 228(?). *BAM* 333 is broken and may have contained a ritual instruction, and N4 no. 228 remains unpublished.

12 According to Frankena (1960: 174) several lines in the ritual can be found in parallel passages in *Šurpu* tablet 3 and 8. However, the relevant lines in *Šurpu* concern *māmītu*-curse. It is possible that AMC line 87 had to do with *arratu lemuttu* (Steinert 2018d: 256).

TABLE 12 Texts without Kiṣir-Aššur's professional title

Group	Text	Content	Format and description
Medical texts	*BAM* 9	(See Sections 3 and 5.4)	
	BAM 78	Obverse: two prescriptions against a hurting spleen (*ṭulīmu*) where the patient cannot sleep, his body has a fever, he eats and drinks increasingly less and he continually seeks out Marduk's sanctuary (obv. 1–3, 7) where the patient on an empty stomach is to suck down a liquid (obv. 1–6) or eat a remedy (obv. 7–9) Reverse: one prescription (rev. 10–17)	Portrait; [...]
	BAM 121	Obverse: ten prescriptions against the upper (SAG) [...] (obv. 1–3(?), 4, 5, 6, 7, 8) and a man's feet (obv. 9, 10–11), which are specified later to be swollen (obv. 11, 12); several prescriptions are anointed (obv. 4, 5, 6, 7) or applied as a poultice (obv. 13) Reverse: two prescriptions treating a man's feet (rev. 14) and feet swollen with fever (rev. 18) to be applied as a poultice (rev. 23)	Landscape; *ṭuppu*
	BAM 131	Obverse: two longer prescriptions treating a patient ill with *šaššaṭu* (obv. 1) and one whose eyes(?) are dried up, who trembles on repeated occasions and is scared or farts(?) (obv. 9–10); the first involves an innkeeper and later washing and anointing the patient (obv. 1–8), the other applying a substance from the neck to the shoulder blades, fumigating(?) the patient's bed and washing the patient (obv. 9–15) Reverse: three prescriptions for bandages against winter stiffness	Portrait; [*ṭuppu*?]

TABLE 12 Texts without Kiṣir-Aššur's professional title (*cont.*)

Group	Text	Content	Format and description
		(rev. 1'–3'), regular stiffness (rev. 4'–6') and to soften up stiffness (rev. 7'–8')	
	BAM 351	Obverse: (broken) Reverse: a single prescription divided into two entries (rev. 1–6, 7–12) listing stones, which are threaded onto plaited red wool and bound around the left hand of the patient against an eye illness (*bir-rat* IGI^{II})	Portrait; N/A
Ritual texts	*BAM* 333	Obverse: a fragmentary incantation (obv. 1–8+[...]) mentioning Ea having established the (healing) plant(s) in the netherworld(?) Reverse: fragmentary, only colophon preserved (rev. 1'–4')	Portrait(?); N/A
	KAL 10 no. 1	Obverse: ritual instructions for performing libations, applying remedies to the patient and a figurine of the "Curse" (obv. 1'–18') and other actions (22'–24'), as well as incantation incipits with brief ritual instructions (19', 20', 21', 25') Reverse: incantation incipits with brief ritual instructions (rev. 1', 2', 3', 4', 5'–6', 7', 8', 9', 10'–11', 12', 13', 14'–15', 16', 17'–18', 19', 20'–21'), ritual instructions for the patient (rev. 22'–23') and for dealing with a figurine of the "Curse" in order to release evil (rev. 24'–27')	Portrait(?); [...]
	KAL 10 no. 5	Obverse and reverse: diagnostic statement and ritual instruction (obv. 1–11), fragmentary incantations (obv. 12–13, 14–(breaks off), rev. 1'–3', 5'–10'), fragmentary ritual instructions (rev. 4', 11') and a rubric (rev. 12')	Portrait; *ṭuppu*

TABLE 12 Texts without Kiṣir-Aššur's professional title (*cont.*)

Group	Text	Content	Format and description
	KAR 21	Obverse: two incantations against seeing dead people (obv. 1–13, 18–24) and a ritual instruction (obv. 14–17) Reverse: one incantation (rev. 7–18) and a ritual instruction (rev. 1–6), presumably against the same problems	Portrait; N/A
	KAR 171	Obverse and reverse: diagnosis concerning an adversary *bēl dabābi* (obv. 1–3) and a ritual instruction with built in words to be spoken (obv. 4–rev. 18)	Landscape; N/A
	KAR 267	Obverse: diagnoses for ghost and confusional states (obv. 1–2), prayers for Šamaš (obv. 12–26) and Girra (obv. 27–30) and ritual instructions (obv. 3–11, 31–38) Reverse: incantation (rev. 1–24)	Portrait; *ṭuppu*
	LKA 40	Obverse (fragmentary) and reverse: *šu'illa*-prayer for Tašmētum (rev. 1'–8')	Portrait; *ṭuppu*
	N4 no. 224	Obverse and reverse: *namburbi*-ritual against various types of "curses" (*arratu*) (obv. 1–3) consisting of incantations and prayers (obv. 10–14, 16–17, 20–26, 27–60+rev. 1–17), a rubric (rev. 18), as well as ritual instructions (obv. 4–9, 15, 18–19, rev. 19–21, 22(?), 23–30)	Portrait; *ṭuppu*
	N4 no. 228	Obverse and reverse: Sumerian-Akkadian bilingual recitation for performing mouth washing of a statue depicting the king made from various materials (obv. 1–rev. 9'). The text ends with a rubric (rev. 10'11')	Portrait; N/A
Other texts	*BAM* 307	Obverse: (broken) Reverse: commentary-like explanatory text (rev. 1–27)	Portrait; [...]

Noticeably, *KAR* 267 is the only dated text among Kiṣir-Aššur's tablets. The text contains a date formula dating it to the 9th of the month *Ulūlu* (August–September) in 658 BCE.[13] As this tablet is the only one of Kiṣir-Aššur's texts that can be isolated to a specific moment in time, it is crucial to discuss *KAR* 267 in relation to Kiṣir-Aššur's career (see Section 7.5).

7.2.1 *Text-internal Features Useful as Allocating Criteria*

Several features within the texts and their colophons can be used to argue for a distribution of the texts in Table 12 to career phases. Nine tablets contain a purpose statement similar to several of Kiṣir-Aššur's *mašmaššu* and *mašmaš bīt Aššur* tablets[14] and they probably served a similar purpose. *BAM* 307 also states that someone other than Kiṣir-Aššur copied this tablet at the request of Kiṣir-Aššur, which is a feature only found among his *šamallû ṣeḫru, mašmaššu,* and *mašmaš bīt Aššur* tablets.[15]

Considering that Kiṣir-Aššur did not copy prescriptions in attested tablets between his *šamallû ṣeḫru-* and *mašmaššu ṣeḫru*-phase, several of the tablets above may belong to the earliest or later phases based on their content. However, this remains speculative. *Namburbi*-rituals are not attested with certainty before Kiṣir-Aššur's *mašmaššu*-phase, and N4 no. 224 may therefore belong to this or subsequent phases (see Section 6.4.1). Furthermore, Kiṣir-Aššur's texts related to the palace or the Aššur cult can be argued to originate in his *mašmaššu-* or *mašmaš bīt Aššur*-phases (see Sections 7.3.1 and 8.6). Thus, it seem plausible that the ritual N4 no. 228 for washing the mouth of a statue of the king himself would belong to one of these phases. Regardless, there are tablets without titles, which seem to resemble tablets copied by Kiṣir-Aššur as *šamallû ṣeḫru,* such as the *šu'illa*-prayer copied on *LKA* 40.[16] However, the addition of a purpose statement in the case of *LKA* 40 argues against assigning this text to Kiṣir-Aššur's earlier phases.[17]

---

13 Maul 2010a: 205.

14 These tablets are: *BAM* 78, *BAM* 121, *BAM* 333, *BAM* 351, *KAL* 10 no. 1, *KAR* 21, *KAR* 171, *LKA* 40, N4 no. 228.

15 One of Kiṣir-Aššur's *mašmaššu*-phase tablets was likely copied by another well known N4 individual, Aššur-šākin-šumi, and is published as the tablet *KAL* 4 no. 7 (see Maul 2010a: 216; Section 6.4). For a recently published tablet from the hand of Aššur-šākin-šumi, see Fadhil 2018.

16 The *šu'illa*-prayer *LKA* 40 was copied without a ritual and directed towards Tašmētum (Frechette 2012: 263, 273). The tablet layout and text are similar to Kiṣir-Aššur's *LKA* 43 copied as *šamallû ṣeḫru.*

17 Other examples from N4 of prayers for preparation of a ritual contain the names of the patient, e.g., *LKA* 51. However, the majority of such tablets do not contain a colophon (Maul 2010a: 213 note 82).

At least *BAM* 9 seems to be from Kiṣir-Aššur's *šamallû ṣeḫru*-phase as argued in Section 5.4. Both *BAM* 9 and *BAM* 121 contain the *ša Nabû tuklassu*-phrase, and *BAM* 121 also contains a purpose statement. As discussed in Section 5.4, the *ša Nabû tuklassu*-phrase was an addition that Kiṣir-Aššur, according to present evidence, added to tablets during his *šamallû ṣeḫru*- and *šamallû mašmaššu ṣeḫru*-phases. It is therefore possible that *BAM* 9 and *BAM* 121 were copied at this time.[18] If this is correct, *BAM* 121 would be the earliest tablet with a purpose statement copied by Kiṣir-Aššur, and furthermore it would have been copied before his *mašmaššu*-phase while including medical prescriptions, which are otherwise not observed in the *šamallû* and *šamallû mašmaššu ṣeḫru* phases. The assignment of *BAM* 121 thus remains uncertain.

7.3 Tablets with Broken Colophons

A group of seven tablets contain breaks in the colophon and consequently these texts cannot be attributed to a specific career phase, regardless of whether or not the colophon originally contained a title. An additional 11 texts contain breaks in the names, preventing their distribution between Kiṣir-Aššur or Kiṣir-Nabû. However, all these texts are listed in what follows to enable the fullest possible overview of texts that may be attributed to Kiṣir-Aššur. Furthermore, several of these texts contain features that are useful for distributing them to phases of Kiṣir-Aššur's career.

The diagnostic-therapeutic texts concern illnesses affecting the respiratory system and the arms (*BAM* 40), various types of stiffness, muscle and internal illnesses (*BAM* 68), various demons affecting the state of mind and epigastrium or abdomen (*BAM* 311), insanity (*BAM* 202), witchcraft (*BAM* 206), and a text for making a patient drunk or thirsty (*BAM* 260), possibly aimed at improving the effect of alcohol and alleviating pain in connection to medical procedures (Scurlock and Andersen 2005: 361; Geller and Cohen 1995: 1813 and note 26). Noticeably, *BAM* 202 concerns various symptoms of insanity and the manuscript contains a previously unnoticed elaborate drawing of a demonic figure (Arbøll 2019).

The incantations and rituals concern a demon or ghost (*KAL* 4 no. 37), a "Curse" (*KAL* 10 no. 13), some part of the ritual *bīt mēseri* (N4 no. 254), ritual instructions accompanying incantations for appeasing an angry god (*ilī ul īde*, "My god, I did not know"; *KAR* 90; Lambert 1974), transgressions (*KAL* 9 no. 41),

18 Kiṣir-Aššur's *šamallû* manuscript N4 no. 175 is also the only text besides *BAM* 121, which contains the writing ᵖZÚ.KEŠDA-AN.ŠÁR/ᵈ*aš-šur* of his name.

TABLE 13 Texts with broken colophons

Group	Text	Content	Format and designation
		Kiṣir-Aššur [*broken title/no title*]	
Medical texts	*BAM* 40	Obverse: five preserved prescriptions (obv. 1–6, 7–11, 15–17, 18–21+[...]) for treating someone who is ill (obv. 1), a slackening chest with swelling and continually twitching and standing(?) eyes infused with blood (obv. 12–14, cf. obv. 15), or grinding lungs (obv. 18). All application methods are largely broken Reverse: four preserved prescriptions (rev. 1'–5', 6'–9', 10'–12', 13'–17'), two of which are relatively broken but concern problems in the left (rev. 10'–12') and right arm (rev. 13')	Portrait; *ṭuppu*
Ritual texts	*KAL* 7 no. 24	Obverse: two incantations for gaining an audience (É.GAL.KU$_4$.RA) (obv. 1–9, 12–15) and at least one ritual instruction (obv. 10–11) Reverse: at least one incantation for gaining an audience (É.GAL.KU$_4$.RA) (rev. 1'–4') and a ritual instruction (rev. 5'–7')	Portrait; *u'iltu*(?)
	KAL 10 no. 13	Obverse: fragmentary diagnostic statement and ritual instruction for treating a "Curse" (obv. 1–12) Reverse: fragmentary ritual instruction(?) (rev. 4'–5')	Portrait(?); *u'iltu*
	LKA 137	Obverse: prayer to Šamaš for taking an omen with two stones (obv. 1–29)	Portrait(?); *u'iltu*

TABLE 13 Texts with broken colophons (*cont.*)

Group	Text	Content	Format and designation
		Reverse: three columns with a ritual instruction for making the stone omen as well as a diagram for how to cast the stones	
	(N4 no. 254, unpublished)	(*Bīt mēseri*?)	(Uncertain)
Other texts	N4 A 2362	(Unclear due to damage)	(Fragmentary); [...]
	(N4 no. 401, unpublished)	(Literary?)	(Uncertain)
		Kiṣir-[*Aššur/Nabû + broken title/no title*]	
Medical Texts	*BAM* 68[a]	Obverse and reverse: one prescription for someone who is ill with *šibiṭ šāri, ḫimiṭ ṣēti, šimmatu, ri*[*mûtu*], *šaššaṭu*, "Hand of ghost", "Hand of Curse", or any illness, and the prescription is to be issued as an enema (obv. 1–rev. 17)	Landscape; [...]
	BAM 202	Obverse and reverse: six prescriptions (obv. 1–6, 7–8, 9–12, 13–16, 17–24+[...]) against various types of insanity to be administered as fumigation and anointment (obv. 1–6), fumigation alone (obv. 13–16)), drunk on an empty stomach (obv. 7–8), ritual actions with figurines (obv. 9–12, 17–24+rev. 1'–4'), and three prescriptions against a man	Portrait; N/A

a Maul (2019: 287) notes that the tablet upon collation can be distributed to Kiṣir-Aššur and likely assigned to his *mašmaššu*-phase. However, he transliterates ᴾ*Ki-ṣir*-AN.[ŠÁR MAŠ.MAŠ(?)]. I have therefore chosen to designate *BAM* 68 as a tablet copied by either Kiṣir-Aššur or Kiṣir-Nabû during an uncertain phase.

TABLE 13 Texts with broken colophons (*cont.*)

Group	Text	Content	Format and designation
		suffering from "Hand of *bennu*" (rev. 5'–11', 12', 13') all supplying him with neck amulets	
	BAM 206	Obverse: (broken) Reverse: a single prescription of various ingredients to be drunk on an empty stomach (rev. 1'–15')	Portrait; IM.GÍD.DA
	BAM 260	Obverse/reverse(?): six prescriptions, likely all for drinking, to make a man drunk (obv. 1–3, 4, 5–6), to make a man thirsty (obv. 7–10) and related to a coughing man (obv. 12–15)	Portrait; *u'iltu*
	BAM 311	Obverse: 41 prescriptions (obv. 1'–50') for producing *mêlu* neck amulets against *ḫūṣ ḫīp(i) libbi*, Lugal-urra, *mimma lemnu*, and the alû-demon Reverse: at least 26 prescriptions (rev. 51'–93') for producing *mêlu* neck amulets treating a terrified man crying like a goat in his bed, a man crying out, Antašubba, Lugal-urra, and a man grinding his teeth in bed	Portrait; N/A
Ritual texts	*KAL* 4 no. 37[b]	Obverse (fragmentary): remains of a ritual instruction (obv. 1'–9') and a prayer(?) (obv. 10'–14') Reverse (fragmentary): remains of a ritual instruction (rev. 1'–6')	Portrait(?); [...]

b Maul and Strauß (2011: 85–86) reconstruct this text as Kiṣir-Nabû's, presumably based on the fact that both broken ancestor names carry the title *mašmaš bīt Aššur*. In Kiṣir-Aššur's colophons, the last ancestor, Bāba-šuma-ibni, would normally be *zabardabbi Ešarra*, whereas both Kiṣir-Nabû's ancestors are frequently *mašmas bīt Aššur*. However, in Kiṣir-Aššur's LKA 119 from his *mašmaš bīt Aššur*-phase, he provides the *mašmaš bīt Aššur* title for his father and grandfather. Therefore, the name cannot be reconstructed with certainty.

TABLE 13 Texts with broken colophons (*cont.*)

Group	Text	Content	Format and designation
	KAL 9 no. 41[c]	Obverse and reverse(?): fragmentary prayer to various gods concerning transgressions (obv. 1–9+ rev. 1'–2') and a ritual instruction (rev. 3')	(Fragmentary, Portrait(?)); N/A
	N4 no. 443	Obverse and reverse: prayer to Girra(?)	Portrait(?); N/A
	KAR 90	Obverse and reverse: header stating the content is related to the ritual actions of *ilī ul īde* (obv. 1), thereafter follows one long ritual instruction (obv. 2–rev. 15) and four brief ones (rev. 16, 17, 18, 19); the final line states that the ritual actions of *Šurpu* are performed afterwards (rev. 20)	Portrait; N/A
Other texts	*ACh Supp.* 2 24	Obverse and reverse (broken around the middle): commentary on individual lines of at least the 20th tablet of the astrological-astronomical omen series *Enūma Anu Enlil*	Portrait; *malsûtu*
	BAM 366	Obverse (col. i–ii) and reverse (col. iii–iv): list containing various types of stones and how many are in the collection; runs from highest to lowest number and produces a total of the inventory	Two-columned; [...]

c Jakob (2018: 91) reconstructs the name as Kiṣir-[Aššur] in rev. 4' and the title [*mašmaš bīt Aššur*] in rev. 5'. Such a division of name and title across two lines is attested in, e.g., *BAM* 164 and *BAM* 177, although I avoid restoration in *KAL* 9 no. 41 as nothing indicates that a title was written in rev. 5'.

incantations and instructions in preparation of going to an audience in a palace (*KAL* 7 no. 24; Stadhouders 2013: 305–11), and a prayer to a divinity who may have been Girra (N4 no. 443). Furthermore, *LKA* 137 consists of a prayer, a ritual and an illustrative drawing for preparing a stone omen ritual (*psephomancy*).[19]

Additionally, there are three texts that cannot be categorized properly within the previous groups: an unpublished literary extract or text (N4 no. 401), a slim two-columned list of amulet stones with designations in the margins of the number available within the collection (*BAM* 366; Schuster-Brandis 2008: 189f. with notes, 218 note 512), and *ACh Supp.* 2 24 from Nineveh that provides a commentary on the first paragraph of the 20th tablet of *Enūma Anu Enlil* concerning eclipses (Rochberg 1988: 176, 225–27; see Section 7.6). N4 A 2362 is presumably too broken to determine the content.

7.3.1 *Text-internal Features Useful as Allocating Criteria*

Several of the tablets discussed above cannot be attributed to a career phase with any certainty, and must be classified as tablets written by either Kiṣir-Aššur or Kiṣir-Nabû at an uncertain stage of their career.[20] Other texts can be argued to stem from certain phases based on text-internal features. As in the group without titles, a number of the tablets with broken colophons include purpose statements that enable a distribution to later career phases.[21] Similarly, *BAM* 206 was labelled as an IM.GÍD.DA, which were only used during Kiṣir-Aššur's *šamallû mašmaššu ṣeḫru-* and *mašmaššu*-phases in the surviving evidence.

KAL 7 no. 24 likely had a broken title after Kiṣir-Aššur's name. Meinhold (2017: 62) reconstructed his title as [MAŠ.MAŠ], and it is relatively certain that the tablet cannot have contained more than two broken signs (ibid.: 164–65, 194–95). The content concerns "entering the palace" (É-gal-ku$_4$-ra) and such incantations generally focus on how to get access to legal authorities and averting any dangers by doing so (Stadhouders 2013: 305–11; see Stadhouders and Panayotov 2018 for similar texts from N4).

Considering that rituals against an "Adversary" (*bēl dabābi*), be it magically or legally, appear on a tablet without a title (*KAR* 171) that also contains a purpose statement, and that such legal connotations are found associatively through

19 Lambert 2007: 19–20; Finkel 1995; Horowitz and Hurowitz 1992; cf. Reiner 1960a. *LKA* 137 obv. 29: [K]A.INIM.MA EŠ.BAR ^{na4}GIŠ.NU$_{11}$.GAL ^{na4}KUR.NU.[DIB], "Incantation for an oracle (using) alabaster and haemati[te] stones" (Finkel 1995: 272).

20 Kiṣir-Aššur's broken unassigned texts: *BAM* 40, N4 no. 401. Broken unassigned texts from either Kiṣir-Aššur or Kiṣir-Nabû: *BAM* 260, *KAL* 4 no. 37, *KAR* 90.

21 The broken tablets with purpose statements are: *BAM* 68, *BAM* 202, *BAM* 311, *KAL* 9 no. 41, *KAR* 90, N4 no. 443. It is unclear if the intitial line in the colophon of *BAM* 206 is a purpose statement, see Ch. 8 note 84.

"Seizing-of-the-mouth" *kadabbedû* in Kiṣir-Aššur's *BAM* 28 from his *mašmaš bīt Aššur*-phase, it is likely *KAL* 7 no. 24 stems from at least his *mašmaššu*-phase.[22] However, it is unclear if *KAL* 7 no. 24 was designed to grant Kiṣir-Aššur himself or his clients an audience.[23]

Other texts provide clues for their distribution as well. Section 6.3 discusses the use of house demarcating rituals during Kiṣir-Aššur's *mašmaššu*-phase. Therefore, the text relating to *bīt mēseri* (N4 no. 254) may belong to Kiṣir-Aššur's *mašmaššu*-phase, although he also copied guidelines for this ritual as *šamallû* (N4 no. 175). Kiṣir-Aššur's ritual for obtaining a stone omen *LKA* 137 is listed in the first section of the EM.[24] However, it is uncertain during what phase Kiṣir-Aššur copied the text, although the content was copied from a certain Nabû-[…]'s IM.GÍD.DA, possibly pointing towards Kiṣir-Aššur's *šamallû mašmaššu ṣeḫru-* or *mašmaššu*-phase.[25] The commentary *ACh Supp.* 2 24 is discussed in Section 7.6.

7.3.2 *Excursus: Inventory Texts from the N4 Collection*

BAM 366 is a two-columned list of amulet stones wherein each entry is marked with a number, which possibly indicates how many stones were present in the stock taker's collection (Schuster-Brandis 2008: 189f. with notes). Unfortunately, the colophon is too broken to determine if the tablet was written by Kiṣir-Aššur or Kiṣir-Nabû, and whether or not it contained a title. I have chosen to discuss this manuscript here alongside two similar texts in relation to Kiṣir-Aššur's tablets without titles or with broken colophons.

It remains uncertain if *BAM* 366 was written at some stage of apprenticeship, in which the apprentice took note while his father took stock, or if the stock taker was a fully educated specialist. The text likely lists the stones and numbers available at a specific point in time. In total, the list states that the N4 collection included 315 stones (*BAM* 366 rev. 18'), divided into many types, and there were as many as 14 stones of some types (*BAM* 366 obv. 5). The colophon totals the entire tablet and states:

22 Note that *kadabbedû* was also treated in Kiṣir-Aššur's *šamallû ṣeḫru* manuscript *BAM* 201.

23 Kiṣir-Aššur was likely not involved in the Aššur cult before he became *mašmaš bīt Aššur* (Section 8.1). If *KAL* 7 no. 24 was designed to grant him entrance to, e.g., the palace and the king, the text may have belonged to his late *mašmaššu*-phase, as this use of the text would indicate he was partially involved in rituals pertaining to the state during this phase.

24 *KAR* 44 rev. 25: "(Omen) decision by stars, birds, oxen, goats (and) stone oracular utterance of all god(s)", EŠ.BAR MUL.MEŠ MUŠEN.MEŠ *u* GU_4.MEŠ MÁŠ.ANŠE.MEŠ INIM.GAR ^{na4}DÚR.NA.DE_5 DINGIR.DÙ.A.BI.

25 *LKA* 137 rev. 8: *ki-i pi-i* IM.GÍD.DA $^{p.d}$PA-[…].

> A total of 315 stones (for) 'neck-(amulet(s))' of Marduk, which *are suitable for use*, placed [*in*? …], the tablets [x(?)] Kiṣir-[Aššur/Nabû …].[26]

As discussed in Section 7.4, the tablets with purpose statements must have been used in relation to preparing rituals. If so, practical application must have required access to the material prescribed in the texts. Comparable sources from other periods illustrate that specific (prepared) drugs could be kept in jars upon which the name of the malady it cured was incised (Walker 1980). Inventory texts, such as *BAM* 366, may therefore reflect items kept in the N4 house at some point in the 7th century. Although the few objects found in the N4 house cannot presently be connected to performative practices, *BAM* 366 and one additional text attest to these aspects of the family trade.[27] Furthermore, a third text can be added, which illustrates that the family also had an interest in taking stock of texts.

The second text is *KADP* 36. The manuscript was excavated in the N4 collection and does not contain a colophon (Pedersén 1986 N4 no. 136). This six-columned text lists an impressive 177 drugs whereof 159 are of vegetable origin (Böck 2011: 702). The tablet was likely organized to provide an overview of what medicaments were in store by giving running totals, and adding specific references to where the ingredients were located (Böck 2010d: 164). A few examples read: "[A total] (of) 15 (different) ingredients, (located) on the first *wooden beam* from above", and "A total of 17 (different) ingredients, (located) on the third *wooden beam*".[28] Clearly, the owners of the N4 house kept track of their supplies and had the necessary medicaments to perform the rituals needed.[29]

---

26 BAM 366 col. iv 18'–22': PAP-*ma* 3 ME 15 NA_4.MEŠ ${}^{19'}$ GÚ *šá* ${}^{\text{p(sic)}}$*Mar-duk* ${}^{20'}$ [*š*]*á*? *ana* $ŠU^{II}$ *šu-ṣu-u* ${}^{21'}$ [(x) x] GAR-*an* DUB-*pa-ni* ${}^{22'}$ [x] ${}^{\text{p}}$*Ki-ṣir*-[…] (Schuster-Brandis 2008: 61–62 and note 172). For the translation of *ša ana qāti šūṣû*, see *CMAwR* 2: 416 with further references; *CMAwR* 1: 64, 121; Reiner 1961: 10 note 1; see discussion in Ch. 6 note 25. It seems likely that the DIŠ is a mistake for ${}^{\text{d!}}$*Mar-duk*, possibly indicating a cultic context.

27 For the archaeological finds in N4, see Miglus 1996: 236–41.

28 *KADP* 36 col. i 18: [PAB] 15 *ina* ${}^{\text{giš}}$PA 1 AN.[T]A-*te* (cf. *CAD* H: 155). See also col. i 36: [PA]B 20 *ina* ${}^{\text{giš}}$PA 2-*te*. Col. ii 11: PAB 17 *ina* ${}^{\text{giš}}$PA 3-*te*. In col. iv 25 storage vessels are mentioned. The drugs are described as stored in the upper, second, third, etc. shelf (*ḫaṭṭu*), roasting vessel (*qālītu*/*karpat qalīte*) or placed in bowls (*qabūtu*) (see Böck in press; Köcher 1955: 10). The term *ḫaṭṭu* is commonly translated as "shelf" in relation to this text, although the term has a range of literal meanings, such as "sceptre, staff, stick, branch" (*CAD* Ḫ: 153). Therefore, Böck (in press) argues that *ḫaṭṭu* should be translated into German as "stock", referring to wooden beams that likely provided support for the roof as part of the house. The various ingredients would possibly have been hung from these to dry. In lack of a better term, I translate it as "wooden beam" here.

29 A study of the correlation between both texts and the ingredients used in the N4 rituals and prescriptions is beyond the scope of the present work, but is worthy of future

A third text (VAT 13723+) from N4 lists various text series and their individual tablets by incipits, and in the margins the scribe presumably provided notes on the number of manuscripts kept in the collection (Geller 2000: 226ff., text A). As such, this text illustrates that multiple copies likely existed in the N4 collection of several tablets within a series, but that the users were perhaps not always aware of the numbers until they took stock (see Maul 2010a: 215 note 93).[30]

7.4 The *mašmaššu*-phase and Purpose Statements

Kiṣir-Aššur's *mašmaššu* tablet *LKA* 115 is the first tablet from a career phase that contains a purpose statement. However, such statements also occur in his *mašmaš bīt Aššur*-phase tablets and on tablets without titles. All these texts are discussed in what follows in order to argue why several of Kiṣir-Aššur's tablets without titles can be assigned to his *mašmaššu*- or *mašmaš bīt Aššur*-phases. *LKA* 115 was also copied at the request of Kiṣir-Aššur (*ú-šaš-ṭir-ma*), and such tablets are also discussed as an allocating criterion.

This study refers to phrases expressed as *ana ṣabāt epēši* "for undertaking a (ritual) procedure" as purpose statements.[31] In general, such phrases are especially attested in Assur and they are frequently coupled with statements that refer to the content as "quickly, hastily extracted" (*ḫanṭiš*/*zamar nasāḫu*).[32] This expression likely designates that the content of the tablet was copied in order to ensure the correct preparation and performance of a specific ritual

research. Equally interesting is the possible economic aspect of such ingredients, which also requires further investigation, but see preliminarily Myer 1975: 137ff.

30 Although the text is not a catalogue, as such, it does list numbers of individual texts of series in relation to the N4 collection (Schwemer 2017: 50–51; Koch 2015: 325; cf. Robson 2013: 56). See Section 3.6.1.

31 Couto-Ferreira 2018: 157, 162 and note 43; Maul 2010a: 212–13; Geller 2010: 100–101; Böck 2008: 296; Maul 2003: 180–81; Maul 1994: 159 note 16; Bottéro 1983: 159; Hunger 1968: 12; Leichty 1964: 153; Eilers 1933: 325. The phrase was typically written in either of the following ways: *a-na*/*ana ṣa-bat*/DAB *e-pe-ši*/DÙ-(*ši*). The individual phrase in Kiṣir-Aššur *KAR* 38 (*mašmaš bīt Aššur*) differs slightly, but relates to the purpose of the text. *KAR* 38 rev. 41: *a-na mu-še-piš-ú-ti ḫa-an-ṭiš* ZI-[(*ḫa*?)]. Maul translates *ana ṣabāt epēši* as: "für die Durchführung des Rituals", "für die Durchführung/Anwendung (eines Rituals)", "für die Vorbereitung der Durchführung (der Behandlung)"; Couto-Ferreira: "in order to apprehend the procedure"; Geller: "for use"; Bottéro: "rapidement prises pour usage immediate"; Hunger: "für die Durchführung eines (bestimmten) Rituals"; Leichty: "for performance of the ritual". The use of the term "purpose statement" here differs slightly from the largely didactic and votive examples illustrated by Peace (1993).

32 The exact nuances of *ḫanṭiš* and *zamar*/*ṣamar* in relation to *nasāḫu* are difficult to evaluate.

or treatment (Maul 2010a: 212–13, 216; Bottéro 1983:159; Hunger 1968: 12).[33] However, the exact role of the tablet in relation to a ritual context cannot be specified.[34] Contemporary letters corroborate that tablets were in fact copied in order to perform certain rituals:

> I shall now look up, collect and copy numerous – 20 to 30 – canonical and non-canonical tablets, (but) perform (the prayers) (only) tomorrow evening and on the night of the 15th day.
>
> *SAA* 10 no. 240[35]

The quoted letter also suggests that relevant tablets could be copied quickly and in great quantity.[36] Other letters from Nineveh suggest that several tablets with rituals were copied in their entirety as concrete instructions for some performances (Robson 2019: 118–119). When such tablets were quickly copied in preparation for a ritual, an assistant may have copied the tablet(s) needed for the ceremonial supervisor (see Section 6.1).

7.4.1 *Kiṣir-Aššur's Tablets with Purpose Statements*

A total of 19 tablets with a purpose statement can be assigned to Kiṣir-Aššur throughout his career, which can be divided into three groups: at least one text from Kiṣir-Aššur's *mašmaššu*-phase, eight texts from his *mašmaš bīt Aššur*-phase, nine without a title, and and an additional text with a broken

---

33 The verb *ṣabātu* was also used to describe the actions associated with editorial activities. Esagil-kīn-apli's and Assurbanipal's editorial activities were described as SUR.GIBIL (= *zarû*, *zâru* or *ṣa-ra-a*(?)) *ṣabātu*, understood literally as: " to undertake a new plying, spinning, weaving" and relates to the process of producing or receiving a "new edition" of a text (Frahm 2018a; Steinert 2018a: 66–72; Wee 2015: 254 and note 27; Wee 2012: 31–32, 303–4; Frahm 2011a: 327–28; Rutz 2011: 294 and note 3; Heeßel 2010a: 143 note 11; Stol 2007b: 241–42; Finkel 1988: 148, [S]UR.GIBIL DAB.MEŠ-*ma*; Hunger 1968: 98–99, no. 321 line 3; see also this term in the AMC line 125; Geller 2018a: 46–47, 49ff.; Panayotov 2018b: 113; Steinert 2018c: 166ff.; Steinert 2018d: 277–278). Therefore, the verb *ṣabātu* here likely refers to the act, i.e., "to undertake work" (*CAD* Ṣ: 21,5). Thus, *ana ṣabāt epēši* becomes "for the execution of a specific performance" in *CAD* (E: 195,1c1').

34 Some N4 tablets for preparation of rituals included the name of the patient, e.g., *LKA* 51 without a colophon, and these examples indicate that such tablets played a concrete purpose in the ritual preparations (see Maul 2010a: 213 note 82).

35 *SAA* 10 no. 240 obv. 23-rev. 2 in Parpola 1993: 191. See also Maul 1994: 31–32, 34; *SAA* 10 no. 245 rev. 12–18 in Parpola 1993: 195.

36 The letter *SAA* 10 no. 255 states that "the tablets are too numerous" to be copied in time for the ritual, which argues against the idea of quickly copying tablets in great quantity (Parpola 1993: 201–2).

title.[37] Furthermore, six texts written by either Kiṣir-Aššur or Kiṣir-Nabû during uncertain career phases contain purpose statements.[38] Generally, Kiṣir-Aššur's *ana ṣabāt epēši* tablets also contain a statement conveying that they were "(quickly) extracted", attesting to the urgency of their production.[39]

Section 6.2 suggested that Kiṣir-Aššur likely began supervising healing ceremonies during his *mašmaššu*-phase, when he copied *KAR* 230. Additionally, *namburbi*-rituals seem to appear in his corpus of texts around this time, possibly indicating a connection. *LKA* 115 represents a *namburbi*-ritual with a purpose statement and stems from Kiṣir-Aššur's *mašmaššu*-phase. As a result, the purpose statements seem to designate that the tablet in question was copied when Kiṣir-Aššur was at a level at which he was allowed to supervise a ritual performance. By extension, he must have been around the level of *mašmaššu*. As discussed above, it is likely that writing his title on tablets was not always a necessity for Kiṣir-Aššur. However, he is assumed to have included it regularly until his *mašmaššu*-phase.

Maul (2010a: 213) commented on N4 tablets with purpose statements and emphasized: "Kein einziges dieser Manuskripte wurde von einem 'jungen Assistenten', einem 'Assistenten' oder einem 'assistierenden jungen Beschwörer' geschrieben". He adds that the reason was probably because it was the master's domain to provide the cure and that it was his responsibility to ensure that mistakes in the text did not induce fatal consequences. Maul's suggestion supports the hypothesis formulated here.[40] In relation to this hypothesis, it is therefore noteworthy that Maul and Strauß (2011: 49) reconstructed the final line in Kiṣir-Aššur's *šamallû ṣeḫru* tablet *KAL* 4 no. 19 with a purpose statement:

37 *Mašmaššu*: *LKA* 115; *mašmaš bīt Aššur*: *BAM* 99, *BAM* 164, *BAM* 177, *BAM* 186, *BAM* 188, *BAM* 300, *KAR* 38 (see Ch. 8 note 84), *KAR* 374; without titles: *BAM* 78, *BAM* 333, *BAM* 351, *KAL* 10 no. 1, *KAR* 21, *KAR* 171, *LKA* 40, N4 no. 228; without title, but including the *ša Nabû tuklassu*-phrase: *BAM* 121; possibly broken title: *KAL* 10 no. 13. See Appendix 1. It remains uncertain if *KAR* 298 contained a purpose statement (cf. Wiggermann 1992: 41; Hunger 1968: 70 no. 201 ms I).

38 *BAM* 68, *BAM* 202, *BAM* 311, *KAL* 9 no. 41, *KAR* 90, N4 no. 443. It is unclear if the first line in the colophon of *BAM* 206 is a purpose statement, see Ch. 8 note 84. For *BAM* 68, see Table 13 note a.

39 The phase is usually written (*ḫanṭiš*/*zamar*) *issuḫa*/*nasḫa* (ZI-*ḫa*) or simply *zamar* before other statements (see Section 9.2).

40 The first of Kiṣir-Nabû's texts with this phrase also stem from his *mašmaššu*-phase (*KAR* 22, *KAR* 56). However, Maul (1994: 159 note 18) suggests that tablets with the *ḫanṭiš nasḫa* "hastily extracted" remark could also have been used to perform the ritual inscribed, although such tablets could also have been copied to enhance the collection (ibid.: 160). In relation to a discussion of the *šamallû ṣeḫru* tablets that were "quickly" copied, Maul (2010a: 216) proposed that such tablets could have played a role in the preparation of the ritual. This remains uncertain.

KAL 4 no. 19 rev. 8': [(*ana ṣabāt epēši*) *ḫanṭiš*] *is-su-ḫa*[41]

In my view, there is insufficient space on the tablet for this reconstruction. Considering the original size of the tablet, I doubt the line would have held more than four smaller signs before *is-su-ḫa*.[42] Thus, I would suggest reconstructing [*ḫa-an-ṭiš*].[43] As a result, no surviving Kiṣir-Aššur colophon with a title indicates that purpose statements were used by Kiṣir-Aššur before he became *mašmaššu*.[44]

Following these hypotheses, the implication is that Kiṣir-Aššur would typically have copied tablets with purpose statements, but excluding titles, somewhere around his *mašmaššu*- or *mašmaš bīt Aššur*-phases, likely after the implementation of *KAR* 230. This observation can be applied to the tablets with purpose statements in general, i.e., they are assigned to Kiṣir-Aššur's *mašmaššu* and *mašmaš bīt Aššur* tablets. However, *BAM* 121 contains both the *ša Nabû tuklassu*-phrase as well as a purpose statement.[45] Section 5.4 suggests that Kiṣir-Aššur used the *ša Nabû tuklassu*-phrase before he became *mašmaššu ṣeḫru*. Therefore, *BAM* 121 may have been the first purpose statement tablet copied by Kiṣir-Aššur before he became *mašmaššu*. This issue cannot be resolved.

7.4.2 *Tablets Copied on Behalf of Kiṣir-Aššur*

LKA 115, containing a ritual against any evil omen observed in a man's house, stems from Kiṣir-Aššur's *mašmaššu*-phase and it is also the first of three tablets from Kiṣir-Aššur's later phases that were likely copied by someone other than Kiṣir-Aššur, perhaps an assistant at some unknown career stage,[46] and thereafter checked by Kiṣir-Aššur himself:

LKA 115 rev. 10': *ki-ma la-bi-ri-šú šà-ṭir bà-*[*ri*? (x)]
LKA 115 rev. 11': *a-na ṣa-bat e-pe-ši* ᵖ*Ki-ṣir-Aš-šur* MAŠ.MAŠ
LKA 115 rev. 12': ⌜*ú*⌝*-šaš-ṭir-ma íb-ri*

---

41 Alternatively, they propose the reading *ana mušēpišūti* (Maul and Strauß 2011: 49). This possibility is also dismissed here.

42 I collated the tablet (VAT 14005) in Berlin during the summer of 2016.

43 Kiṣir-Aššur has several examples of colophons in which the last line only contains the phrase *ḫanṭiš*/*zamar nasāḫu*, see *BAM* 81, *BAM* 186, *BAM* 188, *BAM* 333(?), *BAM* 351, *LKA* 43, *LKA* 89+(?).

44 Note again the problematic *BAM* 121 with a purpose statement, and possibly from before Kiṣir-Aššur's *mašmaššu*-phase (Section 5.4).

45 The tablet is labelled a *ṭuppu*, but it is the only one among Kiṣir-Aššur's *ṭuppu*s that is in landscape format (see Appendix 1). Tablets with landscape format are only missing from Kiṣir-Aššur's *šamallû*-phase.

46 Maul 2010a: 216–17; Maul 1994: 32.

> Written (and) checked like its original. For undertaking a (ritual) procedure (of) Kiṣir-Aššur, the *mašmaššu*. He had *someone* copy (the text), and he checked (it).

The Š-stem of *šaṭāru* and G-stem of *barû* indicates that Kiṣir-Aššur had the content copied on his request and he checked it himself. Considering all of Kiṣir-Aššur's tablets, someone copied at least three further tablets on behalf of Kiṣir-Aššur: N4 no. 241 from Kiṣir-Aššur's *šamallû ṣeḫru*-phase, *BAM* 307 without a title, and *BAM* 99 from Kiṣir-Aššur's *mašmaš bīt Aššur*-phase.[47] While N4 no. 241 was argued in Section 3.7.3 to represent Kiṣir-Aššur's duties as a tutor during his earliest phase, both *BAM* 99 and *LKA* 115 contain *mašmaššu* and *mašmaš bīt Aššur* titles and they were provided with purpose statements, which, as argued above, are an indicator for a later career phase.[48] These later texts likely attest to Kiṣir-Aššur being in a position in which junior assistants would aid him in the preparations (and performance?) of rituals. Additionally, *BAM* 307 can also be assigned to at least Kiṣir-Aššur's *mašmaššu*-phase on the basis of its content and the lack of a title (Section 7.6).

Whether the later texts copied on behalf of Kiṣir-Aššur also functioned as exercises for the younger copyist remains uncertain, although this seems to have been the case in N4 no. 241 (cf. Clancier 2014: 56). Nonetheless, it is noteworthy that Kiṣir-Aššur still labelled the text as his own and that it did not include the copyist's name. Based on the discussions above, it therefore seems unlikely that tablets without titles that include purpose statements should belong to Kiṣir-Aššur's earliest phases. Whatever tablets Kiṣir-Aššur may have copied for his father's performances are therefore not regarded here as being those with Kiṣir-Aššur's name and purpose statements.

7.4.3 *Purpose Statements and Notes on Breaks*

Kiṣir-Aššur copied at least three tablets with notes in the text stating that the original copied from contained breaks. Such notations appear as *ḫepi*/*ḫīpi* "it is broken" or "break" as well as *ḫepi*/*ḫīpi eššu* "it is broken; new" or "new break" (Gabbay and Jiménez 2019: 60; Monroe 2019; Clancier 2014: 53–55; Worthington

47 N4 no. 241: rev. 13: [*ḫa*$^{?}$-*a*]*n*$^{?}$-⸢*ṭiš*$^{?}$⸣ *ú-šá-áš*-⸢*ṭir*⸣ *{*ma*}*; *BAM* 99 rev. 57–58: *a-na ṣa-bat e-pe-ši* ^{p}*Ki-ṣir-Aš-šur* MAŠ.MAŠ É *Aš-šur* [58] *za-mar ú-šaš-ṭir-ma íb-ri* …; *BAM* 307 rev. 28–29: […] ^{p}*Ki-ṣir*-AN.ŠÁR DUMU $^{p.d}$PA-*be-sún* [29] [… *ú-š*]*aš-ṭir-ma ib-ri*. *BAM* 307 was not necessarily an *ana ṣabāt epēši* tablet, as the signs before Kiṣir-Aššur's name are broken.

48 No texts copied on behalf of Kiṣir-Nabû are known. Kiṣir-Nabû may not have reached the level *mašmaš bīt Aššur*, perhaps because Assur fell to the Babylonians and Medes during his *mašmaššu*-phase, i.e., around 614 BCE (see Maul 2010a: 204, 209–11). See Section 2.3.3.

TABLE 14 Kiṣir-Aššur's and Kiṣir-Nabû's texts with notes on breaks

Text	Phase	Purpose/Label	Type of breaks
		Kiṣir-Aššur	
BAM 99	*mašmaš bīt Aššur*	*ana ṣabat epēši*	Rev. 40 *ḫe-pí eš-šú*
BAM 129	*šamallû ṣeḫru*	[...]	Col. i 8, *10, 31 ḫe-pí eš-šú*
N4 no. 237	*šamallû ṣeḫru*	*u'iltu*	Rev. 6, 7, 8, (10?) *ḫe-pí eš-šú*
		Kiṣir-Nabû	
BAM 33	*mašmaššu ṣeḫru*	[...]	Obv. 7, 9, 11 *ḫe-pí*
KAR 44	[...]	*u'iltu*	Obv. 21 *ḫe-pí eš-šú*
KAR 56	*mašmaššu*	*ana ṣabat epēši*	Obv. 7', 8', 10' *ḫe-pí eš-šú*
		Kiṣir-[Aššur/Nabû]	
BAM 311	(No title)	*ana ṣabat epēši*	Obv. 26', 31', rev. 73', 75' *ḫe-pí*

2012: 25–27). In comparison, Kiṣir-Nabû copied at least three such tablets with similar notes. These texts are presented in Table 14.

Considering all of Kiṣir-Aššur's and Kiṣir-Nabû's texts listed above, manuscripts with *ḫepi*-notes appear in the *šamallû ṣeḫru*- (*BAM* 129, N4 no. 237), *mašmaššu ṣeḫru*- (*BAM* 33), *mašmaššu*- (*KAR* 56), and *mašmaš bīt Aššur*-phases (*BAM* 99). Furthermore, several of the texts from later phases include purpose statements (*BAM* 99, *BAM* 311, *KAR* 56). As shown in Section 3.3.1, the passage with these notes on breaks in Kiṣir-Aššur's N4 no. 237 duplicate the same passage in Kiṣir-Nabû's *KAR* 56, and the notes on breaks are almost identical. Thus, the texts were likely copied from the same original, which may have been a damaged writing-board.

Clancier (2014: 53–55) considered the LB Uruk texts with *ḫepi*-notes as examples illustrating a student's ability to copy accurately, although such texts were essentially difficult to implement in practice.[49] Worthington (2012: 26), on the other hand, has questioned the argument that *ḫepi*-statements represent careful transmission in order to avoid restoration, and he argued the existence of several examples of ancient careless restorations from especially the first millennium. Kiṣir-Aššur's *šamallû ṣeḫru*-phase tablet *BAM* 129 contains consecutive rows of entries that are also found on a tablet possibly related to the therapeutic Ugu series (Section 9.3.4). Perhaps one purpose of this tablet was to illustrate Kiṣir-Aššur's ability to copy precisely. However, Kiṣir-Aššur's

49 See also Gabbay and Jiménez 2019: 60–61 and note 32, 63 note 43, 69 note 69; Monroe 2019: 131–132; Cancik-Kirschbaum and Kahl 2018: 190; Gabbay 2016: 63–64.

BAM 99 was copied by an assistant with a purpose statement (Maul 2010: 214 note 85). The assistant may therefore be responsible for the *ḫepi*-note, if we assume Kiṣir-Aššur would himself fill out the blanks when preparing the ritual. *BAM* 99 could have functioned as both an exercise for the student copying the manuscript, and a text for practical implementation by Kiṣir-Aššur. However, it is difficult to account for Kiṣir-Nabû's *KAR* 56, which was copied by himself with a purpose statement when he was *mašmaššu*. As a *mašmaššu*, Kiṣir-Nabû must have been able to fill out such breaks himself when copying the text.

While Kiṣir-Aššur's *šamallû ṣeḫru*-phase tablet *BAM* 129 could support Clancier's hypothesis described above, the use of purpose statements in some manuscripts argues against such a general interpretation. Therefore, the purpose(s) of all these notations cannot be properly evaluated presently. Regardless whether a copyist wrote from writing-boards or clay tablets, it is likely they would occasionally encounter a break in the original. Considering the few N4 tablets with *ḫepi*-notes, it is reasonable to assume that some copies contained unmarked restorations by the copyist.

7.5 A Discussion of the Dated Tablet *KAR* 267

In August (9th of the month *Ulūlu*) of 658 BCE, Kiṣir-Aššur "quickly extracted" the single columned vertical tablet (*ṭuppu*) *KAR* 267 that he "copied and checked according to its original".[50] This text contains a ritual against a ghost and it is the only dated tablet by Kiṣir-Aššur (Maul 2010a: 205 and note 52).[51] Unfortunately, the manuscript was not supplied with a title, and it therefore remains unclear during which part of his career Kiṣir-Aššur copied *KAR* 267. Unlike later NB and LB texts, the NA learned texts from especially N4 were rarely equipped with a date formula.[52] Therefore, the addition of a date to *KAR* 267 is not only important to us, but may also have marked a special occasion for Kiṣir-Aššur.

In general, the ritual in *KAR* 267 intends to dispel a ghost or "confusional states" (*ḫa(y)yattu*) from a man's body to the netherworld.[53] Stol (1993: 42–44)

---

50 *KAR* 267 rev. 28: ^iti^KIN UD. 9^(abbreviation)^.KÁM *lim-mu* ^p^*ša*-^d^PA^?^-[*šu-u*(?)]. See Maul 2010a: 205 and note 52; Hunger 1968: 69, no. 199 ms B. The *limmu* can be found in Millard 1994: 53, 120.

51 Edited in Scurlock 2006 as no. 119–120 and Scurlock 1988b. See Ebeling 1931a: 138–42, no. 30C; Farber 1987: 260–61; Foster 1996: 554–55.

52 Gesche 2001: 50–51, 56; Pedersén 1986: 44; Hunger 1968: 16, 21.

53 Translation according to Scurlock 2006: 257; see *KAR* 267 obv. 2. The ritual may have been associated with the final prayer in *bīt rimki* (Scurlock 1988b: 203; Læssøe 1955: 101), have

translated the latter as a "fit" acting as a demon. Furthermore, a "fit" could produce symptoms such as flowing saliva, bending hands and feet, confused speech, fever and aching "strings", and it is connected to the expression for epilepsy, Antašubba (ibid.: 7–8, 44; see also Avalos 2007).

In accordance with the content, the month and date may relate to ghosts. However, a traditional ritual connected to ghosts occurring on the 9th of *Ulūlu* does not exist. An OB *kispu* ritual may have been performed on the 9th of *Abu* (Tsukimoto 1985: 48–49 with references), a MA ritual against a "fit" was performed on the 29th of the month *Du'ūzu* (Stol 1993: 43; Farber 1977: 141, 189; see Bottéro 1983: 193–96), another NA reference states that ghosts should be supplied with offerings on the 29th of *Abu* (Tsukimoto 1985: 79; Farber 1977: 211–13, text III line 14), and in general a *kispu* ritual was performed in relation to the second New Year celebration in the month *Tašrītu* (Ambos 2013a: 45–46, 57–58; Tsukimoto 1985: 201–4).[54]

The month *Ulūlu* was related to an aspect of Ištar and cleansing in Assyria,[55] possibly through the word *ullulu* "to purify" (Cohen 1993: 322).[56] Various examples of intercalated second *Ulūlu*s are known from the 7th century NA court, but not for the year 658 (Parpola 1983a: 45, 187, 381–82, 482). Noticeably, Kiṣir-Nabû's commentary on "Marduk's Address to the Demons", N4 no. 163, states: "I am Asalluḫi, who was created by his own decree, am I (*to be interpreted*) as follows: he is called Anšar (i.e., Aššur) on account of (the month) *Ulūlu*".[57]

---

been performed in connection to the "Substitute King Ritual" (Parpola 1983a: XXVI), or have been related to the removal of a "curse" (Zilberg and Horowitz 2016: 182–83).

54 On the 1st–3rd of Tašrītu, a ritual called *šumma amēla eṭemmu iṣbassu* was performed (Ambos 2013a: 57ff., 201ff.). *KAR* 267 actually opened with the (admittedly generic) line obv. 1–2: DIŠ NA GIDIM$_4$ DAB-*su ina* SU-*šú il-ta-z*[*a-az-ma* NU DU$_8$-*ár*] ² *ù ḫa-a-a-at-ti* GIDIM$_4$ TUKU.MEŠ ⸢x x⸣[(ca. 4 signs)], "If a ghost afflicts a person, stays continu[ously] in (his) body [and cannot be dispelled], and he continually has confusional states (caused by) a ghost [...]" (Scurlock 2006: 352, 357). Although these were not exactly the same rituals, they both included a prayer to Šamaš (Ambos 2013a: 204–6; Scurlock 2006: 358), and they concern some of the same problems. Although impossible to investigate completely here, *KAR* 267 may have been used similarly. For the New Year celebration(s) in Assyria, see Ambos 2013a: 181ff.; Siddall 2013: 20–21; Annus 2002: 90–94; Maul 2000; Parpola 1983a: 324; van Driel 1969: 162.

55 Also recorded in an inscription of Assurbanipal (Cohen 1993: 323; Borger 1996: 103, 225; cf. ibid.: 38, 226). The Assyrian Astrolabe B describes *Elūlu* as "the work of the Elamite Ištar ..." (Wee 2016: 141 and note 82; Kolev 2013: 159; Cohen 1993: 322).

56 For *Ulūlu*'s possible relationship to Enlil or Ninurta, as well as the work song *alālu* or the word *ulāla* "the feeble", see Wee 2016: 127–28 note 4, 140–41, 143, 149.

57 Ass. 13955/gt; Frahm et al. 2016; Geller 2016: 393; Frahm 2011a: 124–25; *Iraq* 62 no. 35 obv. 1–2: *ana-ku* ᵈ*usal-lú-ḫi šá ina ra-ma-ni-šú* DÙ-*u* ⸢*ana*⸣-[*ku*] ² *ma-a ina* UGU *ú-lu-lu* AN.ŠÁR *qa*-⸢*bi*⸣.

The tablet does not contain a purpose statement, and was likely not aimed at a particular performance. Tanret (2011) argued in connection with the OB chief lamenter Ur-Utu that certain tablets were kept for the sake of remembrance and for creating a family identity, even though they had lost value and purpose. In line with the idea that tablets could hold commemorative purposes, I suggest the date attached to *KAR* 267 was (also) intended to commemorate a special day for Kiṣir-Aššur. The connection between *Ulūlu* and Aššur may supports this, although this remains conjecture. The present chapter argues that Kiṣir-Aššur's titles were important for his texts that are supplied with names until some time around the *mašmaššu*-phase. It is therefore plausible that *KAR* 267 was written during or after this phase. While it is unknown for what occasion the tablet was copied, we can entertain the idea that this text marked a special event for Kiṣir-Aššur in relation to copying a ritual suitable for a variety of private and official cultic duties. This situation may resemble the NB school texts dedicated under special circumstances to the *Nabû-ša-ḫarê* temple in Babylon (Cavigneaux 1999a: 385–86, 388–91)

7.6 Other Technical Literature: *BAM* 307 and *ACh Supp.* 2 24

Perhaps following the instructions laid out in the EM, the lexical list *CT* 37 pl. 25 from Kiṣir-Aššur's *mašmaššu*-phase represents an aspect of his training towards becoming an "expert" (*ummânu*), as suggested in Section 9.4.1. It is therefore expected that he would also copy commentaries during this training phase. However, the only commentary certainly belonging to Kiṣir-Aššur is *BAM* 307 without a title and possibly *ACh Supp.* 2 24 with a broken colophon.[58] The latter text was excavated in Nineveh (K. 3145, see below).

The left side of *BAM* 307 is completely broken, but some lines provide alternative readings, suggesting that the composition had a commentary-like content.[59] The focus was likely pharmacological, as the text lists plants and

58 Frahm (2011a: 144–45) suggests the text could have been written by Kiṣir-Nabû.

59 An example is rev. 25: […]⌜x⌝-u : *ṣu-pur an-zi-i* : *mur-din-nu*, "[…] : the sheepfold of Anzû : *amurdinnu*-bramble" (see *CAD* A/2: 90–91); rev. 19 refers to: […] *rit-ti an-zi-i* ^na4^[GÍR.TAB(?)], "the claw of Anzû (*is*) the [scorpion?]-stone" (see *CAD* R: 386; *CAD* Z: 164); rev. 26 states: […]⌜x⌝ : *ga-bi-id* UR.BAR.RA : ^giš^*bi-nu*, "[…] : "wolf's liver"-plant : *bīnu*-tamarisk". The text may be a mythological commentary similar to Livingstone 1986: 176–79, which also mentions "cedar resin : the fat of Anzû", line 59: ÚŠ ^giš^ERIN Ì.GIŠ *an-zi-i*. For commentaries in the first millennium BCE, see Gabbay 2016; Frahm 2011a.

stones.[60] The relationship between pharmacopeia and commentaries are possibly echoed in a LB text from Borsippa, which states: "When you perform (a treatment of) plant, stone, and wood (for fumigation?), or the art of *āšipūtu* for the sick man – one does (it) in accord with its explanatory comment$^{(?)}$".[61] However, unlike other N4 commentaries, *BAM* 307 does not use the *mā* particle to introduce explanations (Gabbay 2016: 31–34, 52–54; Frahm 2011a: 121–23, 269 and note 1278). Two aspects indicate that the tablet stems from at least Kiṣir-Aššur's *mašmaššu*-phase, although the purpose of the text is uncertain. Firstly, as the only commentary-like text from Kiṣir-Aššur, the text fills the space occupied by commentaries foreshadowed to exist as part of the *ummânu* training via the EM (see Section 9.4). Secondly, the text was copied on behalf of Kiṣir-Aššur whereupon he checked it ([*ú-š*]*aš-ṭir-ma ib-ri*). Although Kiṣir-Aššur likely had a younger pupil copy an exercise as *šamallû ṣeḫru* (see Section 3.7.3), such uses of junior assistants have been suggested in this chapter as generally belonging to Kiṣir-Aššur's *mašmaššu-* and *mašmaš bīt Aššur*-phases. An unresolved question is why Kiṣir-Aššur used someone to copy a tablet with esoteric content.

Additionally, Kiṣir-Aššur could have been the copyist of the commentary *ACh Supp.* 2 24. The colophon states: "for the 'reading' of Kiṣi[r-…]".[62] Perhaps this Kiṣir-[…] was our Kiṣir-Aššur or Kiṣir-Nabû (Frahm 2011a: 144–45). Kiṣir-Aššur has previously been suggested as a possible candidate, supplying manuscripts to the royal libraries (Maul 2010a: 205 and note 53; Villard 1998: 19). However, many NA individuals are attested with this name (cf. Baker 2000: 621ff.), and the content of the commentary concerns astrology, on which the N4 collection contains relatively few tablets (Pedersén 1986: 51; Frahm 2011a: 270 and note 1279). It therefore remains uncertain if the tablet was copied by Kiṣir-Aššur and whether or not he studied astrology at all.[63]

---

60 Several lines refer to illness and cure, rev. 7: […] KUR ^{d}UTU-*ši ana* IGI^{II}.GIG.MEŠ SIG$_5$, "[…] the rising of the sun is good for (*damāqu*) ill eyes" (see *CAD* N/1: 267); rev. 11: [… *ana* (body part with dual)^{I}]^{I}.G[I]G.MEŠ SIG$_5$, "[…] is good [for] ill [(body part)]s"; see rev. 12: […] NU TE, "[…] will not approach".

61 Rochberg 2015: 229 and note 88; Livingstone 1986: 73, cf. p. 7, 61–62, 96–97, 172–73, 163 255–56, 258. BM 34035 rev. 39–40 (on the copy by Epping and Strassmaier 1891: 243): *ki-i* Ú NA$_4$ *u* GIŠ *ù* ^{lú}MAŠ.MAŠ-*ú-tu a-na* GIG *te*$^{!}$*-pu-šú* ^{40} *it-ti ṣi-ti-šú e-pu-uš*. As noted by Rochberg, Livingstone took *ṣītu* as a singular of *ṣâtu* "explanatory word list(s)", which is always in plural. Rochberg (2015: 229 note 89) refers to a similar statement in another LB text. See also Heeßel 2008a: 9–12.

62 Rochberg 1988: 227, rev. 14'–15': (*catch-line*) $^{15'}$ ⌜*ana*? *mal-su*⌝*-ut* ^{p}*Ki-ṣi*[*r-*…]. For this phrase, see Section 9.2.3. See also Frahm 2004: 47 note 18.

63 The text ends with two peculiar lines on the bottom of rev. 17'–18' stating: […]⌜x⌝ *su-bar-tú* $^{18'}$ […] *su-bar-tú ana ma-šu-šú-nu* (Rochberg 1988: 227).

7.7 Summary

This chapter has provided an overview of Kiṣir-Aššur's colophons without titles or possibly broken titles. Within these groups, internal features within the texts and colophons are useful for roughly allocating the tablets to various phases of Kiṣir-Aššur's career. Kiṣir-Aššur was probably more inclined towards writing comprehensive colophons earlier in his career, at which time he may have provided his title in a majority of colophons. Alternatively, as suggested in Section 5.4, the apprentice Kiṣir-Aššur would have provided the devout *ša Nabû tuklassu*-phrase.

An important feature is Kiṣir-Aššur's use of the so-called "purpose statements", which were used to designate the texts as part of a specific ritual or healing ceremony. These statements do not occur in colophons with titles before Kiṣir-Aššur's *mašmaššu*-phase, and colophons with purpose statements, but without titles, must largely be assigned to Kiṣir-Aššur's *mašmaššu*- and *mašmaš bīt Aššur*-phase. Kiṣir-Aššur was likely in a position to head rituals during these phases, and the possible accumulation of tablets with purpose statements during these phases would support this hypothesis. Kiṣir-Aššur's simultaneous use of assistants to copy tablets on his behalf for specific performances underlines this suggestion.

The present chapter also discussed Kiṣir-Aššur's sole dated tablet without a title, *KAR* 267, and suggested it may have been copied in connection to an important event in Kiṣir-Aššur's career, possibly around his *mašmaššu* or *mašmaš bīt Aššur*-phases. If *KAR* 267 truly belonged to either of these phases, it would imply that Kiṣir-Aššur functioned as *mašmaššu* or *mašmaš bīt Aššur* in 658 BCE. However, this remains hypothetical. Finally, two examples of technical literature in the form of commentaries were discussed in relation to content.

CHAPTER 8

Kiṣir-Aššur's *mašmaš bīt Aššur*-phase

This chapter investigates the texts written by Kiṣir-Aššur during his *mašmaš bīt Aššur*-phase, during which he copied the majority of surviving texts that have titles in the colophons (24+). Three groups of tablets are distinguished among these manuscripts. The first and second groups comprise medical and ritual texts respectively, of which a substantial portion are designated as extracts (*nisḫu*, see below). Furthermore, a third group of texts possibly relates to Kiṣir-Aššur's affiliation with the Aššur temple, as witnessed by his title. What follows provides an overview of the text groups copied by Kiṣir-Aššur during his *mašmaš bīt Aššur*-phase, a discussion of his title *mašmaš bīt Aššur*, and a description of the individual texts in each group. Specific features are also investigated. Kiṣir-Aššur copied and possibly formulated several prescriptions labelled as "tested prescriptions" (*bulṭu latku*) during this period. These are analysed in relation to the predominantly medical texts, together with at least one possible panacea, i.e., a universal drug. The present chapter also discusses Kiṣir-Aššur's duties in connection to the Aššur temple.

The career phase "exorcist of the Aššur temple" (*mašmaš bīt Aššur*) is the last identifiable phase to which Kiṣir-Aššur, his brother Šamaš-ibni and their father Nabû-bēssunu progressed. The title *mašmaš bīt Aššur* could therefore mark the pinnacle of Kiṣir-Aššur's career (see Maul 2010a: 206–208, 210–11). All of the texts in Table 15, except for *PKTA* pl. 39–40, are explicitly stated as deriving from his *mašmaš bīt Aššur* phase.

The number of Kiṣir-Aššur's texts with colophons, especially medical and ritual texts, increases markedly during his *mašmaššu*-phase and even more so in his *mašmaš bīt Aššur*-phase. The texts written by Kiṣir-Aššur as *mašmaš bīt Aššur* attest to a variety of subjects, including: prescriptions against illnesses, a number of more broadly defined rituals against ghosts, witchcraft and evils, three *namburbi*-rituals, and a group of texts associated with the Aššur temple.

Of Kiṣir-Aššur's eight medical healing texts that he copied as *mašmaš bīt Aššur*, at least six were copied with a purpose statement that emphasizes their practical dimension.[1] It is worth noting that several of his medical texts from this phase concern internal illnesses (see Section 9.1). Among the rituals designed to remove malevolent causes of illness, three were also supplied

1 *BAM* 99, *BAM* 164, *BAM* 177, *BAM* 186, *BAM* 188, *BAM* 300.

TABLE 15 Texts assigned to Kiṣir-Aššur's *mašmaš bīt Aššur*-phase[a]

Group	Text	Content	Format and designation
Medical texts	*BAM* 99	Obverse and reverse: prescriptions for suppositories (obv. 1–5, 6–12, 13–16, 17–18, 19–24, 25–26, rev. 42–51), potions (obv. 27–29, 30–32, 33, 34, 35, 36, 37, 38, 39, rev. 40–41, 42–51), and baths (rev. 42–51), an enema (rev. 54–55), as well as a bandage (rev. 42–51)	Portrait; N/A
	BAM 164	Obverse and reverse: prescriptions for *mašqītu*-potions for treating a swelling (obv. 1–4), kidneys (obv. 5–9), throbbing inside(s) (obv. 10–12), discharge (obv. 13–17), repeated erection due to urine (obv. 18–21), "Anus illness" (obv. 22–rev. 25), anus (rev. 26–28), and hips (rev. 29–32)	Portrait; N/A
	BAM 177	Obverse: a tested prescription against *apišalû*(?) (obv. 1–7) Reverse: a *naṣmattu*-bandage against *ṣētu*-fever (rev. 8–12)	Landscape; N/A
	BAM 186	Obverse and reverse: Enema rinse good against *aḫḫāzu*- and *amurriqānu*-jaundice, administered against *ḫimiṭ ṣēti* (obv. 1–13), broken prescription "to give relief" (obv. 14–rev. 23), enema (rev. 24–31)	Portrait; N/A

a *PKTA* pl. 39–40 was from the "hand(s) of" either Kiṣir-Aššur or Kiṣir-Nabû, col. iv 16'–17': ⸢ŠU[II]⸣ [p]*Ki-ṣi*[*r* ...] 17' ⸢MAS[!]⸣.MAŠ ⸢É⸣ [AN.ŠÁR] (Parpola 2017: 145). The dual writing of body parts was perhaps a writing convention in N4, see Section 3.3. Section 8.6 suggests that the text could be from Kiṣir-Aššur's *mašmaš bīt Aššur*-phase due to its relevance for the Aššur temple. *PKTA* pl. 10–11 does not preserve a name, but contains an unusual version of the *mašmaš bīt Aššur* title, rev. 25: [MAŠ.MAŠ] ⸢*šá* É⸣ AN.ŠÁR (Parpola 2017: 102). Although this does not resemble Kiṣir-Aššur's usual title, MAŠ.MAŠ É *Aš-šur*/AN.ŠÁR, the text was excavated in the N4 collection (N4 no. 98) and could have been written by him.

TABLE 15 Texts assigned to Kiṣir-Aššur's *mašmaš bīt Aššur*-phase (*cont.*)

Group	Text	Content	Format and designation
	BAM 188	Obverse: (broken) Reverse: enema against *martu*-bile, *aḫḫāzu*- or *amurriqānu*-jaundice (rev. 1–10)	Portrait; N/A
	BAM 300	Obverse: (broken) Reverse: broken prescription (rev. 1–5), considered good against all ailments	Landscape; *u'iltu*
	BAM 303	Obverse and reverse: tested prescriptions for general softening up (obv. 1'–4', 5'–8', 9'–10', 11'–13') and one for softening up feet (obv. 14'–rev. 23')	Portrait; *ṭuppu*
Ritual texts	Beckman and Foster 1988 no. 21	Obverse and reverse: unknown incantation ritual; one long entry of uncertain content(?) (col. i 1–26'); col. ii (broken); two broken entries of uncertain content (col. iii 1'–3'+4'–7')	Two-columned; [...]
	KAR 38	Obverse and reverse: *namburbi*-ritual against divine anger from poorly executed ritual and preparation (obv. 1–8), prayers and incantations (obv. 9–23, obv. 32–rev. 10; rev. 18–27), ritual instructions (obv. 24–31, rev. 11–17, rev. 28–39)	Portrait; *ṭuppu*
	KAR 62	Obverse and reverse: ritual against someone angry consisting of an incantation and rubric (obv. 1–rev. 1) and a ritual instruction (rev. 2–15)	Portrait; *u'iltu*
	KAR 63	Obverse and reverse: ritual against an angry person or anger directed at a man; incantations and rubrics (obv. 1–7, 19–30, rev. 4'–16'), ritual instructions (obv. 8–18, rev. 17'–21'), and a broken section (rev. 1'–3')	Portrait; *u'iltu*

TABLE 15 Texts assigned to Kiṣir-Aššur's *mašmaš bīt Aššur*-phase (*cont.*)

Group	Text	Content	Format and designation
	KAR 80	Obverse and reverse: diagnosis of and ritual against witchcraft (obv. 1–11), prayers, incantations and a rubric (obv. 12–rev. 14'; rev. 20–24; rev. 25–37), ritual instruction (rev. 15–19)	Portrait; *ṭuppu*
	KAR 374	Obverse and reverse: divine anger or turmoil(?); incantation (obv. 1–22 (breaks off)), ritual instruction (rev. 1'–16')	Portrait; *ṭuppu*
	LKA 70+ (*KAR* 57)	Obverse and reverse: second tablet of an incantation ritual for Ištar and Dumuzi; "diagnosis" (col. i 1–2), ritual instructions (col. i 3–13, 14–27; col. iv (7'), (8')+1–7, 13–17), incantations and rubrics (col. i 28–col. ii (10'); col. ii (11'–26'); col. iii (1–8), (9–24), (25–30?) (breaks off); col. iv (broken entry), 8–12), catch-line (col. iv 18)	Two-columned; *ṭuppu*
	LKA 77	Obverse and reverse: Sumerian incantations with Akkadian translations against *mimma lemnu* (col. i 1–4, 5–7, 8–11, 12–21, 22–24, 25–27, 38–43, 44–56, 57–59(?); col. ii 1'–6', 7'–19', 20'–27', 28'–34', 35'–47', 48'–52', 53'–56'; col. iii 1'–12', 13'–21', 22'–30', (break of ca. 8 lines), 40'–42', 43'–55'; col. iv 1–4, 5–7, 8–13', 14'–20', 21'–27', 28'–50', 51'–54' (breaks off); col. v 1–7, 8–33, 34–46, 47–53; col. vi 1–7, 8–24), rubric (col. vi 25)	Three-columned; *ṭuppu*
	LKA 83	Obverse and reverse: incantations against a ghost (obv. 1–12, obv. 13–rev. 14, rev. 15–21)	Landscape; *u'iltu*

TABLE 15 Texts assigned to Kiṣir-Aššur's *mašmaš bīt Aššur*-phase (*cont.*)

Group	Text	Content	Format and designation
	LKA 113	Obverse: *namburbi*-ritual against evil portended by a bow (obv. 1), ritual instruction (obv. 2–12), prayer (obv. 13–17 (breaks off) Reverse: only colophon preserved	Portrait; *ṭuppu*
	LKA 119	Obverse and reverse: *namburbi*-ritual against contagion by dust from an evil place and preparation (obv. 1–11), prayer (obv. 12–rev. 7), ritual instruction (rev. 8–14)	Portrait; *ṭuppu*
Other texts	*KAR* 307	Obverse and reverse: mystical text (obv. 1–29), mythological description of the world (obv. 30–rev. 19), the king's paraphernalia and incense (rev. 20–25), secrecy formula (rev. 26–27)	Portrait; [*ṭuppu*(?)]
	KAV 42	Obverse and reverse: list of gods (obv. col. i–iii 1–119), list of city gates (obv. col. iii 120–33), list of temples with Sumerian names (rev. 14–32+lo.e.), section on the three ziggurats (rev. 33–35), list of gates from Sennacherib's renovation of the *Ešarra* temple complex (rev. 36–40)	Generally three-columned, although see Appendix 1
	N4 no. 110	Obverse: a heading (obv. 1), list of various cultic materials (obv. 2–28), individually ruled off lines possibly describing the cultic circumstances of the list (obv. 29–31) Reverse: a list of obscure deities related to various gods (rev. 1–24)	Portrait: *u'iltu*

TABLE 15 Texts assigned to Kiṣir-Aššur's *mašmaš bīt Aššur*-phase (*cont.*)

Group	Text	Content	Format and designation
		Possibly Kiṣir-Aššur; *mašmaš bīt Aššur* title preserved	
Medical texts	*BAM* 28	Obverse and reverse: symptom description concerned with *kadabbedû*, swollen tongue, troubled breath, running saliva and teeth oozing with blood (obv. 1–3), ritual instructions (obv. 4–6, 10–12, 19–20, rev. 1'–2', 12'–13', 16'), incantations (obv. 7–9, 13–16, 17–18, rev. 3'–11', 14'–15')	Portrait; *ṭuppu*(?)
Ritual texts	*BAM* 321	Obverse and reverse: prayers (obv. 1–9, 27–31), incantations (obv. 18–23) and ritual instructions (obv. 10–17, 24–26, rev. 32–51) concerning a man's god and goddess	Portrait; [...]
	LKA 157	Obverse and reverse: witchcraft diagnosis (col. i 1–13), prayers and incantations (col. i 14–20(?); col. ii 1'–6'; col. iii 1'–17'), ritual instructions (col. i 21–22 (breaks off); col. iv 1'–5'), subscript (col. iv 6')	Two-columned; [...]
		Possibly Kiṣir-Aššur; possibly from the *mašmaš bīt Aššur*-phase	
Other texts	*PKTA* pl. 10–11	Obverse and reverse: temple service rites and instructions for Assyrian temples (obv. 1'–8', 9'–31', rev. 1–23)	Portrait; [...]
	PKTA pl. 39–40	Obverse and reverse: decree by a king Shalmaneser regarding the Aššur temple personnel (col. i 1–4, i 5'–ii 17'; iii 1'; iii 2'–iv 14')	Portrait; (see Section 8.6)

with purpose statements.[2] All these tablets with purpose statements, plus one more, were designated as extracts,[3] seemingly indicating that at least ten out of possibly 26 tablets from Kiṣir-Aššur's *mašmaš bīt Aššur*-phase served largely pragmatic purposes.

Furthermore, two of Kiṣir-Aššur's tablets from this phase were numbered as "7th extract" (*BAM* 99) and "final extract" (*KAR* 63), indicating that Kiṣir-Aššur organized certain extracts during this phase (see Section 9.2.3). *BAM* 99 was written by someone else on the request of Kiṣir-Aššur (*ú-šaš-ṭir-ma*) and supplied with a purpose statement, which suggests that apprentices could have copied some of Kiṣir-Aššur's extracts with purpose statements without explicitly stating so. At least one text (*KAV* 42) was described as "written by Kiṣir-Aššur" (*šà-ṭír* ᵖ*Kiṣir-Aš-šur*) and contains evidence of editing (see Section 8.6).

8.1 The Title *mašmaš bīt Aššur*

The title "exorcist of the Aššur temple" (*mašmaš bīt Aššur*) ran in the Bāba-šuma-ibni family as well as other families attested in the N4 collection (Fadhil 2012: 38). Bāba-šuma-ibni, his son Nabû-bēssunu, Nabû-bēssunu's sons Kiṣir-Aššur and Šamaš-ibni, Nabû-bēssunu's brother Abu-erība, and Abu-erība's son of unknown name, all claimed the title at some point.[4] Whether the title was hereditary, served a practical or honorary purpose, or if individuals claimed the title in relation to specific duties or during particular periods is largely unknown.[5] Furthermore, it is uncertain if individuals claiming this title were counted among the regular temple staff, although they may have been

2 *KAR* 38, *KAR* 374, *LKA* 157.

3 *KAR* 63 does not have a purpose statement, but is designated as a "final extract" (*nis-ḫu qí-ta-a-a-ú*). See Section 9.2.3. *BAM* 321's colophon is largely broken.

4 See Section 2.3.3. The reconstruction by Baker (2017: 18) in *LKA* 141 of Kiṣir-Aššur's title as *šamallû mašmaššu ṣeḫru* ⸢*šá*⸣ [É *Aš-šur*] is disregarded here (see Appendix 1).

5 In the LB colophons investigated by Ossendrijver (2011: 643), titles for copyists frequently represented a mix of traditional clan or qualification titles, but not necessarily temple offices. Villard (2007: 328–29 and note 77) suggested that the title *zabardabbû* may have designated a treasurer (cf. Lafont 1987: 51–52 with comparative third and second millennium BCE material). This prompted Villard (2007: 329) to suggest that exorcists could have served as treasurers before the reign of Esarhaddon. However, this remains uncertain, and Villard (ibid.) points out that we know nothing about this for Kiṣir-Aššur. If Nabû-bēssunu is actually the individual mentioned in *SAA* 13 no. 39, he would have been involved in affairs of the temple administration (ibid.: 328–29). See also May 2018: 66–67.

involved in the performance of various cultic rituals.[6] Contemporary evidence suggests that numerous people within Assur were associated with the Aššur temple during the 7th century BCE (Radner 2017b: 225). Thus, as implied by the title, there is a close association with the Aššur temple, even though the exact nature of it still eludes us.

Different designations for the Aššur temple complex and its various parts were used during the NA period (George 1992: 172, 177, 183, 185–191; van Driel 1969: 34ff.). The two most common names, likely referring to the whole temple complex were É ᵈ*Aššur* and É.ŠÁR.RA.[7] Kiṣir-Aššur and others claimed association with the former in their titles, whereas the latter is attested in Bāba-šuma-ibni's title *zabardabbi Ešarra* (Maul 2010a: 200 note 40, 203). Prebends or leftovers from divine meals may have supported the Bāba-šuma-ibni family, but the evidence is tenuous (cf. Robson 2019: 109; Frame and Waerzeggers 2011: 129; Geller 2010: 50).[8]

Generally, it has been suggested that exorcists in the first millennium BCE acted as "temple enterers" (*ērib bīti*), a priestly title indicating access to the inner temple and association with the temple staff (Frame and Waerzeggers 2011: 132; Geller 2010: 50; Jean 2006: 139). However, it is unknown if this applied to Kiṣir-Aššur and his family,[9] and it is unclear to what extent the N4 family exorcists were allowed into the sanctuary of Aššur.[10] Evidence for some

---

6 Maul 2010: 200–201, 206–207; Jean 2006: 140, 142; Maul 2000: 391; Menzel 1981: 247; cf. Pongratz-Leisten 2015: 331, 394, 396–97.

7 Maul 2010a: 200 and note 40; George 1993a: 145; van Driel 1969: 34; see also Ermidoro 2017: XXVIII; Menzel 1981: 247.

8 Although the context is uncertain, Jean (2006: 141 and note 552) refers to Urad-Gula's "The Forlorn Scholar" letter, in which he states that he received "leftovers" (*riḫātu*) (*SAA* 10 no. 294 obv. 17; see *CAD* R: 340).

9 Priests presumably had shaved heads (Waerzeggers 2008; Löhnert 2007; Sallaberger and Vulliet 2005: 618; Borger 1973: 172–74; Menzel 1981: 189–90, 239–40; cf. Robson 2011b: 605 note 7 concerning NA *bārûs* at court). The exorcist appearing in a dream before the sufferer Šubši-mešrê-Šakkan in *Ludlul bēl nēmeqi* is described as "bearded" (Annus and Lenzi 2010: 39). See also *SAA* 10 no. 96 rev. 1ff. and no. 97 obv. 5′ff. for cultic shaving.

10 The N4 home was connected to individuals in high positions in various temples (Fadhil 2012: 39–42; Maul 2010a: 212, 216–17). NA exorcists are, however, rarely attested directly in relation to the performance of rituals in temples, see, e.g., *SAA* 13 no. 71. They were part of the renovation or production of cultic statues in the temple workshop (*bīt mummi*) (Walker and Dick 2001: 8ff., 15–16, 52 note 34). For a discussion of NA exorcists connected to temples, see Koch unpublished: 7; Jean 2006: 139–43; Sallaberger and Vulliet 2005: 632. Ermidoro (2017: XIX–XX) has recently emphasized that the entire "Inner City" (*libbi āli*), another name for the city Assur, was presented in rituals as "a single cultic place". As such, the city itself may have functioned as a macro-temple complex, meaning that a resident may have had some access to temples. Esarhaddon indicates "his people" had access to the outer courtyard of the Aššur temple (Pongratz-Leisten 2017: LV).

measure of access to the Aššur temple is perhaps implied when water from the cistern (*būrtu*) of a Marduk temple is prescribed in two ritual instructions in *BAM* 28, which was probably copied by Kiṣir-Aššur as *mašmaš bīt Aššur*.[11] This water may have been associated with the *apsû* via an incantation in the text to be recited in connection to using the water.[12] The connection to the *apsû* in the Aššur temple could have been established through an *apsû* water tank, which Sennacherib installed in the inner courtyard.[13] Although *BAM* 28 specifies water from the Marduk temple cistern, Kiṣir-Aššur may have been able to draw *apsû*-water from, e.g., the Aššur temple as a substitute. As such, he may have had access to at least some inner temple courtyards.

8.2 Medical Texts from Kiṣir-Aššur's *mašmaš bīt Aššur*-phase

Kiṣir-Aššur did not copy out medical prescriptions between his *šamallû ṣeḫru*- and *mašmaššu ṣeḫru*-phases. Although a number of medical texts were copied without a title that may belong to his *mašmaššu*- or *mašmaš bīt Aššur*-phases, the prescriptions copied during his *mašmaš bīt Aššur*-phase represent the principal group of medical texts that can certainly be attributed to any of his educational and career phases. What follows provides a brief discussion of the content of the relevant texts.

BAM 28 contains one initial diagnosis separated by lines for *kadabbedû* or *bu'šānu* and afterwards at least five ritual instructions and five incantations.[14] Because the text contains a diagnosis, I have included it in this section. Prescriptions related to *kadabbedû* were already copied by Kiṣir-Aššur as *šamallû ṣeḫru* (see Section 3.1), but *BAM* 28 is the first of Kiṣir-Aššur's texts with colophons to mention the *bu'šānu*-illness. This illness is described by Scurlock

11 *BAM* 28 obv. 5 and 10: A.MEŠ/A PÚ *šá* É ᵈAMAR.UTU, "water of the Marduk temple's well". Such water was also employed in several *namburbi*-rituals (Maul 1994: 41 and note 45). For the word *būrtu*, see Dalley 2013: 65. *BAM* 28 is discussed in Section 8.2.

12 *BAM* 28 obv. 11 and 13ff.: ÉN ÈŠ ZU.AB NÌ.NAM MÚ.A …, "In the abode of the Abzu, which produced all that there is …" (Kinnier Wilson and Reynolds 2007: 73).

13 Gries 2017: 39, 86–87, pls. 70 and 165; Andrae 1938: 13, 26, 155, tafel 2b. The inscription on Sennacherib's *apsû* water tank also mentions the word PÚ/*būrtu* "well" (Gries 2017: 87 with references). The tank was damaged and the pieces were excavated mainly in a cistern in the so-called "Ostanbau", see Gries 2017: pl. 7.

14 One additional fragment of this tablet was published in Beckman and Foster 1988 no. 7, which adds the previously missing title to the colophon. Furthermore, a piece of the tablet was collated in Durand 1982 pl. 120. The text has only been partially edited. See Scurlock and Andersen 2005: 784 with internal references; Kinnier Wilson and Reynolds 2007: 73–74; Collins 1999: 191ff.; Farber 1990b: 313ff.; Scheil 1921: 17–17 no. 13.

and Andersen (2005: 40–42) as a syndrome, which can occur in the "windpipe", among the teeth or in the hard and soft palates or soft cheek pockets (*nurzu* and *narbu*).[15] Several of the incantations in BAM 28 are in (pseudo) Sumerian and the repetitive incantation "Mouth-seizing, mouth-seizing, mouth-seizing seiz[ed …], bite, bite, bite […]" appears to be a form of mumbo-jumbo.[16] As discussed above, at least two instructions use water from the cistern (*būrtu*) of the Marduk temple. Notably, temples are rarely mentioned in medical texts, and the only other example among Kiṣir-Aššur's texts is BAM 78 without a title. This text describes how a patient with specific internal pains of the *tulīmu* should "visit Marduk's sanctuary (*ešertu*) and he will recover".[17]

Originally, Köcher (1963a: XVI) and later Beckman and Foster (1988: 1–3) suggested that the text was copied by Kiṣir-Nabû, based on the fragmented signs in the theophoric element of the copyist's name. Now, the last line of the colophon comprising BAM 28 and Beckman and Foster 1988 no. 7 reads:

> *BAM* 28 rev 18': [DU]B *p**Ki-ṣir-*$^{d!}$[x (x)] ^{lú}MAŠ.MAŠ É AN.⸢ŠÁR⸣
> "[Tabl]et of Kiṣir-[Aššur], the *mašmaš bīt Aššur*".[18]

Considering that Kiṣir-Nabû probably did not reach the phase *mašmaš bīt Aššur* (Maul 2010a: 211), it is reasonable to assume that the name should be reconstructed as *Ki-ṣir*-AN$^{!}$.[ŠÁR] or $^{d!}$[*Aš-šur*], but this requires further collation (cf. May 2018: 65, 71; Ch. 8 note 18). However, it cannot be excluded that the name should be reconstructed as Kiṣir-Nabû. The text was designated as "quickly extracted".

BAM 99 contains several diagnoses and prescriptions concerning internal maladies of the gastro-intestinal system, as well as various illnesses of the anus

15 Scurlock 2014: 289–90; cf. Farber 1990b: 315 and note 59. The name *bu'šānu* likely refers to the verb *ba'āšu* "to stink", possibly referring to a symptom of the illness (Böck 2014a: 157, 166). The illness is regularly identified as "diphtheria" by modern researchers, although this remains uncertain (Scurlock 2014: 390; Scurlock and Andersen 2005: 40; Köcher 1978: 20–21; cf. Cadelli 1997: 32; Kinnier Wilson 1996: 138; Kämmerer 1995: 157; Kinnier Wilson 1966: 52–54).

16 BAM 28 obv. 17–18: ÉN KA.DAB KA.DAB KA.DAB DA[B (*ca. five signs missing*)] ^{18} ZÚ.KUD ZÚ.KUD ZÚ.KUD [(*ca. four signs missing*)]. For a discussion of such incantations, see Böck 2014a: 189–90; Veldhuis 1999: 46–48.

17 BAM 78 obv. 3: [x x b]i$^{?}$ ud ⸢*aš*⸣-*rat* ⸢^{d}⸣[AMAR.U]TU KIN.KIN-*ma* TI; see a translation of a duplicate passage from BAM 77 in Stol 2006: 113.

18 In Köcher's copy, the name could be read *p**Ki-ṣir-*^{d}A[G$^{(\text{ligature})?}$]. Ligatures of ^{d}AG in Kiṣir-Nabû's name can be found in, e.g., BAM 101 rev.$^{?}$ 13, BAM 106 rev. 9', and KAR 223 rev. 14. Furthermore, the lú of the title looks like a Babylonian form on Beckman and Foster's copy.

and ritual instructions for producing enemas and suppositories, for drinking potions, and for bathing the patient.[19] *BAM* 99 is listed as a "7th extract", includes a purpose statement, and states that it was copied hurriedly on behalf of Kiṣir-Aššur (*ú-šaš-ṭir-ma*), as discussed in Section 7.4.2.

BAM 164 contains several prescriptions for potions concerning a variety of maladies, which are specified as being against swelling (*dikšu*), the kidney(s) (ÉLLAG), the spleen (ŠÀ.GI$_6$), discharge (*mūṣu*), continually "rising" due to urine,[20] and "Anus illness" (DÚR.GIG).[21] After the majority of prescriptions, the text specifies the number of plants to be used and in one example that the ingredients are "tested" (*latkūti*). After these notations, the patient is instructed to drink the concoction in water, beer or wine. Kiṣir-Aššur copies several "tested" prescriptions during his *mašmaš bīt Aššur*-phase, and these are discussed in Section 8.3. The colophon designates the text as "hurriedly extracted" and supplies it with a purpose statement.

BAM 177 is a brief text containing two prescriptions, of which the latter is against "sun-heat" (*ṣētu*).[22] The first prescription may have been designated as "tested", although the final signs of the sentence are broken (*lat-ku* ⸢x⸣[x], see below). The latter prescription is the only one to specify an application method, namely a "poultice" (LAL-*ti*). The colophon contains a purpose statement and states that the text was "hurriedly extracted".

---

19 The text is edited in Geller 2005: 212ff. no. 35. See also Scurlock and Andersen 2005: 786 with internal references. Identified illnesses include: "Ill inside(s)" (*qer-be-nu* GIG; Scurlock and Andersen 2005: 121–22), "'Overflow' of the intestines illness" (*ter-di-it ir-ri* GIG), and "Anus illness" (DÚR.GIG; Scurlock and Andersen 2005: 150–53).

20 *BAM* 164 obv. 20: 5 Ú.MEŠ DIŠ NA *ana* GÌŠ.MEŠ-*šú ma-gal* ZI.ZI-*bi*, "If a man repeatedly 'rises' greatly because of his penis[(pl.)] [*sic*]" (see Geller 2005: 62–63, 80–81 "If a man repeatedly rises/has an erection because of his urine"). The verb *tebû* indicates "sexual arousal, erection" (*CAD* T: 317–18), and Scurlock and Andersen (2005: 110–111) consider this to be an example of priapism: "If a person continually has an erection when he tries to urinate …". The other comparable examples have KÀŠ.MEŠ over GÌŠ.MEŠ. This is perhaps a mistake in *BAM* 164 that could have occurred due to the purpose statement.

21 The text is partially edited in Geller (2005: 80–83, 124–25 ms zz) and Scurlock and Andersen (2005: 787 with internal references).

22 The first prescription states obv. 7: PAB 18 *a-pi-is-lat lat-ku* ⸢x⸣[x], "total: 18 (drugs) …(?), tested […]". The writing *a-pi-is-lat* may be related to *apišalû*, which may refer to a deformity, perhaps regarded as an illness from the country Apišal (*CAD* A/2: 170; *CDA*: 20; see Steinert 2015: 125). However, due to the meagre number of references, Scurlock (2014: 462 note 51) disregards this reading and suggests a reading *a-pi-iš$_6$-šat* related to *apišītû* "portion, agreed proportion" (*CAD* A/2: 197). The interpretation remains uncertain. The reading "Sun-heat" *ṣētu* in the second prescription is that of Scurlock 2014: 462 note 51; cf. Scurlock and Andersen 2005: 788 with internal reference. However, it is also possible to interpret the signs *ṣe-ti* as ZÍ-*ti* "bile" (*martu*).

BAM 186 contains three prescriptions for oils to be administered as enemas.[23] The first is a lavage for the anus and the prescription is designated as "good and tested" against *aḫḫāzu-* or *amurriqanu*-jaundice (see Section 9.1). After the prescription follows a single line in obverse line 13, before and after which is a horizontal ruling line, stating: "rinse of oils (against) 'sun-heat'".[24] Two prescriptions follow, of which the first is fragmentary and the second is for an enema. The function of obverse line 13 as a subscript to the first prescription or a heading for the second (and third?) prescription remains uncertain (see Section 8.3.2). The colophon contains a purpose statement and specifies that the text was "quickly extracted".

The obverse of BAM 188 is completely broken, but the reverse contains a diagnosis and a prescription for a single enema used for a man ill from bile, *aḫḫazu-* or *amurriqanu*-jaundice.[25] The text is a partial duplicate of the first prescription in BAM 186 (see Section 8.3.2 below). The two types of jaundice encountered in BAM 186 and BAM 188 above, *aḫḫāzu*, the "catcher-demon", and *amurriqānu*, "making yellow(?)",[26] are the two common types of jaundice attested in Mesopotamian sources.[27] Among Kiṣir-Aššur's texts with colophons it is notable that jaundice is treated only in these two texts. Although this may be a coincidence, these illnesses are not featured in Kiṣir-Aššur's earlier texts. The colophon of BAM 188 contains a purpose statement and the text is "quickly extracted".

Only a small portion of the reverse remains of BAM 300, but this is sufficient to conclude that it once contained at least one prescription involving fumigation and considered suitable for any malady. The text is treated and discussed in Section 8.4. The colophon contains a purpose statement and the text is designated as an *u'iltu* that was "quickly extracted".

---

23 The text is partially edited in Scurlock and Andersen (2005: 788 with internal reference). See also Steinert 2015: 117 note 50, 125.

24 Obv. 13: *mar-ḫaṣ ša* Ì.MEŠ *ḫi-miṭ* UD.DA.

25 The text is partially edited in Scurlock and Andersen (2005: 788 with internal reference).

26 For *aḫḫāzu* from *aḫāzu* "to seize, hold", see CAD A/1: 185f.; *AHw*: 20. For *amurriqānu* from *warāqu* "to be(come) green-yellow", see CAD A/2: 91f.; *AHw*: 92. For discussions, see, e.g., Böck 2014a: 74, 123–25, 148–51, 179, 183 note 98; Scurlock and Andersen 2005: 32–34, 138–39, 191–92.

27 It seems that *aḫḫāzu* was considered to be more severe than *amurriqānu*, although both cases could be lethal (Böck 2014a: 125 and notes 105–106; see also CAD A/1: 186). Though one would expect a connection between jaundice and the liver and gallbladder (Scurlock and Andersen 2005: 138, 191), only *aḫḫāzu* was really connected to the liver as well as Ninurta (Böck 2014a: 74; Scurlock and Andersen 2005: 32–34, 138, 476, 520). Waste of flesh was thought to be connected to *amurriqānu* (Böck 2014a: 138–39).

BAM 303 contains at least five prescriptions, of which one is largely broken (the beginning of the obverse).[28] The remaining four prescriptions are described as "(sets of) ingredient(s)" (*maššītu*) used "for softening up" (*lubbuku*).[29] The last prescription is longer and designated as a "(set of) ingredient(s) for lubricating [feet] that are inflated with wind and (are) stiff".[30] The manuscript is specified in the colophon as consisting of "tested prescription(s) from the hands of the scholar".[31] The text is without known duplicates (Köcher 1964: XXII) and is unique.

As discussed in the overview above, six of Kiṣir-Aššur's eight medical texts from his *mašmaš bīt Aššur*-phase contain purpose statements attesting to the practical application of this knowledge (BAM 99, BAM 164, BAM 177, BAM 186, BAM 188, BAM 300). These are extracted (*nasāḫu*) and at least one is a numbered extract (*nisḫu*, BAM 99). Additionally, several of the texts from this phase contain "tested prescriptions", which is a feature rarely previously observed (BAM 164, BAM 177, BAM 186, BAM 303). Kiṣir-Aššur's texts contain treatments against previously unencountered illnesses, which appear to involve broadly applicable prescriptions (BAM 300). Notably, Kiṣir-Aššur copied a text that was "from the hands of the scholar" (BAM 303).

8.3 Tested Prescriptions among the Medical Texts

Four of Kiṣir-Aššur's medical texts from his *mašmaš bīt Aššur*-phase (BAM 164, BAM 177, BAM 186, BAM 303), as well as a single *mašmaššu ṣeḫru*-phase manuscript (N4 A 2727), contain statements that individual prescriptions were "tested" (*latku*, Steinert 2015: 125, 128). Furthermore, three of these examples (BAM 164, 177, 186) are specified as excerpted tablets with purpose statements (ibid.: 123). This section investigates these examples to illustrate Kiṣir-Aššur's

28 The text is partially edited in Steinert (2015: 127–28) and Scurlock and Andersen (2005: 789 with internal reference).

29 Obv. 7', obv. 10', obv. 13', rev. 23'.

30 Rev. 20'–22': … *maš-ši-ti šá* [GÌR[II](?)] [21'] *šá* IM *id-*[*p*]*i-t*[*u*] [22'] *ù šá-ag-gi a-na lu-ub-bu-*[*ki*] (following Scurlock and Andersen 2005: 170). The IM *id-*[*p*]*i-t*[*u*] is peculiar. The related word *idiptu* is translated in CAD (I-J: 9) as "wind" that functions like an illness or demon, and derives from *edēpu* "inflated" (CDA: 124). CAD (Š/1: 72) suggests another reading of the line: *šá* IM *ed-pi tu-*[x-(x)] *ù šá-ag-gi*…. However, this remains unclear. Köcher (1964: XXII) described the last prescription as "Herstellung von Streumitteln" on the basis of rev. 19'–20': Ú.ḪI.A *an-nu-t*[*i*] [20'] *ana* IGI *ta-za-ru*. However, it remains unclear if "you scatter these plants" into something or if *ana* IGI refers to scattering the ingredients in front of the patient, possibly written without the third person singular pronominal suffix.

31 Rev. 24': *bul-ṭu lat-ku šá* ŠU[II] UM.ME.A.

use of such "tested" knowledge during his *mašmaš bīt Aššur* phase by discussing the meaning behind the term "tested" (*latku*) and providing an example that could indicate that Kiṣir-Aššur himself was involved in testing during his phase.

In general, the Bāba-šuma-ibni family seems to have used authorized and "tested" knowledge in their practice..[32] Steinert suggests that such phrases indicated a tendency among healers such as Kiṣir-Aššur to use "tested" remedies because they either had greater confidence in them or wanted to confirm the efficacy of a remedy (Steinert 2015: 123, 139 and note 121). Kiṣir-Aššur's five examples are shown in Table 16.

All tablets, except N4 A 2727, were written when Kiṣir-Aššur was *mašmaš bīt Aššur* and is assumed to have been in a position to "test" prescriptions

TABLE 16 Kiṣir-Aššur's tested prescriptions

Text	Prescription(s) on tablet
BAM 164	Obv. 13–17: ^{16} ... 9 Ú.MEŠ ^{17} *mu-ṣi lat-ku-ti ina* GEŠTIN NAG.MEŠ "Nine tried drugs for discharge, he keeps drinking (them) in wine"
BAM 177	Obv. 1–7: ^{7} PAB 18 *a-pi-is-lat lat-ku* ⸢x⸣[x] "Total: 18 (drugs) against *apišalû*-deformity(?), tested [...]"
BAM 186	Obv. 1–13: ^{10} *mar-ḫa-ṣu an-*[*n*]*u-*[*u*] ^{11} *ana aḫ-ḫa-zi u a-mur-ri-q*[*a-ni*] ^{12} *da-mi-iq lat-ku* (dividing line) ^{13} *mar-ḫaṣ ša* Ì.MEŠ *ḫi-miṭ* UD.DA "This "tested" rinse is good for *aḫḫāzu* and *amurriqānu*. Rinse of oils (against) *ḫimiṭ ṣēti*."
BAM 303	Obv. 5'–8': $^{7'}$ ... ḪI-*tú šá lu-u*[*b-bu*]*-ki* $^{8'}$ *bul-ṭu lat-ku*[a] "Set of ingredients for sof[tening] up, a tested prescription" Obv. 10', 13': ... *maš-ši-ti*/ḪI-*tú* KI.MIN "Set of ingredients 'ditto'" Rev. 24': *bul-ṭu lat-ku šá* ŠU^{II} UM.ME.A "Tested prescription(s) from the hands of the *ummânu*"
N4 A 2727	(Unpublished): *bulṭī latkūti ša ina qāti šūṣû*

a Followed by two prescriptions in which the final phrase, *maš-ši-ti* KI.MIN and ḪI-*tú* KI.MIN, perhaps also duplicates the *bulṭu latku* (Obv. 9'–10' and 11'–13').

32 Several examples of "tested" treatments occur in, e.g., the internal illness compendium *BAM* 95 copied by Nabû-bēssunu (Geller 2005: 128–133, 208–11, 230–31 ms v) and among Kiṣir-Nabû's texts (e.g., *BAM* 168 obv. 78–81). The N4 manuscript *BAM* 42, from Aššur-šākin-šumi contains several prescriptions designated as "a secret of kingship" (*BAM* 42 obv. 12, obv. 35). For such labels in N4, see Maul 2010a: 198.

and evaluate their efficacy. In comparison, the only "tested" text besides N4 A 2727 predating Kiṣir-Aššur's *mašmaš bīt Aššur*-phase is *KAR* 230, which was described as a "tested ritual procedure" (*ne-pi₅-šam lat-ku*). However, it is certain that this phrase does not refer to a test performed by Kiṣir-Aššur (Section 8.3.2).

The tested prescriptions in *BAM* 164, *BAM* 177, and *BAM* 186 are found in the N4 collection in duplicate prescriptions that are also labelled "tested", and in some instances in duplicate prescriptions listed as non-tested.[33] The last tablet, *BAM* 303, was a *ṭuppu* specified as: "tested prescription(s) of the hands of the scholar" (Steinert 2015: 123, 127–28).[34] Accordingly, all prescriptions on this tablet may have been considered "tested" (ibid.: 127–28).[35] Phrases referring to "scholars" have been interpreted as an indication that the knowledge was regarded as "handed down from an anonymous scholarly source" (ibid.: 123). The prescriptions in *BAM* 303 are without known duplicates.

8.3.1 *Meaning of the Phrase "Tested Prescription"*

The term *latku* "tested" was generally used to describe individual prescriptions as a "tested prescription" (*bulṭu latku*).[36] The verbal root *latāku* means "to test, check, verify" (*CAD* L: 111–112, 216–17; Steinert 2015: 105). The term *latku* therefore implies "that knowledge of effective drugs and remedies had been acquired through practical experience" (ibid.: 104). The phrase was probably used to indicate that prescriptions regularly produced the desired results and evidence for testing by specialists can be found in the contemporary NA royal

33 *BAM* 164 is duplicated by the N4 manuscripts *BAM* 116 (broken colophon) and the eight-columned *BAM* 161, as well as the four-columned Nineveh manuscript *BAM* 431; all examples are labelled as "tested" (Steinert 2015: 137–38 with score transliteration). *BAM* 177 is partly duplicated in the N4 manuscript *BAM* 124 col. iii 38–40, which is not labelled as "tested". *BAM* 186 is duplicated in the N4 manuscripts *BAM* 188 rev. 1–10 and *BAM* 189 col. iv 1–16, neither of which are labelled as "tested" (see below). *BAM* 303 is without known duplicates.

34 It remains uncertain if Kiṣir-Aššur is the *ummânu* mentioned testing the prescriptions (see Geller 2010: 193 note 178). *BAM* 303 is also one of only three instances in which the theophoric element of Kiṣir-Aššur's name is written ᵈ*Aš-šur* rather than *Aš-šur*. The other two examples are Kiṣir-Aššur's *šamallû ṣeḫru* texts N4 no. 237 and N4 no. 289.

35 The two prescriptions that are not explicitly labelled as "tested" contain the statement: ḪI-*tú*/*maš-ši-ti* KI.MIN (*BAM* 303 obv. 10', 13'), which supports them being tested.

36 Steinert 2015; Geller 2010: 17–18. Another type of efficacy phrase used is *ana* X *damiq* – "(a drug) is good for X", perhaps meaning "effective" (Steinert 2015: 116–18), which was also used in the NA royal correspondence by healers (ibid.: 117 and note 51). The term could be used as well to qualify, e.g., rituals against various non-medical things (ibid.: 118 and note 53–54). For the use of *latāku* in relation to witchcraft, see Schwemer 2007a: 89.

archives (ibid.: 111–13, 139).[37] However, minor variation occurs between manuscripts of the same "tested" remedies (ibid.: 138), and in some cases the same prescription that was considered as "tested" can also occur without this phrase (ibid.: 135 note 104).

Steinert has recently argued that the *latku*-phrases "had a communicative function" in that they improved "the user-friendliness of the text", although they rarely occur in a standardized way (Steinert 2015: 115–16). Little is known about the historical development of the "tested remedies" and it is difficult to determine when and by whom efficacy phrases were added (ibid.: 120–21). This is partly because Mesopotamian healers never added indications if they or others confirmed a remedy (ibid.: 121). Note that Adad-šumu-uṣur, the famous chief exorcist of Esarhaddon, tested at least one treatment on slaves before it was administered to the royal family (Geller 2010: 88). Sadly, we do not know the prescription. However, the combination of the low frequency of attestations and that "tested" remedies occur on tablets with purpose statements may indicate that the "tested" remedies had special status for the healers (Steinert 2015: 123; Geller 2010: 17–18).

8.3.2 *An Example of Kiṣir-Aššur as Investigator of Efficacy?*

The "tested" prescription in *BAM* 186 from Kiṣir-Aššur's *mašmaš bīt Aššur*-phase is mostly duplicated by a similar prescription in his *mašmaš bīt Aššur* manuscript, *BAM* 188, which was not deemed tested.[38] Furthermore, a non-tested prescription in the slim, multi-columned text *BAM* 189 from N4 also duplicates the prescription in *BAM* 188 and possibly the tested prescription in *BAM* 186.[39] *BAM* 189 does not contain a colophon and the copyist is unfortunately unknown. The situation in these three prescriptions therefore differs from the known duplicates of the "tested prescription" in *BAM* 164, all of which were labelled as "tested" (Steinert 2015: 137–38). The three prescriptions are transliterated here, followed by a translation of the relevant passages:

A = *BAM* 188 (rev. 1–10);
B = *BAM* 186 (obv. 1–13);
C = *BAM* 189 (col. iv 1–16):

---

37 Steinert uses *BAM* 95 rev. 26 to argue that drugs provided regular results via the phrase *bulṭu latku ša ina qāti kayamā*[*nti šūṣû*?], "A tested remedy that [*was established*] *by regular practice* (lit. 'hand')" (Steinert 2015: 139 note 121; Geller 2005: 133–34 no 21 ms v). However, see Ch. 6 notes 25–26 with references and further discussion of similar phrases.

38 Unfortunately, the obverse of *BAM* 188 is almost completely broken (Köcher 1963b: XXI).

39 *BAM* 189 = N4 no. 326. The format resembles the stone inventory list *BAM* 366, written by either Kiṣir-Aššur or Kiṣir-Nabû (see Appendix 1).

A1–2	DIŠ NA *lu* ZÉ *lu aḫ-ḫa-zu* ^{2} *lu a-mur-ri-qa-nu* GIG *ana* TI-*šú*
A3	^{šim}GÚR.GÚR ^{šim}LI ^{šim}BAL
B1–2a	2 GÍN ^{šim}GÚR.GÚR 2 GÍN ^{ši}[^{m}LI] ^{2} 2 GÍN ^{šim}BAL →
C1–3	^{giš}[x x] ^{2} ^{giš}LI ^{3} ^{giš}BAL
A4	^{šim}MAN.DU GI DÙG ^{ú}*úr-nu-u*
B2b–3	½ GÍN ^{šim}[MAN.DU] ^{3} 2 GÍN GI DÙG.GA 1 GÍN ^{giš}*ú*[*r-nu-*(*u*)]
C4–6	^{giš}MAN.DÙ ^{5} GI DÙG ^{6} *úr-nu-u*
A5	^{ú}KUR.KUR ^{ú}GEŠTIN.KA$_{5}$.A ^{ú}*kar-šú*
B4–5	½ GÍN ^{ú}KUR.KUR 1 GÍN ^{ú}GEŠTI[N.KA$_{5}$.(A)] ^{5} [x GÍN]⸢x x x x⸣ ½ GÍN ^{ú}*k*[*ar-šú*]
C7–10a	^{ú}KUR.KUR ^{8} GEŠTIN.[KA]$_{5}$.A ^{9} kar-[x x (x)][40] ^{10} *kar-*[*šú*? →
A6	^{ú}ḪAB ^{giš}*tar-muš*$_{8}$ ^{giš}IGI-*lim* ^{giš}IGI-20
B6–7	½ ^{ú}ḪAB 2 GÍN ^{ú}*tar-muš*$_{8}$ ^{7} 1 GÍN ^{ú}IGI-*lim* 1 GÍN ^{ú}IGI-20
C10b–13	x? Ḫ]AB? ^{11} 1(aš) *tar-muš*$_{8}$ ^{12} 1(aš) IGI-*lim* ^{13} 1(aš) IGI-20
A7	^{ú}*er-ru-u* 14 Ú.MEŠ *an-nu-ti*
B8a	2 GÍN ^{ú}*er-ru-u* →
C14–16	1(aš) *er-ru-u* ^{15} PAP 14 *mar-ḫaṣ* ^{16} *aḫ-ḫa-zu*
A8	*mal-ma-liš* LAL *ina* KAŠ SAG ŠEG$_{6}$-*šal*
B8b	*ina* KAŠ ŠEG$_{6}$-*šal*
A9	*ina* MUL$_{4}$ *tuš-bat ta-šá-ḫal*
A10	Ì.GIŠ LÀL *ana* IGI ŠUB-*di ana* DÚR-*šú* DUB
B9	Ì LÀL *ana* IGI ŠUB-*di ana* DÚR-*š*[*ú* DUB]

40 The line below also opens with the sign KAR. Furthermore, *BAM* 189 col. iv 10 seems to end with ḪAB, and the opening KAR likely spells out *kar-šú*. As a result, col. iv 9 must list another plant, but then the total of 14 plants in line 15 does not fit with the amount of plants. Perhaps the young student wrote *karšu* twice, maybe in both forms: *karašu* and *karšu*.

B10–12 *mar-ḫa-ṣu an-*[*n*]*u-*[*u*] 11 *ana aḫ-ḫa-zi u a-mur-ri-q*[*a-ni*] 12 *da-mi-iq lat-ku*

B13 *mar-ḫaṣ ša* Ì.MEŠ *ḫi-miṭ* UD.DA

A If a man is ill with "bile", *aḫḫāzu*-jaundice, or *amurriqānu*-jaundice, to cure him:
3–7 … (*list of plant-based ingredients*) …
7b You weigh out these 14 plants equally (and) boil (them) in premium beer. You leave (the blend) outside overnight by the star(s). You sieve it (and) add plant oil and honey into it. You pour (it) into his anus.

B 1–8 … (*list of plant-based ingredients with varying measurements*) …
8b You boil (them) in beer. You add oil (and) honey into it. [You pour (it) into] his anus. This "tested" rinse is good against *aḫḫāzu*-jaundice and *amurriqānu*-jaundice.

Rinse of oils (for) *ḫimiṭ ṣēti*.

C 1–14 … (*list of plant-based ingredients, from line 7 supplied individually with a measure of one*) …
15 Total: 14 (plants), an *aḫḫāzu* rinse.

I propose that the three prescriptions transliterated and translated above represent the same prescription.[41] This is based on the roughly similar list of ingredients and the partial overlap in illnesses treated by the prescriptions. The ingredients used in all three prescriptions are generally identical and presented in the same order, with the exception of the addition of a single broken ingredient in B (obv. 5) and perhaps also C (col. iv 9). All three prescriptions are against *aḫḫāzu*-jaundice, which suggests a similar aim. However, B can be directed against both *aḫḫāzu*-jaundice and *amurriqānu*-jaundice, and A can be used against bile (*martu*), *aḫḫāzu*-jaundice, or *amurriqānu*-jaundice. Additionally, the illnesses are listed at different places in the texts. A opens with diagnoses, whereas B and C identify the illnesses at the end of the prescription.

---

41 Erica Couto-Ferreira (2018) has recently published a similar argument concerning these three texts, and she reached the same conclusion. My study was written independently of Couto Ferreira's, and I was not aware of her publication before my dissertation, on which this monograph is based, was submitted in August 2017.

Furthermore, B and C identify the prescription as a "rinse" (*marḫaṣu*), and C also totals the number of ingredients. Notably, B specifies that it is a "tested rinse" considered "good for *aḫḫāzu*- and *amurriqānu*-jaundice" at the end of the prescription. Perhaps the measurements in B could indicate that specificity was required to be considered "tested", although, e.g., the so-called "tested eye salve of Ḫammurabi" is found in duplicates with and without measurements (Steinert 2015: 134). We shall return to this below.

A number of other differences can also be observed. B contains individual weight measurements for each ingredient, C does not specify the measurements in the first half and adds the generic 1(aš) as the weight measurement for each ingredient in the second half, and A instructs the reader to weigh out the ingredients equally. Additionally, A and B contain instructions for preparing the prescription after the lists of ingredients, which are omitted in C. The instructions also differ between A and B, with A containing more specific instructions than B. Nonetheless, the almost identical ingredient lists and shared use against *aḫḫāzu*-jaundice in all three instances suggest that these prescriptions can be regarded as the same. The differences could indicate that the prescriptions are from different recensions or the result of personal variation. However, another hypothesis is possible.

To reiterate, A and B are from Kiṣir-Aššur's *mašmaš bīt Aššur*-phase, whereas C is by an unknown copyist from N4. Furthermore, A and B are both from tablets with purpose statements, suggesting a practical application of the knowledge contained therein. The duplicate prescriptions in A and B could be applied against several related illnesses, although only B was labelled as "tested".[42] Speculatively, B may have been labelled as "tested" by Kiṣir-Aššur and the addition of weight measurements and an additional ingredient are the result of his test of the prescription.[43] If so, Kiṣir-Aššur perhaps verified the effect of the prescription in A against *aḫḫāzu*- and *amurriqānu*-jaundice, but maybe not against bile (cf. Geller 2010: 17–18). Following this line of reasoning, Kiṣir-Aššur would have copied A before B. The final separating line in B makes such a difficult hypothesis slightly more probable, if it is interpreted as

42 For the relationship between "bile" and the various types of jaundice, see Böck 2014a: 122–28 with further references.

43 Couto-Ferreira (2018: 158 and note 30) notes that *BAM* 186 rev. 23 contains the unusual phrase "I have collected (18) oils", 18 Ì.MEŠ *aš-bu-uš*. However, there are at least one sign following *aš-bu-uš* not treated by Couto-Ferreira. The sign appears to add Š[U$^{(II?)}$ (x)], possibly referring to "(*in*) [(my$^{?}$)] hand", although a preposition before ŠU would have been preferable (see *CAD* Š/1: 6f.). The reading is therefore uncertain. This line could be a further indication that *BAM* 186 represents an experimental text.

a subscript to the first prescription.[44] After having specified that the "tested" prescription is considered good against *aḫḫāzu* and *amurriqānu*, the prescription states its true purpose, which is separated from what precedes it by a horizontal line: "a rinse of oils (for) 'inflammation by sun-heat' (*ḫimiṭ ṣēti*)" (Stol 2007a: 22ff., 37–38). Thus, the prescription was used in this particular case to treat *ḫimiṭ ṣēti*, an illness not specified elsewhere as treatable by this particular rinse.[45] Regardless of the interpretation, the appearance of this prescription in two *mašmaš bīt Aššur* texts containing few prescriptions could indicate that the remedy was among Kiṣir-Aššur's preferred prescriptions.

8.4 Panaceas among the Medical Texts

At least one of Kiṣir-Aššur's *mašmaš bīt Aššur* texts (*BAM* 300) suggests that he may have employed certain panaceas, i.e., widely applicable treatments used to cure various maladies.[46] It is likely that certain cures were preferred by individual healers (Steinert 2015: 123, 139; Geller 2010: 17–18). One panacea may be the so-called "tried eye salve of Ḫammurabi", which Steinert (2015: 134–35) argued in the LB Uruk recension likely functioned "as a panacea for all eye ailments", i.e., a remedy for every problem affecting the eye. In relation to Kiṣir-Aššur, it was hypothesized above that the first prescription in *BAM* 186 may have been a tested version of a prescription similar to the extract found in *BAM* 188. This prescription may therefore have been used on numerous occasions by Kiṣir-Aššur against certain internal maladies. Similarly, Section 6.2 argued that *KAR* 230 was a multipurpose ritual, which could be used during most house calls.

Additional texts may corroborate Kiṣir-Aššur's preference for a limited number of prescriptions for certain maladies. *BAM* 300 was "quickly extracted" (*ḫa-an-ṭiš* ZI-*ḫa*) with a purpose statement as an *u'iltu* when Kiṣir-Aššur was *mašmaš bīt Aššur*. The text only contains a broken treatment for anointing and

---

44 However, it remains uncertain how to interpret this line. B contains three prescriptions. As the second and third prescription in B do not contain preserved passages specifying what illnesses against which they were directed, it is also possible that obv. 13 functioned as a header. The second prescription is designated in rev. 23 as: "18 oils *for* relaxi[ng(?)]", 18 Ì.MEŠ *ina pu-uš-šu-*[*ḫi*?]. Note that *puššuḫu* mostly occurs in prescriptions in relation to *ana* (*CAD* P: 231). The third prescription is broken at the relevant passage in rev. 28: "Total: 8 plant[s for(?) …]", PAB 8 Ú.[MEŠ …].

45 Yet, *BAM* 186 states that it is "extracted" (*nasāḫu*), indicating that it was copied from a manuscript. How to understand this situation remains uncertain.

46 See Steinert 2015: 134–35; Geller 2010: 25, 104. For another panacea found in Nineveh and Sultantepe, see *CMAwR* 2: 435ff.

fumigating a patient, as well as a description of the prescription that is delineated by ruling lines and placed directly before the colophon:

Rev. 1': [... *traces of three signs* ...] MUN
Rev. 2': [... x] [túg]NÍG.DÁRA ŠU.LAL [x-ṣ]a[?]-⌈x[147]
Rev. 3': [...]⌈x *ina*[?]⌉ Ì EŠ.MEŠ-*su ina kal-li gul-gu*[*l-li*[?]][48]
Rev. 4': *ina* NE SAR-*šu-ma* TI-*uṭ*[49]

Rev. 5': [*šu*]-*ut bu-luṭ gim-ri ka-la-ma* SIG_5-*iq*[50]

[...] salt [2'] [...] a soiled rag [... [3'] ...] you continually anoint him in oil, you fumigate him with embers in a *kallu*-bowl of a sku[ll] and he will get well.
This is a 'universal' prescription good for all (illnesses).

The sole prescription in *BAM* 300 could therefore be used against most maladies and was designated in its subscript as a panacea (Köcher 1964: XXII). Incidentally, while the EM lists few "prescription" types (*bulṭus*), and few of these are specific, one type mentioned in the second section is the generic "prescription for all of every (illness)" (EM rev. 35: *bul-ṭi kal gim-ri*; cf. Steinert 2018c: 186). This is reminiscent of the description in *BAM* 300 and could indicate that this passage of the EM reflects some knowledge concerning specific types of medicine that was acquired by exorcists in practice.

Kiṣir-Aššur copied several tablets with few prescriptions as *mašmaš bīt Aššur* and without titles, although only *BAM* 300 contains a subscript that labels the

---

47 The "soiled rag", *ulāp lupputi*, is used in a variety of ritual and medical contexts (*CAD* U–W: 71–72).

48 The *kallu*-bowl is described as made of clay or wood, although *CAD* (K: 83) also lists the word as part of descriptions of the "crown (*kallu*) of the human skull (*qaqqadu*)" or "shell (*kallu*) of a turtle" (see *AHw*: 426). The *gulgullu* is listed as a "skull" or a "container shaped like a human skull" (*CAD* G: 127–28; *AHw*: 297). In the majority of examples, a skull refers to human remains. In at least one example a patient is fumigated using a human skull, see *AMT* 98,1 obv./rev.[?] 9': ... *ina gul-gul* NAM.LÚ.U_{18}.LU *ina* NE *tu-qat-tar-š*[*u* ...], "... you fumigate hi[m] with embers in a human skull [...]" (*CAD* G: 128). Presumably, *BAM* 300 describes a similar situation.

49 For fumigation, see Böck 2009a: 117; Finkel 1991; Golz 1974: 83–85; Herrero 1984: 109–110.

50 The translation is not literal. The word *gimru* designates "totality" or "everything", and in relation to divine epithets, e.g., *bēl gimri*, it can be translated "lord of the universe" (*AHw*: 289; *CAD* G: 76–77; *CDA*: 93). Thus, *buluṭ gimri* becomes "universal prescription" here. Similarly, *kalāma* means "all (of it)" or "everything" and is generally used indeclinable as object of verbs, in genitive constructions, and in apposition to a preceding substantive to stress totality (*AHw*: 423–24; *CAD* K: 65–66; *CDA*: 142; see von Soden 1995: 106 §65h; cf. *SAAS* 13: 53).

prescription as "universal".[51] Other tablets with few prescriptions were found in multiple copies in N4, attesting to their use in the collection.[52] Furthermore, Kiṣir-Aššur may have had a number of "favourite" prescriptions for a selection of maladies, such as the "tested prescription" in *BAM* 186.[53] As a result, it is possible that Kiṣir-Aššur regularly used several of the prescriptions on tablets that bear only a few prescriptions.

8.4.1 *Excursus: Kiṣir-Aššur's Possible Multipurpose Medical Incantations*

Kiṣir-Aššur's medical tablets from his various phases contain relatively few incantations. In addition to groupings of incantations against *kadabbedû* and *bušānu* in *BAM* 28 and *abracadabra* incantations against *sagallu* in *BAM* 129,[54] individual incantations related to medical healing occur in *BAM* 102 against "Anus illness", perhaps in *BAM* 333 as a (microcosmic) creation myth (see Köcher 1971: XI),[55] in N4 no. 24 for "Child calming",[56] and in the unpublished N4 A 400.[57] In general, Geller (2007b: 389–92) has suggested that medical incantations, i.e., incantations occurring in medical texts, serve ancillary functions, increasing the effectiveness of prescriptions or serving to induce positive psychological effects on the patient.

Although Kiṣir-Aššur's medical tablets with incantations were copied for varying purposes, such as the possible pedagogical purpose behind the *imgiddûs* *BAM* 102 and N4 no. 24, it is conceivable that Kiṣir-Aššur's few medical incantations – because of their low number – were broadly applicable against the maladies they treat (as with the prescription *BAM* 300 discussed above), or that they were rarely employed medically. The incantation against "Anus illness" in *BAM* 102 is unfortunately mostly broken and the ritual instruction

51 Single prescription tablets, e.g., *BAM* 177.

52 Multiple duplicated tablets, e.g., *BAM* 68 (Kiṣir-Aššur or Kiṣir-Nabû), which is duplicated in *BAM* 69 obv. 1–17 (= N4 no. 18) and *BAM* 70 obv.? 1'–9' (breaks off) (= N4 no. 536).

53 Whether or not some form of anaesthetics was available to ancient healers remains uncertain, but it is noteworthy that *BAM* 260, copied by either Kiṣir-Aššur or Kiṣir-Nabû at an uncertain stage, may contain instructions for getting the patient drunk enough that he may pass out (Scurlock and Andersen 2005: 361; Heeßel 2002b: 104–105; Geller and Cohen 1995: 1813 and note 26). If so, these prescriptions could have been part of the *ad hoc* prescriptions of these healers.

54 See also *BAM* 321. The left edge of the tablet is broken, but obv. 1–9 and rev. 27–31 seem to be magical recitations.

55 The incantation mentions Ea and possibly some healing plants related to the netherworld, see *CAD* Š/1: 318.

56 I consider N4 no. 24 here, although it could be argued that this incantation served a prophylactic purpose. However, a crying child may have heralded the presence of Lamaštu, and therefore it indicated a negative situation related to illness (see Section 5.2.2).

57 Likely, the two unpublished incantations in N4 A 2727 also belong in this discussion.

is explicitly "not written" (Section 6.1). However, it is not impossible that the incantation was similar to other incantations against "Anus illness" from N4, such as those found on Kiṣir-Aššur's N4 A 2727 and the anonymously copied *BAM* 105 (N4 no. 239). The latter text contains two incantations (obv. 1–6, 8–11?) and a ritual instruction to the first incantation reads:

> *BAM* 105 obv. 7: DÙ.DÙ.BI *ina* UGU *al-la-ni nap-šal-ti maš-qí-ti* \ DÚR GIG ŠID-*nu*
> "Its ritual: you recite (the incantation) over (*any*) suppository, ointment (or) enema for 'Anus illness'" (see Geller 2005: 231).

The first incantation of *BAM* 105 could therefore be used as a "*Kultmittelbeschwörung*" to activate or enhance the effect of almost any kind of remedy designed to cure "Anus illness", and perhaps related illnesses.[58] The first incantation in *BAM* 105 does therefore seem to be universally applicable against rectal problems. If we assume that a somewhat similar incantation was copied onto *BAM* 102, this incantation could have served a comparable purpose for Kiṣir-Aššur.[59] Noticably, the first incantation of Kiṣir-Aššur's N4 A 2727 duplicates the initial incantation of *BAM* 105, and both recitations and accompanying instructions in the manuscript are said to be "tested prescriptions, which are *suitable for use*(?)" (see Section 5.3).

Comparatively, there are only two similar medical incantations among the LB school texts published by Finkel (2000: 148), which address problems in the kidney and epigastrium, as well as a fever (nos. 50–51).[60] In general, Geller (2007b: 391–92) found it problematic to explain why some medical texts include medical incantations whereas the majority of medical texts do not

58 It may have been possible to activate or enhance the effect of specific ingredients and cures with an incantation, perhaps pointing to a belief that drugs and cures could be used for evil effects as well, mirroring the Greek *pharmakon*, which refers to various healing drugs and poisons. For examples, see *CAD* Š/1: 320; Böck 2014a: 91; Geller 2007b: 397–98. For the duality of *pharmakon* see Nutton 2004: 98, 328 note 6, 348 note 82. This duality may be another reason why the NA royal court used divination to determine if specific drug were to be applied (Koch 2015: 129 and note 340; *SAA* 10 no. 185 and no. 187). The question of the negative effects of medication should be investigated further.

59 See also Kiṣir-Aššur's fragmentary tablet *KAL* 10 no. 5 without a title containing treatments against *māmītu*, in which two single-line instructions can be found on the reverse after incantations (rev. 4': [...] 3-*šú* ŠID-*n*[*u* ...]; rev. 11': [K]A.INIM.MA *ana* UGU ḪU? 3-*šú* [...]). This may be reminiscent of the example from *BAM* 105 quoted above.

60 Again, Gesche's school texts largely excluded medical material and Gesche (2001: 213–15) discussed such material in relation to the professional specialization process.

(cf. Geller 2010: 91ff.). In connection to Kiṣir-Aššur, it is therefore not surprising that he copied relatively few medical incantations among his tablets with colophons. Whether the low number of medical incantations indicates that Kiṣir-Aššur regularly used only a limited number of them, or that he simply used them infrequently remains unresolved.

8.5 Ritual Texts from Kiṣir-Aššur's *mašmaš bīt Aššur*-phase

The second group of Kiṣir-Aššur's *mašmaš bīt Aššur* texts comprise ritual texts with incantations, prayers and ritual instructions. What follows presents a brief discussion of the content of each relevant text in order to provide an overview of this group.

BAM 321 likely opens on the obverse with a prayer (obv. 1–9) and moves into a ritual instruction alongside another incantation (obv. 10–23).[61] Afterwards, the obverse contains an additional ritual instruction (obv. 24–26) and another prayer (obv. 27–31). The reverse, most of which is fragmentary, contains a large ritual instruction referencing another incantation (rev. 32–51). The initial prayer pretitions a man's god and goddess to be favourable towards the supplicant,[62] the second mentions Enlil, Enki and Asalluḫi,[63] and the third prayer is directed towards Nabû and Tašmētu.[64] The colophon is broken and only Bāba-šuma-ibni's name remains. However, two broken names before Bāba-šuma-ibni's name end with the preserved titles *mašmaš bīt Aššur*, suggesting that the names should be reconstructed as Kiṣir-Aššur and Nabû-bēssunu. Notably, the text is a duplicate of the first part of *BAM* 322, which is designated as "a copy *from* the palace of Ḫammurabi".[65] *BAM* 322 was copied by a high priest of the Aššur temple and for reasons unknown placed in the N4 collection (Steinert 2015: 129). If Kiṣir-Aššur's *BAM* 321 represents a copy of the

---

61 The text remains unedited (see Böck 2014a: 78–79 note 8).

62 Obv. 1.

63 Obv. 19–20, obv. 23.

64 Obv. 27.

65 Part of the text is duplicated by the peculiar manuscript *BAM* 322 obv. 1–28 (Köcher 1971: IX–X; see Lenzi 2008a: 196 note 302; Steinert 2015: 128–29; Maul 2010a: 212 and note 78). Interestingly, *BAM* 322 contains a dividing line after obv. 28, after which obv. 29 states: GABA.RI É.GAL ᵖ*ḫa-am-m*[*u-r*]*a-bi* LUGAL ŠÁR, "copy *from* the palace of Ḫamm[ur]abi, king of the world". The latter half is later designated in rev. 91 as: GABA.RI É.GAL ᵖ*Aš-šur*-ŠEŠ-SUM-*na* LUGAL Š[ÁR], "copy *from* the palace of Esarhaddon, king of the world". Robson (2019: 133) has recently expressed doubt about the claim regarding the text's provenance.

relevant section of *BAM* 322, it could signify that he purposely copied ancient knowledge thought to be derived from Ḫammurabi's palace.

The text copied by Beckman and Foster (1988: 4) as no. 21 contains an unknown incantation ritual and it remains unedited. The colophon is fragmentary, and nothing further can be added here.

KAR 62 contains an incantation and a ritual that is stated in the incipit to be "If an angry man is to be reconciled (with someone)" (Pedersén 1986: 54, N4 no. 104; Ebeling 1931b: 22–23).[66] Furthermore, the ritual instruction prescribes making an "ox" (*alpu*) of clay, which is possibly buried by the river.[67] However, the sign for "ox" (GU$_4$) can also be read "ghost" (*eṭemmu*), and the *eṭemmu* was described in the underworld vision of an Assyrian prince as having the head of an ox, but the hands and feet of a human (Ambos 2013a: 60 note 177; Livingstone 1989: 72 line 6). As a result, it is possible that the text was connected to ghosts.[68] The text was labelled as an *u'iltu* of Kiṣir-Aššur.

KAR 63 consists of several incantations and ritual instructions concerned with soothing an angry or furious man (Pedersén 1986: 54, N4 no. 101; Ebeling 1931b: 16–20).[69] The text is labelled as a "hurriedly extracted" *u'iltu* of Kiṣir-Aššur and designated as a "final extract" (see Section 9.2.3). Interestingly, all entries are duplicated with only minimal variation by *KAR* 43, which was designated as: "written and checked [ac]cording to the wording of an *imgiddû*-tablet, an 'Akkadian' copy".[70] Notably, *KAR* 43 contains the note "new break" (*ḫe-pí eš-šú*) in rev. 17, but this line is copied with (reconstructed?) text in *KAR* 63 rev. 15. The question is if these tablets were copied from the same original, and if they were contemporary copies. This remains uncertain.

KAR 80, edited and republished as *KAL* 2 no. 8, concerns a ritual with prayers for a man with various symptoms who is suffering because of witchcraft (*kišpu*)

66 Rev. 1: KA.INIM.MA DIŠ *zi-na-a ana* SILIM!-⌈*me*⌉. The verb *zenû* "to be angry" is well attested in connection to men and gods (*CAD* Z: 85–86). The tablet is edited in Ebeling 1931b: 20–24.

67 Rev. 2: DÙ.DÙ.BI GU$_4$ *šá* IM DÙ-*uš*; rev. 14–15: … ⌈NU⌉ *ina* ÍD [15] *te-tem-mir-ma* … (see *CAD* T: 336).

68 For a ghost as an ox, see George 1991: 148–49, 157 line 18.

69 See also Scurlock 1997: 82 and note 32; Ebeling 1915: 92–95, edition of the duplicate *KAR* 43; *KAR* 63 obv. 7: KA.INIM.MA DIŠ NA *mám-ma* U[GU]-*šú sa-bu-us*, "If someone is angry with a man" (*CAD* Š/1: 5); rev. 16': [K]A.INIM.MA DIŠ NA *ra-a'-ba-ni-iš i-šá-su-šú*, "If they cry out in anger to a man".

70 *KAR* 43 (= N4 no. 71) rev. 25: [*ki*]-*i* MURÚB IM.GÍD.DA GABA.RI URI^{ki} SAR È (*BAK* no. 275; cf. *CAD* P: 454 for MURÚB as *pû*). Variations occur in individual signs, e.g., *KAR* 43 obv. 12 ending -*tu*/ *KAR* 63 obv. 12 ending -*tu*$_4$, as well as line divisions, e.g., *KAR* 43 obv. 13ff./*KAR* 63 obv. 13ff. with varying line endings.

by his "adversary" (*bēl dabābi*). The last incantation is designated as "*ušburrudû* (to undo witchcraft), for burning figurines".[71]

KAR 374 consists of an incantation possibly addressed to Venus on the obverse and a ritual instruction for producing figurines on the reverse, both of which were possibly connected to (divine) anger (*rūbu*).[72] The text was "hurriedly extracted" with a purpose statement.

LKA 70(+*KAR* 57) consists of the second tablet in the Nineveh recension of the incantation ritual *nēpeš Du'ūzi-Ištar* "the (ritual) procedure(s) of Dumuzi (and) Ištar".[73] These ritual actions were formally directed towards ghosts (*eṭemmu*), the *sagḫulḫaza*-demon, and *mimma lemnu* "Any evil",[74] although the ritual refers to *ḫa(y)yattu* "fit" and *mimma lemnu*, as well as various demons.[75] Farber (1977: 24–26), however, noted differences between the Nineveh and Assur recensions concerning how the tablets are ordered, and while *LKA* 70+ should formally be the second tablet, a tablet before is not known in Assur. The ritual was probably performed around the end of the month *Tammuz* (June–July) (ibid.: 122–23).[76]

71 Rev. 37: KA.INIM.MA UŠ$_{11}$.BÚR.RU.DA.KAM *ša* NU.MEŠ *qa-li-i*. *CMAwR* 1: 293ff. no. 8.4A, 306ff. 8.5B; Schwemer 2007b: 31–36, 143–47; Seux 1976: 396–399; Abusch 1974: 258; Ebeling 1918: 27–34. Obv. 6–7: LÚ BI EN D[U$_{11}$].DU$_{11}$-*šú kiš-pi* NIGIN-*š*[*u*] [7] *kip-di* Ḫ[UL.MEŠ *ik-p*]*u-du-šú* …, "his adversary has encircled that man with witchcraft, ev[il] schemes [have been pl]otted against him …" (*CMAwR* 1: 301). Furthermore, Nabû-bēssunu is supplied with the title [lú]ME.ME É AN.[ŠAR] in the colophon. ME.ME can be read *āšipu*, although it is unusual in the N4 colophons. The writing may be an intentional reference to the writing [d]ME.ME for the healing goddess Gula.

72 Unedited, see Reiner 1995: 23 note 85; Maul 1994: 75 note 35; *CAD* N/1: 266. *KAR* 374 rev. 16: *ana ru-ub-bi* ŠUB-*di*, "(in order) to throw *off* anger". The term *rūbu*/*rubbu* for "anger, wrath" is not well attested, although at least two SB examples address Ištar, which mirrors the incantation that here possibly addresses Venus (*CAD* R: 400; *AHw*: 992). The production of figurines are mentioned in *KAR* 374 rev. 5: 2 NU IM DÙ, "you make 2 clay figurine(s)". For anger and fury in connection to the god Erra, see Machinist 1983: 224.

73 Farber 1977: 127ff. ms b and pl. 14; Scurlock 1988a no. 86; see also Wiggermann 2010. Concerning such rituals and their setting, see Leick 2003: 225–26.

74 Farber 1977: 140–41. The rituals play on the well-known relationship between the netherworld and Dumuzi as well as Ištar, as known from Ištar's Descent (Lapinkivi 2010). By extension, the Ištar-Dumuzi cult was related to Dumuzi's relationship to the harvest and a ritual was performed for the dead Dumuzi during the month Tammuz, i.e., in the summer when the harvest was done (Cohen 1993: 477, 479–481).

75 Farber 1977: 9; 144–45, 148–51; see Section 7.5. Noticeably, Farber's "Hauptritual B" was against various acts of sorcery and took place in a man's house (Farber 1977: 218–60; Wiggermann 2010: 342–343).

76 See von Soden 1936: 259. Additionally, Farber (1977: 124) argues for this ritual being part of the heading found in the EM obv. 5, see Geller 2000: 244, 252 note 5; Jean 2006: 64.

LKA 77 belongs to the series Ḫulbazizi, meaning "to eradicate evil", and the various rituals are directed towards removing the generic evil *mimma lemnu* "any evil".[77] The incantations are bilingual and each of the three columns on each side of the tablet comprise two columns with Sumerian and Akkadian in each. The incantations were apparently widely applicable.[78] The relationship between *mimma lemnu* and the patient's bed seems pivotal to several treatments of illnesses by Kiṣir-Aššur's family.[79] The Ḫulbazizi series is also mentioned in the EM as a work within *āšipūtu*.[80] The colophon of *LKA* 77 contains a curse and an instruction not to remove Kiṣir-Aššur's name.

LKA 83 consists of two incantations and a brief recitation to ensure that the ghost, possibly of a recently deceased, went to the underworld and took various evils with it.[81] The text is labelled as an *u'iltu* of Kiṣir-Aššur. It is noteworthy that two of three entries on *LKA* 83 duplicate passages found in two non-consecutive and broken entries in the substitute king ritual.[82] Scurlock suggests that this may have been influenced by a desire in the substitute king ritual to ensure that the king was not haunted by the ghost of the substitute king (Scurlock 1988a: 343).

Three of Kiṣir-Aššur's *mašmaš bīt Aššur* manuscripts consist of *namburbi*-rituals. *KAR* 38 comprises several ritual instructions accompanied by prayers for a *namburbi*-ritual to keep away evil from a man and his house in connection to incorrectly followed cultic guidelines and imperfectly performed rituals.[83]

---

77 *LKA* 77 col. vi 25: KA.INIM.MA ḪUL.BA.ZI.Z[I.K]E$_4$. See the edition in Ebeling 1953b; see also Farber 2014: 32, 39 and note 2, 242; Maul 2010: 195 and note 26; Jean 2006: 78 and notes 284–85; Heeßel 2002a: 113 note 20, 169 no. 163; Wiggermann 2000: 220 and note 15–16; Farber 1989: 114–15; Hunger 1968: 71 no. 203 ms B. Irving Finkel is preparing a complete edition of Ḫulbazizi texts.

78 One such incantation, although not found in *LKA* 77, is *ša maldi eršīya ittiqu* "He who transgressed the 'privacy' (lit.: edge(?)) of my bed", which occurs on several Lamaštu amulets. See Wiggermann 2007b: 106–7 and note 3; Wiggermann 2000: 220 and note 15–16, 223 and note 28, 242, 246; Wilhelm 1979; Appendix 3; for *maldu*, see *CAD* M/1: 363.

79 See also the discussion in Arbøll 2019. The focus on the bed during illness and the significance of being bedridden require further investigation.

80 *KAR* 44 obv. 7: ... *u* ḪUL.BA.ZI.[ZI $^{\text{si-la}}$]$^{\text{-⸢e-ri⸣-m}}$[^{a}]. The note represents the opening incipit of the series (Geller 2000: 252 note 7).

81 Scurlock 1988a: 343, 344–350 no. 83; Tsukimoto 1985: 173ff.

82 The two duplicate passages appear in Lambert 1957–58 pl. 10 columns B 1'–4' (entry continues until line 8') and D 1'–5'. The entries are almost identical, disregarding variantions in signs and Sumerograms. See Scurlock 1988a: 343; Lambert 1957–58: 109; Parpola 1983a: XXII–XXXII; Ebeling 1953a: XI. See also Ambos 2013b on the substitute king ritual.

83 Maul 1994: 421–431 ms A; Caplice 1970: 124–32; Ebeling 1955b: 184–89; Ebeling 1954a: 5; Ebeling 1931b: 47–52. Although Maul (1994: 421) stresses that the ritual could be used by

Kiṣir-Aššur's father Nabû-bēssunu also copied this ritual (*RA* 18 pl. 28). Maul (1994: 421) suggested, correctly in my opinion, that this could indicate that the ritual was particularly important for this family. The text was labelled as "quickly extracted for a (ritual) performance", and is the only tablet from Kiṣir-Aššur with this purpose statement.[84] *LKA* 113 is a *namburbi*-ritual with instructions and incantations against any kind of evil portended by a bow [*sic*].[85] The colophon is fragmentary and can be interpreted as either tracing the text back to three previous copies or as inferring that the text was compiled from three different sources.[86] *LKA* 119 is a *namburbi*-ritual to avert the bad effects of dust derived from an evil place and to ensure that it does not come near a man.[87] These three rituals are discussed in Section 6.4.2.

LKA 157, edited and republished as *KAL* 2 no. 25, contain prayers and ritual instructions addressing Šamaš on behalf of a man with various symptoms resulting from witchcraft (*kišpu*).[88] The colophon ends with a purpose statement and by stating that the tablet was "quickly extracted".[89]

---

the exorcists when performing rituals for the king, the text itself emphasizes that it is to keep the evil from "a man and his house" (obv. 2: … ⸢*ana*! NA⸣ *u* É-*šú* NU TE-*e*).

84 *KAR* 38 rev. 41: *a-na mu-še-piš-ú-ti ḫa-an-ṭiš* ZI-[*ḫa*/*ḫi*]. For this variant, see *CAD* M/2: 267; Maul 2010a: 212 and note 80; Hunger 1968: 12, 69 no. 198. The statement in *BAM* 206 rev. 16': *a-na pi-še-er-ti kiš-pi šá ina* UZ[U GU$_7$.MEŠ(?)] is perhaps also a purpose statement (Hunger 1968: 12, 75 no. 219), although it may be a generic formula describing the function of such material (see *CMAwR* 1: 53–55, note to line 15').

85 Reiner 1995: 88 notes 365 and 376; Maul 1994: 207f. and note 407; Ebeling 1955a: 137–38 no. 21; Ebeling 1954a: 4–5; Lambert 1956: 164.

86 Rev. 1': GABA.R[I …]
Rev. 2': *aná* KA IM.[GÍD?.DA? …]
Rev. 3': GABA.RI [giš]*li*$_9$-*u*$_5$ ⸢x⸣[x KA?.D]INGI[R.RA?[ki?] …]
"Cop[y of …], according to an [IM.GÍD.DA]-tablet [of …], copy of a writing-board [from Ba]byl[on? …]" (cf. Maul 1994: 207f.).
It is unclear how these lines should be interpreted, although they likely attest to three different sources upon which the copied text is based. If the three sources consisted of the same text or differing recensions thereof remains uncertain. Regardless, LKA 113 seems to be indicative of a level of active redaction in relation to what text ended up on the actual tablet. Similarly, Kiṣir-Nabû wrote a single prescription with a purpose statement during an uncertain phase, which opened with the following ruled-off statement: "I excerpted (the following) from among many tablets (and) I collected (them) together". Geller 2005: 230–31. *BAM* 101 obv. 1–3: TA ŠÀ-*bi* DUB.M[EŠ] MEŠ-[*tim*] [2] *ú-na-as-si-ḫa* ⸢x⸣[x] [3] *a-na a-ḫa-meš ú-qa*[*r-rib*]. Such indications of redaction should be investigated further.

87 Maul 1994: 8 note 67, 52 note 86, 90 note 64, 445 note 15; Ebeling 1954b: 178–181.

88 *CMAwR* 1: 2–4, 293–305 no. 8.2 ms A, 306–317 no. 8.5 ms B; Schwemer 2010b: 130–31; Schwemer 2007b: 68–71, 176–77.

89 Additionally, col. iv 6' contains a subscript designating the cause as witchcraft. This resembles a catch-line, although the line does not end EGIR-*šú* "(it is written) after this".

The group of ritual texts in this section can be subdivided into texts dealing with hostility (*KAR* 62, *KAR* 63, *KAR* 374(?)), witchcraft (*KAR* 80, *LKA* 157), ghost rituals (*LKA* 70+, *LKA* 83), rituals to treat *mimma lemnu* (*LKA* 70+, *LKA* 77) and *namburbi*-rituals (*KAR* 38, *LKA* 113, *LKA* 119). Notably, Kiṣir-Aššur copied a text that, on a duplicate from N4, is stated as originating from Ḫammurabi's palace (*BAM* 321). Unlike the prescriptions discussed in Section 8.2, only three texts contain purpose statements (*KAR* 38, *KAR* 374, *LKA* 157) and three ritual texts were said to have been extracted (*KAR* 38, *KAR* 374 and *KAR* 63, see Appendix 1).[90] Because several ritual texts do not contain purpose statements, they may have served purposes other than immediate practical implementation. Furthermore, Kiṣir-Aššur copied most texts related to witchcraft, hostility, and "adversaries" during his *mašmaš bīt Aššur*-phase. However, he did copy related texts earlier, such as the *namburbi*-ritual *KAL* 4 no. 7 against witchcraft from the *mašmaššu*-phase or the prescription against *kadabbedû* in *BAM* 201 from his *šamallû ṣeḫru*-phase. Nonetheless, what is preserved from Kiṣir-Aššur's *mašmaš bīt Aššur*- and *mašmaššu*-phases could indicate that rituals against witchcraft and other similar evils were copied and practiced at a more advanced stage of his career.[91]

8.6 Texts Connected to the Aššur Temple

A number of Kiṣir-Aššur's texts from his *mašmaš bīt Aššur*-phase show that he may have had official cultic duties in connection to the Aššur temple. In general, N4 texts such as the "Marduk Ordeal" (*SAA* 3 no. 34; N4 no. 453) and Sargon's letter to Aššur concerning his 8th campaign against Urartu (=N4 no. 477; Thureau-Dangin 1912; see Mayer 1983; Weidner 1937–39: 144 with references) indicate that the Bāba-šuma-ibni family had access to knowledge of state rituals that were associated with the Aššur temple (Pongratz-Leisten 2017: xxxv; Maul 2010a: 200–201; Pedersén 1986: 56–57). Whether these texts always represent this family's involvement is not entirely clear (cf. Pongratz-Leisten 2015: 391), although Maul (2010a: 200–201) emphasized that persons serving as Aššur temple exorcists must have been connected to the arrangement and performance of cultic and royal rituals in the city of Assur. This section discusses

90 *LKA* 157 was probably also stated to be "quick[ly extracted]".

91 In general, rituals aimed at gaining control over other individuals, such as the É-gal-ku$_4$-ra rituals, were not mentioned in the EM (*CMAwR* 1: 4; Schwemer 2011: 431–32; Schwemer 2007a: 67, 127–31, 159–61). Possibly, rituals for calming angry people or hostility (e.g., *KAR* 62, *KAR* 63) are to be included in this category, although they could also be interpreted as countermeasures on par with anti-witchcraft rituals.

Kiṣir-Aššur's various texts related to the Aššur temple in order to review the evidence for his attachment to the temple in connection to his title *mašmaš bīt Aššur.*

KAR 307 likely contains part of a mythological description of a ritual connected to the New Year ritual cycles (Livingstone 1989: XXIV–XXV; *SAA* 3 no. 39; Livingstone 1986: 82ff.), which were celebrated in Assur during the months Šabaṭu (11), Addaru (12) and Nisānu (1) when the Assyrian king dwelled in Assur and participated in a number of rituals.[92] The text possibly explains the mythological reasoning behind elements of a ritual cycle performed in Šabaṭu, connecting the king to the warrior aspect of Ninurta.[93] The colophon contains a secrecy statement and the text is not dated.[94]

KAV 42 is a version of the "Götteradressbuch of Assur" and describes the various gods that were resident in Assur according to their temples, a list of city gates, city shrines, the ziggurats of the city, and Sennacherib's new gates of the Aššur temple (*SAA* 20 no. 49; George 1992: 173ff. ms d, pl. 37–38; Menzel 1981: T 146ff.).[95] Almost all duplicates were excavated in the N4 collection, although

92 Ermidoro 2017: XVIII–XX; Pongratz-Leisten 2017: XLVII–XLVIII; Pongratz-Leisten 2015: 407–426; Ambos 2013a: 181–183; Maul 2000. See also Tsukimoto 1985: 218–227.

93 Pongratz-Leisten 2017: XLIX; Annus 2002: 6, 27, 93–94, 100–101; Maul 1999a: 211–212; Livingstone 1986: 146–48. One associated act was perhaps the execution of the "enemy" that may have been a prisoner (Maul 1999a: 211).

94 This text, *KAV* 42, *LKA* 137, N4 no. 110, and possibly N4 A 2727 contain a peculiar addition to the colophon, *KAR* 307 rev. 28: [MU] PA-*ṭu-u* GIM SUMUN-*ma*; *KAV* 42 rev. 42: PA-[*ṭ*]*u-u* GIM SUMUN-*ma*; *LKA* 137 rev. 7: MU PA[!]-*ṭu-u* GIM SU[MUN-*ma*(?)]; N4 no. 110 rev. 25: PA-*ṭu-u* GIM SUMUN-*m*[*a*] (see *BAK* no. 205–207). N4 A 2727 has a row of very damaged and faint signs, which may have read: ⸢PA-*ṭu-u* GIM SUMUN-*ma*⸣. The meaning of the phrase remains uncertain and it is only attested in a handful of texts from Assur (Hunger 1968: 8), see in addition to the texts here *BAK* 228 = *KAR* 178; *BAK* 279 = *KAR* 164; *BAK* 283 = *LKA* 106; *BAK* 287 = *LKA* 114 (N4 no. 507); *KAL* 4 no. 53. *AHw*: 852 regards the term PA-*ṭu-u* as a possibly unclear designation for a tablet, and *CAD* (P: 310) simply states that the meaning is unknown. Maul and Strauß (2011: 108 note 15) regarded the statement as a reference to the copy in question commenting on either "äußere Gestaltung oder auf gewisse Mängel der Textvorlage", which were intentionally repeated by the copyist in the present manuscript. Hunger discussed possible readings such as *ḫaṭṭû* for PA-*ṭu-u* originating from *ḫaṭû* "to make a mistake, neglect, omit" (*CAD* Ḫ: 156–58), in which MU would then designate "line, entry" (*šumu*), i.e., "faulty (entries) like the original". This would have the implication that the original was already considered faulty. Considering that three of five tablets with this phrase were written during Kiṣir-Aššur's *mašmaš bīt Aššur*-phase (*KAR* 307, *KAV* 42, N4 no. 110), it is possible *LKA* 137 should be assigned to his later phases as well.

95 For differences between *KAV* 42 and the *tākultu*-rituals in such stylized lists of divinities in Assur, see Pongratz-Leisten 2017: XXXIX–XL; Pongratz-Leisten 2015: 397–99.

not all necessarily were written by the Bāba-šuma-ibni family.[96] Notably, no recensions of the text are completely identical (George 1992: 167; Menzel 1981: T 146–47). As such, *KAV* 42 is the only NA source that includes a list of the gates from Sennacherib's extension to the *Ešarra* temple complex (rev. 36–40).[97] The text is designated as "written (by) Kiṣir-Aššur …".[98] The first line of the colophon further specifies: "the old gates are not listed" (George 1992: 183).[99] This may denote that Kiṣir-Aššur edited the copied text. In general, such "topographical texts" are believed to have provided theological and cosmological glorification of the respective city (Pongratz-Leisten 2017: XXVIII; George 1992: 1–4, 167). Kiṣir-Aššur's text may represent a wish to create an updated version that identifies himself as a foremost scholar in such cultic matters while celebrating the city of Assur.

The unpublished tablet N4 no. 110 contains "cultic" material (see Ebeling 1954c: 115). The obverse contains several individual lines, as well as a long list of cultic materials and objects related to one or more rituals, presumably described separately as "rites" (*parṣū*, *CAD* P: 195ff.) in obverse line 30.[100] A section of the reverse equates various peculiar gods with common divine names and titles, and this part of the text seems to function as a theological commentary.[101] It remains uncertain which ritual(s) and what cult the content of N4 no. 110 is connected to. The manuscript attests to Kiṣir-Aššur's initiation into esoteric knowledge during his *mašmaš bīt Aššur*-phase, which is presumably related to one or more cults in Assur.

PKTA pl. 10–11 (= *SAA* 20 no. 37) contains temple service instructions for the Assyrian temples throughout various cities.[102] It is possible that Kiṣir-Aššur copied the text, even though his name is not preserved in the colophon. The

96 George 1992: 168, 173; ms c (N4 no. 458), d (*KAV* 42, N4 no. 138), e (unknown), f (N4 no. 491), g+i = one tablet (N4 no. 604 and 612), h (N4 no. 608), j+k = one tablet(?) (unknown). However, ms f was written by a *šangû*-priest of Adad (*BAK* no. 270) and ms g+i was written by an unnamed *šangû*-priest(?) of *Ešarra*.

97 Pongratz-Leisten 2017: LVI-LVII; George 1992: 167–72; see also Pongratz-Leisten 2015: 396–97.

98 *KAV* 42 rev. 43: *šà-ṭír* ᵖ*Ki-ṣir-Aš-šur* …

99 *KAV* 42 rev. 41: KÁ.MEŠ SUMUN.MEŠ NU SAR (George 1992: 184, *BAK* no. 207). This resembles the writing in Kiṣir-Aššur's *BAM* 102 rev. 3: DÙ.DÙ.BI-*šú la šaṭ-ru*, "its ritual is not written".

100 Obv. 30: GARZA.MEŠ te x x […].

101 E.g., rev. 5: "The 'Divine fox' (*is*) Nergal of the funerary offe[rings]", ᵈKA$_5$.A ᵈU.GUR *šá ki-i*[*s-pi*], and rev. 8: "The 'Divine mayor' (*is*) Mar[du]k, king of the go[ds]", ᵈ*ḫa za-nu* ᵈAMAR.[UT]U LUGAL DIN[GIR.MEŠ].

102 Ermidoro 2015: 125–26; Menzel 1981: T 110–12, no. 53.

ritual may be an abbreviated version of the *tākultu*-ritual,[103] which involved the participation of the king in providing offerings in the form of a ceremonial banquet for the gods of the various Assyrian temples (Pongratz-Leisten 2015: 392–99, 394; Pongratz-Leisten 2017: XXVI–XXVII). *PKTA* pl. 10–11 was excavated in N4 and the remains of the second line of the colophon read "[…] of the Aššur temple".[104] Based on these two observations, Parpola (2017: 102) and Pongratz-Leisten (2015: 394) have reasonably suggested that the text was copied by Kiṣir-Aššur. If Kiṣir-Aššur is identified as the copyist of this text, his use of this version of the *tākultu*-ritual remains uncertain.

PKTA pl. 39–40 (= *SAA* 20 no. 51) was likely copied by either Kiṣir-Aššur or Kiṣir-Nabû and is a copy of a decree by a king Shalmaneser (possibly Shalmaneser V, ca. 726–723).[105] The text concerns rations for and the duties of the Aššur temple personnel, although it does not list exorcists.[106] The colophon states: "The hands of Kiṣi[r-…]",[107] which is not observed in other Kiṣir-Aššur texts. In other contexts, phrases in the colophons related to the "hand" (*qātu*) of someone occur as (*ina*) *qāt* PN "hand of PN",[108] possibly designating the copyist (*CAD* Q: 194; Hunger 1968: 8).[109] Perhaps the formulation can be considered similar in meaning to *šà-ṭír*, as observed in *KAV* 42. The text's purpose remains unclear. Although the text does not formally list a title, I consider it likely that it was part of Kiṣir-Aššur's *mašmaš bīt Aššur*-phase tablets because of its association with the Aššur temple.[110]

In general, the texts suggest a familiarization with the cult of Aššur and cultic topography of Assur. However, none of the texts demonstrate that Kiṣir-Aššur prepared such rituals or participated as performer, although cultic

103 Pongratz-Leisten 2017: XXXVII; Pongratz-Leisten 2015: 394; cf. Ermidoro 2015: 125–26 and notes 18–20; Menzel 1981: 151–53; van Driel 1969: 60–75, 165.

104 Rev. 25: [x x x x x] ⸢*šá* É⸣ AN.ŠÁR.

105 Considering the text's relationship to the Aššur temple, it is reasonable to assume that the name was Kiṣir-Aššur and his title was *mašmaš bīt Aššur*. The text may also mention Sennacherib (Parpola 2017: 144–145 col. iii 1').

106 Menzel 1981: T 18–19, text no. 16; van Driel 1969: 179–82. Shalmaneser V likely abolished certain privileges for the elites of Assur, which resulted in a conflict mentioned in the "Assur Charter" (Saggs 1975: 14–15 rev. 31–33).

107 *SAA* 20 no. 51; Menzel 1981: T 18–19, no. 16. N4 no. 330 col. iv 16': ⸢ŠU^{II}⸣ ^{P}*Ki-ṣi*[*r-*…].

108 See, e.g., *BAK* 10, 43, 48, 50, 92, 94–104, 107, 116, 128, 146–47, 231, 385, 425, 457–58, 464–65.

109 See *BAK* 137 line 3: *ina* ŠU^{II}-*šú iš-ṭur-ma*, "he copied it with his hands (i.e., personally)", and *BAK* 171 line 2 and *BAK* 172 line 1: *ina* ŠU^{II}-*šú im-šuḫ-ma*, "he performed the computations personally" (*CAD* Q: 194).

110 A connection between N4 and temple personnel is attested in several administrative and legal texts excavated in room 11 of the N4 house (Maul 2010a: 201 and notes 41–42).

materials and ceremonies are mentioned in the manuscripts.[111] Furthermore, several influential families, such as Aššur-šākin-šumi's family of *šangû*-priests of Aššur and Nergal, are associated with the N4 collection (Fadhil 2012: 39; Maul 2010a: 216–17). The suggestion by Maul (ibid.: 200–201) concerning the Bāba-šuma-ibni family's involvement in state rituals was further developed by Pongratz-Leisten (2017: XXXV), who described the family as organizers of "the cult of the Aššur temple" and saw Kiṣir-Aššur as the "author of several state rituals" (also Pongratz-Leisten 2015: 391, 394, 396).[112] However, the crucial evidence needed to connect Kiṣir-Aššur and his family to actual performances in the Aššur cult is currently lacking.[113] Kiṣir-Aššur may have been initiated into exclusive knowledge regarding these rituals, but anything beyond the possible involvement of Kiṣir-Aššur's family in these rituals is at present ambiguous.

8.7 Summary

The majority of Kiṣir-Aššur's tablets with colophons derive from his *mašmaš bīt Aššur*-phase. As suggested by his title, he may have had duties in connection to the Aššur temple during this phase. Several texts suggest that he was familiar with the cult of Aššur, cultic topography of the city of Assur and various stately rituals, although they cannot be connected directly to active participation in the Aššur cult. Kiṣir-Aššur's possible duties to the temple in connection to his title therefore remain uncertain. Regardless of any possible official duties, Kiṣir-Aššur could have continued to have private clients as *mašmaš bīt Aššur*, which may be indicated by the purpose statements on manuscripts relating to

111 Reportedly, the administrative texts excavated in N4 do not show a clear link between the Bāba-šuma-ibni family and the Aššur temple cult (see Section 2.3.1). However, the results of Henrietta Cseke's unpublished dissertation *Die Wirtschafts- und Verwaltungsurkunden aus dem sog. "Has des Beschwörungspriesters" in Assur* from 2002 have not been available to me.

112 Maul has on several occasions suggested that the Aššur temple exorcists were involved in performing rituals for the Assyrian king (e.g., Maul 1994: 421). Additionally, texts from N4 suggest that the exorcists copied *šu'illa*-prayers originally designed for, e.g., Sîn-šarra-iškun, although it remains uncertain if they performed these rituals (see references in May 2018: 78 and note 127; Maul 2010a: 204 and note 50). Note that Geller proposes that "the *mašmššu* was first and foremost a temple priest" on the basis of his analysis of the EM (Geller 2018b: 292).

113 As shown in Villard 1998, only one NA royal letter may indicate a connection between Kiṣir-Aššur and the royal court (see Section 2.3.5). Furthermore, only Aššur-nādin-aḫḫē's text *SAA* 20 no. 17 relates directly to a stately ritual among the family's tablets with colophons (see May 2018: 69 with references).

healing. The same seems to have been the case for Adad-šumu-uṣur at the royal court (Robson 2019: 109).

Kiṣir-Aššur's group of medical texts contain a number of treatments for illnesses not previously encountered, mainly connected to internal illnesses. Furthermore, the texts attest to the active practice of this knowledge through his frequent use of purpose statements and extracts. A number of his texts with purpose statements make use of prescriptions labelled as "tested". The label "tested" may refer to a drug's ability to regularly produce wanted results. It remains uncertain if Kiṣir-Aššur tested prescriptions himself, but two texts discussed in Section 8.3.2 could represent an example of this. Additionally, Kiṣir-Aššur copied *BAM* 300 with a prescription labelled as a panacea, i.e., a widely applicable drug. Therefore, several of Kiṣir-Aššur's medical texts from his *mašmaš bīt Aššur*-phase seem to attest to practiced knowledge. This practiced knowledge was occasionally considered "tested" or widely applicable, indicating that Kiṣir-Aššur may have relied on trustworthy prescriptions or perhaps tested the effect of certain prescriptions himself.

Finally, Kiṣir-Aššur's ritual texts from his *mašmaš bīt Aššur*-phase attest to the treatment of various sources of evil, such as ghosts, *mimma lemnu*, witchcraft, and "adversaries" (*bēl dabābi*), as well as hostility, and various *namburbi*-rituals. Especially texts connected to witchcraft and hostility appear to be related to Kiṣir-Aššur's later phases. The *mašmaš bīt Aššur* ritual manuscripts themselves may not necessarily represent practice in all instances, but Kiṣir-Aššur still acquired knowledge about certain rituals for various purposes during his *mašmaš bīt Aššur*-phase.

CHAPTER 9

Situating Kiṣir-Aššur's Knowledge Production

The *mašmaš bīt Aššur*-phase represents the final stage of Kiṣir-Aššur's career, according to the surviving evidence. Based on the discussion of Kiṣir-Aššur's surviving tablets in the preceding chapters, this chapter discusses Kiṣir-Aššur's overall text production to contextualize what he copied and used in relation to the scholarly textual traditions of his time. The first section investigates Kiṣir-Aššur's medical focuses in his healing texts. The following section provides a discussion of Kiṣir-Aššur's extracts (*nisḫus*). Kiṣir-Aššur produced a number of extracts, and these are found especially among tablets from his *mašmaš bīt Aššur*-phase and tablets that cannot be assigned to a specific phase. These extract texts are first discussed in relation to statements in the colophons that designate them as extracts from writing-boards. Other extracts were supplied with numbers and were likely organized. These numbered extracts are discussed in relation to their numbering, their possible organization, and their function. Afterwards follows an investigation of the use of incipits, catch-lines in colophons, and duplicate passages in Kiṣir-Aššur's texts in relation to the therapeutic series *šumma amēlu muḫḫašu umma ukāl* "If the crown of a man's head is feverish" (Ugu), known from contemporary Nineveh, and the so-called "Assur Medical Catalogue", an Assur catalogue of text incipits possibly related to a recension of the Ugu series. This analysis examines to what extent Kiṣir-Aššur drew on a recension of the therapeutic series and navigated according to its incipits. This chapter also addresses Kiṣir-Aššur's text production in relation to the Exorcist's Manual. Finally, Kiṣir-Aššur's textual production is contextualized in the light of the scholarly traditions of Assur, his manuscripts derived from the Gula temple in Assur, and the N4 collection's connection to the Nineveh text collections.

9.1 Kiṣir-Aššur's Overall Medical Focus

Kiṣir-Aššur's medical texts are discussed in relation to his individual career phases throughout the previous chapters. This section discusses all of Kiṣir-Aššur's medical material in order to identify areas of the body upon which Kiṣir-Aššur was particularly focussed. Dividing Kiṣir-Aššur's medical corpus on the basis of the tablets that bear his colophons is not as straightforward as it might seem. This is because most texts contain a number of prescriptions

© TROELS PANK ARBØLL, 2021 | DOI:10.1163/9789004436084_010

that focus on different areas of interest, e.g., a few individual diagnoses afflicting several body parts, one illness with many varied symptoms affecting one or more areas of the body, or various conditions relating to roughly one area of the body. Furthermore, several illnesses are diagnosed without symptom descriptions, and it is therefore difficult to assess what symptoms they were believed to have caused in such generic entries.[1] Additionally, the texts are not of similar length and can contain one (e.g., *BAM* 68) or multiple entries (e.g., *BAM* 9).

What follows is an attempt to group the material according to illnesses and the affected areas of the body described in the symptom descriptions in the texts themselves. A division of texts by body parts decontextualizes the material to some extent, as the various body parts were not always consistently demarcated in ancient terminology or physiological conception (see Sections 4.4 and 4.4.1).[2] Modern anatomical terms are, however, not useful for the present purpose either, as these tend to be too specific. Several illnesses and symptom descriptions are also problematic, as they can affect several areas of the body. Thus, the areas described in Table 17 are somewhat generalized according to the symptom descriptions of afflicted body parts in the texts themselves and as such are only meant to be illustrative. Texts that do not specify body parts, symptom descriptions, illness names, or explicit causes of illness have been excluded.

Table 17 shows that Kiṣir-Aššur's surviving texts relate to many illnesses and symptoms that affect all the major areas of the body. In terms of diagnosed illnesses or causes of illness, a number are listed in more than one text, namely: *aḫḫāzu-* and *amurriqānu-*jaundice, "Anus illness", "adversary", "hand of Curse" or Curse, "hand of ghost" or ghost, "seizing-of-the-mouth" (*kadabbedû*), *ṣētu-*fever (= "sun-heat"), *ḫimiṭ ṣēti* (= "inflammation by sun-heat"), *šaššaṭu*, and witchcraft. Several of the illnesses listed can produce various symptoms that affect several body parts, making them difficult to group. Such illnesses include *aḫḫāzu-* and *amurriqānu-*jaundice, which cause various internal symptoms as well as discolouration of the eyes and skin (Böck 2014a: 122–128; Scurlock and Andersen 2005: 32–34, 138–39), and *ṣētu*, which causes, e.g., headaches, rash, muscle pains, abdominal bloating, vomiting, lung problems, or mental alterations (Stol 2007a: 22–39; Scurlock and Andersen 2005: 53–59). Yet, both these

1 Other afflictions, e.g., *suālu-*cough, function mainly as a symptom, but can also occasionally be described as an illness (e.g., Scurlock and Andersen 2005: 178, 181).

2 Although not all illnesses can be demarcated in relation to body parts, some texts, such as the AMC, state that their content was arranged "from the crown (of the head) to the (toe)nail(s)". This description is also found in the Assurbanipal colophon *BAK* 329 line 4.

TABLE 17 Illnesses and affected parts of the body in Kiṣir-Aššur's texts

Group	Text	Illness/Cause	Affected area(s)
		Kiṣir-Aššur	
Head, eyes, ears, nose, mouth	*BAM* 9	"Hand of ghost"; *sagkidabbû*-migrane; *ṣētu*-fever	Head, ears
	BAM 28	"Seizing-of the-mouth" (*kadabbedû*); ("stinking-illness" (*bu'šānu*))	Nose, mouth, teeth, tongue
	BAM 351	"'Mistiness' of the eyes" (*birrat īnī*)	–
Thorax, epigastrium, abdomen (organs and gastro-intestinal system), renal, rectal, and potency problems	*BAM* 78	–	Spleen (*tulīmu*)
	BAM 99	"Anus illness" (DÚR.GIG); "sick insides" (*qerbēnu* GIG); "'overflow' of the intestines" (*terdīt irrī*)	Abdomen, anus
	BAM 102	"Anus illness" (DÚR.GIG)	–
	BAM 164	"Anus illness" (DÚR.GIG)	Kidney, renal, rectal problems, potency
	BAM 177	*apišalû*(?); *ṣētu*-fever	–
	BAM 186	*Aḫḫāzu*-jaundice; *amurriqānu*-jaundice; *ḫimiṭ ṣēti*	–
	BAM 188	Bile (*martu*); *aḫḫāzu*-jaundice; *amurriqānu*-jaundice	–
	N4 A 2727	("Anus illness" (DÚR.GIG)?)	–
	(*RA* 15 pl. 76)	(see below)	(see below)
	RA 40 pl. 116	*Ašû*; *pašittu*-bile; *lubāṭu*; *suālu*-cough	Respiratory system, stomach, oesophagus

TABLE 17 Illnesses and affected parts of the body in Kiṣir-Aššur's texts (*cont.*)

Group	Text	Illness/Cause	Affected area(s)
Muscles, nerves, tendons, "strings", and the lower body	*BAM* 81	*Maškadu*	–
	BAM 121	–	Upper [...], feet
	BAM 122	*Šimmatu*-paralysis; *šaggu*-stiffness	"Strings", shin, feet
	BAM 129	*Sagallu; šaššaṭu*	"Strings", neck, waist, eyes, motoric system
	BAM 131	*Šaššaṭu; sikkatu*-lesion(?); *ašṭu*-stiffness	"Strings", eyes, motoric system
	BAM 303	*Šaggu*-stiffness; ([GÌR^{II}] *šá* IM *id*-[*p*]*í*-*t*[*u*])	Feet(?)
	N4 A 400	*Maškadu*	–
Skin, wounds (stings, bites)	*KAL* 4 no. 41 (*RA* 15 pl. 76)	[*Garābu*(?)] (see below)	[(Skin?)] (see below)
Complex causes of illness, diagnoses or symptoms affecting several body parts and/or the mind	*BAM* 40	*Dikšu*; MUR.MEŠ GIG	Eyes, thorax, lungs, arms
	BAM 201	"Hand of curse (*māmītu*)"; *kadabbedû*	Eyes, epigastrium/abdomen, feet
	KAL 10 no. 4	"Curse" (*māmītu*)	–
	KAL 10 no. 5	"Curse" (*māmītu*)	–
	KAR 80	"Adversary" (*bēl dabābi*); witchcraft (*kišpu*)	Head, mouth, arms, hands, feet, "strings"
	KAR 171	"Adversary" (*bēl dabābi*)	–
	KAR 267	Ghost; *ḫa*(*y*)*yattu*-fit	–
	LKA 70+	Ghost; *sagḫulḫazû*(?); *mimma lemnu*	–
	LKA 89+ *LKA* 90	Ghost(?)	–
	LKA 157	Witchcraft (*kišpu*)	Head, ears(?), mouth, neck, stomach, "strings", hands, feet

TABLE 17 Illnesses and affected parts of the body in Kiṣir-Aššur's texts (*cont.*)

Group	Text	Illness/Cause	Affected area(s)
	N4 A 2191	(Ghost?)	(Unpublished)
	N4 no. 237	Ghost	–
	RA 15 pl. 76	Snakebite; scorpion sting; a horse illness (colic?)	(Unspecified affected body parts and various systemic symptoms, see Chapter 4)
Other	*BAM* 300	(Universally applicable)	–
		Kiṣir-[Aššur/Nabû]	
Thorax(?)	*BAM* 260	–	Airways(?)
Complex diagnosis affecting several body parts and/or the mind	*BAM* 68	*Šibiṭ šāri*; *ḫimiṭ ṣēti*; *šimmatu*-paralysis; *r*[*imûtu*-numbness(?)]; *šaššaṭu*; "Hand of ghost"; "Hand of curse (*māmītu*)"; any illness	–
	BAM 202	*Demmakurrû*-derangement; insanity (*ṭēmu šanû*); "Hand of *bennu*-epilepsy"	Behavioural change, motoric system
	BAM 311	*Ḫūṣ ḫīp*(*i*) *libbi* ("internal crushing pain"); Lugal-urra (epilepsy demon); *Alû*-demon; Antašubba-epilepsy	Behavioural change, eyes, epigastrium/abdomen, motoric system

examples seem to be situated internally and are therefore grouped in relation to afflictions of the thorax, epigastrium and abdomen. More problematic is the *māmītu* "Curse" that can afflict several areas of the body, although it is frequently diagnosed in the abdomen (Maul 2019: 25ff.; Maul 2010b: 135–41, 145–46; Scurlock and Andersen 2005: 506–508; Maul 2004). I label this illness as complicated, despite *māmītu*'s general focus on the abdomen. An additional problem is that several of the illness names appear in purely ritual texts, such as *LKA* 70+, and if the ghost mentioned therein relates to an illness, it is likely as the cause and not necessarily as the diagnosis. Such illnesses are also labelled as "complex".

In terms of affected areas of the body, as well as illnesses known to affect similar areas diagnosed without symptom descriptions, three groups of texts can be identified that focus on: 1) the thorax, epigastrium, abdomen, its organs, associated processes and illnesses, and the anus, i.e., primarily internal illnesses; 2) the "strings" of the body, its motor system, and the lower body parts; and 3) complex illnesses or causes of illness that affect several bodily areas. However, these groupings remain tentative due to the generalized classification utilized above.

The majority of the relevant material derives from Kiṣir-Aššur's *mašmaššu*- and *mašmaš bīt Aššur*-phases. Yet, Kiṣir-Aššur's focus on the "strings" is apparent from his *šamallû ṣeḫru*-phase onwards (*BAM* 129, N4 A 400). The same may also apply to the abdominal treatments, although the evidence is less explicit. The relevant text *RA* 15 pl. 76 possibly concerns a type of horse colic related to the stomach, although the actual diagnosis or symptom description is poorly understood (see Appendix 2). Cures for internal ailments are likely also found during Kiṣir-Aššur's *mašmaššu ṣeḫru*-phase (N4 A 2727). Both treatments of the "strings" and internal illnesses reappear during Kiṣir-Aššur's *mašmaššu*-phase and are attested in the bulk of material from his *mašmaš bīt Aššur*-phase as well.

It is difficult to estimate whether or not the texts in these groups served pedagogical or pragmatic purposes in Kiṣir-Aššur's training, practice, or personal interests. Several of the tablets may well have fulfilled all purposes to some extent. Nonetheless, several of the tablets listed above include purpose statements connected to practice. If the tablets with purpose statement are disregarded, the groups change. By excluding Kiṣir-Aššur's tablets with purpose statements the group of internal treatments become substantially smaller (around three texts).[3] The texts copied by Kiṣir-Aššur concerning the internal maladies may therefore have been connected particularly with practice. Incidentally, this group relates especially to Kiṣir-Aššur's *mašmas bīt Aššur*-phase, perhaps reflecting the complicated nature of diagnosing and treating such illnesses. However, this suggestion has to remain hypothetical for the time being.

Böck (2010a: 69) estimated that appoximately 70% of the first millennium Mesopotamian medical treatment texts were concerned with internal illnesses

3 The tablets with purpose statements and prescriptions for internal illnesses are: *BAM* 78, *BAM* 99, *BAM* 164, *BAM* 177, *BAM* 186, *BAM* 188.

affecting the thorax, heart, lungs, liver, stomach, abdomen, waist and groin, as well as renal and rectal maladies (see also Pedersén 1986: 53). Internal illnesses may also have taken up large parts of the Nineveh Ugu recension and the AMC (see Steinert 2018a; Scurlock 2014: 295–306; Heeßel 2010b: 32–33), although this was not the main focus in the 2nd subseries of Sa-gig (Heeßel 2000: 24–30). Kiṣir-Aššur's texts appear to have been characterized by an interest in "string" and lower body illnesses associated with the muscles, tendons, and nerves, and a professional need to treat various clients' abdominal, gastro-intestinal, renal, and rectal symptoms. The two text groups discussed here are also mirrored in the "tested" treatments in *BAM* 164, *BAM* 186, perhaps N4 A 2727 primarily against internal maladies, and *BAM* 303, presumably against illness of the feet.

9.2 Numbered *Nisḫu*-extracts

Kiṣir-Aššur's tablets were frequently described as "extracted" (*issuḫa, nisḫu, nasḫa*) or "quickly extracted" (*ḫanṭiš/zamar nasāḫu*), often with a purpose statement (see all attestations in Appendix 1). The word *nasāḫu* literally refers to tearing out body parts, pulling out hair, uprooting plants, and expelling demons or illnesses (*CAD* N/2: 1ff.). In relation to texts, the meaning is therefore to pull something out from a united whole, i.e., a piece of text from a somewhat standardized manuscript, although not necessarily from a series.[4] There are two kinds of extract texts in the N4 collection: 1) those stated to be "extracted" as one or more select parts from a manuscript (e.g., ZI-*ḫa*), and 2) those numbered according to some principle as an extract containing one or more select parts from a manuscript (e.g., 7 *nis-ḫu*). Both types can be supplied with catchlines, which may indicate a wish to be able to locate the extract in the copied manuscript (see Section 9.3).

In total, 16 out of Kiṣir-Aššur's 27 extracted texts, and seven of Kiṣir-Nabû's 12 extracted texts have purpose statements.[5] Such extracts are found among

4 Hunger 1968: 2, 4; Leichty 1964: 148, 151; cf. Black 1985. Frahm (2010b: 177–78 and note 66) argues that *nasāḫu* refers to an excerpt from memory of a series or work, but not necessarily a physical copy in front of the copyist (see also Payne 2010: 293).

5 Kiṣir-Aššur's extracts *ana ṣabāt epēši*: *BAM* 78, *BAM* 99, *BAM* 164, *BAM* 177, *BAM* 186, *BAM* 188, *BAM* 300, *BAM* 333, *BAM* 351, *KAR* 21, *KAR* 38 (*ana mušepišūti*), *KAR* 171, *KAR* 374, *LKA* 40, *LKA* 157, N4 no. 228. Cf. *KAL* 10 no. 1. Kiṣir-Aššur's extracts without a purpose statement: *BAM* 9, *BAM* 28, *BAM* 81, *BAM* 201, *KAR* 63, *KAR* 267, *LKA* 43, *LKA* 89+, *RA* 15 pl. 76. Uncertain if the text contains a purpose statement due to a break: *KAL* 4 no. 19; *KAR* 298. Kiṣir-Nabû's extracts *ana ṣabāt epēši*: *BAM* 101, *BAM* 168, *KAR* 22, *KAR* 56, *LKA* 81, *LKA* 110. Kiṣir-Nabû's extracts without

Kiṣir-Aššur's *mašmaššu*- and *mašmaš bīt Aššur*-phases and on tablets without titles (see Appendix 1). The presence of purpose statements on many of the extracts could indicate that they were used in the preparation of a healing ceremony (Maul 2010: 212). Other texts were presumably extracted as part of Kiṣir-Aššur's training, such as his *šamallû ṣeḫru* manuscripts *BAM* 201 and *RA* 15 pl. 76. Comparatively, Kiṣir-Nabû's *BAM* 52 and *BAM* 106 were extracted for his "reading, lecture(?)" (*malsûtu*), possibly indicating an instructive purpose.[6] Section 3.6 suggests that Kiṣir-Aššur's numbered extracts copied as *šamallû ṣeḫru* may first have functioned as copying exercises and subsequently as teaching material. As such, this use likely mirrored Clancier's proposed use of such text in LB Uruk as exercises, pedagogical texts, or *aide mémoires* (Clancier 2014: 55). A collection of scholarly texts from LB Uruk from a family of *āšipu*s, descending from a certain Šangû-Ninurta, is used for comparison throughout this chapter (Robson 2014: 155–58; Robson 2013: 565–569; Stevens 2013: 216). Although their collection differs in some respect from the 7th century BCE collections investigated here, the collection is useful for comparison because it held an Ugu recension, perhaps differing from the one found at Nineveh, as well as an abbreviated (*pirsu*) numbered series based on the LB Uruk Ugu recension (Heeßel 2010b: 34 and note 50; see Salin 2016). As such, the situation could potentially mirror the numbered *nisḫu*-extracts with medical material from N4.

9.2.1 *Extracts and Writing-boards*

Before discussing the numbered extracts, the evidence for what physical medium these and other extracts were copied from first needs to be evaluated. This serves to elucidate the function of the numbering system of certain extracts. Several of Kiṣir-Aššur's and Kiṣir-Nabû's tablets state that the content was copied from writing-boards. Examples of writing-boards have been found especially at Nimrud, which typically consisted of wooden or ivory frames with a layer of wax that could be inscribed, and several such frames were combined to create at least two surfaces upon which to write.[7] The fragment of at least one ivory writing-board was discovered in the N4 house, attesting to

a purpose statement: *BAM* 52, *BAM* 147, *KAL* 4 no. 44, *KAR* 72. Uncertain due to break: *BAM* 106, *LKA* 118, N4 no. 80, N4 no. 404. Extract from either Kiṣir-Aššur or Kiṣir-Nabû extracted *ana ṣabāt epēši*: *BAM* 202, *BAM* 311. Text by Kiṣir-Aššur or Kiṣir-Nabû, containing a purpose statement, but uncertain if it was an extract: *KAL* 9 no. 41.

6 *CAD* M/1: 171; Clancier 2014: 58; Stevens 2013: 220 note 51; Frahm 2011a: 52; Geller 2010: 141.

7 Wiseman 1955; Mallowan 1954: 98–107 and pls. 12–13; see also Howard 1955 for a technical discussion of the Nimrud writing-boards, as well as the 2nd millennium BCE Ulu Burun writing-board in Payton 1991.

the presence of such manuscripts in the collection (Klengel-Brandt 1975). That exorcists may have brought writing-boards in order to check texts, related to their duties is indicated by both literary and non-literary texts. The literary composition *Ludlul bēl nēmeqi* offers a description of an exorcist who appears to the protagonist in a dream, signalling the end of the protagonist's suffering:

> In the dream Ur-Nintinugga, the *Babylonian*(?) [...], a bearded young man wearing his crown, an exorcist, carrying a writing-[board].[8]

In a NA letter that is part of the royal correspondence between the king and his scholars (*SAA* 10 no. 202), the king's exorcist Adad-šumu-uṣur writes to king Esarhaddon to make excuses for a late reply:

> I had to drive to the palace those rams which the chief cook had brought forth for me, and the writing-board was in my house. Now then, I can look at the board and extract the relevant interpretation.[9]

Administrative records from Nineveh indicate that wooden writing boards (*lēʾu*) were used during the assembling of Assurbanipal's libraries (Parpola 1983b: 6).[10] Although writing-boards in the Nineveh collections were fewer in number than ordinary tablets (ibid.: 8), they often consisted of more than one "page" and could contain more text than an ordinary clay tablet (ibid.; Wiseman 1955: 4, 7–8). Due to the practical aspects of writing-boards, they were employed in some instances to "import" knowledge to Assyria (Fincke 2003–04: 126). Such boards must therefore have been employed throughout the NA cities.[11] Based on the Nineveh evidence, Maul (2010a: 199 and note 37) estimated that writing-boards may have constituted around 15% of the total

---

8 *Ludlul bēl nēmeqi* tablet III lines 39–41 (Lambert 1996: 50–51; see Foster 1996: 317; lines 40–42 in Annus and Lenzi 2010: 24, 39; lines 40–42 in Oshima 2014: 96–97, 285–289, 416): *ina* MÁŠ.GE$_6$ ^{p}*ur-nin-tin-ug*$_5$*-ga* ⌜din?.tir?⌝ [x x x] ^{41} *eṭ-lu ṭar-ru a-pir a-ga-šú* ^{42} MAŠ.MAŠ-*ma na-ši le-*ʾ[*u-um*]. Foster (1991: 27–28) suggests that the writing-board may represent the text of *Ludlul bēl nēmeqi* itself (see also Noegel 2007: 73).

9 *SAA* 10 no. 202 obv. 8–12: *ina* ŠÀ É.GAL *a-na* ⌜UDU!.NITÁḪ⌝.MEŠ *šú-nu* ^{9} *ša* ^{lú}GAL-MU *ú-še-ṣa-an-ni* ^{10} *ú-se-li* ^{giš}ZU *ina* É *šú-u* ^{11} *ú-ma-a an-nu-rig* ^{giš}ZU ^{12} *a-mar pi*!*-šìr-šu a-na-sa-ḫa* (Parpola 1993: 164). It is possible that the letter should be dated to late June 670 BCE (see Parpola 1983a: 133 no. 147).

10 Were these boards used especially for prescriptions? The list provides the numbers 6+ tablets and 24 boards for "medical recipes (*bulṭē*)" (Parpola 1983b: 6). For additional fragments of these administrative records related to Assurbanipal's libraries, see Lambert 1989: 95–96.

11 Comparatively, writing-boards were commonly employed in the NB temple administration at Sippar (MacGinnis 2002 with further references; see also Freydank 2001).

stock of tablets (see Maul 1994: 160–61; Parpola 1983b: 4–5 note 11–12). Kiṣir-Aššur's and Kiṣir-Nabû's texts with colophons stating that they were copied from writing-boards are listed in Table 18.

Both Kiṣir-Aššur and Kiṣir-Nabû extracted texts from writing-boards. In terms of the explicit statements studied here, Kiṣir-Nabû seems to have copied from writing-boards more often than Kiṣir-Aššur. Perhaps instead of elaborate descriptions, Kiṣir-Aššur frequently included the generic copying statement "(written and checked) according to its original" (*kīma labīrišu*) to his colophons, which offers no information about the medium of the original manuscript.[12]

TABLE 18 Kiṣir-Aššur's and Kiṣir-Nabû's texts copied from writing-boards

Text	Writing-board statement	Translation
	Kiṣir-Aššur	
BAM 9	GABA.RI ^{giš}ZU [GN(?)]	Copy of a writing-board [(from GN?)]
BAM 131	[TA$^{?}$] ^{giš}ZU *šá bul-ṭi ša* É ^{d}ME.ME	[From(?)] a writing-board of prescriptions from the temple of Gula
BAM 201	TA ŠÀ ^{giš}ZU *šá bul-ṭi ša* É ^{d}ME.ME	From a writing-board of prescriptions from the temple of Gula
LKA 113	GABA.R[I ...] *aná* KA IM.[GÍD.DA(?) ...] GABA. RI ^{giš}*li*$_9$-*u*$_5$ ⸢x⸣[x KA$^{?}$.DI]NGI[R.RA$^{?\text{ki}?}$ ...]	Cop[y ...] according to an *im*[*giddû*-tablet ...], copy of a writing-board [(from) Bab]y[lon(?)]
RA 15 pl. 76	GABA.RI ^{giš}*le-'i*	Copy of a writing-board
	Kiṣir-Aššur or Kiṣir-Nabû	
BAM 68	[T]A ŠÀ ^{giš}ZU	[Fr]om the middle of a writing-board

12 The tablets in Appendix 1 with such generic copying statements and without information about the manuscript copied from are: *BAM* 28; *BAM* 311; Beckman and Foster 1988 no. 21; *CT* 37 pl. 25; *KAL* 4 no. 19; *KAL* 4 no. 37; *KAL* 7 no. 24; *KAL* 10 no. 4; *KAL* 10 no. 5; *KAL* 10 no. 13; *KAR* 62; *KAR* 63; *KAR* 80 (= *KAL* 2 no. 8); *KAR* 267; *KAR* 307; *KAR* 374; *LKA* 40; *LKA* 43; *LKA* 77; *LKA* 89+; *LKA* 115; *LKA* 119; *LKA* 141; *LKA* 146; *LKA* 157; N4 A 400; N4 A 2191(?); N4 A 2727; N4 no. 110; N4 no. 175; N4 no. 224; N4 no. 237; N4 no. 289; *PKTA* pl. 39–40. Maul (2019: 122) translates the phrase as: "Wie die zugehörige Vorlage". Robson (2011a: 566–67) suggests that such statements may refer to clay tablets, but unlike the writing-boards, the medium clay was not worth recording. The writing-boards originating from specific cities are discussed in Section 9.5.1.

TABLE 18 Kiṣir-Aššur's and Kiṣir-Nabû's texts copied from writing-boards (*cont.*)

Text	Writing-board statement	Translation
	Kiṣir-Nabû	
CMAwR 1 pl. 25–26	*ki-i* ⸢KA⸣ ^{gi}[^{š}L]I.⸢U$_5$⸣.UM URI^{ki} GABA.RI [^{u}]^{ru}[N]IN[A]$^{\text{?ki}}$	According to an Akkadian w[ri]ting-board, a copy from [N]inev[eh](?)
BAM 52	*ki-i pi-i* ^{giš}ZU URI^{ki} GABA.RI UNUG^{ki}	According to an Akkadian writing-board, a copy from Uruk
BAM 106	*ki-i pi-*⸢*i*⸣ [(^{giš}ZU URI^{ki}?) GABA].RI UNUG^{ki}	According to [(an Akkadian writing-board(?)), a cop]y from Uruk
BAM 147	*ki-i* KA ^{giš}ZU URI^{ki}	According to an Akkadian writing-board
(*CT* 15 pl. 43f. = *SAA* 3 no. 37)	GABA.RI ^{giš}ZU NINA^{ki}	A copy of a writing-board (from) Nineveh
KAL 4 no. 44	*ina* ZAG ^{giš}ZU U[RI^{ki}]	According to an Ak[kadian] writing-board
KAR 22	GABA.RI ^{giš}ZU *Aš-šur*^{ki}*-i*	Copy of an Assyrian writing-board
KAR 56	GABA.RI ^{giš}ZU *Aš-šur*^{ki}*-i*	Copy of an Assyrian writing-board
KAR 72	*ina pu-ut* ^{giš}ZU *Aš-šur*^{ki}*-i*	According to an Assyrian writing-board
LKA 79	*ina pi-i* ⸢x⸣[...]	According to ⸢x⸣[...]
LKA 81	[TA$^{?}$ ŠÀ$^{?}$ ^{giš}]ZU [...]	[From the middle of a w]riting-board [(from GN?)]
LKA 112	GABA.RI ^{giš}ZU	Copy of a writing-board
LKA 118	[... *k*]*i-i pí-*[*i lēʾi*(?) ...]	[... accor]ding to [a writing-board(?) ...]
N4 no. 80	[... ^{giš}LI].U$_5$.UM URI$^{⸢\text{ki}⸣}$	[...] an Akkadian [writ]ing-board
N4 no. 247	*ina* ZAG$^{!}$ ^{giš}⸢ZU⸣ [NI]NA$^{\text{!ki}}$ GA[B]A.RI EN.LÍL^{k}[^{i}]	According to a writing-board (from) [Nin]eveh, a co[p]y from Nippur
N4 no. 404	⸢GABA.RI⸣ ^{giš}⸢ZU⸣ *Aš-šur*^{ki}*-i*	Copy of an Assyrian writing-board

Kiṣir-Nabû regularly refers to writing-boards that he copied from as "Akkadian" (URI^{ki}) or "Assyrian" (*Aš-šur*^{ki}*-i*).[13] These designations likely refer to Babylonian ("Akkadian") or Assyrian script, and texts at Nineveh are known to have been copied with Babylonian signs and recopied into Assyrian sign forms.[14] The reason for Kiṣir-Nabû's specifications remains uncertain.[15] However, several of Kiṣir-Nabû's texts with colophons copied from "Akkadian" originals, i.e., tablets in Babylonian script, are found in NA script, which may indicate that the script of his texts was occasionally changed.

9.2.2 *Extract Series*

Long works of scholarly and magico-medical texts comprising multiple tablets were often collected into series (*iškaru*). Such collections are known from a variety of libraries throughout the first millennium BCE. The term *iškaru* (ÉŠ. GÀR) "series" was used to describe a collection of tablets with fixed entries that were created through academic consensus and editing. The opposite term *aḫû* (BAR) "extraneous" seems to indicate scholarly (standardized) traditions that existed in parallel to the series, perhaps with the same "authoritative" status.[16] A few of these works were reedited into so-called *nisḫu*- and *pirsu*-series, i.e., smaller extracted rows of texts presumably aimed at collecting the most convenient passages for the users, perhaps in order to facilitate eased reference or practical application.[17] The word *pirsu* carries some of the same connotations as *nisḫu*, designating a "detachment, section, division" or

13 "Akkadian" writing-boards: *CMAwR* 1 pl. 25–26; *BAM* 52; (*BAM* 106, see Section 9.2.3); *BAM* 147; *KAL* 4 no. 44; N4 no. 80 (Walker and Dick 2001: 227–42). "Assyrian" writing-boards: *KAR* 22; *KAR* 56; *KAR* 72; N4 no. 404 (Maul 1994: 380ff., 546–47).

14 Fincke 2003–4; see also Worthington 2006: 18 and note 2.

15 Note *BAM* 3 (= N4 no. 90) with a colophon including a catch-line and a statement that the content was "extracted according to an 'Akkadian' writing-board". Although difficult to argue with the current evidence, it is possible that the manuscript was copied by Kiṣir-Nabû due to the reference to an "Akkadian" writing-board (see Worthington 2006).

16 Rochberg 2016: 225–26; Koch 1995: 88–93; Rochberg 1984: 137–38 and notes 44–45, 140–41, 143. As Robson (2011a: 571–73) has recently stressed, the standardization of cuneiform literature is extremely problematic, and in many cases local differences between scholarly communities may have existed.

17 See Koch 2015: 35, 41–42; Scurlock 2014: 295, 329; Heeßel 2010b: 34–35; see also Salin 2016. Although a commentary, the astrological *Šumma Sîn ina tāmartīšu* series was used as a practical tool and was quoted frequently in the letters to the Assyrian king (Veldhuis 2010: 81, 84–85; Koch 1999: 150–51). The *nisḫu* and *pirsu* collections of various series are generally poorly studied.

"cutting" of, e.g., threads or texts, and derives from the word *parāsu* "to cut, divide, separate" (*CAD* P: 165, 411; *AHw*: 830ff.; Leichty 1964: 149).[18]

How should the extract texts in Kiṣir-Aššur's collection be evaluated? What can they tell us about the collection and the use of magico-medical knowledge in Neo-Assyrian Assur? Looking into comparative evidence from the first millennium, one can see that there are several examples of both *nisḫu*- and *pirsu*-texts of series, among them a *nisḫu*-series from Nineveh of Uruanna[19] and of *Šumma ālu*.[20] There is also an already abbreviated selection (*liqtu*) of *Enūma Anu Enlil* (Koch 2015: 184 and note 477), as well as a *pirsu*-series of Lamaštu (Farber 2014: 20–22) and *bīt salā' mê* (Ambos 2013a: 211–212; Læssøe 1955: 20).[21] However, most important for the current discussion is the LB Uruk *pirsu*-series of at least ten tablets in a numbered sequence extracted from the Šangû-Ninurta family's 45-tablet recension of Ugu (Scurlock 2014: 329; Heeßel 2010b: 33–34 and note 51; Köcher 1978: 18).[22]

Kiṣir-Aššur's colophons mention a "first extract" (*nisḫu maḫrû*), various numbered extracts (x *nisḫu*), or a "final extract" (*nisḫu qītāyû*). If Kiṣir-Aššur extracted knowledge in a similar manner, as it is known from LB Uruk, one could suggest that some N4 numbered *nisḫu*s functioned as an Assur extract series, likely of a larger series similar to the Nineveh Ugu series (Heeßel 2010b:

18 Among at least one MA scholarly family, literary works were divided into sections, each described as IM.GÍD.DA (Wagensonner 2011: 652 and note 36).

19 Böck 2011: 692–93; Kinnier Wilson 2005: 45–46. Assurbanipal claims in the Nineveh colophons to have edited Uruanna anew and created the *nisḫu*-series (Steinert 2018c: 167 and note 60; Böck 2011: 692–93; Hunger 1968: 98–99 no. 321). For Uruanna in general, see Rumor 2017; Böck 2010d: 163–65; Kinnier Wilson 2005; Stol 2004–05: 504–505; Köcher 1995; Reiner 1995: 28–29.

20 Koch 2015: 258–59; Koch 2013: 243 note 14; Heeßel 2007a: 4 note 35 and 37; Frahm 1998: 13 and note 8; Freedman 1998: 7–8 with references. An extract series of *Šumma ālu* was also known from LB Uruk. In Uruk, an extract could include a single omen, and the majority were designated as "extraneous" (*aḫû*) (Koch 2013: 243 note 14). See also the *nisḫu*s from Nineveh in *CT* 40 pl. 8 (Koch 1995: 139).

21 The only numbered recension of *bīt salā' mê* consisted of "sections" (*pirsu*) (Ambos 2013a: 211). An auxiliary series of *Enūma Anu Enlil* was known as a "guide to (*rikis girri*) *Enūma Anu Enlil*" and consisted of excerpts from the main series (Veldhuis 2010: 81; Hunger and Pingree 1999: 20; Koch 1995: 82). Koch (2015: 117) also refers to a *nisḫu* from Assur of *niṣirti bārûti*. A *nisḫu*-series of *Šumma izbu* was also known at Nineveh (De Zorzi 2014: 235–36; De Zorzi 2011: 44; Leichty 1970: 22; see also Koch 2015: 271).

22 A comparison with the Nineveh Ugu-series is complicated by the fragmentary state of the Uruk material (Heeßel 2010b: 34 and note 50; cf. Köcher 1978: 19–20 and note 20). *SpTU* I no. 59 is the 41st Ugu tablet and no. 48 is the 45th Ugu tablet. *SpTU* I no. 44 is the 9th *pirsu* tablet and no. 46 is the 10th *pirsu* tablet. For the Uruk *pirsu*-series, see also Salin 2016.

35; Böck 2009a: 107; cf. Scurlock 2014: 329).[23] In a LB Uruk *nisḫu* collection of *Šumma ālu* omens (*SpTU* III no. 93), the 72nd and 73rd *nisḫu*s consist of a single omen (Koch 2013: 243 note 14; Heeßel 2007a: 4 notes 35 and 37; Frahm 1998). As such, it is not impossible that even the brief *nisḫu*s in N4 could belong to an organized collection. However, the numbering remains difficult to explain in Uruk as well as Assur.

9.2.3 *Numbered and Organized Extracts*

Several of Kiṣir-Aššur's and Kiṣir-Nabû's extract tablets have additional numerical notations (e.g., 7 *nisḫu*). In Kiṣir-Aššur's case, they were copied at least at the very beginning and the very end of his career, in his *šamallû ṣeḫru*- and *mašmaš bīt Aššur*-phases, but possibly also during his *mašmaššu*-phase. Furthermore, two of Kiṣir-Aššur's examples, and all three of Kiṣir-Nabû's, do not provide a title and only append the *ša Nabû tuklassu*-phrase, likely indicating that the texts were written before the *mašmaššu*-phase and perhaps even earlier (Section 5.4). The numerical notions are difficult to interpret, however, and warrant discussion. What follows discusses one problematic notation (*qītāyû*), the numbering of extracts, and, finally, how these numbered extracts should be interpreted in relation to the extracts in general. Table 19 provides an overview of Kiṣir-Aššur's and Kiṣir-Nabû's numbered extracts.

TABLE 19 Kiṣir-Aššur's and Kiṣir-Nabû's numbered extracts[a]

Text	Title	Extract-phrase	Translation
		Kiṣir-Aššur	
BAM 9	([*ša*] *Nabû tuklassu Tašmētum* [...])	(*catch-line*) [*nis-ḫu*] IGI-*ú* GABA.RI ^{giš}ZU [...]	First [extract], a copy of a writing-board [...]

a *BAM* 40 may have been designated as a numbered extract, although almost nothing remains of the left side of the colophon, rev. 20: [x]-*ú* [(*nis-ḫu*?) x x] ⸢x IM⸣ ^{p}*Ki-ṣir*-AN.ŠÁR [x x (x) x x]. The reconstructed *nis-ḫu* in combination with a number is entirely hypothetical, and as such the tablet is disregarded for now.

23 Heeßel (2011: 35 note 56) provides the examples *BAM* 52, 99, 106, *RA* 15 pl. 76 and a text published by Labat (1959: 10–13). Böck (2009a: 107) emphasizes that many extracts without numbers were "for *ad hoc* use". For another *nisḫu maḫrû* from Assur, see Geller 2007d.

TABLE 19 Kiṣir-Aššur's and Kiṣir-Nabû's numbered extracts (*cont.*)

Text	Title	Extract-phrase	Translation
BAM 99	*mašmaš bīt Aššur*	*7 nis-ḫu* GABA.RI *É-sa-bad šá* BAL.TI^{ki} ... *za-mar ú-šaš-ṭir-ma íb-ri*	7th extract, a copy (from) the Esabad-temple in Assur ... He had it hurriedly copied and he checked it
KAL 7 no. 24	[*mašmaššu*(?)]	⸢4$^{?}$-*ú*⸣ *niš-ḫu* GIM SUMUN-*šú* ⸢SAR⸣ [*b*]*a*-⸢*ri*⸣	4th(?) extract written and checked like its original
KAR 63	*mašmaš bīt Aššur*	*nis-ḫu qí-ta-a-a-ú ki-ma* SUMUN-*šú* SAR-*ma bà-rì za-mar* ZI-*ḫa*	Final extract written and checked like its original, hurriedly extracted
RA 15 pl. 76	*šamallû ṣeḫru* (*ša Nabû tuklassu*)	(*catch-line*) 32$^{?}$-*ú nis-ḫu* GABA.RI ^{giš}*le-ʾi*	32nd(?) extract, a copy of a writing-board
		Kiṣir-Nabû	
BAM 52	(*ša Nabû tuklassu*)	(*catch-line*) 6 *nis-ḫu liq-ti šá bul-ṭi ki-i pi-i* ^{giš}ZU URI^{ki} GABA.RI UNUG^{ki} SAR-*ma bà-rì* ... [*ana mal-su*?]-*ti-šú* ZI.MEŠ-*ḫa*	6th extract, a selection of prescriptions according to an Akkadian writing-board, a copy (from) Uruk, written and checked ... (repeatedly?) extracted [for] his [readi]ng
BAM 106	(*ša Nabû tuklassu*)	(*catch-line*) [7] *nis-ḫu liq-ti bul-ṭi ki-i pi*-⸢*i*⸣ [...] ... ⸢*a*⸣-*na mal-su-ti-šú za-mar* Z[I-*ḫa*]	[7th(?)] extract, a selection of prescriptions, according to [...] ... hurriedly extracted for his reading
BAM 147	(*ša Nabû tuklassu*)	(*catch-line*) *nis-ḫu* 2-*ú ki-i* KA ^{giš}ZU URI^{ki} *šà-ṭir bà-rì* + ... *ḫ*[*a-a*]*n*-[*ṭi*]*š* Z[I]-*ḫa*	2nd extract written and checked according to an Akkadian writing-board ... q[ui]c[kl]y ext[r]acted

As pointed out above, a *nisḫu* refers to a text created from "tearing" out one or more pieces of text from a united whole, e.g., a series found on tablets or writing-boards. The numbers written in connection to the word *nisḫu* are commonly interpreted as the number of the *nisḫu*-text in question in relation to a set of excerpts (e.g., Heeßel 2010b: 35 and note 56; Böck 2009a: 107; Leichty 1964: 149). The question is if the extracts were organized or serialized, and if so how, or if the same text was copied multiple times.[24]

In *BAM* 9 and *KAR* 63, the numerical notations were substituted with words indicating the first (*maḫrû*, *BAM* 9 rev. 70: [*nis-ḫu*] IGI-*ú*) and final or end (*qītāyû*, *KAR* 63 rev. 22': *nis-ḫu qí-ta-a-a-ú*) in a sequence (Hunger 1968: 2). The latter is especially problematic. The word *qītāyû* is only attested twice, and it is translated as "final" from *qatû* "to finish, complete, bring to an end" (*CAD* Q: 281), "zum Ende führend" (*AHw*: 924), or "concluding" (*CDA*: 290).[25] In connection to extracts (*niḫus*), Hunger (1968: 8) translates it as "Abschließender Auszug". The form AL.TIL for *qatû* is found several times in colophons, which designate that the copy is complete (*CAD* Q: 179; Hunger 1968: 5).[26] The question is whether *qītāyû* designates that the manuscript in question is finished with the correct amount of entries, or if the word should be analysed in connection to numbered extracts as the final one in a set of extracts.[27] Although the idea of copying several extracts for pedagogical purposes in order to master certain knowledge is appealing, it should be emphasized that *KAR* 63 derives from Kiṣir-Aššur's *mašmaš bīt Aššur*-phase, which argues against a primarily pedagogical interpretation.

The majority of Kiṣir-Aššur's and Kiṣir-Nabû's organized extracts, however, contain numbers. The syntax of the numbers occasionally differed, although

24 The famed NA astrologer Nabû-zuqup-kēnu (Baker 2001: 912–13) seems to have had students copy out the same tablet of a composition several times with different tablet numbers (Koch 2015: 330 and note 922).

25 See *KAR* 63 (*BAK* 199) and *ACh Supp.* 2 no. 72 rev. 9 (*BAK* 508).

26 *ACh Supp.* 2 no. 72 rev. 9 reads: 13$^{?}$ *nis-ḫu* TIL-*a-a-u* GABA.RI ^{giš}ZU *šá liq-ti šà-ṭir* [*bari*], "13th (and) final extract, a written and checked copy of a writing-board with a collection of omen excerpts" (*CAD* L: 270; Hunger 1968: 138). The word *liqtu* is also found on Kiṣir-Nabû's *BAM* 52 and *BAM* 106, and it is translated as "collection (of omens or prescriptions)" in *CAD* (L: 206–207), and is often translated as "selection" (e.g., Koch 2015: 184), although Hunger (1968: 138) translates it as "Exzerptzeilen". Noticeably, *ACh Supp.* 2 no. 72 was excavated in Nineveh (K. 6478), but it was copied by the *šamallû* [*ṣeḫru*(?)] Marduk-šallim-aḫḫē presumably from a family of Aššur temple *ṭupšarrus*, and this family is attested by several tablets in the N4 collection (Fadhil 2012: 40–41). As a result, both uses of *qītāyû* can be said to come from an environment connected to N4.

27 Section 8.5 identified *KAR* 43 as a duplicate manuscript of *KAR* 63, with one major difference being the notice of a "new break" in *KAR* 43. Perhaps Kiṣir-Aššur copied *KAR* 43 first and thereafter reconstructed the break in *KAR* 63, making it a "complete" copy.

they were probably meant to convey the same notion of numbering. Some numbers were written with phonetic complements that mark them as ordinal numbers (e.g., 2-*ú*, 32-*ú*), preceding and following the items counted. Other numbers were written without phonetic complements and preceded the items counted. Both groups must refer to ordinal numbers, since for example *BAM* 52 was labelled as extract number six without a phonetic complement (6 *nis-ḫu*).

The texts seem to have been extracted for different purposes. Only one of Kiṣir-Aššur's tablets was supplied with a purpose statement and was designated as being copied on the request of Kiṣir-Aššur (*BAM* 99). This could indicate that the numbered extracts generally served a different purpose from unnumbered extracts with purpose statements. Other texts seem to have had a pedagogical purpose, such as Kiṣir-Aššur's earlier tablets *BAM* 9 and *RA* 15 pl. 76 discussed in Chapter 3. Similarly, two of Kiṣir-Nabû's tablets were labelled as extracted for his "reading" (*ana malsûtišu*) (*BAM* 52, *BAM* 106), which could highlight their pedagogical context.[28] The numbered extracts from Kiṣir-Aššur's later phases less likely had a pedagogical purpose.[29]

Several of the numbered extracts are concerned with medical texts.[30] This has led several researchers to suggest that the numbered *nisḫu*s functioned as an extract series from a recension of the Nineveh Ugu series, comparable to the LB *pirsu*-series of the Uruk Ugu series.[31] However, this interpretation requires the organized extracts from N4 to appear in a numbered sequence. Table 19 shows that, although Kiṣir-Aššur copied a "first extract" (*BAM* 9) earlier in his career, possibly around the *šamallû ṣeḫru*-phase, and a "final extract" as *mašmaš bīt Aššur*, he did not have a running total of extracts throughout his career. Several texts reveal this lack. *BAM* 99 was a "7th extract" copied when Kiṣir-Aššur was *mašmaš bīt Aššur* and *RA* 15 pl. 76 a "32nd(?) extract" from his *šamallû ṣeḫru*-phase.[32] Therefore, other principles may have governed their arrangement.

---

28 *Malsûtu* is also frequently translated as "lesson" or "lecture". For this term, see Gabbay 2016: 21–22, 51–52, 273, 293; Stevens 2013: 220 note 51; Frahm 2011a: 52–54, 144–45; Geller 2010: 141.

29 *BAM* 99 may have functioned pedagogically for the assistant copying the tablet on behalf of Kiṣir-Aššur, or perhaps the pedagogical purpose for Kiṣir-Aššur – if any – lay in him familiarizing himself with these prescriptions.

30 The exceptions are *KAL* 7 no. 24 and *KAR* 63, which do not contain medical prescriptions. *KAR* 63 contains an incantation against someone angry, but should be included in this category as per the inclusion of such material in, e.g., the AMC (see Section 9.3.2).

31 Heeßel 2010b: 35; Böck 2009a: 107; cf. Scurlock 2014: 329. See also Steinert 2018b: 15. For the later *pirsu*-series from Uruk, see above.

32 Although, the colophon is problematic, see discussion in Appendix 2.

Two of Kiṣir-Aššur's and all of Kiṣir-Nabû's numbered extracts were supplied with catch-lines.[33] Such lines could be used to position the extract within the manuscript from which it was copied, and may indicate a wish to be able to retrace from where within a certain manuscript the *nisḫu* was extracted (Hunger 1968: 1; see Section 9.3). The catch-lines and colophons or especially Kiṣir-Nabû's *BAM* 52 and *BAM* 106 are useful for understanding the numbering of extracts. *BAM* 52 likely ended with a catch-line opening *BAM* 106:

The colophon of *BAM* 52
Rev. 101: DIŠ NA ŠÀ.MEŠ-*šú* MÚ.MEŠ-*ḫu i*[*r*]-*ru-šú i-ár-ru-ru* IGI.MEŠ-*šú* NIGIN.MEŠ-⸢*du*⸣
Rev. 102: 6 *nis-ḫu liq-ti šá bul-ṭi ki-i pi-i* ^{giš}ZU URI^{ki} GABA.RI UNUG^{ki} SAR-*ma bà-rì*
Rev. 103: DUB-*pi* ^{p}*Ki-ṣir-*^{d}PA *šá* ^{d}PA *tuk-lat-su*
Rev. 104: [D]UMU $^{\text{p.d}}$UTU-*ib-ni* ^{lú}MAŠ.MAŠ É AN.ŠÁR
Rev. 105: [*ana mal*$^{?}$-*s*]*u*$^{?}$-*ti-šú* ZI.MEŠ-*ḫa*

'If a man's insides are continually bloated, his intestines rumble, his face seems continually to spin' (is the next entry). Sixth extract, a selection of prescription(s), written and checked according to an 'Akkadian' writing-board, a copy (from) Uruk. The tablet of Kiṣir-Nabû whose trust is Nabû, the son of Šamaš-ibni, the *mašmaš bīt Aššur*. (Repeatedly(?)) extracted [for] his [*'readi*]*ng'*.

The opening line of *BAM* 106
obv. 1: [DIŠ NA ŠÀ].⸢MEŠ⸣-*šú* MÚ.⸢MEŠ-*ḫu ir-ru*⸣-*šú* ⸢*i-ár*$^{?}$⸣-[*ru* IGI.MEŠ-*šú* NIGIN.MEŠ-*du*]

If a man's insides are continually bloated, his intestines rumble, his face seems continually to spin ...[34]

BAM 52 is also described as an extract of a Babylonian writing-board copied from Uruk and as a selection of prescriptions. These statements are repeated in the colophon of *BAM* 106, which could indicate that *BAM* 106 was a continuation

33 Kiṣir-Aššur: *BAM* 9, *RA* 15 pl. 76. Kiṣir-Nabû: *BAM* 52, *BAM* 106, *BAM* 147.

34 The catch-line also occurs in other manuscripts, see citations in Scurlock and Andersen 2005: 59–60, 126 no. 6.51.

of the extracts begun in *BAM* 52. Unfortunately, the colophon of *BAM* 106 is fragmentary and an amount of reconstruction is necessary:

The colophon of *BAM* 106

Rev. 6':	[(x) $^{\text{na4}}$*g*]*a-bi-i* ^{šim}GÍR U_5 ARGAB^{mušen} Ú.BABBAR [x x x x]
Rev. 7':	[7] *nis-ḫu liq-ti bul-ṭi ki-i pi-*⸢*i*⸣ [^{giš}ZU$^?$ URI$^{\text{ki?}}$]
Rev. 8':	[GABA].RI UNUG^{ki} AB.SAR [*bari*]
Rev. 9':	⸢DUB x$^?$ x$^?$⸣ ^{p}*Ki-ṣir-*^{d}AG *ša* ^{d}AG *tuk-*[*lat-su*]
Rev. 10':	DUMU ^{d}UTU-DÙ ^{lú}MAŠ.MAŠ DUMU ^{d}PA-*be-sún* ^{lú}MAŠ.[MAŠ É *Aššur*]
Rev. 11':	DUMU $^{\text{p.d}}$*Ba-ba$_6$-šum-*DÙ ^{lú}ZABAR.DAB.BA [*É-šár-ra*(?)]
Rev. 12':	⸢*a*⸣*-na mal-su-ti-šú za-mar* Z[I-*ḫa*]
Rev. 13':	[(x) x] *e-rib* É [*ar-ḫ*]*i-iš li-ṣa-am-ma* [x x x (x)?]

(*Catch-line*). [Seventh] extract, a selection of prescription(s), written and [checked] according to [*an 'Akkadian' writing-board*(?)], a [co]py (from) Uruk. The tablet x x(?) of Kiṣir-Nabû whose tr[ust] is Nabû, the son of Šamaš-ibni, the *mašmaššu*, son of Nabû-bēssunu, the *maš*[*maš bīt Aššur*], son of Bāba-šuma-ibni, the *zabardabbû*-priest [of *Ešarra*(?)]. Hurriedly ex[tracked] for his 'reading'. […] let the enterer of the house [qui]ckly go out and […].

Kiṣir-Nabû's *BAM* 106 opens with the catch-line of the "6th extract" *BAM* 52. Both tablets were likely designated as "a selection of *bulṭus* according to the mouth of an 'Akkadian' writing board, a copy from Uruk", and extracted for Kiṣir-Nabû's "reading". On the basis of the preserved parts of similar colophons, as well as the catch-line of *BAM* 52 opening *BAM* 106, it seems that *BAM* 106 can tentatively be reconstructed as the "[7th] extract". If so, these two extracts consequently were numbered in a sequence. These two texts may therefore derive from the same writing-board, and they could have been numbered and supplied with catch-lines for eased continued extraction.[35] This could mirror Kiṣir-Aššur's *šamallû ṣeḫru* tablets that are designated as "first [extract]" (*BAM* 9) and "32nd(?) extract" (*RA* 15 pl. 76).[36] Although *BAM* 52 and *BAM* 106 were consecutive tablets labelled as *malsûtus* for Kiṣir-Nabû, indicating a

35 Note that Šamaš-ibni was referred to as *mašmaš bīt Aššur* in *BAM* 52 and *mašmaššu* in *BAM* 106. However, the different titles for Šamaš-ibni in Kiṣir-Nabû's *mašmuššu ṣeḫru*- and *mašmaššu*-phase manuscripts indicate that Šamaš-ibni's titles may occasionally have been used in a non-linear manner, see Ch. 2 note 37.

36 As stated in Section 3.6, several of Kiṣir-Aššur's *šamallû ṣeḫru* colophons are too broken to determine if they were numbered extracts.

pedagogical purpose not explicitly found in Kiṣir-Aššur's extracts, Kiṣir-Aššur's BAM 9 and RA 15 pl. 76 may have been copied as part of a group of consecutive extracts from one or more writing-boards to collect desired entries for a given purpose during his *šamallû ṣeḫru*-phase.

It is, however, unclear how to interpret the remaining numbered extracts. BAM 99 may have been considered the "7th extract (of) a copy (from) the *Esabad*-temple in Assur", much as BAM 52 and BAM 106 were possibly derived from the same writing-board (cf. Hunger 1968: 71).[37] However, BAM 99 was copied by someone for Kiṣir-Aššur (*ú-šaš-ṭir-ma*) with a purpose statement, and as such it likely did not serve a pedagogical function for Kiṣir-Aššur. It remains uncertain if KAL 7 no. 24 was the 4th extract and KAR 63 the concluding extract in various rows of extracts. KAR 63 is, however, the only example for which an interpretation of this text as the last extract in a row of copies of the same text may be applicable. This is based on the sole observation that the N4 manuscript KAR 43 without a number duplicates KAR 63 (see Section 8.5).

At least some numbered extracts may have occurred in series that were organized according to the order of extraction, and in at least one instance may have been extracted from the same manuscript. What remains unclear is if all extracts in a row or from a certain manuscript were numbered. If they were, many are now missing and this cannot be explained. Regarding their function, it is possible that several of the brief and unnumbered extracts with or without catch-lines and purpose statements may have been part of a collection of preferred material of numbered and unnumbered *nisḫu*s. These may have been extracted for eased reference of relevant passages from a longer text and could potentially have been used more than once, some perhaps pedagogically and maybe later practically, some only for practice.

As argued in Section 3.6, Kiṣir-Aššur probably copied a row of extracts during his training as *šamallû ṣeḫru*. Although any interpretation of these extracts has to remain hypothetical, I regard them as a sourcebook that he drew upon during his training, although it may have remained a handy reference tool during the later stages of his career.[38] In general, regardless of why the numbered extracts were copied, I consider it likely that they functioned as reference works during Kiṣir-Aššur's later phases. A tentative parallel could be the NA court

37 The syntax, however, is not clear.

38 In his study of ancient medicine, Nutton (2004: 4–5) emphasized that institutional priorities would have been different from those of practicing physicians: "An erudite philosophical disquisition on medical theory on the model of Galen or a multi-volume survey of the whole of medicine was irrelevant when what was most needed was a short compendium that reduced medicine to a manageable compass and provided a restricted range of practical therapies within a single volume."

astrologers' use of the explanatory series *Šumma Sîn ina tāmartīšu* for practical application over the main series *Enūma Anu Enlil*.[39] Although *Šumma Sîn ina tāmartīšu* was a series and functioned explanatorily,[40] the *nisḫus* discussed here, regardless whether they were drawn from a single writing-board or used as an organized handbook, could have functioned as practical tools containing useful material that was utilized *ad hoc*. Although this does not explain how the numbers functioned, a single authoritative therapeutic extract series does not seem to have existed in N4, despite the existence of several individual rows of extracts for various purposes. It is possible that numbering systems for extracts were used differently throughout the various collections according to practice and scholarly traditions. For now, it is not possible to posit a hypothesis that is applicable to all examples.

9.3 Catch-lines and Duplicate Passages in Kiṣir-Aššur's Texts in Relation to the Therapeutic Series Ugu

Scurlock (2014: 329) suggested that Assur extracts of medical texts often commence with a recognizable entry from the beginning of a tablet within a recension of the therapeutic series "If the crown of a man's head is feverish …" (*šumma amēlu muḫḫašu umma ukāl*, abbreviated Ugu) and proceed into various less obviously chosen passages.[41] The Ugu series consisted of medical therapeutic prescriptions and incantations with diagnostic and symptom descriptions. It is therefore necessary to discuss the possible attested recensions of the Ugu series in order to contextualize Kiṣir-Aššur's medical texts and examine how his extracts relate to the possible recensions of the Ugu series.

Scurlock used two examples from N4 to exemplify her hypothesis.[42] Therefore, the opening entries of Kiṣir-Aššur's extracts, as well as consecutive rows of duplicated entries, can be useful for understanding the textual relationship to the texts from which they were copied. Furthermore, Kiṣir-Aššur's colophons were occasionally supplied with catch-lines (see Appendix 1). Such lines quote the first entry on the manuscript copied from, which follows the

39 Veldhuis 2010: 81ff.; for this series, see Koch 2015: 182–84; Frahm 2011a: 155ff.; Koch 1999: 149–151.

40 For a comparable case of a serialized commentary on a medical text, likely *šumma amēlu muḫḫašu umma ukāl*, see LB tablet 11N–T4, which was designated as a 24th *pirsu* (Civil 1974: 336–38; see also Jiménez 2014b).

41 For this series, see directly below. For extracts and the Ugu series, see also Böck 2008: 298; Worthington 2003: 2–3.

42 Scurlock 2014: 329. *BAM* 3 = N4 no. 90; *BAM* 156 = N4 no. 166.

last entry copied onto the extract. The assumed purpose of catch-lines was to facilitate the transition from one tablet to the next in a series or row of connected texts, as well as to be able to retrace the place at which one stopped within a manuscript when copying (Hunger 1968: 1–2; Leichty 1964: 148–49). At least 17 of Kiṣir-Aššur's tablets, including those with partly broken colophons, include catch-lines. Notably, one of Kiṣir-Aššur's tablets (*BAM* 201) and one of either Kiṣir-Aššur's or Kiṣir-Nabû's tablets (*BAM* 68) have generic catch-lines: "If 'Ditto' …" and "[10] shekels of …".[43] Unlike catch-lines that quote specific diagnoses or symptom descriptions, these generic catch-lines are not easily recognizable. Their purpose may therefore have differed from the more recognizable catch-lines.

At the current stage of our knowledge, there may have existed at least two NA Ugu recensions. One is the Nineveh Ugu series, the other is represented by a catalogue consisting of incipits of therapeutic works arranged into overarching groups known as the Assur Medical Catalogue (abbreviated AMC). Unfortunately, the Ugu series is fragmentary and a complete reconstruction is still ongoing. Before discussing Kiṣir-Aššur's texts in relation to this therapeutic series, it is necessary to describe the Ugu series and the AMC in greater detail.

9.3.1 *The Therapeutic Series Ugu*

Many fragmented and multi-columned tablets excavated at the Nineveh libraries contain symptom descriptions, diagnoses, prescriptions, and incantations. These tablets are numbered according to a series opening with the incipit "If the crown of a man's head is feverish" (DIŠ NA UGU-*šú* KÚM *ú-kal*), here abbreviated Ugu.[44] This series is arranged head-to-toe, consists of a number of subseries with accompanying tablets, and appears to be an attempt to serialize

43 *BAM* 201 rev. 42': DIŠ KI.MIN ^{ú}ḪAB ^{ú}GÌR.NAGA.GA^{mušen} ^{ú}SIKIL EGIR-*šú iš-šaṭ-ṭar*; *BAM* 68 rev. 18: [10] GÍN ^{ú}NU.LUḪ.ḪA 10 GÍN ^{ú}*am-ḫ*[*a-ra*]. Note the broken catch-line of *BAM* 129 col. iv 22': […] ⸢^{ú}⸣ÚKUŠ GAZI^{sar} ^{giš}[…]. The catch-line of *BAM* 68 opens col. iii of the 5th tablet of the 5th subseries of Ugu, see Section 9.3.4.

44 The series is also referred to as the Nineveh Medical Compendium (Steinert 2018e). However, I have chosen not to adopt this terminology here in order to differentiate the possible different recensions of the Ugu series. See Salin 2016; Scurlock 2014: 11–12, 295, 297–98, 300–302, 304–7; Wee 2012: 229 and note 77; Böck 2010a: 69–70; Heeßel 2010b: 31–35; Attinger 2008: 25–27; Böck 2008: 295–300; Geller 2005: 14–15 no. 22–24, cf. 15 no. 25; Worthington 2005: 6; Attia and Buisson 2003: 1–2; Worthington 2003; Cadelli 2000: 52–60; Fincke 2000: 6–7; Heeßel 2000: 110–11; Haussperger 1997: 201–202; Köcher 1980a: VII, IXff.; Köcher 1980b: VII, IXff.; Köcher 1978: 17–20; see also Panayotov 2018b: 108–109. Concerning the Akkadian name of this series, see Steinert 2018d: 219–220.

select therapeutic texts.[45] Köcher suggested that Ugu was generally composed and standardized in Nineveh under Assurbanipal, although clear evidence is lacking and earlier material hints at a possible serialization in Babylonia.[46]

At Nineveh, the series was divided into at least eight subseries and included 33+ tablets in a relatively fixed sequence.[47] Comparatively, a later 45-tablet Ugu recension existed in LB Uruk and perhaps differed from NA Nineveh Ugu (Heeßel 2010b: 33–34). Other contemporary scholarly series were known in various recensions throughout Assyria (see Section 9.5.3), and, as discussed in the following section, the Assur Medical Catalogue indicates another (serialized)

45 The most important magico-medical texts of the Ugu series are available in copy in *AMT* and *BAM* (see Heeßel 2010b: 35). For editions of individual series, see Ch. 9 note 47.

46 Heeßel 2010b: 33 and note 45; Köcher 1978: 20 and note 32. Possibly, "extraneous" *aḫû* prescriptions existed in Nineveh as well (Rochberg 1987: 329 and note 12). For the concept *aḫû*, see Section 9.2.2.

47 Scurlock 2014: 296; Heeßel 2010b: 32–33. The reason for the difficulty in establishing the series is that tablets were numbered according to subseries in Nineveh, and they were counted according to the overall series in Uruk (Heeßel 2010b: 33–34 and note 49). Following Heeßel (2010b), the Nineveh recension of the series was built up of at least the following subsections:

1. *šumma amēlu muḫḫašu umma ukāl* – "If the crown of a man's head is feverish"; 5+ tablets (see Attia and Buisson 2003; Worthington 2005; cf. Worthington 2007).
2. *šumma amēlu īnāšu marṣā* – "If a man's eyes are ill"; 3+ tablets (see Geller and Panayotov in press; Fincke 2000: 6–7).
3. *šumma amēlu šinnīšu marṣā* – "If a man's teeth are ill"; 2 tablets.
4. *šumma amēlu napīš appišu kabit* – "If a man's breath is troubled"; 6+ tablets (see Haussperger 1999).
5. *šumma amēlu suāla maruṣ ana kīs libbi itâr* – "If a man is ill with *suālu*, which turns into *kīs libbi*"; 5+ tablets (see Johnson in press; Cadelli 2000: 67–288; cf. Köcher 1978: 19; Haussperger 2000; Haussperger 2002; Heeßel 2010b: 32 note 43; Johnson 2014).
6. *šumma amēlu šer'ān kišādišu ikkalšu šugidimmakkû* – "If a man's neck tendon hurts (it is) *šugidimmakkû*"; 4+ tablets (see Köcher 1964: xii note 10; Heeßel 2010b: 32 note 44).
7. *šumma amēlu kalīssu ikkalšu* – "If a man's kidney(s) hurt him"; 3 tablets (see Böck 2008: 297–300). The fragment K. 3661 (*CMAwR* 1: 126ff. no. 7.5 ms A) ends with the catch-line col. iv 17': DIŠ NA ÉLLAG-⸢*su* GU$_7$-*šu*⸣ *lu* ŠU an [... *lu* ŠU ... DAB-*su*], "If a man's kidney causes him a nagging pain either the hand of ...[... or the hand of ... has seized him]", and afterwards the fragment may state col. iv 18': DUB.8.KÁM [DIŠ NA SA]G ŠÀ-*šú* [*na-ši*], "Tablet 8 (of the series) [*If a man's epi*]*gastrium is* [*'risen'*]". Abusch and Schwemer (*CMAwR* 1: 128) suggested this name for a previously unknown subseries consisting of eight tablets, and they hypothesized that it could be listed in the AMC before *šumma amēlu kalīssu ikkalšu* in a broken entry (cf. AMC line 45–46 and Steinert 2018d: 236–237).
8. *šumma amēlu ina lā simānišu qablīšu ikkalāšu* – "If a man's waist hurt him before his time"; 5+ tablets (see Geller 2005: 14–15 no. 22–24, cf. 15 no. 25).

Preliminary tranliterations of the majority of the medical material published in copy can be found on the BabMed website.

collection of therapeutic tablets was known in Assur. As a result, the Nineveh Ugu recension may not have served as the only standardized series across all of contemporary Assyria.

9.3.2 *The Assur Medical Catalogue* (AMC)

The so-called "Assur Medical Catalogue", abbreviated AMC, is a catalogue comprising the incipits of therapeutic works arranged into overarching collections, and these may collectively represent a recension of Ugu or the incipits of non-serialized individual tablets.[48] The text was excavated in Assur and was written by a "young physician" (*asû ṣeḫru*).[49] The AMC arrange incipits of individual tablets into groups or subseries, providing individual totals of the amount of tablets within individual groups, alongside additional texts such as incantations.[50]

The AMC consists of two parts: a first section listed "[from] the top (of the head) to the (toe)nails" ([TA] UGU EN *ṣu-up-ri*), listing 50+ tablets, and a second section focusing on other areas such as divine anger, birth, and veterinarian prescriptions listing 30+ tablets. Furthermore, the opening of the AMC may have had an introduction similar to the EM, possibly indicating a pedagogical purpose behind the tablet.[51] As a result, the AMC could have been used to provide an overview of the healing texts available and their titles.

---

48 Panayotov 2018b: 90, 92–93, 95ff., 116; Steinert 2018a: 77ff.; Steinert 2018b: 13, 15; Steinert 2018c: 172ff., 189ff.; Steinert 2018d: 203ff.; Scurlock 2014: 295–306; Heeßel 2010b: 34–35; Böck 2010c: 99–100; Attinger 2008: 26–27; Böck 2008: 297–300, 345; Geller 2005: 247 no. 48; Beckman and Foster 1988: 3. A new edition can be found by Steinert et al. 2018. Beckman and Foster (1988: 3) originally labelled it a "catalogue of medical texts", and Scurlock (2014: 295) titled it an "Ugu Catalog". The second part of the AMC is unattested in series tablets from the Nineveh collections (Steinert 2018d: 206). Geller (2018a: 52) tentatively suggested the AMC should be attributed to Esagil-kīn-apli, although this remains uncertain (cf. Steinert 2018c: 178). For an overview of headings and number of tablets attested in the AMC, see Steinert 2018c: 199–200.

49 AMC lines 126–29: [*kīma labīrīšu*? *ša-ṭir-ma*] BA.AN.È ^{127} [DUB? ...]⌜x x⌝ ^{lú} *{lú?}* A.ZU TUR ^{128} [DUMU ^{m}... ^{lú}SAN]GA? ^{d}*Ba-*⌜*ba*$_6$⌝ *šá* ⌜*qé*⌝*-reb* BAL.TIL^{ki} ^{129} [(*tākil-ki ul ibâš*? ...)] ^{d}*Gu-la*. May (2018: 71) has recently argued that the copyist of the AMC may have been related to Kiṣir-Aššur's family and that the AMC could have originated from the N4 collection (cf. Steinert 2018d: 278–279).

50 Panayotov 2018b: 94, 112–113; Steinert 2018d: 221–222, 235; Scurlock 2014: 295–96. After each tally of tablets additional material is listed with *adi* (EN) "including".

51 AMC line 1: [DUB SAG.MEŠ? ...] MU.⌜NE⌝, see also Panayotov 2018b: 93–94, 114; Steinert 2018d: 219–220; cf. Scurlock 2014: 295. This may also resemble the opening line of the catalogue of Sa-gig, the physiognomic series *Alamdimmû*, and associated series (Schmidtchen 2018: 313; Finkel 1988: 146).

Current hypotheses suggest that the AMC represents a recension of the Ugu series (Panayotov 2018b: 95–96; Steinert 2018b: 13; Steinert 2018c: 189; Steinert 2018d: 205–206; Scurlock 2014: 295, 301–302) or a catalogue of more or less standardized therapeutic texts (Heeßel 2010b: 34–35 and notes 53 and 55) that are related to the city of Assur and are possibly distinct from the Nineveh Ugu recension (Steinert 2018c: 173ff.; Böck 2010c: 99 and note 213; Geller 2005: 9; Köcher 1964: XII note 10; cf. Panayotov 2018b: 95–97, 101–102, 106ff.; Steinert 2018b: 15; Steinert 2018d: 206; see discussion in Steinert 2018c: 189–190). The AMC and Nineveh Ugu differ in the number of subseries and the sum of tablets associated with them (Steinert 2018d: 205–206; Scurlock 2014: 305–6; Heeßel 2010b: 31–35), as well as in the inclusion of prescriptions in the AMC that are not known to have been part of the Nineveh Ugu recension (e.g., veterinarian texts). Regardless of whether or not the AMC represents an Ugu recension, Heeßel (2010b: 34–35 and note 55) has pointed out that an Ugu recension different from the Nineveh recension may have been known in Assur (see also Heeßel 2018: 316; Heeßel 2008b). The AMC seems to have listed recognizable incipits representing therapeutic texts, and healers could use these incipits to navigate the corpus of medical texts. It remains unknown if these therapeutic texts were standardized. These incipits are therefore useful for understanding Kiṣir-Aššur's extracts from therapeutic texts in terms of incipits and catch-lines.

9.3.3 *The AMC and Kiṣir-Aššur's Incipits and Catch-lines*

Since the AMC may represent an Assur recension of Ugu and since it may have functioned as a catalogue of titles, it is important to compare Kiṣir-Aššur's opening incipits and catch-lines to the AMC to preliminarily evaluate to what extent Kiṣir-Aššur's texts drew upon these recognizable incipits. This comparison produced only two parallels: Kiṣir-Aššur's *BAM* 131, concerned with *šaššaṭu* and various types of stiffness, and Kiṣir-Aššur or Kiṣir-Nabû's *LKA* 146, a mythological incantation and a ritual for producing phylacteries to be hung around the neck. Kiṣir-Nabû does not seem to have any preserved lines among his texts that parallel the AMC.[52] The parallel incipits of *BAM* 131's catch-line state:

BAM 131 rev. 9': [DIS NA *b*]*ur-ka-a-šú mun-ga* DIRI EGIR-*šú iš-š*[*aṭ*?-*ṭar*?]
AMC line 53: DIŠ NA ⸢*bur*!⸣-*ka-šú mun-ga* DIRI
AMT 51,4+32,5+43,3 col. iv 26': DIŠ NA *bur-ka-šú* [...][53]

52 *KAR* 90, copied by either Kiṣir-Aššur or Kiṣir-Nabû, mentions in obv. 1: *ì-lí ul i-de*. This text is mentioned in AMC line 85: ⸢ÉN⸣ DINGIR.MU ⸢*ul i*⸣-[*di* ...].

53 This text has recently been joined, but is yet to be edited in its new format. The line numbers are derived from the original picture found on CDLI no. P394437.

The catch-line in *BAM* 131 is attested as the third of three associated incipits in the AMC,[54] but it is also attested in Nineveh as a catch-line in *AMT* 51,4+, which is the "2nd tablet" of a partially preserved subseries, perhaps from the Nineveh recension of Ugu.[55] Both the AMC and *AMT* 51,4+ therefore agree that this catch-line marked the 3rd tablet of this subsection. Consequently, the catch-line could refer to a standardized tablet. *BAM* 131 was copied from "a writing-board of prescriptions from the Gula temple",[56] which indicates that the text represented by the catch-line was perhaps available on this writing-board.

The choice to cut off the extract at this catch-line may have been influenced by its status as a known incipit among scholars of healing. Therefore, this particular writing-board may have contained the content of several somewhat standardized tablets related to an Assur treatment tradition. The opening incipit of *BAM* 131, "[If a man] is ill with [*ša*]*ššaṭu*-illness ...",[57] however, is not attested as an incipit of an Ugu tablet in the AMC or at Nineveh, although the prescription is known from Nineveh.[58]

The parallel incipit of *LKA* 146's catch-line is found in the AMC and likely also the N4 manuscript *BAM* 315 (Steinert 2018d: 253; Pedersén 1986 N4 no. 555):

LKA 146 rev. 25:	[*ana*] ⸢DIB⸣-*tì*		^{d}*A-num* BÚR-*ri* EGIR-*šú*
AMC line 84:	*ana* DIB		^{d}*A-nim* B[ÚR$^{?}$ ...]
BAM 315 col. i 43:	[*ana* DI]B-*ti*	{A}	^{d}*A-nim* B[ÚR]

The catch-line occurs in the AMC in a section concerning divine anger (Steinert 2018a: 216). The content of *LKA* 146 revolves around the production of "phylacteries" or leather bags hung around the neck (*mêlu*; Stol 1993: 102), and the text contains a mythological incantation involving sages (*apkallū*) and Ea providing 21 of these bags or "poultices" to humanity (Lambert 1980: 78–79, 82). The incipit of *LKA* 146, "As Ea was in the river 'House of Peace where the *mušḫuššu*-monster gathers eggs/gemstones'",[59] is only otherwise attested on a LB tablet (BM 33999). The colophon of *LKA* 146 provides no clues as to its origins.

54 AMC line 53: ⸢DIŠ NA⸣ S[A.GAL GIG$^{?}$ (...): DIŠ NA SA] ÚR.MEŠ-*šú* 1-*niš* GU$_{7}$.MEŠ-*šú* : DIŠ NA ⸢*bur*!⸣-*ka-šú mun-ga* DIRI.

55 *AMT* 51,4+ col. iv 27': DUB.2.KÁM [...]. Perhaps the second tablet of a *sagallu*-subseries, see Scurlock 2014: 305; AMC line 53. The number likely marked *AMT* 51,4+ as the 2nd tablet, and therefore the catch-line refers to the 3rd tablet.

56 *BAM* 131 rev. 10': [TA] ^{giš}ZU *šá bul-ṭi ša* É ^{d}ME.ME ...

57 *BAM* 131 obv. 1: [DIŠ NA *šá-á*]*š-ša-ṭa* GIG ...

58 *BAM* 131 obv. 1–8 is duplicated in *CT* 23 pl. 5–14 col. iv 11–17 and *AMT* 4,5 col. iv$^{?}$ 1'–4'.

59 *LKA* 146 obv. 1: ÉN ^{d}*É-a ina* ^{id}É.SILIM.MA MUŠ.ḪUŠ NUNUZ UR$_{4}$.UR$_{4}$.A.DÈ.

The incipits found in the AMC may represent known titles, which could be used to navigate the corpus of prescriptions. It cannot be verified if these tablets were standardized.[60] As mentioned above, the presence of generic catch-lines could indicate that Kiṣir-Aššur did not always navigate texts according to easily recognizable incipits. And as shown here, Kiṣir-Aššur and Kiṣir-Nabû rarely seem to have navigated according to the titles of the AMC in their preserved incipits or catch-lines. This does not exclude the possibility that individual texts or writing-boards were arranged in accordance with the AMC. Kiṣir-Aššur certainly copied veterinarian prescriptions, which were probably listed in the AMC, and such material is not known at present to have been part of the Nineveh Ugu recension (see the section above). As a result, the sources indicate that Kiṣir-Aššur may have copied material included in the AMC, albeit rarely according to the various incipits.

9.3.4 *Kiṣir-Aššur's Texts and Nineveh Ugu*

Several of Kiṣir-Aššur's manuscripts, including extracts as well as other texts, duplicate passages in tablets of the Nineveh Ugu series. These duplicate passages are investigated here to visualize to what extent rows of prescriptions were copied according to the Nineve Ugu recension.[61] Kiṣir-Nabû's tablets *BAM* 52 and *BAM* 168 are also included because of their importance for establishing the relationship between extracts and writing-boards in Section 9.2.3. Several of Kiṣir-Aššur's texts are duplicates of passages in Nineveh manuscripts, although these are not included, as the tablets cannot be placed within the Ugu recension.[62] Table 20 presents the passages in Kiṣir-Aššur's texts that are duplicated in a tablet containing the Nineveh Ugu series.

This table makes it clear that Kiṣir-Aššur's tablets do contain several passages that also occur in the Nineveh Ugu series. However, they are rarely in any clear order, and do not have recognizable incipits or catch-lines that open the individual Ugu tablets. The only two tablets that contain consecutive entries from presumed Ugu manuscripts are *BAM* 129 and *BAM* 131. Incidentally, *BAM*

60 However, the tablets listed in the AMC were serialized, as implied by the total of counted tablets, which are said to have been "edited anew" (AMC line 125: [NÍGIN x x D]UB.MEŠ [*sa-di-ru šá* S]UR.GIBIL *ṣab-tu*, see Ch. 7 note 33).

61 There is an inherent problem in the fact that several of the tablets represent Kiṣir-Aššur's extracts and could therefore have been extracted according to different principles, as suggested by Scurlock (2014: 329).

62 Several fragments published in *AMT* and *BAM* vol. 5–6 likely derive from the Nineveh Ugu recension. Duplicate passages between these and Kiṣir-Aššur's texts are occasionally found, e.g., the catch-line of *BAM* 351 rev. 13: DIŠ NA *bir-ṣa* IGI.MEŠ EGIR-*šú*, listed in the middle of *AMT* 87,3 col. ii 6′: DIŠ NA *bir-ṣa* IGI.IGI [...]. However, many fragments cannot be identified safely as sections of Ugu and are therefore disregarded here.

TABLE 20 Passages in Kiṣir-Aššur's texts duplicated in Ugu[a]

Ugu Text → K.-A. Text ↓	1st tablet of the 1st subseries (Worthington 2005)	2nd tablet of the 1st sub-series (Attia and Buisson 2003)	3rd tablet of the 1st subseries (*AMT* 102,1+ *BAM* 484+*BAM* 486)
BAM 9			
Obv. 1–8	–	Lines 169'–76'	–
Obv. 12–13	Lines 220'–21'	–	–
Obv. 14–20	–	Lines 84–89	–
Obv. 23–30	Lines 141'–46'	–	–
Obv. 33–34	Line 148'	–	–
Obv. 35–41	–	Lines 7–8+68–69	–
Obv. 42–46	–	–	Col. i 1–6
Obv. 51–54	–	–	Col. i 52'–54'
Obv. 61–63	–	Lines 66–67	–

Ugu Text → K.-A. Text ↓	2nd tablet of the 3rd subseries (*BAM* 543)	Related tablet (*BAM* 523+ *AMT* 24,1+ *AMT* 28,7+ *AMT* 76,5+ *AMT* 77,1+ *AMT* 77,2+ *AMT* 77,5+ *AMT* 78,1)
BAM 28		
Obv. 4–6/10–12	–	(Cf. col. iv 4'–6')
Obv. 7–9	–	Col. iv 1'–3'
Obv. 13–16	–	Col. iv 14'–16'
Obv. 17–18	–	Col. iv 17'–18'
Rev. 3'–11'	(Col. iii 65'–73'+iv 1–2)	–
Rev. 12'–13'	Col. iv 4–5	–

a Items in parenthesis are only partial or possible duplicates. The various tablets are edited in Geller 2005 and Cadelli 2000; *BAM* 574 = Cadelli 2000: 68–123; *BAM* 575 = Cadelli 2000: 124–86; *BAM* 579 = Cadelli 2000: 252–89; *AMT* 40,5 = Geller 2005: 144–48 no. 23 ms X; *AMT* 43,1+57,6 = Geller 2005 136–43 no. 22 ms W; *BAM* 99 = Geller 2005: 212–17 no. 35 ms II; *BAM* 168 = Geller 2005: 202–11 no. 34 ms HH. For the tablets of the first subseries of Ugu, see Worthington 2005; Attia and Buisson 2003.

TABLE 20 Passages in Kiṣir-Aššur's texts duplicated in Ugu (*cont.*)

Ugu Text → K.-A. Text ↓	**1st tablet of the 5th subseries (*BAM* 574)**	**2nd tablet of the 5th subseries (*BAM* 575)**	**3rd tablet of the 5th subseries (*BAM* 578)**	**5th tablet of the 5th subseries (*BAM* 579)**
***BAM* 68**				
Obv. 1–rev. 17	–	–	–	(Col. ii 54'–64')
Rev. 18 (=catch-line)	–	–	–	Col. iii 1
***RA* 40 pl. 116**				
Obv. 1–3	–	–	(Col. ii 13)	–
		Two Comparative Kiṣir-Nabû Tablets		
***BAM* 52**				
Obv. 35–37	–	–	–	Col. ii 54'–55'
Obv. 39–44	–	–	–	Col. i 40–44
Rev. 63–65	–	Col. i 21–22	–	–
Rev. 78–79	Col. ii 5–6	–	–	–
Rev. 97–100	–	–	Col. i 70+col. ii 1	–
***BAM* 168**				
Obv. 18–32	–	–	–	Col. ii 54'–64'

Ugu Text → K.-A. Text ↓	**1st tablet of the 8th subseries (Geller 2005 pls. 15–18)**	**3rd tablet of the 8th subseries (Geller 2005 pls. 19–20)**
***BAM* 99**		
Rev. 40–42	(Col. iii 13')	–
Rev. 42–51	Col. iii 14'–19'	–
[Rev. 53]	(Col. iv 1(?))	–
Rev. 54–55	Col. iv 2	–
	Two Comparative Kiṣir-Nabû Tablets	
***BAM* 106**		
Rev. 1'–5'	–	Col. iii 9'–12'
***BAM* 168**		
Obv. 70–75	Col. i 1–4	–
Obv. 76–77	(Cf. col. i 5–6)	–

TABLE 20 Passages in Kiṣir-Aššur's texts duplicated in Ugu (*cont.*)

Ugu Text → **K.-A. Text ↓**	**1st/2nd tablet of a subseries (*CT* 23 pl. 5–14)**[b]	**2nd tablet of a subseries (*AMT* 51,4+32,5 +43,3)**
***BAM* 129**		
Col. i 1–7	Col. ii 4'–8'	–
Col. i 8–11	Col. ii 9'–14'	–
Col. i 12–17	Col. ii 15'–17'	–
Col. i 18–19	Col. ii 18'–19'	–
Col. i 20–23	Col. ii 20'–23'	–
Col. i 25(?)–33	[Col. ii 27'–35']	–
Col. ii 4'–7'	Col. ii 44'–47'	–
Col. ii 8'–16'	Col. ii 48'–col. iii 2'	–
Col. ii 17'–22'	Col. iii 3'–5'	–
Col. ii 23'–29'	Col. iii 6'–10'	–
[Col. ii 30']	Col. iii 11'–12'(?)	–
[Col. iii broken]	(?)	(?)
Col. iv 1'–2'	(Col. iv 8'–10'?)	–
***BAM* 131**		
Obv. 1–8	Col. iv 11–17	–
Obv. 9–15	Col. iv 18–23	–
[Breaks off]	(?)	(?)
Rev. 1'–3'	–	Col. iv 20'–21'
Rev. 4'–6'	–	Col. iv 22'–23'
Rev. 7'–8'	–	Col. iv 24'–25'
Rev. 9' (=catch-line)	–	Col. iv 26' (= catch-line)

b The tablets published as *CT* 23 pl. 1–14 are presumed to have contained sections of the second tablet of an uncertain subseries of the Nineveh Ugu related to *sagallu*-illness named in *CT* 23 pl. 1 obv. 1 as: DIŠ SA.MEŠ uzuÚR-*šú* 1-*niš* GU_7.MEŠ-*š*[*ú*], "If the 'strings' of his (i.e., the patient's) thigh all hurt at once" (Scurlock 2014: 303–304; Scurlock and Andersen 2005: 257).

129 and *BAM* 131 are not explicitly labelled as "extracts".[63] Kiṣir-Aššur may therefore have intended for these texts to function as copies of the original by copying consecutive sections of therapeutic texts on them.

Several of Kiṣir-Aššur's manuscripts, such as *BAM* 9, contain numerous duplicate prescriptions, occasionally duplicated on more than one tablet within a subseries of the Nineveh Ugu recension. *BAM* 9 was described as: "[The] first [extract], a copy of a writing-board", and therefore this writing-board may have contained several tablets related to the first subseries of Ugu.[64] The same could have been the case with Kiṣir-Nabû's *BAM* 52 and *BAM* 106, both of which may have been extracted from a "selection of prescriptions" on a writing-board from Uruk. The duplicate passages from these two texts span two subseries and *BAM* 52 draws its entries from various tablets of the 5th subseries of Ugu in a non-consecutive order. As a result, the writing-board referred to in the colophons may represent an Uruk tradition related to the 5th and 6th subseries of Nineveh Ugu. It may have been arranged similarly to the Nineveh tradition, but extracted on *BAM* 52 and *BAM* 106 according to unknown principles, or, alternatively, the writing-board was arranged differently than the Nineveh Ugu recension.

BAM 68 was extracted with a purpose statement, and the catch-line corresponds to the prescription following the duplicate in the Ugu manuscript.[65] As a result, the limited evidence presented by *BAM* 68 is that the writing-board copied from contained at least these two prescriptions in the order of the Nineveh Ugu recension.

The Assur and Nineveh texts related to Ugu probably do not represent a single series.[66] Similarly, Kiṣir-Aššur's texts do not appear to be derived from a completely standardized Assur recension, although the individual writing-boards from which they were copied may have contained somewhat standardized sections, perhaps arranged according to well-known incipits.[67] However, the fact that many of Kiṣir-Aššur's texts were extracts confuses the evidence in

63 The colophon of *BAM* 129 is broken, and it is unclear if the text was labelled as an extract.

64 *BAM* 9 rev. 70: [(*nis-ḫu*)] IGI-*ú* GABA.RI ^{giš}ZU [...].

65 *BAM* 68 rev. 18: [10] GÍN ^{ú}NU.LUḪ.ḪA 10 GÍN ^{ú}*am-ḫ*[*a-ra* ...].

66 Cadelli (2000: 53 note 3) referred to *BAM* 3 as an example of a separate recension of the first subsection of Ugu in Assur. Scurlock (2014: 329) stressed that the text was an extract and thus cannot be used as an example of a separate recension (see also Worthington 2006: 18).

67 Heeßel notes that the Nineveh tradition of Ugu must have been known in Assur, since, e.g., *BAM* 209 is listed as the third tablet of the subseries *šumma amēlu šer'ān kišādišu ikkalšu šugidimmakku*, although the tablet does not contain the entire text from the third tablet of the Nineveh recension (Heeßel 2010b: 34–35 and note 55; see also Panayotov 2018b: 99; Steinert 2018c: 175 note 99; Steinert 2018d: 224, 287; Scurlock 2014: 329).

terms of consecutive rows of entries. It is clear, however, that the tablets with colophons rarely begin with recognizable incipits or end with well-known catch-lines.[68]

9.4 The Exorcist's Manual (EM)

The so-called "Exorcist's Manual",[69] abbreviated EM, is a collection of text incipits or overarching titles referring to series and groups of texts of the exorcist's craft (*āšipūtu*). The EM opens: "Titles of the series of the exorcist's craft (*iškar āšipūti*) which have been established for learning and reading (*ana iḫzi u tāmarti kunnū*), a complete list".[70] It has therefore been suggested that the EM functioned as a pedagogical tool providing a reference list that defined the ideal range of exorcistic knowledge,[71] a work on how to become an *āšipu* and expert (*ummânu*),[72] as well as a work celebrating the *āšipu* profession's status.[73] The title *ummânu* designated a "master" of any craft, and in connection to the scholarly disciplines the title is usually translated as "scholar" or "expert".[74]

Seven manuscripts of the EM are known: three from the NA period and four from the NB and LB periods.[75] The earliest datable copy is *KAR* 44 from the

68 Geller (2005: 14 no. 21) also made this observation about Nabû-bēssunu's *BAM* 95, although Köcher (1963a: XXII-XXIII) noted that many entries are duplicated in the relevant Ugu subsection.

69 Occasionally also referred to in Assyriological literature as the "*āšipu*'s curriculum" or the "vademecum of the exorcist". See Geller 2018b; Frahm 2018a; Bácskay and Simkó 2012; Frahm 2011a: 324–25; Schwemer 2011: 421; Heeßel 2010a; Hecker 2008: 76–79; Jean 2006: 62ff.; Geller 2000: 226, 242ff.; Bottéro 1985: 65–112; Zimmern 1915–16: 204ff.

70 Schwemer 2011: 421; Jean 2006: 62; Bottéro 1987–90: 224; cf. Bottéro 1985: 66. *KAR* 44 obv. 1: SAG.MEŠ ÉŠ.GÀR MAŠ.MAŠ-*ti šá a-na* NÍG.ZU *u* IGI.DU$_8$.A *kun-nu* PAP MU.NE. The translations often vary, see Schwemer 2011: 421; Frahm 2011a: 325; Lenzi 2008a: 85; Jean 2006: 63.

71 E.g., Frahm 2018a: 36–37; Schwemer 2011: 421; Jean 2006: 62; Maul 1994: 32.

72 E.g., Clancier 2014: 42–48, 62; Jean 2006: 62; see Geller 2018b: 292.

73 E.g., Lenzi 2008a: 85; Bottéro 1985: 65–66, 87.

74 Verderame 2014: 713–14 and note 2; Radner 2011: 364, 366; Verderame 2008: 52–53 and note 3, 55ff.; Parpola 1993: XIII–XV, XVII–XVIII; Lambert 1962. See also Lenzi 2008b with further references. The title was regularly used for the king's chief advisor. However, the exact rendering of the term is problematic (Verderame 2014: 713 note 2).

75 NA tablets: ms A = VAT 8275 (*KAR* 44; Geller 2000 Text E ms A = Jean 2006 sigl. A; Assur, N4 no. 132); ms F = A 366 (unpublished; see Geller 2000: 242 note 9; Jean 2006 sigl. F; Assur, N4 no. 310), the colophon is damaged (Jean 2006: 63 note 259); ms B= 79-7-8,250 (Geller 2000 Text E ms B = Jean 2006 sigl B; Nineveh). NB and LB tablets are: ms C= BM 55148 (82-5-22,1480)+BM 68411 (82-9-18,8409)+BM 68658 (82-9-18,8657)+other fragments (Geller

N4 collection, copied by Kiṣir-Nabû (Schwemer 2011: 421), and an additional NA example from the N4 collection.[76] The difficult text comprises 44 lines including the colophon, with many titles written in complex Sumerograms, phonetic Akkadian, or pseudo-Sumerian phrases, and a few individual entries are provided with glosses (Frahm 2011a: 329; Schwemer 2011: 421; Geller 2000: 242; Bottéro 1985: 65–66). The EM, as represented by *KAR* 44, is structured as follows:

- **Heading**, obv. 1: "Titles of the series of the exorcist's craft (*āšipūtu*) which have been established for instruction and study, a complete list" (see Schwemer 2011: 421)
- **First section of text titles**, obv. 2–rev. 26
- **Heading/subscript**(?), rev. 27: "Titles of the series of the exorcist's craft of Esagil-kīn-apli"
- **Second section of additional scholarly knowledge, instructions addressing the reader and a blessing**, rev. 28–36, rev. 37–40, and rev. 41–42[77]
- **Colophon**, rev. 43–44

In general, many individual titles, particularly within the first section of the EM, refer to multi-tablet exorcistic series or text groups related to, e.g., the temple, cult, or court (Schwemer 2011: 421–22). The second part is more general in its text descriptions and lists various additional works that are needed to uncover the secrets behind the texts, works to familiarize oneself with scholarship beyond exorcism, and finally a prayer on behalf of the reader.[78] The lines are intentionally cryptographic and likely instruct the reader how to gain

---

2000 Text E MS c = Jean 2006 sigl. c; Sippar); ms D= Rm 717+BM 34188 (Sp I 294)+BM 99677 (83-1-21,2039)+BM 140684 (1987-11-3,1) (Geller 2000 Text E ms d = Jean 2006 sigl. d; Babylon); ms E= BM 36678 (80-6-17,410) (Geller 2000 Text E ms e = Jean 2006 sigl. e; Babylon), the reverse contains an esoteric astrological text, possibly a commentary (Frahm 2018a: 16–17, 41–42; cf. Geller 2000: 242); ms G= *SpTU* V no. 231 (Jean 2006 sigl. G; Clancier 2014: 63–64; Uruk). *SpTU* V no. 231 was classified as an IM.GÍD.DA, and RM 717+ may have been labelled as *gì-ṭu* [p]GI-*im*-⌈[d]EN⌉ (see Frahm 2018a: 11–15 with a discussion; cf. Jean 2006: 72). Al-Rawi and George (2006: 54) associated Esagil-kīn-apli and *Enūma Anu Enlil*, which may explain the association between the EM and the astrological text in BM 36678 (cf. Frahm 2018a: 16–17, 30ff.).

76 A 366 (= N4 no. 310). The colophon of A 366 is reportedly badly damaged and remains unpublished (Frahm 2018a: 10–11; Maul 2010a: 197 note 30; Jean 2006: 63 note 259; Geller 2000: 242 note 9).

77 Frahm (2018a: 21–24) argues that the second section can be subdivided into three subsections (rev. 28–36, 37–38, and 39–40), and the passage in rev. 41–42 constitutes a third section in the EM.

78 Frahm 2018a: 23. The prayer is still partly incomprehensible (Frahm 2011a: 327 note 1561). For a discussion of works overlapping the EM and the AMC, see Steinert 2018c: 182–183.

access to his craft's hidden dimension (Frahm 2011a: 325–26; cf. Lenzi 2008a: 94). The section containing instructions in *KAR* 44 states:

Rev. 36:	"(*A list of works*), up to the point where you master all of the *exorcist*'s craft (*išippūtu*) and see the secret.
Rev. 37:	Afterwards, (through) *ṣâtu*-commentaries, *translations*, and *lišānu*-lists/*Emesal*-texts (bilingual word lists),
Rev. 38:	you will learn how to explore the rituals (in) Sumerian (and) Akkadian.
Rev. 39:	Liver omens(?), 'head-to-head' *Enūma Anu Enlil* (astrological omens) (and) (*Šumma*) *ālu ina mēlê šakin* (terrestrial omens),
Rev. 40:	ponder (and) discuss *in conjunction with each other*(?)."[79]

The works enumerated in lines 37–38 were perhaps "not meant to be studied for their own sake, but with the intention of achieving a better understanding of the ritual texts listed in the 'manual'" (Frahm 2011a: 329). Additionally, terrestrial and astrological omens were associated with *āšipūtu*, although they were not commonly considered part of the discipline (Al-Rawi and George 2006: 54). Finally, the EM instructs the reader to interpret the texts and arrange

79 Individual parts of the translation follows Frahm 2018a. *KAR* 44 rev. 36–40: EN *ri-kis i-šip-pu-ti ta-kaš-šá-du tam-ma-ru* NÍG.ŠEŠ 37 EGIR$^{!}$-*nu* NÍG.ZI.GÁL.EDIN.NA GÙ BAL.E.DÈ *u* EME.SAL.MEŠ 38 KI.DU.DU.MEŠ EME.GI$_7$ EME.URI^{ki} *ši-te-ʾa-a ta-aḫ-ḫa-zu* 39 ZÀ$^{!}$.GAR.RA.ZU.DÈ.E.GIN$_7$ A.ZA.AD A.ŠU.UŠ.MA U$_4$ AN ^{d}EN.LÍL.LÁ URU *ina* SUKUD GAR 40 *kit-pu-du*$^{!}$ *šu-ta-du-nu mit-ḫur-ti*. Frahm (2018a: 21) suggests that the 2nd person singular present verbal forms and perhaps infinitives or imperatives in rev. 40 may be non-subordinated verbal forms indicating three sections with individual sentences. This interpretation is followed here. The final *mit-ḫur-ti* from *maḫāru* may also indicate that the discussants should come to an agreement or oppose each other. Although teamwork was advised, in order to achieve an answer through discussion, the scholars at court also disagreed (e.g., Verderame 2014; Radner 2011: 363). The word ZAG.GAR(.RA) may refer to dream interpretation or less likely to the esoteric and poorly attested terrestrial omen series Tukumbi Apindua instead of liver omens (Frahm 2018a: 22; Jiménez 2014a: 109–10; cf. Geller 2000: 251; Jean 2006: 71). A.ZA.AD and U$_4$.ŠÚ.UŠ are known from *Nabnītu* (*MSL* 16: 52) as Sumerian renderings of the Akkadian *qaqqadu* "head" and may refer to the lexical tradition, suggesting that the two series mentioned were aligned "head to head", or even refer to an unknown illness list (Frahm 2018a: 23). Why *Enūma Anu Enlil* and *Šumma ālu* are mentioned in the last section, whereas Sa-gig and *Alamdimmû* are listed in the first section, is unclear (Koch unpublished: 13–14).

scholarly discussions of the knowledge, which mirrors a situation also known from the so-called "Examination text" and Assurbanipal's colophons.[80]

The EM continually stresses comprehensiveness (Lenzi 2008a: 86–90, 92). Still, it lacks genres of *āšipūtu*, such as "aggressive rituals" that enforce control over others without explicit consent, the therapeutic series Ugu, and the series *muššu'u*.[81] This may be because the EM represents the "ideal range of knowledge an *āšipu* should acquire according to standards established in the late second millennium BC" (Schwemer 2011: 423), but not necessarily the entirety of 7th century BCE *āšipūtu* in general or variants thereof (see also Bottéro 1985: 98–99). Nonetheless, the EM still includes titles, which may refer to prescriptions.[82]

Two lines, obv. 1 and rev. 27, each with rulings demarcating the individual lines from the remaining text, structure the EM.[83] The former is commonly regarded as a header, although there is no consensus on whether the latter is a header of the second section[84] or a subscript to the first.[85] The two sections are disproportionate to one another (Bottéro 1985: 92–93). Notably, reverse lines 27

80 Gesche 2001: 198; Sjöberg 1972. Although the examination text likely reflects OB practices, the text is found in NA copies (ibid.). See *BAK* 318 and one of Assurbanipal's early inscriptions concerning the *tapḫurti* (UKKIN) *ummânī* "assembly of scholars" (Novotny 2014: 77, 96 col. i 17–22; Zamazalová 2011: 314, 316–18; Livingstone 2007: 100; Villard 1997: 135–39; Pongratz-Leisten 1999: 311–12; see also Frahm 2011a: 272–73; Lieberman 1990: 319). An active oral environment likely existed alongside the written traditions, as attested by phrases such as *ša pî ummâni* "from the mouth of the scholar" (Elman 1975; see Frahm 2011a: 43–45).

81 Schwemer 2011: 432; Böck 2007: 23–29; Lenzi 2008a: 86 and note 109; Jean 2006: 83–109; Bottéro 1985: 128–29.

82 E.g., *KAR* 44 obv. 16–17: IGI.GIG.GA.KE$_4$ ZÚ.GIG.GA.KE$_4$ *u* KIR$_4$.ḪAB.DAB.BA [17] ŠÀ.GIG.GA.KE$_4$ MUR.GIG.GA.KE$_4$ *u* TU$_6$.TU$_6$ GIG DÙ.A.BI, "'Eye illness', 'Tooth illness', and *bušānu*-illness, 'Ill inside(s)', 'Lung illness', and incantations (against) every illness"; *KAR* 44 rev. 33: *bul-ṭi* AN.TA.ŠUB.BA [d]LUGAL.ÙR.RA ŠU.DINGIR.RA ŠU [d]INANNA ŠU.GIDIM.MA.⸢KE$_4$?⸣, "Prescription(s) for *miqit šamê*, 'Lord of the roof', 'Hand of god', 'Hand of Ištar', 'Hand of ghost'"; *KAR* 44 rev. 35: *ù bul-ṭi kal gim-ri* ..., "and prescriptions for all of every (illness)". However, it is unclear how to understand all these titles (cf. Wee 2012: 136–37). The titles in *KAR* 44 obv. 16–17 may have been thematic rubrics usually found after incantations, which could perhaps be combined with prescriptions (see Steinert 2018c: 181 and note 122).

83 *KAR* 44 rev. 27 was ruled before and after this line. BM 55148+ and Rm 717+ do not have a ruling after the equivalent line in *KAR* 44 rev. 27, and *SpTU* V no. 231 does not seem to have rulings at all (Frahm 2018a: 18 and note 19).

84 Clancier 2014: 47; Schwemer 2011: 422; Schwemer 2010a: 211–212; Heeßel 2010a: 160; Jean 2006: 72–73; Al-Rawi and George 2006: 54–55; Beaulieu 2000: 15; Finkel 1988: 150; Bottéro 1985: 93–100; Lambert 1962: 68; Zimmern 1915–16: 224. Geller (2012: 44, 49) ascribes the first section to Esagil-kīn-apli, but he defines rev. 27 as a heading.

85 Frahm 2011a: 325–26; Lambert 2008: 94–95; Lenzi 2008a: 86–87.

refers to the scholar Esagil-kīn-apli (see Section 9.5.3). Frahm (2011a: 325–26) and Lenzi (2008a: 87) identified this as a subscript to the first section,[86] in part because Esagil-kīn-apli's works Sa-gig and *Alamdimmû* appear in the first section of the text.[87] The EM may have served as a reference work and perhaps a pedagogical tool for training *āsipus*,[88] and the second section could illustrate the process towards becoming an expert (*ummânu*).[89] However, it remains uncertain if the text functioned as a curriculum (cf. van der Toorn 2007: 58). Considering the many hypotheses concerning the EM's purpose, the following section will discusses the content of Kiṣir-Aššur's texts in light of current arguments concerning the EM's possible purpose.

9.4.1 *Kiṣir-Aššur's Texts in Light of the Exorcist's Manual*

As already mentioned, there were two copies of the EM in the N4 collection. One manuscript, *KAR* 44, was copied by Kiṣir-Nabû, but the other remains unpublished. It is therefore unknown if Kiṣir-Aššur read or copied the EM. This is a problem for any discussion evaluating the importance of the text.

Pedersén (1986: 58) and Jean (2006: 147–153, 165–67) have suggested that the N4 collection held many copies of the series and text groups mentioned in the EM, although there are some difficulties in identifying some of these titles.[90] The N4 collection was not restricted to the *āšipūtu* described in the EM, however, and it included texts that were not listed in it (Schwemer 2011: 423). Furthermore, several of Kiṣir-Aššur's texts are extracts and not copies of entire manuscripts within series, as discussed above. This complicates any comparison between Kiṣir-Aššur's texts and the EM, as it is not always clear under what title in the EM a given manuscript would have belonged.

According to current consensus, we would expect titles in the first section of the EM to appear during Kiṣir-Aššur's earlier phases and represent his training towards becoming an *āšipu*, whereas works from the second section should appear later during his training and represent advanced knowledge for becoming an expert. However, at least two of Kiṣir-Aššur's texts indicate that the EM

86 Lenzi (2008a: 86–87) analysed other subscripts and found that reverse line 27 in other manuscripts of the EM state SAG.MEŠ and ŠU.NIGIN, and he argued that such "totals" were typically found as subscripts in lists.

87 Jean's (2006: 72–75) tripartite division into *āšipūtu* of Esagil-kīn-apli (obv. 1–rev. 27), *kakugallūtu* (rev. 28–30) and *išippūtu* (rev. 31–36) with additional knowledge (rev. 37–42) was perhaps influenced by Bottéro (1987–90: 226). It is disregarded here because the text itself does not support such a division (see Frahm 2018a: 21 note 36).

88 See Ch. 9 notes 71–72.

89 Clancier 2014: 48; see Frahm 2018a: 21–23, 24, 38–40; Schwemer 2011: 422; Lenzi 2008a: 94; Bottéro 1985: 98.

90 See also Heeßel 2017: 374; Clancier 2014: 47; Lenzi 2008a: 86 note 109.

should be dismissed as a curriculum that was followed sequentially or as two separate sections for consecutive stages of training. Kiṣir-Aššur copied *BAM* 129 with incantations, rituals, and treatments for *sagallu*- and *šaššaṭu*-illness and N4 A 400 with an incantation and a ritual instruction for treating *maškadu*-illness as *šamallû ṣeḫru*. The *sagallu*-illness was listed alongside *šimmatu*-paralysis and perhaps *maškadu*-illness in the second section of the EM.[91] *BAM* 129, as well as several other of Kiṣir-Aššur's *šamallû ṣeḫru* texts, may, however, stem from an Ugu recension (Section 9.3.4). Yet, if the focus of these texts must be reconciled with the EM, it is interesting that another early manuscript (*BAM* 9) contains at least two references to prescriptions against ŠU.GIDIM.(MA), and this entry is also found in the second section of the EM in the line after *sagallu*-illness.[92] Other of Kiṣir-Aššur's *šamallû ṣeḫru* texts could potentially be listed in the first section of the EM, such as snakebites and scorpion sting prescriptions, as well as veterinarian knowledge in *RA* 15 pl. 76,[93] and the *šu'illa*-prayer *LKA* 43.[94] As a result, Kiṣir-Aššur copied knowledge listed in both sections of the EM during his earliest traceable phase.

Kiṣir-Aššur's *šamallû* manuscripts N4 no. 175 and *KAL* 10 no. 4 contain instructions on how to perform sections of *bīt mēseri* and ritual means for removing a "Curse" (*māmītu*). Both these texts were likely listed in the first section of the EM in successive lines.[95] As discussed in Section 5.2, only Kiṣir-Aššur's *šamallû mašmaššu ṣeḫru* texts N4 no. 24, a "child calming incantation", can be adequately connected to the EM in the first section.[96] Kiṣir-Aššur's

---

91 *KAR* 44 rev. 32: "The craft of (curing those) ill with paralysis, numbness and *sagallu*, *maškadu*(?)", *ši-pir šim-mat ri-mu-ti u* SA.GAL SA.GIG GIG (see Arbøll 2018a: 275 note 55; Jean 2006: 70; Geller 2000: 251, 254 note 32, 258; Bottéro 1985: 82–83). If SA.GIG is interpreted as *maškadu* (e.g., *CAD* M/1: 368), this would fit the content of Kiṣir-Aššur's *mašmaššu* manuscript *BAM* 81.

92 *KAR* 44 rev. 33, see Ch. 9 note 82. Similarly, N4 no. 237 from Kiṣir-Aššur's *šamallû ṣeḫru*-phase provides treatments for ghostly afflictions, and the unpublished N4 A 2191 contains a ritual against a ghost.

93 *KAR* 44 obv. 19: ZÚ.M[U]Š TI.LA GÍR.TAB TI.LA ..., "To cure a snakebite, to cure a scorpion (sting) ..."; rev. 24: TÙR ÁB.GU$_4$.ḪI.A *u* U$_8$.UDU.ḪI.A ANŠE.KUR.RA SIKIL.E.DÈ, "To purify the pen of cattle and sheep, (as well as) horses".

94 Listed in the first section of *KAR* 44 obv. 4: ŠU.ÍL.LA.KAM. It is unclear if N4 no. 289 was listed in the EM. Possibly the manuscript N4 no. 228 should be included in the category "mouth washing" (*mīs pî*) mentioned in *KAR* 44 obv. 2.

95 *KAR* 44 obv. 11–12: *e-piš-tù* É *rim-ki* É *me-se-ri*.MEŠ *u* KA.L[U]Ḫ.Ù.DA 12 UŠ$_{11}$.ḪUL.GÁL.MEŠ ÁŠ.ḪUL.GÁL.MEŠ UŠ$_{11}$.BÚRU.DA *u* NAM.ÉRIM.BÚR.RU.DA [*ma-mi-t*]*a a-na pa-šá-ri*, "ritual *bīt rimki*, *bīt mēseri*, 'mouth-washing', 12 'evil spells', 'evil *arratu*-curses', *ušburrudû* and *namerimburrudû* for undoing a *māmītu*-curse".

96 *KAR* 44 obv. 15: LÚ.TUR.ḪUN.GÁ. *LKA* 89+ treats ghost and *mimma lemnu* and *LKA* 141 reconciles a man with the god of his house. Treatments related to "Hand of ghost" appear

single manuscript from the *mašmaššu ṣeḫru*-phase, N4 A 2727, may have concerned "Anus illness", which is not explicitly listed in the EM.[97] Although the limited evidence from Kiṣir-Aššur's *šamallû*-phase belongs to the first section of the EM, the texts from other stages prior to the *mašmaššu*-phase suggest that Kiṣir-Aššur was trained according to principles other than the hypothesized curricular structures of the EM.

Kiṣir-Aššur may not have been fully trained until somewhere during his *mašmaššu*-phase (Chapter 6). During this phase, he copied texts identified in both sections of the EM, e.g., *namburbi*-rituals[98] and rituals for keeping evil out of a man's house (*KAR* 298).[99] The only lexical text copied by Kiṣir-Aššur (*CT* 37 pl. 24f.) is also from his *mašmaššu*-phase. His commentary-like pharmaceutical text (*BAM* 307) and perhaps a commentary on *Enūma Anu Enlil* from Nineveh (*ACh Supp.* 2 24) may be from his *mašmaššu*-phase (Section 7.6).[100] If this reconstruction is correct, these texts are the only ones that can be related to the last instructions of the EM (see above). However, only Kiṣir-Aššur's *šamallû ṣeḫru* text N4 no. 241 is described as a *ṣâtu*-commentary, although this manuscript appears during his earliest phase and Kiṣir-Aššur had a younger pupil copy it on his behalf. Furthermore, the *šamallû* manuscript N4 no. 175 was copied "for his (own) 'reading'" *ana tāmartīšu*, although the nuances of the expression remain uncertain (see Section 5.1). None of Kiṣir-Aššur's manuscripts are labelled explicitly as *lišānu-/Emesal*-texts, as is the case with the EM, and *ACh Supp.* 2 24 was probably not copied by Kiṣir-Aššur. Furthermore, *BAM* 307 was copied on behalf of Kiṣir-Aššur ([*ú-š*]*aš-ṭir-ma ib-ri*), and may not have been for instructional purposes. Yet, it is significant that several texts connected to the commentaries and lexical lists probably occur during Kiṣir-Aššur's *mašmaššu*-phase, around the time he was finishing his training.

---

in *KAR* 44 rev. 33: *bul-ṭi* AN.TA.ŠUB.BA ᵈLUGAL.ÙR.RA ŠU.DINGIR.RA ŠU ᵈINANNA ŠU.GIDIM.MA.⸢KE$_4$?⸣. Perhaps ŠU.DINGIR.RA treatments were related to *LKA* 141, although the manuscript does not contain *bulṭus*.

97 Note the mentioning of "to cut off diarrhoea" in *KAR* 44 obv. 18: … ŠÀ.SUR.KU$_5$.RU.DA …

98 *KAR* 44 rev. 29: NAM.BÚR.BI Á.MEŠ AN *u* KI-*tim*. Note, however, that Geller (2000: 257) and Bottéro (1985: 71–72) suggest *KAR* 44 obv. 14: ḪUL *ka-la* may also relate to *namburbi*-rituals.

99 For *KAR* 298 in *KAR* 44 obv. 20, see Section 6.3. Kiṣir-Aššur's unpublished text related to *bīt mēseri* (N4 no. 254), a work also found in the first section of the EM, may also stem from his *mašmaššu*-phase, or earlier. See *KAR* 44 obv. 11: É *me-se-ri*.MEŠ.

100 Kiṣir-Aššur also copied the commentary-like text N4 no. 110 during his *mašmaš bīt Aššur*-phase.

Comparatively, Kiṣir-Nabû copied a number of commentaries and instructive works, although none of these are described as *ṣâtu*-commentaries.[101] The commentaries include *AfO* 12 pl. 13–14 from his *mašmaššu ṣeḫru*-phase,[102] possibly *Iraq* 62 no. 35 without a title,[103] N4 no. 163 with the *ša Nabû tuklassu*-phrase,[104] and N4 no. 220, possibly from his *mašmaššu ṣeḫru*-phase.[105] Tentatively, Kiṣir-Nabû's commentaries seem to be from around his *mašmaššu ṣeḫru*-phase. As such, his commentaries are from a phase in which he was in the process of becoming an exorcist.

In the case of Kiṣir-Aššur, such training patterns as might have existed in the EM do not appear. However, the lines addressing the reader in the second section may relate to lexical and commentary texts occurring during Kiṣir-Aššur's *mašmaššu*-phase. Therefore, Kiṣir-Aššur does not seem to have depended for his initiation into *āšipūtu* on the EM as a curriculum.[106] Kiṣir-Aššur's training may have been based on other principles. The conclusions drawn throughout this study support this hypothesis. Nonetheless, the EM as a whole can be said to represent a traditional catalogue of the *āšipu*'s craft. Furthermore, the discrepancies between entries listed in the EM and specific texts copied by Kiṣir-Aššur could indicate the professional profile of the *āšipu* had undergone changes since the time the EM was composed, perhaps to include lore of neighbouring crafts, such as that of the *asû*. The EM was probably a learned text worthy of scholarly analysis, and the second section may illustrate how expert exorcists practiced scholarship and were encouraged to study beyond the discipline. Unfortunately, Kiṣir-Nabû's title in the colophon of *KAR* 44 is broken, but he may have been *mašmaššu* when he copied the text.[107] If

101 For the various types of commentaries, their setting within the scholarly environments and the terminology employed, see most recently the Cuneiform Commentaries Project website; Gabbay 2016; Frahm 2011a.

102 Frahm 2018b; Frahm 2011a: 121–123, 269; Reiner 1958: 51.

103 This text's origin in N4 and the name of Kiṣir-Nabû is not entirely certain (cf. Frahm 2011a: 269). Frahm et al. 2016; see Geller 2016: 393; Frahm 2011a: 32, 123–26, 269.

104 Frahm et al. 2016; Geller 2016: 394–96; Frahm 2011a: 121–123, 269.

105 Rev. 12': M[AŠ?.M]A[Š? (TUR?)]; Abusch 2016: 393–95; Frahm et al. 2013a; Frahm 2011a: 121–123, 269. It has also been suggested that Kiṣir-Nabû was the copyist behind the Nineveh manuscript *CT* 15 pl. 43f. (= *SAA* 3 no. 37), although Livingstone's reconstruction of Kiṣir-Nabû's name remains uncertain. Note the commentary on Udug-ḫul tablet 2–4, VAT 8286 (*LKA* 82, N4 no. 39), copied in Geller 2016 as pl. 137, which contains a colophon consisting of one fragmentary line (Frahm 2015).

106 Whether or not the inhabitants of the N4 house all depended on an overarching curriculum remains uncertain, although some individuals copied similar texts (cf. May 2018: 63, 77).

107 E.g., Frahm (2018a: 10), Hecker (2008: 79), and Bottéro (1985: 86) translated him as *mašmaššu*, although Frahm adds (junior?). See also Schwemer 2011: 421–22.

Kiṣir-Aššur copied or read the EM, the evidence suggests that this would have happened around his *mašmaššu*-phase, and the text could have been used to reflect on how the profession and its approaches to scholarship was traditionally conceptualized. As such, the EM may have been part of advanced scholarly training, but it does not seem to have functioned as a curriculum in the case of Kiṣir-Aššur. Whether or not the EM actually relates to the training of *ummânu*s remains uncertain, as the EM itself does not explicitly refer to this title (cf. Clancier 2014: 62) and Kiṣir-Aššur never claims it.[108]

9.5 Kiṣir-Aššur and the Scholarly Traditions in Assur

Kiṣir-Aššur copied a number of texts throughout his career that derive from various locations, such as the Gula temple in Assur (see below). Kiṣir-Aššur therefore seems to have had access to scholarly knowledge from various cities. This section examines to what extent Kiṣir-Aššur drew on the dominant scholarly traditions of his time in Assur and what access he may have had to text collections in other cities. The results situate Kiṣir-Aššur's knowledge production within the 7th century BCE scholarly environment.

9.5.1 *Texts Derived from Geographical Locations*

Kiṣir-Aššur's colophons occasionally include information concerning the city or text collection from which the manuscript copied originated. The examples are listed in Table 21, which includes Kiṣir-Nabû's relevant texts, for comparison. These texts provide a starting point for discussing the scholarly traditions in Assur, which Kiṣir-Aššur used in his textual production. In total, 17 texts contain information concerning the geographical origin of the knowledge.

Only a small group of the tablets from Kiṣir-Aššur and Kiṣir-Nabû contain geographical information. Of these, half of Kiṣir-Aššur's and all of Kiṣir-Nabû's tablets were explicitly copied from writing-boards. Interestingly, their collective geographical span is limited, including only three Babylonian cities (Babylon, Nippur via Nineveh, Uruk), the Gula temple in Assur, and Nineveh. What follows is a discussion of this geographical spread in terms of access to textual traditions.

108 However, see *BAM* 303 and the discussion of a reference to an unspecified *ummânu* in this text.

TABLE 21 Kiṣir-Aššur's and Kiṣir-Nabû's colophons with geographical information[a]

Region	City or Place	Name, Text, Copying Statement
Babylonia	Babylon	– **Kiṣir-Aššur, *KAR* 230** GABA.RI KÁ.DINGIR.RA^{ki}
		– **Kiṣir-Aššur, *LKA* 113** GABA.RI $^{giš}li_9$-$u_5^?$ ⌜x⌝[x KA.DI]NGI[R.RA$^{ki?}$]
	Nippur	– **Kiṣir-Nabû, N4 no. 247; Farber 2.5.3. K** *ina* ZAG$^!$ ^{giš}⌜ZU⌝ [NI]NA$^{!ki}$ GA[B]A.RI EN.LÍL^{k}[^{i} ...]
	Uruk	– **Kiṣir-Nabû, *BAM* 52** 6 *nis-hu liq-ti šá bul-ṭi ki-i pi-i* ^{giš}ZU URI^{ki} GABA.RI UNUG^{ki}
		– **Kiṣir-Nabû, *BAM* 106** [7(?)] *nis-hu liq-ti bul-ṭi ki-i pi-*⌜*i*⌝ [^{giš}ZU(?) URI^{ki}(?)/ GABA].RI UNUG^{ki}
Assyria	The Gula Temple in Assur	– **Kiṣir-Aššur, *BAM* 99** 7 *nis-ḫu* GABA.RI *É-sa-bad šá* BAL.TI^{ki}
		– **Kiṣir-Aššur, *BAM* 131** [x] ^{giš}ZU *šá bul-ṭi ša* É ^{d}ME.ME
		– **Kiṣir-Aššur, *BAM* 201** TA ŠÀ ^{giš}ZU *šá bul-ṭi ša* É ^{d}ME.ME
	Nineveh	– **Kiṣir-Aššur, *LKA* 70+(*KAR* 57)** GABA.RI URU NINA^{ki}
		– **Kiṣir-Nabû, *CMAwR* 1 pl. 25–26** *ki-i* ⌜KA⌝ ^{gi}[^{š}L]I.⌜U$_5$⌝.UM URI^{ki} GABA.RI [^{u}]^{ru} [N]IN[A]$^{?ki}$
		– **(Kiṣir-Nabû(? Broken), *CT* 15 pl. 43f.)** [(LIBIR.RA.BI?)].GIM GABA.RI ^{giš}ZU NINA^{ki}
		– **Kiṣir-Nabû, N4 no. 247; Farber 2.5.3. K** *ina* ZAG$^!$ ^{giš}⌜ZU⌝ [NI]NA$^{!ki}$ GA[B]A.RI EN.LÍL^{k}[^{i} ...]

a The copy by Köcher of *BAM* 68, a tablet copied by either Kiṣir-Aššur or Kiṣir-Nabû, contain the following line in the colophon: [T]A$^!$ ŠÀ ^{giš}ZU [*ša*$^?$ É(?)].MAŠ.MAŠ [x x x x]. One reconstruction could be [*šá* É ^{d}]MAŠ.MAŠ or [*šá* URU ^{d}]MAŠ.MAŠ[$^{ki?}$ ...]. The god written ^{d}MAŠ.MAŠ is Nergal (Borger 2004: 274). However, his city, Kutha, does not appear to be written as URU ^{d}MAŠ.MAŠ$^{(ki)}$. George (1993: 121 no. 742; George 1992: 178 line 150) lists an É.MAŠ.MAŠ as Ištar-Ninlil's temple at Nineveh. The tablet is currently unavailable for collation, but if the signs read [É ^{d}]ME$^!$.ME$^!$, the text may be from the Gula temple. However, according to Maul's recent collations from an excavation photo, the text now reads: [T]A ŠÀ ^{giš}ZU [*ḫ*]*a-an-ṭiš* ZI-*ḫ*[*a*] (Maul 2019: 285). I have followed this reading in Appendix 1 and here, which is why the text is not included in Table 21.

9.5.2 *The Gula Temple Library in Assur*

Maul has emphasized that to copy a text "quickly" (*ḫanṭiš, zamar*), if taken literally, the text must be available nearby (Maul 2010a: 213). Three of Kiṣir-Aššur's tablets (*BAM* 99, *BAM* 131, *BAM* 201) were copied from manuscripts in the "Gula Temple" (*Esabad* or *bīt* ᵈME.ME), which in *BAM* 99 is specified as being in Assur.[109] The implication is that Assur had a Gula temple, which has yet to be discovered and excavated, with a scholarly library of healing texts to which scholars such as Kiṣir-Aššur could go to copy or borrow the required text.[110] Several temples in the city Assur were dedicated to Gula, as witnessed by Kiṣir-Aššur's *KAV* 42 from his *mašmaš bīt Aššur*-phase. The relevant passage states:

> "*Egal-maḫ* : magnificent and exalted house : the temple of Gula;
> *E-sa-bad* : house of (the lady) whose ear is open : the temple of Gula; …
> *E-namtila* : house of life : the temple of Gula".[111]
>
> GEORGE 1992: 180–81

According to Wiggermann (2008: 303–4) there was a Marduk temple called "House of Life" (*É-nam-ti-la*) that was established in Assur around the time of Aššur-uballiṭ (1353–1318 BCE), which possibly was located in the northern part of the city.[112] This precinct existed throughout the MA period and into the NA period, when it was associated with the temple of Gula (ibid.: 204; George 1992: 180–81). Gula's temples *É-gal-maḫ* and *É-sa-bad* are documented in Assur from the MA period onwards (Wiggermann 2008: 204 notes 9–11; George 1992: 180–81). Thus, the Marduk temple *É-nam-ti-la* and Gula's temples could have been merged at some point, perhaps into a single complex (Wiggermann 2008: 204, 211; George 1988: 34).

Assur was therefore home to at least one temple associated with Gula, although the generic *bīt Gula* (É ᵈME.ME), mentioned in *BAM* 131 and *BAM* 201, is not attested as one of the official names of her temples (George 1993a). To my knowledge, there is only one reference to a specific geographical location

---

109 Other references to the *Esabad* or Gula temples include, e.g., *STT* 73 (*BAK* no. 380) and *BAM* 322 (see Steinert 2015: 129 and note 84). However, not all Gula temples contained libraries (Stol 1997: 408–9) and the Gula temple in Assur has not been excavated.

110 Maul 2010a: 214; Wiggermann 2008: 211; Maul 1994: 161. Tablets could likely be borrowed, as some colophons stress the urgency to return them (e.g., Stevens 2013: 214–15; Maul 1994: 161–62).

111 *KAV* 42 rev. 25–28: [É].GAL.MAḪ: É *ra-bu-u ṣi-*⌜*i*⌝*-*[*ru*]: É ᵈ*Gu-l*[*a*] ²⁶ [É].SA.BAD: É *pe-ta-at uz-*[*ni*]: É ᵈ*Gu-l*[*a*] ²⁷ … ²⁸ [É.N]AM.TI.LA: É *ba-lá-ṭi* : É ᵈ*Gu-*[*la*].

112 On the question of Tukulti-Ninurta I's import of tablets for Assur, see the following section.

called É ᵈME.ME: a settlement possibly of this name in the vicinity of Uruk (Beaulieu 2003: 314–15). Although positing a connection to Uruk would at present be conjecture, it is interesting that Kiṣir-Nabû's *BAM* 52 and *BAM* 106 were copied from an Uruk writing-board. Furthermore, Farber cautiously suggested that an overlap in traditions could have existed between Assur and Uruk in relation to the child calming incantation copied by Kiṣir-Aššur and Kiṣir-Nabû.[113] Moreover, we know of the existence of a temple for the god Aššur in Uruk after the fall of the city of Assur in 614 BCE (Radner 2017a: 83–84; Beaulieu 2003: 331–333; Beaulieu 1997).[114] However, the spelling É ᵈME.ME probably constitutes a generic reference to Gula's temple in Assur called *Esabad*, as specified in *BAM* 201. The *Esabad* temple presumably contained the manuscript collection referenced in Kiṣir-Aššur's texts.

9.5.3 *Textual Traditions in Assur*

Assur may have maintained certain local textual traditions by the 7th century. Tukulti-Ninurta I (ca. 1243–1207 BCE) brought cuneiform tablets related to exorcism (*āšipūtu*) and medicine (*malṭarāt asûti*) from Babylonia to Assur during his Babylonian campaigns in the 13th century.[115] Likewise, a MA "Babylonian quarter" may have contained text collections (Wiggermann 2008: 203–4, 215). As such, it is probable that the MA scholarly traditions were based often on contemporary Babylonian material (Veldhuis 2014: 351–53; Wagensonner 2014a; Heeßel 2012: 10–11, 13–15; Heeßel 2007a: 6, 9). These MB scholarly traditions were possibly standardized, before or upon arrival to Assur, and used as building blocks comprising standardized rows of entries that Heeßel calls "Textbausteine",[116] upon which the first millennium BCE standardized series were likely based (Heeßel 2011: 171, 174–75, 192).

Heeßel has stressed that one or more partly standardized MA recensions of *Šumma ālu* and *bārûtu* were circulated alongside their differing first millennium standard recensions in early NA Assur.[117] Additionally, a separate

113 Farber 2014: 35. An Assurbanipal colophon was also discovered among the LB Uruk tablets (Beaulieu 2010: 4–5, 17).

114 Both Babylon and Uruk played a role in safekeeping Assyrian knowledge after the fall of the NA empire (Da Riva 2014: 115; Frahm 2011a: 295; Beaulieu 2010; Clancier 2009: 385–87; Beaulieu 1997: 66–67).

115 Foster 1996: 228–29; Machinist 1978: 128–29 ms B rev. iv 2'–8'. See also Heeßel 2017: 369–71; Veldhuis 2014: 322–24; Heeßel 2012: 11 note 134; Frahm 2011b: 523; Weidner 1952–53.

116 See also Veldhuis 2014: 320. However, innovation did appear in Assur during the MA period, see, e.g., Heeßel 2017: 372; Geller 1990.

117 Heeßel 2012: 10–15; Heeßel 2007a: 4–7; cf. Koch 2013: 242–43; Koch 2005: 25–26; Freedman 1998: 6–7, 13. E.g., *KAL* 1 no. 37, which was labelled as the 210th tablet of *Šumma ālu*, contains a tablet number not known in the standard recension of *Šumma ālu*, although the

recension of *Enūma Anu Enlil* also existed in Assur.[118] As such, the scholarly communities of Assur perpetuated distinct textual traditions that differ from those found at Nineveh. It is therefore of note that not a single copy of Sa-gig nor perhaps of Esagil-kīn-apli's physiognomic omen series *Alamdimmû* has been excavated at Assur.[119]

Esagil-kīn-apli was presumably the *ummânu* of the king Adad-apla-iddina (1068–1047 BCE),[120] although it is unclear if he was a historical figure and editor of the texts ascribed to him[121] or part of an invented tradition.[122] He is, however, generally accepted as the editor of the standard recensions of Sa-gig and *Alamdimmû*.[123] Esagil-kīn-apli may also have composed the royal inscriptions of Adad-apla-iddina, and he or his students may have authored the EM and the so-called "Sa-gig/*Alamdimmû* catalogue".[124] Based on the independent textual traditions found in Assur and the discovery of a text fragment referring to Esagil-kīn-apli, Heeßel (2010a) hypothesized that scholars in Assur rejected Esagil-kīn-apli's diagnostic-prognostic and physiognomic omen series.[125] The text is VAT 10493+ and it contains physiognomic omens from *Alamdimmû*. The first section (col. iii) ends with the following subscript:

---

number may be a scribal error (Heeßel 2007a: 4 and note 41; see also the *Enūma Anu Enlil* and *Šumma ālu* catalogue from Assur and a discussion of this text in Rochberg 2018; Freedman 1998: 322–23 provides a partial edition).

118 Fincke 2001: 35–39; see Rochberg 2018; Steinert 2018c: 170; Veldhuis 2010: 81. Individual MA fragments of *Maqlû* also suggest a pre-Nineveh recension (see Schwemer 2017: 51).

119 Heeßel 2010a: 157–67. For an example of a differing recension of *Alamdimmû* in Assur, see Böck 2000: 19. For the lack of Sa-gig in N4, see Section 3.6.1.

120 Geller 2018a: 44ff.; Frahm 2011a: 324 and note 1547; Heeßel 2011: 193–95; Heeßel 2010a: 162–64; Lenzi 2008b: 142–43 and note 18. A LB list of kings and scholars presents Esagil-kīn-apli as the *ummânu* of a broken king, after which, in incorrect chronologically order, occur Esagil-kīna-ubbib as the *ummânu* of Adad-apla-iddina (1068–1047 BCE) and Nebuchadnezzar I (1125–1104) (Helle 2018: 233 obv. 16 and rev. 17, 234 note 77; Wee 2015: 252 note 19; Frahm 2011a: 324; Lenzi 2008b: 141–43). Esagil-kīna-ubbib was known as the author of the Babylonian Theodicy (Lambert 1962: 66–67). Perhaps Esagil-kīna-ubbib and Esagil-kīn-apli were contemporary exorcists (Beaulieu 2007b: 14; cf. Wee 2012: 252 note 19; Rutz 2011: 295 note 5). The list may indicate that Adad-apla-iddina had two *ummânus*, Esagil-kīna-ubbib and Esagil-kīn-apli, who succeeded each other (Frahm 2011a: 324; cf. Heeßel 2010a: 163).

121 E.g., Frahm 2018a: 29–33; Heeßel 2010a: 166–67; Charpin 2010: 51–52; Lambert 2008: 95; Heeßel 2000: 104; Finkel 1988: 144; cf. Geller 2012: 44.

122 Rutz 2011: 299 note 21; Robson 2008: 477.

123 E.g., Wee 2012: 27–35, 223, 272, 279; Heeßel 2010a: 143, 157–59; Böck 2000: 14–15; Heeßel 2000: 104–107; Finkel 1988.

124 Frahm 2018a: 32–33. For this catalogue, see Frahm 2018a: 24–26; Schmidtchen 2018; Frahm 2011a: 326–28; Heeßel 2000: 104–10; Finkel 1988.

125 Heeßel 2010a: 154–64; cf. Frahm 2018a: 40–41; Wee 2012: 252; Frahm 2011a: 220.

> The old version of *Šumma alamdimmû*, which Esagil-kīn-apli had not 'voided' (lit.: 'released', NU DU$_8$.MEŠ-*šú*); first tablet of *Alamdimmû*.[126]

Heeßel (2010a: 154–57) interpreted the phrase NU DU$_8$.MEŠ-*šú* (*lā upaṭṭirušu*) as a statement referring to Esagil-kīn-apli's editorial activities. As such, the phrase likely indicates that Esagil-kīn-apli had not edited, and thereby cancelled the authoritative effect of, the older first section of *Alamdimmû* found on VAT 10493+.[127] The preserved omens from this section, designated as part of the 1st tablet of *Alamdimmû*, are not listed in the preserved parts of the 1st tablet of Esagil-kīn-apli's *Alamdimmû* (Heeßel 2010a: 155; see Böck 2000: 71). However, the second section of VAT 10493+ largely duplicates the second tablet of Esagil-kīn-apli's *Alamdimmû* recension, though it also includes commentaries (Heeßel 2010a: 155; see Böck 2000: 72–89). As such, VAT 10493+ may indicate that an older version of *Alamdimmû* was transmitted in Assur (see Heeßel 2010a: 159).

Esagil-kīn-apli's traditions were closely connected with politics.[128] His editorial work was possibly connected to his role as advisor to Adad-apla-iddina (Frahm 2011a: 324–25), and the Sa-gig/*Alamdimmû* catalogue explicitly states that the user of these series should place his knowledge at the disposal of the king.[129] Furthermore, it seems that the 7th century Assyrian kings venerated Esagil-kīn-apli's textual innovations.[130] Although it is uncertain when

126 Heeßel 2010a: 143–53 col. iii 6–7: DIŠ ⌜*alam*⌝-*dím-mu-u* LIBIR.RA *šá É-sag-gíl*-GIN-A NU DU$_8$.MEŠ-*šú* [7] DUB.1.KÁM *alam-<dím>-mu-ú*.

127 See *CAD* P: 300. D-stem *paṭāru* is used in relation to "void" with *riksu* "band, bond, joint, package, collection (of tablets), structure, contract, decree" in several examples, which may relate to the serialization, as Sa-gig is also called *rikis murṣi u rikis kūri* "the compilation of illness and the compilation of distress" (Wee 2012: 303 and note 137; Heeßel 2010a: 154–55 and note 17; *CAD* R: 347ff.). Frahm (2011a: 329–31) questioned Heeßel's interpretation, understanding the line as an indication that Esagil-kīn-apli was perhaps involved in providing commentaries found in the second section of the text, but he has since retracted part of his critique (see Frahm 2018a: 40–41).

128 Frahm 2011a: 324 and notes 1545–46; Heeßel 2010a: 166–67; Charpin 2010: 51–52; Heeßel 2000: 91–92.

129 See Finkel 1988: 148, 150. ND 4358+4366 and BM 41237+ lines 31'–33': [*a-ši-pu*(?)] TAR-*is* EŠ.BAR *ḫa-a'-iṭ* ZI-*tì* UN.MEŠ [32'] [*sa-k*]*ik-ka u alam-dím-ma-a ka-liš* ZU-*ú li-ḫi-iṭ lib-ri lìb-bi* [33'] [*liš-ta-bil*]-*ma ana* LUGAL ME-*a liš-kun*, "[Let the *āšipu*] who makes the decisions, and who watches over people's lives, who comprehensively knows Sa-gig and *Alamdimmû*, inspect (the patient) and check (the appropriate series), [let him ponder], and let him put his diagnosis at the disposal of the king".

130 E.g., by referring indirectly to him in their royal inscriptions, see Frahm 2018a: 38–40. Assurbanipal also refers indirectly to Esagil-kīn-appli in his colophons (Frahm 2011a: 332 note 1588).

Esagil-kīn-apli's editions were introduced at the Assyrian court, it is possible that Assurnaṣirpal's relocation of the royal residence to Kalḫu during the 9th century BCE prompted an import of contemporary Babylonian scholarly knowledge. Academic rivalry would subsequently have forced the Assur scholars to reject Esagil-kīn-apli's corpus.[131] Therefore, the Assur scholars may have attempted to retain their own and older traditions in order to maintain authority in the interpretation of knowledge (Heeßel 2010a: 165–66).[132] Interestingly, several exorcists within the Bāba-šuma-ibni family claimed the title "Assur(-city) exorcist" (*mašmaššu aššurû*(?)),[133] which may indicate a particular type of exorcist. If correct, the title could support the hypothesis that Assur scholars circulated particular traditions.[134]

9.5.4 *Exchange of Knowledge between Assur and the Nineveh Text Collections*

Certain manuscripts indicate that knowledge was exchanged between Assur and Nineveh, despite a presumed rejection of Esagil-kīn-apli's traditions at Assur.[135] Nineveh was the centre of 7th century Assyrian scholarship

---

131 Heeßel 2010a: 167. Esagil-kīn-apli also was not listed as *ummânu* in the Assur "Synchronistic King List" (Frahm 2018a: 41; Heeßel 2010a: 159).

132 An unresolved issue in relation to the Assur scholars' textual traditions is the effect that Marduk's exile in Assyria and Sennacherib's *akītu*-house may have had on the Assur scholarly communities. See, e.g., Maul 2017: 352; Pongratz-Leisten 2015: 417–18; Livingstone 1989: XXIX, 81ff.; Livingstone 1986: 205ff.; Frymer-Kensky 1983.

133 Fadhil 2012: 46; Maul 2010a: 208–209. E.g., Abu-erība *KAL* 2 no. 34 col. iv 14': ^{lú}MAŠ.MAŠ BAL.TIL^{k}[^{i}]; Nabû-bēssunu *LKA* 109 rev. 15': ^{lú}MAŠ.MAŠ BAL.TIL^{ki} (cf. Gelb 1954: 223 col. iv 29: ^{lú}MAŠ.MAŠ URU BAL.TIL^{ki}-*u* = *mašmaššu aššurû*). The titles *ṭupšarru aššurû* (e.g., *BAM* 1 col. iv 28: ^{lú}DUB.SAR URU BAL.TIL^{ki}-*u*; see Fadhil 2012: 14, 29–30, 32–33, 41–42, 45–46, 47, 50–51, 59) and *asû aššurû* (Matouš 1933 no. 44 col. vi 32': ^{lú}A.ZU BAL.T[IL^{ki}]) are also attested. See Section 2.3.4.

134 Or perhaps the title refers to the exorcist having duties in relation to the city itself (cf. Maul 2010a: 210–11). May (2018: 66) has recently suggested that the title *zabardabbû* was used in the Bāba-šuma-ibni family because it was employed in Esagil-kīn-apli's geneology. However, clear evidence in support of this hypothesis is still lacking.

135 Future research into the N4 text collection and the Nineveh libraries in general should be contextualized within the discussion of textual traditions specific to Assur and Oppenheim's hypothesis on the so-called "stream of tradition" (Oppenheim 1960: 410–11; Oppenheim 1977: 13–14). Oppenheim's hypothesis considers the Mesopotamian scholarly and literary traditions as static texts, which were handed down faithfully, anonymously, and conservatively for centuries. However, during recent years Robson (2011a) especially has argued strongly against this view. The same text had different meanings in relation to time and place, textual traditions were localized, various users used texts differently, and innovation as well as creativity played a role in the transmission of knowledge (see, e.g., Heeßel 2011: 171, 174–75, 192; Heeßel 2010a: 154–67; George 2003: 31–33;

par excellence (e.g., Fincke 2017). Although earlier NA kings had collected scholarly writings (ibid.: 382–83), Esarhaddon (680–669 BCE) appears to have begun assembling scholarly tablets and initiating a copying program of learned texts at Nineveh (Frahm 2011b: 523; Frame and George 2005: 278–79). Assurbanipal (668–627 BCE) assembled tablet collections throughout the first half of his reign in the South-west Palace, the North Palace, and the Nabû temple on the Kuyunjik mound, collectively referred to as "Assurbanipal's library".[136] These collections consisted of knowledge gathered in Babylonia,[137] obtained through scholars' private libraries,[138] and assembled through textual production within the Nineveh scriptoriums.[139] Assurbanipal's collections were largely contemporary to Kiṣir-Aššur.

In general, scholars could travel in pursuit of knowledge or particular works, although it is unclear if this was the norm (Robson 2014: 156, 159; cf. Robson 2011a: 566, 570; see also Fadhil 1998). Regardless, the need for access to important collections, such as the royal libraries, must have been pivotal for scholars working outside of the court.[140] A few royal letters may indicate a relationship between the Bāba-šuma-ibni family and the Assyrian court (Section 2.3.5),[141] and it is possible that Kiṣir-Aššur and/or Kiṣir-Nabû supplied manuscripts to Assurbanipal's libraries.[142] Furthermore, Kiṣir-Aššur may have performed rituals for the king during the winter months, while he dwelled in Assur (Section 8.6).

One of Kiṣir-Aššur's texts (*LKA* 70+) and two of Kiṣir-Nabû's texts (*CMAwR* 1 pl. 25–26; N4 no. 247)[143] are stated as being copied from Nineveh texts, although

Fincke 2001; Frahm 1999). The present study provides a partial solution to this situation, although a discussion of the "stream of tradition" without considering the entire N4 text collection is not desierable. I therefore refer the reader to Robson (2019), who has recently problematized Oppenheim's hypothesis broadly in the NA period.

136 Frahm 2011b: 523; Pedersén 1998: 158–65; Parpola 1986.

137 Frahm 2011b: 523; Frame and George 2005; Fincke 2004: 57.

138 *SAA* 7 no. 49–56; Fincke 2004: 55, 57; Parpola 1983b.

139 Fincke 2017: 387; Frahm 2011b: 523; Frame and George 2005: 280; Lieberman 1990: 309–12.

140 See Robson 2011a: 570–71. It is unclear if scholarly tablets were ever sold (ibid.: 566).

141 Some of the influential scholarly families from Assur associated with the Bāba-šuma-ibni family may have had connections to the royal court (see May 2018: 68, 74–76; Frahm 2011a: 270).

142 See Frahm 2011a: 269–70 and note 1279 concerning *ACh Supp.* 2 24; Maul 2010a: 205 and note 53; Villard 1998; Livingstone 1989: 95 no. 37.

143 *CT* 15 pl. 43f. was excavated at Nineveh, but the colophon is very fragmentary (see Livingstone 1989: 95). It is therefore unclear if the text was written by Kiṣir-Nabû, as suggested by Livingstone. Additionally, *ACh Supp.* 2 24 was perhaps copied by Kiṣir-Aššur, and this text was also excavated at Nineveh (see Section 7.6). The evidence for assigning these texts to Kiṣir-Aššur and Kiṣir-Nabû remains tenuous.

not necessarily copied at Nineveh (see Villard 1998). *LKA* 70+ was copied when Kiṣir-Aššur was *mašmaš bīt Aššur* and is connected to the Ištar-Dumuzi ritual series that addresses the removal of demonic influences (Farber 1977: 10). Kiṣir-Nabû copied N4 no. 247 "according to a Nineveh writing-board, a copy (from) Nippur" as *mašmaššu*, which is a partial duplicate to Kiṣir-Aššur's incantation N4 no. 24 (Section 5.2.1). Kiṣir-Nabû's text published in *CMAwR* 1 pl. 25–26 is largely against the "adversary" (*bēl dabābi*) and it was copied from a writing-board in Babylonian script from Nineveh.[144] None of the texts specify they were copied at Nineveh, and both Kiṣir-Nabû's texts comprised Babylonian knowledge and not standardized Nineveh texts. Furthermore, Kiṣir-Aššur's *LKA* 70+ does not agree with the order of tablets in the series found at Nineveh (Farber 1977: 24–26).

Maul (2010a: 204) placed Kiṣir-Nabû in the last third of the 7th century BCE during a period presumably marked by decentralization and a decline of royal influence (Oates 1991: 164). Although the effects of decentralization may have strengthened some local traditions, Assur's hypothesized individuality may have required scholars to import the textual tools of rulers at the time, such as the Esagil-kīn-apli traditions flourishing at Nineveh. Kiṣir-Nabû may therefore have studied the Nineveh textual traditions, also represented by the EM (*KAR* 44), in order to accommodate a new need within the Assur community.[145]

The N4 tablet *BAM* 322 is a one columned tablet copied by a high priest (*šangû*) of the Aššur temple and consists of two sections, the first designated as "a copy (from) the palace of Ḫammurabi" and the second as "a copy (from) the palace of Esarhaddon".[146] The second section is described as follows, before the statements concerning Esarhaddon's palace:

> Remedies (and) ritual pro[cedures? from the temple of] Gula. Tried, selected and checked procedures, which are *suitable for use*. (Whenever) you perform (them), they (the patients) will be alright. Guard the secret exorcism corpus so that no one may disclose (it)!
>
> STEINERT 2015: 129 and note 84[147]

144 For the relevant passage in N4 no. 247 rev. 24 and *CMAwR* 1 pl. 25–26 rev. 24–25, see Table 21 in Section 9.5.1.

145 Note that another example of the EM was excavated in N4 (A 366), but remains unpublished (Jean 2006: 63). Whether this predates Kiṣir-Nabû remains unknown.

146 See Ch. 8 note 65; Steinert 2015: 128–29; cf. Frahm 2011b: 523.

147 *BAM* 322 rev. 89–90: *bul-ṭi né-*[*pe-ši šá* É ^{d}]ME.ME *né-pe-ši lat-ku-ti am-ru-ti ba-ru-ti šá ana* ŠU^{II} *šu-*[*ṣu-u*] ^{90} DÙ-*uš-ma i-šal-*[*li*]*-mu ni-ṣir-ti* MAŠ.MAŠ-*ti* ŠEŠ-*ma man-ma* NU DU$_{8}$.

According to Steinert (2015: 129), this subscript indicates that the second section of *BAM* 322 was originally located on a manuscript at the Assur Gula temple. From there, it was copied and subsequently integrated into Esarhaddon's palace. Finally, the high priest of the Aššur temple copied it alongside other material in Esarhaddon's palace and made it available to the Bāba-šuma-ibni family. Therefore, it seems that the Aššur temple clergy and plausibly also the Bāba-šuma-ibni family had (controlled) access to Nineveh texts.[148] However, this access may have been through sources already located within Assur (cf. Robson 2014: 158–59).

9.6 Summary

Kiṣir-Aššur's medical tablets contain prescriptions for treating all the major areas of the body. However, three groups indicate a particular medical focus. These consist of diagnoses, symptom descriptions, and prescriptions, as well as incantations and ritual instructions against internal illnesses and their symptoms, "string" and lower body maladies, as well as complex disorders affecting several body parts. The first group in particular may have been linked to his practice.

Kiṣir-Aššur produced a number of *nisḫu*-extracts throughout his career. Several of the extracts contain purpose statements, date especially to his later phases, and may reflect practical application. A number of *nisḫu*s are extracted from writing-boards, providing insights into the role of such manuscripts in NA scholarship. Finally, a group of extracts whose content is mainly medical contain numbers or structural remarks. In at least one instance, two Kiṣir-Nabû manuscripts appear to have been extracted consecutively from the same writing-board and numbered accordingly. Kiṣir-Aššur copied at least two numbered *šamallû ṣeḫru* manuscripts from a hypothesized consecutive row of training material, which could have been extracted from a single writing-board. The numbered extracts from N4 do not presently attest to a *nisḫu*-series, but instead to texts presumably extracted for various purposes in relation to training and practice.

148 Maul 2010a: 205 and note 53, 218–20; Villard 1998; see May 2018: 76; Heeßel 2017: 375. Current theories propose the association of the royal court, temples, and scholars hindered critical and individual thought (e.g., Frahm 2011b: 525–26). When more of the relationships between the Assur, Kalḫu and Nineveh libraries have been examined, such ideas should be discussed further.

Kiṣir-Aššur's texts were also analysed in relation to the Nineveh Ugu series and the possibly differing Assur recension represented by the incipits catalogued in the AMC. In relation to the AMC, Kiṣir-Aššur rarely copied these incipits. His occasional use of generic and hardly recognizable catch-lines indicates that his texts were copied according to other principles. Furthermore, a comparison between Kiṣir-Aššur's texts and the known portions of the Nineveh Ugu series revealed that Kiṣir-Aššur's extracts are rarely extracted in any discernable order. This could indicate that the manuscripts from which Kiṣir-Aššur copied were not standardized according to the Nineveh Ugu recension. Yet, some manuscripts not explicitly labelled as extracts, such as *BAM* 129, duplicate consecutive entries from a manuscript possibly belonging to the Nineveh Ugu series. At present, it is therefore unclear what determined the structure of Kiṣir-Aššur's extracts. Nonetheless, it is clear that they represent knowledge that was utilized for pragmatic purposes. Finally, Kiṣir-Aššur does not seem to have followed the EM as a curriculum for becoming an *āšipu*. Therefore, by following the microhistoric approach Chapter 9 has challenged and contrasted numerous theories concerning the training of exorcists and their use of knowledge.

CHAPTER 10

Synthesis and Conclusion

This study has provided the first detailed analysis of a particular *āšipu*'s education and practice. A number of surprising features have been illuminated through the analysis of Kiṣir-Aššur's education, which indicates that it was different from what we would expect. Kiṣir-Aššur copied prescriptions related to the treatment of snakebites, scorpion stings and horses as *šamallû ṣeḫru*. All three areas of healing consist of prescriptions and they are usually regarded as uncommon in Mesopotamian healing. The study showed that these areas of healing likely provided Kiṣir-Aššur with a conceptual framework for interpreting the overwhelming powers of venomous liquids, which could be used for understanding the physiological processes of the human body. The venoms were generally compared to the bile found in mammals, which may have provided an explanatory physiological framework. In relation to the veterinarian prescriptions, it is possible that Kiṣir-Aššur used knowledge about animal anatomy to gain an understanding of the internal mechanisms of the human body. Additionally, it was proposed that he could have practiced horse treatments and it may be possible to extrapolate from this that Kiṣir-Aššur also acted as a veterinarian. Kiṣir-Aššur also copied several medical manuscripts with diagnoses, symptom descriptions, and treatments of various illnesses. These therapeutic texts appear to have been copied according to assignments focusing on an anatomical or physiological area of the body, according to a specific ailment, or handpicked sections from a collection of prescriptions. Concerning his diagnostic capabilities, Kiṣir-Aššur may have been trained in diagnostics through a combination of the therapeutic texts from his *šamallû ṣeḫru*-phase and oral teachings. Significantly, according to the surviving evidence he never copied Sa-gig, which is assumed to have been the primary tool with which to learn diagnostic principles. The numbered extracts that he produced as *šamallû ṣeḫru* may have provided him with the most useful text passages for acquiring all the abovementioned skills. Additionally, Kiṣir-Aššur was trained in methods for treating causes of illness by petitioning or influencing the responsible deity through prayer, ritual actions, and substitution. Surprisingly, he also seems to have taught basic scribal skills to at least one younger pupil.

After his *šamallû ṣeḫru*-phase, Kiṣir-Aššur copied rituals for removing the affliction "Curse" and gaining an overview of the confinement ritual *bīt mēseri*. As *šamallû mašmaššu ṣeḫru*, he copied texts intended to soothe ghosts or personal gods in a domestic setting. During this phase, he also copied a text for prophylactically calming a baby or child. It is possible that the texts he copied provided a continuous focus on knowledge related to understanding and learning how to practice healing. I presented evidence to suggest that Kiṣir-Aššur may himself have acted as a paediatrician during this phase. Although child calming rituals are known to have been part of the *āšipu*'s proficiencies, it is interesting that it appears at this point in his training, after a period in which he studied texts related first primarily to medicine and afterwards aimed at performing and understanding more advanced rituals. During the *mašmaššu šamallû ṣeḫru*-phase he also copied texts for treating possible domestic causes of misfortune. This process, I suggested was intended to widen the young *āšipu*'s scope from individual, to house, to cult, to family, and following the *mašmaššu ṣeḫru*-phase, to entire households. Kiṣir-Aššur, while probably trained under his father's supervision, may therefore have experienced increased autonomy in certain areas of practice during some phases. It is possible that he treated animals as *šamallû ṣeḫru* and later infants, babies, or children as *šamallû mašmaššu ṣeḫru*, with increased autonomy in order to gain more experience. Additionally, it is also possible that this sequence of medical training was the result of an intrinsic ethical and economic system, which allowed greater room for medical errors on animals and to some extent on young children. This suggestion is based on the observation that animals could be replaced through economic compensation, whereas the failed treatment of an infant, baby, or child could perhaps damage the healer's social reputation. It is therefore possible that medical incompetence in relation to adult healing was the only form of negligence that could potentially terminate a healer's practice.

The *mašmaššu ṣeḫru*-phase was the first time since the *šamallû ṣeḫru*-phase that he copied prescriptions (*bulṭu*). Furthermore, these were described as "tested" procedures. When Kiṣir-Aššur became *mašmaššu*, he surprisingly does not seem to have been fully trained. It is likely that he was not allowed to supervise rituals and perform house calls on his own until sometime during this phase. Yet, the material attests to an increase in authority, as he copied rituals designed for conducting house calls and rituals for protecting entire households during this phase. He had previously acquired insight into such rituals as *šamallû*. Furthermore, the fact that purpose statements and *namburbi*-rituals generally do not appear before this phase indicates that these were elements connected with supervising rituals and conducting house calls without supervision.

A significant result of this monograph relates to practical, as opposed to abstract, theoretical knowledge. Many of Kiṣir-Aššur's tablets appear to be extracts in some form. Some tablets were numbered according to obscure principles, possibly numbering excerpts extracted from larger texts, whereas other manuscripts were simply mined for Kiṣir-Aššur's practice. What is clear, however, is that Kiṣir-Aššur's texts often seem to have been copied and extracted for specific purposes, such as training and practice. They therefore reflect practiced knowledge. Kiṣir-Aššur's use of tested prescription, and perhaps his own test of at least one prescription, during his *mašmaš bīt Aššur*-phase, coupled with many purpose statements on medical and ritual tablets from the *mašmaššu*- and *mašmaš bīt Aššur*-phases, as well as on tablets without titles, attest to the practical implementation of this knowledge. It appears that as *mašmaš bīt Aššur* he may have depended on fewer but more trustworthy prescriptions, of which at least one prescription was universally applicable. Furthermore, the evidence suggests that rituals connected to witchcraft and hostility were related to Kiṣir-Aššur's later career phases.

Overall, Kiṣir-Aššur's medical texts may be assigned to three major groups relating to: internal, renal, and rectal illnesses; illnesses affecting the "strings", the motoric system, and the lower extremities; and a limited number of complex illnesses or causes of illness. In particular, the group concerning internal, renal, and rectal illnesses seems to be part of Kiṣir-Aššur's practice. Whether or not these areas reflect his personal specialization(s), or whether he even had an area of specialization, remains uncertain. Furthermore, if the majority of his texts had a practical dimension, it is probable that the texts from his *mašmaš bīt Aššur*-phase related to the Aššur temple were practical tools used in connection to specific duties, to familiarize Kiṣir-Aššur with the cult of Aššur, or as models that were modified according to need.

From a microhistorical point of view, this study provides a foundation for further in depth analyses of individual healers' training and practice. Surprisingly, Kiṣir-Aššur rarely produced exact copies with colophons of the established series, and some texts are only known from his manuscripts or from duplicates in the N4 collection. Although this is not necessarily proof of an idiosyncratic scholarly environment in N4, it does indicate that the texts Kiṣir-Aššur copied and used occasionally fell outside the parameters we know from the royal collections in Nineveh. It is possible that his texts reflect textual traditions specific to the scholarly environments of the city of Assur. However, Kiṣir-Aššur's copies of texts from these traditions indicate that they were part of his training and practice. Kiṣir-Aššur does not appear to have been trained according to current interpretations of the Exorcist's Manual, although the limited number of scholarly texts from around his *mašmaššu*-phase may reflect the wider range of advanced scholarship that was encouraged in the second part of the EM. Thus, the evidence presented cautiously speaks in favour of abandoning the EM as a verbatim curriculum for becoming an *āšipu*. The inclusion in Kiṣir-Aššur's training and practice of texts of other and different types of medical knowledge than are explicitly listed in the EM may indicate that the professional profile of the exorcist had undergone changes since the time the EM was composed. However, this question requires further analysis, ideally combined with a discussion of the development of the *āšipu* profession in later periods.

By investigating the small mysteries of medical practice that individual manuscripts presented, this study has examined the wider use of veterinarian and paediatric knowledge in Mesopotamia. Furthermore, physiology has rarely been discussed in relation to whether or not a Mesopotamian conception of internal underlying processes existed. Building on previous research, I hypothesized that a system concerning fluids, such as venom and bile, may have been used in metaphoric relationships to establish a conception of how some aspects of the internal parts of the body functioned.

Therefore, by considering all of a single *āšipu*'s texts from his entire career, it is possible to achieve a more diverse understanding of the purposes that individual texts may have served, independent of genre labels. This monograph has provided a well-rounded and holistic analysis that emphasises emic perspectives with the added etic background where necessary. The publication of further tablets will potentially modify these results, yet such modifications will not significantly change the conclusions drawn concerning Kiṣir-Aššur as a case study of a practitioner working at a specific time, in a certain location. This study has striven towards not overemphasizing particular individual features, as well as accounting for the amount of unattainable knowledge, such as oral teachings. However, both the fragmentary material and the method have their limits and many of the results remain, unavoidably, hypothetical. Therefore, this study does not hold all the answers regarding Kiṣir-Aššur's magico-medical focuses or the impact they had on his career. Further research into the orthography and spelling habits of Kiṣir-Aššur and his family may enable additional N4 texts to be assigned to specific members of the Bāba-šuma-ibni family. However, a comprehensive examination of such features is beyond the scope of the present analysis. Nonetheless, comparative texts and general theories have provided the necessary background and supporting information, in accordance with the microhistoric approach, to support my observations about Kiṣir-Aššur.

In a broader perspective, a number of preliminary observations regarding the similarities and differences between Kiṣir-Aššur and contemporary *āšipu*s at the royal court might highlight possible areas for future studies. A few exorcists at the royal court in Nineveh may have overseen the treatment of children in addition to adults (see Section 5.2.2). The arguments presented here, regarding Kiṣir-Aššur's hypothesized practice as a paediatrician, indicate that such duties may have been part of some exorcists' professional obligations.

However, we currently know little about the concrete development in patient groups or changing responsibilities of other individual healers. The letters and reports from Nineveh suggest that court *āšipu*s never quoted Sa-gig, and at least one exorcist tested a prescription before use on patients (see Sections 3.6.1 and 8.3.1). Therefore, current research tentatively implies that some *āšipu*s at court depended on, e.g., experience in their practice. Kiṣir-Aššur did not copy Sa-gig, as far as we know. Furthermore, Kiṣir-Aššur also depended on experience to some degree, as well as pragmatism, which is evidenced by his use of fewer trusted prescriptions in later phases and the proposed test of a prescription during his *mašmaš bīt Aššur*-phase. Yet, other aspects of Kiṣir-Aššur's practice perhaps contrast that of exorcists in Nineveh. While rituals at court could be copied in their entirety for what may have been strict performances (see Section 7.4), Kiṣir-Aššur's manuscripts demonstrate how relevant sections of both medical and ritual texts were chosen and copied for concrete purposes. Some such texts likely served as *aide mémoires*, and rituals were perhaps adapted according to specific circumstances.

While Kiṣir-Aššur and his family perhaps had occasional professional contact with the Assyrian kings, little evidence suggests he had direct access to the Nineveh court and its scholarly knowledge. Like one exorcist at court, Kiṣir-Aššur perhaps had private clients as *mašmaš bīt Aššur* in addition to his possible duties at the Aššur temple (see Section 8.7). Unlike the letters and reports from the Nineveh exorcists, Kiṣir-Aššur's manuscripts provide us with scholarly texts copied for specific professional purposes, and they show how he operated within a local and distinctive scholarly environment. Thus, Kiṣir-Aššur primarily acquired texts via the local learned community and its institutions. Although Kiṣir-Aššur was not part of the inner circle of scholars at Nineveh, certain aspects of how he practiced his profession seem to be roughly similar to some of the routines of the *āšipu*s at the royal court. Yet, other aspects of his practice do not appear to be comparable. It remains possible, however, that the conclusions drawn regarding Kiṣir-Aššur's training and career are not generally applicable to wider medical practices in Mesopotamia, and perhaps not even in the NA period. These questions require further research, and they will hopefully be addressed in the future. Yet, this study has shown that Kiṣir-Aššur's texts reveal a localized tradition of medical knowledge.

By focusing on practical rather than abstract knowledge, the case of Kiṣir-Aššur provides a contextualized and comprehensive study of how medical knowledge in all forms was used by a specific ancient healer. Consequently, this work not only adds to our knowledge of how ancient texts were used, but differs significantly from some contributions on Mesopotamian medicine. It is therefore my hope that it serves as a step towards gaining a deeper understanding of medical practices in ancient Mesopotamia.

APPENDIX 1

Catalogue of Texts

The following catalogue lists the texts in which the colophon includes Kiṣir-Aššur's name, the remains of his name (Kiṣir-[…]), or texts that are discussed in relation to Kiṣir-Aššur throughout this monograph. All the N4 numbers refer to the numbers in Pedersén's catalogue of the N4 text collection (Pedersén 1986: 59–76). Additional transliterations of the majority of *BAM* texts can be found on the BabMed and CDLI websites.

The following overview presents information on the tablet format, how the tablet was investigated by the present author, the CDLI numbers where applicable, relevant bibliographical entries, and the content of the individual texts listed according to the entries on each tablet in more or less detail. The manuscripts are listed alphabetically according to the first letter in the acronym:

ACh Supp. **2 24** (K. 3145; Nineveh)

Tablet:	Single-column tablet in portrait format; collated via the CDLI photograph
Content:	Commentary on tablet 20 of *Enūma Anu Enlil*
CDLI no.:	P394833 (photograph)
Bibliography:	Rochberg 1988: 225–227 (transliteration and commentary) Virolleaud 1912: 42–43 no. 24 (copy)
Discussion:	Frahm et al. 2013b with additional bibliography Frahm 2011a: 144–145 Frahm 2004: 47 note 18

Obv. 1–20	Commentary on individual lines of at least the 20th tablet of *Enūma Anu Enlil*
(*Breaks off*)	
Rev. 1'–13'	(Same as above)
Rev. 14'–17'	Colophon:

DIŠ ⸢MUL.ŠUDUN⸣ A.AB.B[A] a-dir ⸢x⸣[(x x x x x x?)] 15' ⸢*ana*? *mal-su*⸣-*ut* ᴾ*Ki-ṣi*[*r*-(x x x x x x?)] 16' [(x x x x?)] :? *su-bar-tú* 17' [(x x x x x?)] *su-bar-tú ana ma-šu-šú-nu*

BAM **9** (VAT 13785; Assur N4 no. 607)

Tablet:	Single-column tablet in portrait format; collated during the summer of 2015; H 164mm/W 96mm/T 24mm

Content: Prescriptions against afflictions of the head predominantly caused by ghosts

CDLI no.: P285113 (photograph)

Bibliography: Worthington 2005 ms G (treatment of individual lines)
Hunger 1968: 70 no. 200 ms A (colophon)
Köcher 1963a: XIII–XIV and pl. 18–20 no. 9 (copy)

Discussion: Steinert 2018c: 175 note 100
Steinert 2018d: 220–221, 286
Scurlock and Andersen 2005: 174 no. 8.46, 311–12 no. 13.145 no. 13.149 no. 13.157, 497 no. 19.276, 784 (treatment and discussion of individual lines)

Obv. 1–8	Prescription against a ghost and throbbing temples applied onto the temple(s)
Obv. 9–11	Prescription applied onto the temple(s)
Obv. 12–13	Fragmentary prescription
Obv. 14–15	Fragmentary prescription for treating pains in the right temple and a weeping right eye (IGI^{II} ZAG-*šú* ÉR)
Obv. 16–17	Prescription for treating pains in the left temple and a weeping left eye applied onto the temple
Obv. 18–20	Fragmentary prescription for treating pains of the temples and weeping [eyes]
Obv. 21–22	Fragmentary prescription for treating a headache (*sagkidabbû*)
Obv. 23–25	Prescription applied [to the head] in the case of a man's head burning with *ṣētu*-fever (UD.DA TAB-*ma*) and his hair falls out
Obv. 26–30, 31–32	Fragmentary prescriptions
Obv. 33–34, 35–39	Fragmentary prescriptions applied to the head(?)
Obv. 40–41	Fragmentary prescription to soothe (*nu-úḫ-ḫi*) throbbing temple(s)
Rev. 42–46	Prescription for removing a headache (*sakidabbû*) from a man's body
Rev. 47–50	Prescription for anointing to treat a ghost that has seized a man
Rev. 51–54	Prescription for anointing to treat a stinging and roaring head, ringing ears and stinging fingers caused by a ghost
Rev. 55–57	Prescription for fumigation to remove a persistent ghost that the *āšipu* does not know how to remove ([*a-n*]*a* KIN ŠU.GIDIM.MA ZAL.ZAL ⌜*ša*⌝ $^{lú!}$MAŠ.MAŠ ZI-*šú* NU ZU-*e*)
Rev. 58–60	Prescription against a throbbing head applied onto the head
Rev. 61–63	Prescription to soothe [throbbing] temple(s) applied (onto the head)

Rev. 64–65	Fragmentary prescription for bandaging the head
Rev. 66–68	Fragmentary prescription applied onto the head
Rev. 69–76	Catch-line; colophon:

[(*nis-ḫu*)] IGI-*ú* GABA.RI ^{giš}ZU [x x x x x x x x x x(?)] ^{71} [D]U[B (*blank*)] ^{p}*Ki-ṣir*-AN.ŠÁR DUMU $^{\text{p.⌜d⌝}}$AG-*bé*-[*sun* ^{lú}MAŠ.MAŠ É AN.ŠÁR(?)] ^{72} [(x x?) *šá* ^{d}A]G *tuk-lat-su* ⌜^{d}⌝[*T*]*aš-me-tu*$_4$ ⌜x⌝[(x x x x x?)] ^{73} [DUMU $^{\text{p.d}}$*B*]*a-ba*$_6$-MU-DÙ ^{lú}ZABAR.DAB.BA *É*-[*šár-ra*] ^{74} [(*nīš* ^{d}PA$^{?}$ *u*$^{?}$) ^{d}AM]AR.UTU *šu-mì šaṭ-rù la t*[*a-pa-šiṭ*] ^{75} [(x x x?) ^{d}]AG ⌜*ù*⌝ ^{d}A[MAR.UTU] ^{76} [(x x x x?)]⌜x x x x x-*šú*⌝-*m*[*a* (x x x?)]

***BAM* 28+Beckman and Foster 1988 no. 7** (EHE 333+YBC 2120; Assur N4 no. 626)

Tablet:	Single-column tablet in portrait format; *BAM* 28 not collated, Yale fragment collated via private photographs
Content:	Incantations and ritual treatments for *kadabbedû* and associated illnesses of the nose and mouth
CDLI no.:	P285130 (copy of EHE 333)
Bibliography:	*Unedited*
	Kinnier Wilson and Reynolds 2007: 73 (partial edition)
	Beckman and Foster 1988 no. 7 (copy of YBC 2120)
	Durand 1982 no. 333 (collated copy of parts of EHE 333)
	Hunger 1968: 74 no. 213 ms A (colophon)
	Köcher 1963a: XVI and pl. 30–31 no. 28 (copy)
	Scheil 1921: 16–17 no. 13
Discussion:	Steinert 2018d: 225–226
	Scurlock and Andersen 2005: 40 no. 3.61, 287 no. 13.19, 784
	Collins 1999: 191–195

Obv. 1–3	Symptom description: "[If a ma]n's [...] is seized and there is c[ontinually] *kadabbedû*, his [tongu]e swells up, his breath is troubled, his salvia runs, (and) all his [t]eeth are week and ooze blood"
Obv. 4–6, 10–12	Ritual instructions involving water from the cistern of Marduk's temple and washing of the patient's mouth
Obv. 7–9, 13–16, 17–18	Incantations in (pseudo) Sumerian
Obv. 19–20 (*breaks off*), 1'–2'	Fragmentary ritual instructions
Rev. 3'–11', 14'–15'	Incantations in Akkadian and Sumerian
Rev. 12'–13', 16'	Ritual Instructions involving washing(?) the patient's mouth and a potion for drinking
Rev. 17'–18'	Colophon:

[(x)?] GIM SUMUN-*šú šà-ṭír bà-rì* [*ḫ*]*a-an-ṭiš na-às-ḫa* 18' [DU]B $^{*\text{p}*}$*Ki-ṣir*-$^{\text{d!}}$-[x (x)] ^{lú}MAŠ.MAŠ ⌜É AN.ŠÁR⌝

BAM 40 (VAT 13773(+)14073; Assur N4 no. 607)

Tablet:	Single-column tablet in portrait format; collated during the summer of 2016; H 71mm/W 69mm/T 22mm
Content:	Prescriptions with treatments of the chest, lungs and arms
CDLI no.:	P285140 (photograph)
Bibliography:	*Unedited*
	Köcher 1963a: XVIII and pl. 41–42 no. 40 (copy)
Discussion:	Table 19 note a
	Steinert 2018d: 229
	Scurlock and Andersen 2005: 189–90 no. 9.24, 713 note 34 (treatment and discussion of individual lines)

Obv. 1–6	Fragmentary diagnosis and prescription for applying (LÁL-*su-ma*) ingredients, measured according to a half mina, to an uncertain part of the body
Obv. 6–11	Fragmentary prescription
Obv. 12–14	Diagnosis: "If a man's chest (GABA.MEŠ-*šú*) [repeatedly] slacken (DUḪ.[MEŠ(?)]) [...] his innards ([...] ŠÀ-*šú*), there is a swelling (*dikšu* TUKU) [...], constantly [his] arm[s] [?], [con]stantly [...], his eyes continually turn (IGI.MEŠ-*šú* NIGIN.MEŠ] and st[and(?)] (DU.[BA(?)]) [...], (and) are infused with blood (MÚD *šu-un-u'-a*$^{!}$) [...]"
Obv. 15–17	Fragmentary prescription for "If a man's chest [repeatedly s]lacken [...]"
Obv. 18–21 (*breaks off*)	Fragmentary prescription for "[if a man]'s [...], an illness of the lungs (MUR.MEŠ GIG)
Rev. 1'–5', 6'–9'	Fragmentary prescriptions
Rev. 10'–12'	Prescription for seven bandages (NÍG.LAL) for a patient with an affected left arm
Rev. 13'–17'	Fragmentary prescription for a man with [...] in either the [left] or right arm
Rev. 18'–20'	Catch-line; fragmentary colophon:

[(x x x x x?)]⌜tab⌝ [(x x x x?)] 20' [(x) x] ú [x x x x] ⌜IM⌝ ^{p}*Ki-ṣir*-AN.ŠÁR [x x x (x)]

BAM **68** = ***KAL*** **10 no. 73** (A 258; Assur N4 no. 45)

Tablet: Single-column tablet in landscape format; not collated
Content: Prescription against a variety of afflictions
CDLI no.: P285167 (copy)
Bibliography: Maul 2019: 284–287 ms A (edition)
Cadelli 2000: 257–262 ms D (edition)
Hunger 1968: 76 no. 220 (colophon)
Köcher 1963a: XX and pl. 64 no. 68 (copy)
Discussion: Sections 9.3.4 and 9.5.1 as well as Table 21 note a

Obv. 1–rev. 17 Prescription consisting of 25 (Köcher's copy reads a total of 26, which must be mistake) ingredients weighted in ten shekels (obv. 4–10) and five shekels (rev. 11–12) to produce an enema (*ana* DÚR-*šú* DUB-*ak-ma*) for a man ill with *šibiṭ šāri*, *ḫimiṭ* [*ṣē*]*ti*, *šimmatu*, *r*[*imûtu*], *šaššaṭu*, *šugidimmakku*, *šunamerimmakku* ["Anus illness" (DÚR.GIG)?] or any illness (*u ka-la* GIG)
Rev. 18–20 Catch-line; colophon:

a-na ṣa-bat e-pe-š[*i*] ᴾ*Ki-ṣir*-an-[x x x (x)] [20] [T]A ŠÀ ᵍⁱˢZU [*ḫ*]*a-an-ṭiš* ZI-*ḫ*[*a*]

BAM 78 (A 261; Assur N4 no. 37)

Tablet: Single-column tablet in landscape format; not collated
Content: Prescriptions for treating the spleen
CDLI no.: P285177 (copy)
Bibliography: *Unedited*
Hunger 1968: 70 no. 201 ms A (colophon)
Köcher 1963a: XXI and pl. 69–70 no. 78 (copy)
Discussion: Stol 2006: 113
Scurlock and Andersen 2005: 135–36, 785

Obv. 1–6 Prescription for seeking out the sanctuary of Marduk (⌜*aš*⌝-*rat* ⌜d⌝[AMAR.U]TU) and sucking down liquid (*ú-na-ṣab-ma*) in case of a hurting spleen (*tulīmu*) where the patient cannot sleep day or night, his body holds fever (KÚM), and his intake of bread(?) and beer(?) decreases
Obv. 7–9 "Ditto" prescription for a substance to be eaten on an empty stomach
Rev. 10–17 Fragmentary prescription consisting of 12 plants
Rev. 18–20 Colophon:

a-na ṣa-bat [*e-pe-ši* ^{p}*Ki-ṣi*]*r-Aš-šur* ^{19} D[UMU $^{\text{p.d}}$PA-*be-sun*(?) $^{(\text{lú})}$]MAŠ.MAŠ É [*Aš-šur*] ^{20} *ḫa-a*[*n-ṭiš* ZI-*ḫa šà-ṭ*]*ir-ma b*[*à-rì*]

BAM **81** (A 240; Assur N4 no. 18)

Tablet: Single-column tablet in portrait format; not collated
Content: Prescriptions for treating *maškadu*-illness
CDLI no.: P285180 (copy)
Bibliography: *Unedited*
Hunger 1968: 68–69 no. 197 ms E (colophon)
Köcher 1963a: XXI and pl. 71 no. 81 (copy)
Discussion: Steinert 2018d: 240
Scurlock 2014: 305
Reiner 1995: 82 note 330

Obv. [Broken]
Rev. 1'–7' Prescription applied (LÁL) to release (*ip-pa-áš-šar*) *maškadu*
Rev. 8'–9' "Ditto" prescription for a potion for drinking
Rev. 10'–16' Prescription for an enema
Rev. 17'–18' Colophon:

ú-ìl-ti ^{p}*Ki-ṣir-Aš-šur* MAS.[MAŠ] $^{18'}$ [*ḫa*]*-an-ṭiš* ZI-[*ḫa*]

BAM **99** (A 274+VAT 13726; Assur N4 no. 161)

Tablet: Single-column tablet in portrait format; collated via the CDLI photograph
Content: Prescriptions for treating rectal maladies
CDLI no.: P285198 (photograph of VAT 13726)
Bibliography: Geller 2005: 212–217 no. 35 ms II (edition)
Hunger 1968: 71 no. 202 ms A (colophon)
Köcher 1963a: XXIII and pl. 87–88 no. 99 (copy)
Discussion: Scurlock and Andersen 2005: 52 no. 3.118, 121–122 no. 6.27, 148–149 no. 6.166, 349 no. 14–22, 786

Obv. 1–5 Prescription for a suppository for "[If a man] passes blood [from] his anus, that man suffers internally" (*qer-be-nu* GIG)
Obv. 6–12, 13–16 Fragmentary prescriptions for suppositories
Obv. 17–18 Prescription for a suppository for "If a man excretes blood (and) the middle of his anus stings him li[ke …]"

Obv. 19–24	Prescription for a suppository, a potion and a bath for "If a man passes blood from his anus like a haemorrhaging woman, […], (but) there is not 'Anus illness' (DÚR.GIG), he is ill with diarrhoea" (*ter-di-it ir-ri* GIG)
Obv. 25–26	Prescription for a suppository for "If a man is ill with 'Anus illness' (DÚR.GIG), defecates blood and the middle of his anus 'hastens'/trembles(?) (*qé-reb* DÚR-*šú i-ḫa-áš*)"
Obv. 27–29	Prescription for a potion to be drunk on an empty stomach for "If a man passes blood from his anus, (as if) struck by a weapon like a (menstruating) woman"
Obv. 30–32	Prescription for a potion to be drunk on an empty stomach for "[If a man] passes [blood from his anus], that man suffers internally"
Obv. 33, 34, 35, 36	Fragmentary prescriptions for potions
Rev. 37, 38, 39	Prescriptions for potions
Rev. 40–41	Prescription for a potion for drinking; noted break ([*ḫe*]-*pí eš-šú*)
Rev. 42–51	Prescription for a suppository, a potion, a bath, and a bandage for "If a man passes blood from his anus like a woman haemorrhaging, … and there is not 'Anus illness' (DÚR.GIG), he is ill with diarrhoea (lit.: overflow of the intestines, *ter-di-it ir-ri*)"
Rev. 52–53	Fragmentary prescription
Rev. 54–55	Prescription for an enema
Rev. 56–59	Colophon:

[56]7 *nis-ḫu* GABA.RI *É-sa-bad šá* BAL.TI[ki] [57] *a-na ṣa-bat e-pe-ši* [p]*Ki-ṣir-Aš-šur* MAŠ.MAŠ É *Aš-šur* [58] *za-mar ú-šaš-ṭir-ma íb-ri* [59] DUMU [p.d]AG-*bi-su-nu* MAŠ.MAŠ É AN.ŠÁR

BAM 102 (A 381+402; Assur N4 no. 21)

Tablet:	Single-column tablet in landscape format; not collated
Content:	An incantation against "Anus illness" (DÚR.GIG)
CDLI no.:	P285201 (copy)
Bibliography:	Geller 2005: 166–67 no. 26 ms AA_2 (edition)
	Hunger 1968: 70 no. 200 ms B (colophon)
	Köcher 1963a: XXIII and pl. 89 no. 102 (copy)
Discussion:	Sections 6.1 and 8.4.1
	Steinert 2018d: 239
	Maul 2009: 74–75
	Biggs 1967: 11

Obv.	[Broken]
Rev. 1	End of incantation continued from the obverse

Rev. 2	Rubric stating the incantation is against "Anus illness" (DÚR.GIG)
Rev. 3	Separate line: "Its ritual instruction is not written" (DÙ.DÙ.BI-*šú la šaṭ-ru*)
Rev. 4–7	Colophon:

IM.GÍD.DA ^{p}*Ki-ṣir-Aš-šur* MAŠ.MAŠ ^{5} DUMU $^{\text{p.d}}$AG-*bi-sún* MAŠ.MAŠ É AN.ŠÁR ^{6} [DUMU $^{\text{p.d}}$*B*]*a-ba*$_{6}$-MU-DÙ ZABAR.DAB.BA *É-šá*[*r-ra*] ^{7} [(x) x x x x x ZAB]AR.DAB$^{!}$.B[A (x x x?)]

***BAM* 121** (VAT 8949; Assur N4 no. 6)

Tablet:	Single-column tablet in landscape format; collated during the summer of 2015; H 63mm/W 108mm/T 20mm
Content:	Prescriptions for treating an uncertain upper body part and the feet
CDLI no.:	P285219 (photograph)
Bibliography:	*Unedited*
	Hunger 1968: 69 no. 198 ms B (colophon)
	Köcher 1963b: IX and pl. 6 no. 121 (copy)
Discussion:	Scurlock and Andersen 2005: 170 no. 8.25, 786

Obv. 1–3	Fragmentary prescription for a man's head, temples or epigastrium(?) (DIŠ NA SAG […])
Obv. 4, 5, 6, 7	Four one-line "Ditto" (DIŠ KI.MIN) prescriptions for anointing (MAR) the affected area
Obv. 8	Fragmentary prescription
Obv. 9, 10–11	Two fragmentary prescriptions for a man's feet (DIŠ NA GÌ[R^{II} …]; DIŠ NA GÌR[^{II}-*šú*(?) …])
Obv. 12	Fragmentary prescription for "If a man's feet are swollen" (DIŠ NA GÌR^{II}-*šú* MÚ.MÚ)
Obv. 13	"Ditto" (DIŠ <KI>.MIN) prescription applied (LÁ) to the affected area
Rev. 14–17	Fragmentary prescription for a man's feet (DIŠ NA GÌR^{II}-*šú i*-[…])
Rev. 18–23	Prescription for applying (LÁ) a remedy in the case "If a man's feet are ill (and) swollen with fever" (DIŠ NA GÌR^{II}-*šú* KÚM *e-sil-tu*$_{4}$ GI[G x])
Rev. 24–26	Colophon:

a-na ṣa-bat e-pe-ši ZI-[*ḫ*]*a*$^{!}$ ^{25} DUB-*pi* ^{p}ZÚ.KEŠDA-AN.ŠÁR *ša* ^{d}PA NIR-*su* ^{26} DUMU $^{\text{p.d}}$AG-*be-sun* ^{lú}MAŠ.MAŠ É AN.ŠÁR

***BAM* 122** (A 264+269; Assur N4 no. 265)

Tablet:	Single-column tablet in portrait format; not collated
Content:	Prescriptions for treating symptoms of the legs and feet
CDLI no.:	P285220 (copy)
Bibliography:	Scurlock 2014: 566–569 (edition)
	Köcher 1963b: x and pl. 7–8 no. 122 (copy)
Discussion:	Steinert 2018d: 240
	Böck 2010c: 103
	Scurlock and Andersen 2005: 249 no. 11.7, 291 no. 13.48, 338 no. 13.267, 517 no. 19.351, 786

Obv. 1–7	"If a man's shin continually slackens" (DIŠ NA *kim-ṣa-šú* DUḪ.DUḪ); prescription for a bandage (*ina* KUŠ *te-ṭer*$_5$*-ri* LÁ-*id*)
Obv. 8–15	"If a man's feet hurt him and there is paralysis, the 'strings' of his feet are stiff (and) his feet continually shift places" (DIŠ NA GÌR^{II}-*šú šim-ma-tú* TUKU GU$_7$.MEŠ-*šú* SA GÌR^{II}-*šú sa-ag-gu-ma* GÌR^{II}-*šú* ⸢BAL.BAL⸣-*šu*); prescription for a concoction that you regularly wash the patient with seven times (*a-di* 7-*šú* TU$_5$-*šú ta-sa-dar-šum-ma*)
Obv. 16–25	"If a man's feet hold paralysis (and) there is heat, and his walking around is difficult" (DIŠ LÚ GÌR^{II}-*šú šim-ma-tú ú-kal-la* KÚM.MA TUKU-*a ù a-na a-tál-lu-ku* DUGUD-*šú*); fragmentary prescription
Rev. 1'	[End of broken prescription]
Rev. 2'–10'	"If a man's 'string(s)' of the feet are stiff and he is not able to walk about" (DIŠ NA ⸢SA⸣ GÌR^{II}-*šú ša-gu-ma a-tál-lu-ka la i-le-ʾi*); prescription "for giving relief to the 'strings' of his feet" (*ana* SA.MEŠ GÌR^{II}-*šú pu-uš-šu-ḫi*)
Rev. 11'–17'	"[If a man]'s feet continually feel 'heavy' (and) [hurt] him, (and) he is not able [to walk about], that man's [feet are ill with(?) ...]" ([DIŠ NA] GÌR^{II}-*šú* DUGUD.MEŠ [GU$_7$]-*šú* [*a-tál-lu-ka*(?)] *la i-le-ʾi* NA BI ⸢x⸣[...]⸢x⸣ [...]-*šú*); prescription for anointing (ŠÉŠ.MEŠ-*ma*)
Rev. 18'–19'	Prescription for a potion
Rev. 20'–23'	Prescription without instructions for administering it
Rev. lo.e. 24'	Colophon:

[*ú-il*]-*ti* ^{p}*Ki-ṣir*-AN.ŠÁR MAŠ.MAŠ [(x x x?)]

***BAM* 129** (VAT 13790+13968(+); Assur N4 no. 588)

Tablet:	Tablet with two columns on each side in portrait format; collated during the summer of 2016
Content:	Abracadabra incantations and ritual instructions for treating *sagallu*-illness on the obverse, and diagnoses and prescriptions for treating *šaššaṭu*-illness on the reverse
CDLI no.:	P285226 (photograph)
Bibliography:	*Unedited* Köcher 1963b: XI and pl. 19–21 no. 129 (copy)
Discussion:	Wee 2012: 156–157, 168, 193, 208, 217–218 and notes 59–60, 254 and note 39, 312, 440, 471 and note 79, 473, 621–622 Scurlock and Andersen 2005: 297 no. 13.78, 786 Farber 2004: 127 note 54 Heeßel 2000: 372

Obv. col. i 1–6, 12–16, 20–23	Abracadabra incantations
Obv. col. 7, 17, 24	Rubrics: "Recitation for *sagallu*-illness" (KA.INIM.MA SA.GAL.LA.KÁM)
Obv. col. i 8–11, 18–19, 25–33	Ritual instructions
(*Breaks off*)	
Obv. col. ii 1'–3'	[Broken]
Obv. col. ii 4'–7', 17'–22', 23'–28'	Broken Abracadabra(?) incantations
Obv. col. ii 8'–16'	Ritual instructions
Obv. col. ii 29'	Broken rubric: "Two r[ecitations …] (2 K[A.INIM.MA …])
Obv. col. ii 30'	Broken ritual instructions
(*Breaks off*)	
[Rev. col. iii]	[Completely broken]
Rev. col. iv 1'–2'	Fragmentary prescription for applying (LÁ-*id*) a substance
Rev. col. iv 3'–5'	Diagnosis for *šaššaṭu*-illness with a stiff [neck] and hips ([DIŠ NA GÚ-*su*] MURUB$_4$^{II}-*šú aš-ṭa šá-áš-šá-ṭa* MU.NI) and a prescription for bandaging the patient (*ina* KUŠ SUR LÁ-*id*)
Rev. col. iv 6'–13'	Diagnosis for a man sick with *šaššaṭu*-illness, twisted neck, and yellow [eyes] ([DIŠ NA *šá-á*]*š-šá-ṭa* GIG GÚ-*su i-zu-ur* [IGI^{II}(?)]-*šú* SIG$_7$ ŠUB-*a* [*ana* TI]-*šú*) and a prescription for a fumigation(?) of the patient's

	bed (NE [ŠURUN GUD] NIGIN GIŠ.NÁ-⌈*šú*⌉ *ta-šár-rap*), relaxing his "strings" (SA.MEŠ-*šú i-pa-ša-ḫu*) and washing the patient (RA-*su-ma*)
Rev. col. iv 14'–17'	Diagnosis for a man ill with *šaššaṭu*-illness with affected neck, Achilles-tendons, hands and feet, and a prescription for bandaging the patient
Rev. col. iv 18'	"Ditto" prescription for anointing the patient continually (ŠÉŠ.MEŠ)
Rev. col. iv 19'–21'	Diagnosis for a man ill with *šaššaṭu*-illness and a fragmentary prescription
Rev. col. iv 22'–28'	Catch-line; colophon:

[(x x x x x)]⌈x a$^{?}$ x⌉[(x x x x x)] $^{24'}$ [(*nothing remains*)] $^{25'}$ [(*nothing remains*)] $^{26'}$ [(x) x ^{p}*Ki-ṣir*-AN].ŠÁR ^{lú}ŠÁMAN.LÁ BÀN.DA $^{27'}$ [DUMU x x x x x] ^{lú}MAŠ.MAŠ É AN.ŠÁR $^{28'}$ [DUMU x x x x x Z]ABAR.DAB.BA *É-šár-ra*

BAM **131** (VAT 13775; Assur N4 no. 601)

Tablet:	Single-column tablet in portrait format; collated during the summer of 2015; H 68mm/W 77 mm/T 25mm
Content:	Prescriptions for treating *šaššaṭu*-illness and various types of stiffness
CDLI no.:	P285228 (photograph)
Bibliography:	*Unedited*
	Hunger 1968: 71 no. 203 ms K (colophon)
	Köcher 1963b: XI and pl. 22 no. 131 (copy)
Discussion:	Steinert 2018d: 240
	Wee 2012: 471–472
	Scurlock and Andersen 2005: 249 no. 11.9 no. 11.10, 787
	Heeßel 2000: 372

Obv. 1–8	Fragmentary prescription against *šaššaṭu*-illness; contains several steps involving getting served by an innkeeper (^{lú}KÚRUN.NA) and being washed (TU$_5$-*šú*)
Obv. 9–15	Prescription for something dried up (*i-ba-al*, cf. BabMed's transliteration), eyes trembling on repeated occasions and being scared or farting; administered by applying (LAL) mixture from the neck to the shoulder blades, doing something to the patient's bed, and washing ([*ta-ra-aḫ*]-*ḫa-su*] the patient(?)

(*Breaks off*)

Rev. 1'–3'	Prescription for a bandage (*na-aṣ-mat-ti*) against a winter skin lesion/stiffness (*sik-ka-te/šig-ga*$_{14}$*-te šá* EN.TE.[NA])
Rev. 4'–6'	Prescription for a bandage (*na-aṣ-mat-ti*) against a skin lesion/ stiffness (*sik-ka-te/ šig-ga*$_{14}$*-te*)
Rev. 7'–8'	Prescription for a bandage (NÍG.LÁ) to soften up stiffness (*aš-ṭa ana lu-bu-ki*)
Rev. 9'–12'	(Catch-line); colophon:

[TA] [giš]ZU *šá bul-ṭi ša* É [d]ME.ME *šà-ṭir bà-rì* [11'] [DUB] [p]*Ki-ṣir*-AN.ŠÁR DUMU [p.d]PA-*be-sun* MAŠ.MAŠ [É AN.ŠÁR] [12'] *šà* IR [d]AG ZÀḪ-*a-šú liq*-[*bi*]

BAM **164** (A 234; Assur N4 no. 367)

Tablet:	Single-column tablet in portrait format; not collated
Content:	Prescriptions for treating renal and rectal problems
CDLI no.:	P285258 (copy)
Bibliography:	*Unedited*
	Geller 2005: 80–83, 124–125 ms zz (treatment of individual lines)
	Hunger 1968: 70 no. 201 ms B (colophon)
	Köcher 1963b: XVII and pl. 67–68 no. 164 (copy)
Discussion:	Steinert 2015: 125
	Scurlock and Andersen 2005: 111 no. 5.58, 787

Obv. 1–4	Potion (*mašqītu*) consisting of five ingredients to be drunk against a piercing pain (*di-ik-ši*)
Obv. 5–9	Potion consisting of 11 ingredients to be drunk for the kidneys (ÉLLAG)
Obv. 10–12	Potion consisting of five ingredients for the spleen (ŠÀ.GI$_6$)
Obv. 13–17	Tested potion consisting of nine ingredients to be drunk against discharge (*mu-ṣi lat-ku-ti*)
Obv. 18–21	Potion consisting of five ingredients for drinking "If a man repeatedly has an erection *when* he urinates[!] (text: because of his penis[(pl.)])" (DIŠ NA *ana* GÌŠ.MEŠ-*šú ma-gal* ZI.ZI-*bi*)
Obv. 22–rev. 25	Potion consisting of seven ingredients for drinking against "Anus illness" (DÚR.GIG)
Rev. 26–28	Potion consisting of five ingredients for the anus (DÚR)
Rev. 29–32	Fragmentary instructions for a potion for the hips (MURUB$_4$.MEŠ)
Rev. 33–35	Fragmentary instructions for a potion
Rev. 36–37	Colophon:

a-na ṣa-bat DÙ-*ši* [p]*Ki-ṣir*-AN.ŠÁR [37] [MAŠ.MAŠ É] *Aš-šur za-mar* ZI-*ḫa*

BAM 177 (A 209; Assur N4 no. 454)

Tablet:	Single-column tablet in landscape format; not collated
Content:	Prescriptions
CDLI no.:	P285269 (copy)
Bibliography:	*Unedited*
	Hunger 1968: 70 no. 201 ms C (colophon)
	Köcher 1963b: XIX and pl. 82 no. 177 (copy)
Discussion:	Section 8.2 and Ch. 8 note 22
	Steinert 2018d: 250
	Steinert 2015: 125
	Scurlock 2014: 462 note 51, 455 (*BAM* 124 col. iii 40)
	Scurlock and Andersen 2005: 788

Obv. 1–7	18 ingredients against *apišalû*-illness(?), tested (*lat-ku* ⸢x⸣[x])
Rev. 8–12	Bandage (*naṣmattu*, LAL-*ti*) of 12 ingredients against *ṣētu*-fever
Rev. 13–14	Colophon:

ana ṣa-bat e-pe-ši ᴾ*Ki-ṣir-Aš-šur* ¹⁴ MAŠ.MAŠ É *Aš-šur za-mar is-s*[*u-ḫ*]*a*

BAM 186 (VAT 8277; Assur N4 no. 124)

Tablet:	Single-column tablet in portrait format; collated during the summer of 2015; H 98mm/W 51mm/T 21mm
Content:	Prescriptions for treating internal illnesses
CDLI no.:	P285278 (photograph)
Bibliography:	*Unedited*
	Section 8.3.2 (treatment of individual lines)
	Couto-Ferreira 2018: 152–53, 158 (treatment of individual lines)
	Hunger 1968: 70 no. 201 ms D (colophon)
	Köcher 1963b: XX–XXI and pl. 90 no. 186 (copy)
Discussion:	Steinert 2015: 125 (treatment of individual lines)
	Scurlock and Andersen 2005: 138 no. 6.114, 788
	Böck 2014a: 125–126 note 106

Obv. 1–12	Tested rinse administered as an enema and considered good against *aḫḫāzu*- and *amurriqānu*-jaundice
Obv. 13	Subscript(?) to the previous rinse stating it is a rinse of oils against *ḫimiṭ ṣēti*
Obv. 14–rev.23	Fragmentary prescription of 18 oils, which "I have collected" (*aš-bu-uš* Š[U$^{(\text{II?})}$ (x)])

Rev. 24–31 Enema consisting of eight ingredients
Rev. 32–34 Colophon:

a-na ṣa-bat e-pe-ši [33] P*Ki-ṣir-Aš-šur* MAŠ.MAŠ É [*Aš-šur*] [34] *ḫa-an-ṭiš na-a*[*s*]-*ḫa*

BAM 188 (A 266; Assur N4 no. 313)

Tablet:	Single-column tablet in portrait format; not collated
Content:	Prescription for treating internal illnesses
CDLI no.:	P285280 (copy)
Bibliography:	Section 8.3.2 (edition)
	Couto-Ferreira 2018: 152–53 (edition)
	Hunger 1968: 70 no. 201 ms E (colophon)
	Köcher 1963b: XXI and pl. 90 no. 188 (copy)
Discussion:	Scurlock and Andersen 2005: 139 no. 6.119, 788

Obv.	[Broken]
Rev. 1–10	An enema consisting of 14 ingredients for "If a man is ill (from) bile (*martu*), *aḫḫāzu*- or *amurriqānu*-jaundice"
Rev. 11–13	Colophon:

a-na ṣa-bat e-pe-ši [12] P*Ki-ṣir-Aš-šur* MAŠ.MAŠ É *Aš-*[*šur*] [13] *ḫa-an-ṭiš is-su-*[*ḫa*]

BAM 201 = ***KAL*** 10 no. 80 (VAT 13787; Assur N4 no. –)

Tablet:	Single-column tablet in portrait format; collated during the summer of 2016; H 122mm/W 60mm/T 22mm
Content:	Prescriptions for treating *māmītu*-curse and associated symptoms
CDLI no.:	P285292 (photograph)
Bibliography:	Maul 2019: 309–312, 530–531 (photo and edition)
	Hunger 1968: 69 no. 199 ms D (colophon)
	Köcher 1964: XI and pl. 2–3 no. 201 (copy)
Discussion:	Schuster-Brandis 2008: 211
	Scurlock and Andersen 2005: 788

Obv. 1'–15'	Fragmentary prescription to make a bandage of cloth (*ina* TÚG SUR-*ri* LÁ-*id*)
Obv. 16'–22'	"Ditto" prescription for inducing vomit and to make a bandage of cloth
Obv. 23'–28'	Prescription for a bandage of the flesh ([… UZ]U.MEŠ-*šú* LÁ-*id*) for "If a man's insides continually becomes swollen and there is a

	hot fever, his(?) [...] is swollen (and) his inside (are) constricted, his fee[t] are raised [...]; that man (suffers from) 'Hand of Curse (or) *kadabbedû*"
Obv. 29'–30'	Prescription for a bandage(?) for a man who is "ill, and he continually throws up blood and pus with his saliva"
Rev. 31'–41'	Prescription for a bandage of the epigastrium (SAG ŠÀ-*šú*), something to be eaten, and a potion for "[If a man]'s eyes are full of yellow, that man (is ill from) 'Hand of Curse"
Rev. 42'–49'	Catch-line; colophon:

TA ŠÀ ^{giš}ZU *šá bul-ṭi ša* É ^{d}ME.ME $^{45'}$ SAR È *ḫa-an-ṭiš na-às-ḫa* $^{46'}$ ⌜*ú-ìl-ti* ^{p}*Ki-ṣir*-AN.ŠÁR ŠÁMAN.LÁ TUR⌝ $^{47'}$ [DUMU $^{\text{p.d}}$A]G-⌜*bi-su-nu* MAŠ.MAŠ É⌝ [AN.ŠÁR] $^{48'}$ [(x) x x x x(?)] i[g]i(?) [x x x x (x)?] $^{49'}$ [(x) x x x x(?)]⌜x⌝[x x x x (x)?] (*breaks off*)

***BAM* 202** (VAT 13739+14130; Assur N4 no. 476)

Tablet:	Single-column tablet in portrait format; collated during the summer of 2015; H 117mm/W 79mm/T 22mm
Content:	Prescriptions for treating psychological and neurological problems
CDLI no.:	P285293 (photograph)
Bibliography:	Arbøll 2019 (new copy and edition) Chalendar 2013 (edition) Hunger 1968: 70 no. 201 ms F (colophon) Köcher 1964: XI and pl. 4–5 no. 202 (old copy)
Discussion:	Steinert 2018d: 249 Böck 2010b: 94 Stol 2009: 2 note 10, 6–7, 11–12 Scurlock and Andersen 2005: 83 no. 3.268, 315 no. 13.169, 375 no. 16.43, 383 no. 16.87, 788 Heeßel 2000: 86 note 61, 223 Stol 1993: 5–7 and note 10, 20–21 and note 163, 49–50 and notes 259 and 261, 149–150 and note 14 Farber 1977: 74–75 note 4

Obv. 1–6	Prescription for fumigation and anointment for "If *dem*[*makurr*]*û* (derangement) has seized a man and his mind a[lters time and again], his speech is incoherent, he [get]s a dep[ression] time and again (lit.: his [min]d continually fa[lls on him]), and he talks a lot, (in order) to res[tore] his mind to him ..."
Obv. 7–8	"Ditto" prescription for a potion to be drunk on an empty stomach

Obv. 9–12	“Ditto” prescription for producing a figurine, providing it with clothing, and eating a substance
Obv. 13–16	Fragmentary prescription for a fumigation ceremony
Obv. 17–rev. 4’	Fragmentary prescription for producing a figurine of the patient’s body and marrying it off to the demon afflicting the patient
Rev. 5’–11’	Prescription for placing ingredients around the patient’s neck for “If a man continually j[er]ks in his bed, he cries like a goat, he groans, he shudders (lit.: he is afraid), (and) he talks a lot: “Hand of *bennu*-epilepsy”, a [*šē*]*du*-demon deputized by Sîn.”
Rev. 12’, 13’	Two “ditto” prescriptions for a leather bag worn around the neck
Rev. 14’–15’	Colophon and final fragmentary statement:

a-na ṣa-bat e-pe-ši ^{p}*Ki-*[*ṣir*-x-x (x x x x?)] $^{15'}$ ⸢*ṣa*$^{!}$⸣-[*l*]*a*[*m*$^{?}$] ⸢$^{\text{d}!?}$(diš)⸣-*be*$^{?}$-*e*[*n*$^{?}$]-⸢*na*$^{!?}$⸣ *šá-n*[*é-e* ^{d}30]

The tablet contains a previously unnoticed drawing of a demon after the colophon. The last line of the colophon is written in a slightly smaller hand and likely relates to this drawing.

BAM **206** (A 245; Assur N4 no. 355)

Tablet:	Single-column tablet in portrait format; not collated
Content:	Prescription for treating witchcraft
CDLI no.:	P285296 (copy)
Bibliography:	*CMAwR* 1: 53–55 no. 1.6. ms A and pl. 129 no. 12–18 (edition and collations) Hunger 1968: 75 no. 219 (colophon) Köcher 1964: XII and pl. 8 no. 206 (copy)

Obv.	[Broken]
Rev. 1’–15’	Fragmentary prescription
Rev. 16’–17’	Colophon:

a-na pi-še-er-ti kiš-pi šá ina UZ[U GU_7.MEŠ(?)] $^{17'}$ IM.GÍD.⸢DA⸣ ^{p}*Ki-ṣi*[*r-*... (*breaks off*)]

BAM **260** (A 215; Assur N4 no. 30)

Tablet:	Single-column tablet in portrait format(?); not collated
Content:	Prescriptions for making a man drunk and thirsty
CDLI no.:	P285344 (copy)
Bibliography:	Heeßel 2002b: 102–103 (partial edition) Köcher 1964: XX and pl. 60 no. 260 (copy)

Commentary:	Scurlock and Andersen 2005: 361 no. 15.15, 789
	Geller and Cohen 1995: 1813 and note 26

Obv./rev.? 1–3	Prescription for a potion for making a man drunk (DIŠ NA *a-na šu-uk-ku-ri*)
Obv./rev.? 4, 5–6	"Ditto" prescriptions for a potion
Obv./rev.? 7–10	Prescription for making a man thirsty (DIŠ NA *a-na ṣu-um-me-e*)
Obv./rev.? 11	Fragmentary prescription
Obv./rev.? 12–15	Fragmentary prescription for "If a man coug[hs ...]" (DIŠ NA *gu-uḫ-*[*ḫa* ...])
Obv./rev.? 16	Colophon:

ú-ìl-ti ᵖ*Ki-*[*ṣir-*x x]

BAM **300** (A 383; Assur N4 no. 312)

Tablet:	Single-column tablet in landscape format; not collated
Content:	Prescription for a universally applicable fumigation procedure
CDLI no.:	P285384 (copy)
Bibliography:	Section 8.4 (edition)
	Hunger 1968: 69 no. 198 ms C (colophon)
	Köcher 1964: XXII and pl. 70 no. 300 (copy)

Obv.	[Broken]
Rev. 1'–4'	Prescription for anointing and fumigating the patient
Rev. 5'	Subscript stating that the prescription is considered good against all maladies ([*šu*]-*ut bu-luṭ gim-ri ka-la-ma* SIG_5-*iq*)
Rev. 6'–7'	Colophon:

[*a-n*]*a ṣa-bat e-pe-ši ḫa-an-ṭiš* ZI-*ḫa* ⁷' [*ú-ì*]*l-ti* ᵖ*Ki-ṣir-Aš-šur* MAŠ.MAŠ É *Aš-šur*

BAM **303** (A 220; Assur N4 no. 430)

Tablet:	Single-column tablet in portrait format; not collated
Content:	Prescriptions for the feet
CDLI no.:	P285387 (copy)
Bibliography:	*Unedited*
	Hunger 1968: 70 no. 200 ms D (colophon)
	Köcher 1964: XXII and pl. 72 no. 303 (copy)
Discussion:	Steinert 2015: 127–128
	Geller 2010: 193 note 178
	Scurlock and Andersen 2005: 170 no. 8.27, 789

Obv. 1'–4'	Fragmentary prescription
Obv. 5'–8'	Tested prescription with ingredients (*maš-ši-ti*/ḪI-*tú*) for softening up (*šá lu-u*[*b-bu*]-*ki*)
Obv. 9'–10', 11'–13'	Two "ditto" prescriptions
Obv. 14–rev.23'	Prescription for "ingredients for softening up [feet(?)], which are stricken with wind and stiffness" (*maš-ši-ti šá* [GÌR^{II}(?)] *šá* IM *id-*[*p*]*í-t*[*u*] *ù šá-ag-gi a-na lu-ub-bu-*[*ki*]) to be scattered (*ana* IGI *ta-za-ru*); the final line designates all four prescriptions as "ingredients which softens up" (4 *maš-šá-a-ti šá lu-ub-bu-*[*ki*])
Rev. 24'–27'	Colophon:

bul-ṭu lat-ku šá ŠU^{II} UM.ME.A $^{25'}$ DUB ^{p}*Ki-ṣir-*^{d}*Aš-šur* MAŠ.MAŠ É *Aš-šur* $^{26'}$ DUMU $^{p.d}$PA-*be-sun* MAŠ.MAŠ É *Aš-šur* $^{27'}$ DUMU $^{p.d}$*Ba-ba*$_{6}$-M[U]-DÙ

BAM **307** (A 257; Assur N4 no. 351)

Tablet:	Single-column tablet in portrait format; not collated
Content:	Commentary-like, possibly pharmacological, text
CDLI no.:	P285391 (copy)
Bibliography:	*Unedited*
	Hunger 1968: 71 no. 202 ms B (colophon)
	Köcher 1964: XXIII and pl. 74 no. 307 (copy)
Discussion:	Section 7.6
	Scurlock and Andersen 2005: 789

Obv.	[Broken]
Rev. 1–27	Individual fragmentary entries providing alternative readings of several ritual ingredients, possibly serving a commentary-like purpose
Rev. 28–29	Colophon:

[(Broken)] ^{p}*Ki-ṣir-*AN.ŠÁR DUMU $^{p.d}$PA-*be-sún* ^{29} [(Broken) *ú-š*]*aš-ṭir-ma ib-ri*

BAM **311** (VAT 8914; Assur N4 no. 141)

Tablet:	Single-column tablet in portrait format; collated during the summer of 2016; H 171mm/W 76mm/T24mm
Content:	Prescriptions for producing leather bags worn around the neck
CDLI no.:	P285395 (copy)
Bibliography:	*Unedited*
	Hunger 1968: 75 no. 218 (colophon)
	Köcher 1964: XXIII–XXIV and pl. 75–77 no. 311 (copy)

Discussion: Arbøll 2019 (discussion of individual lines)
Steinert 2018d: 249, 259–60, 262
Scurlock 2014: 667, 701, 754
CMAwR 1: 49–52
Böck 2010b: 92–93
Schuster-Brandis 2008: 63 and note 179
Scurlock and Andersen 2005: 83 no. 3.268, 315 no. 13.169, 422 no. 18.25, 789
Heeßel 2000: 86 note 61, 223, 316 and note 15
Stol 1993: 6 and note 10, 16 and notes 110–111, 29 and note 49, 30 and note 61, 37 and note 140, 41 and notes 166–167, 82 and note 101, 103–104 and notes 31, 33, 40, and 44, 150 and note 14

Obv. 1', 2', 3', 4', 5', 6', 7', 8', 9, 10'–13', 14', 15', 16', 17', 18'–19', 20', 21'
"Ditto" prescriptions for leather bags worn around the neck

Obv. 22' Subscript: "15 leather bags worn around the neck, if a man has *ḫūṣ ḫīp(i) libbi*" (15 *me-eli* DIŠ NA *ḫu-uṣ* GAZ ŠÀ-*bi* TUKU.MEŠ-*ši*)

Obv. 23'–24' Instruction for a leather bag worn around the neck in the case of Lugal-urra; obv. 24' has a previously unnoticed KÚR sign on the left edge designating a mistake in the line

Obv. 25', 26', 27', 28', 29', 30', 31', 32', 33', 34', 35', 36', 37', 38', 39'–40'
"Ditto" prescriptions for leather bags worn around the neck

Obv. 41' Prescription for a leather bag worn around the neck for a specific fragmentary circumstance

Obv. 42' Prescription for a leather bag worn around the neck to keep *mimma lemnu* from approaching a man (DIŠ *mim-*[*ma* Ḫ]UL *ana* NA NU [T]E-*e*)

Obv. 43', 44', 45' "Ditto" prescriptions for leather bags worn around the neck

Obv. 46' Prescription for a leather bag worn around the neck to keep *mimma lemnu* from seeking out a man's bed (DIŠ *mim-ma* ḪUL *ana* GIŠ.NÚ NA NU DIM$_4$)

Obv. 47' Prescription for a leather bag worn around the neck "If a man is seized by an evil *alû*-demon" (DIŠ NA A.LÁ.ḪUL DAB-*su*)

Obv. 48', 49', 50' "Ditto" prescriptions for leather bags worn around the neck

Rev. 51'–55' Prescription for a leather bag worn around the neck "If a man continually jerks [in] his bed, he cries like a goat, he g[rowls], he shudders, (and) he cries out a lot, "hand" of *bennu*, [a *šedû* deputized by Sîn]" (DIŠ N[A *ina* K]I.NÁ-*šú* ḪULUḪ.⌜ḪULUḪ⌝-*ut* GIM GÙ ÙZ GÙ-*si* ⌜*i*⌝-[*ram-mu-um*] *i-par-ru-ud ma-ga*[*l*] GÙ.GÙ-*si* ŠU *be-en-nu* ^{d}[ÀLAD *šá-né-e* ^{d}30])

Rev. 56'	"Ditto" prescription for a leather bag worn around the neck
Rev. 57'–58'	Prescription for a leather bag worn around the neck "If a man [...] (and) weeps continuously" (DIŠ N[A ..] *ib-ta-na-ki*)
Rev. 59'	Prescription for a leather bag worn around the neck in the case of Antašubba
Rev. 60', 61', 62', 63', 64', 65', 66'–67', 68', 69'–70', 71', 72', 73', 74'–75', 76'	"Ditto" prescriptions for leather bags worn around the neck
Rev. 77'–78'	Prescription for a leather bag worn around the neck in the case of Antašubba, Lugal-urra or [...]
Rev. 79'–80', 81'–82', 83', 84', 85', 86'	"Ditto" prescriptions for leather bags worn around the neck
Rev. 87'–89'	Prescription for a leather bag worn around the neck "If a man grinds his teeth [in] his b[ed]" (DIŠ [N]A [*ina*] K[I.NÁ]-*šú* ZÚ.MEŠ-*šú* ZÚ.GUZ-⌜*aṣ*⌝)
Rev. 90' 91', 92', 93'	Fragmentary prescriptions for leather bags worn around the neck
Rev. 94'–96'	Colophon:

[(x) x x x]⌜x⌝ SAR È *a-na ṣa-bat* DÙ-*ši* ᴾ*Ki-ṣir*-AN.[ŠÁR(?)] 95' [x x x x] ˡᵘ́MAŠ.MAŠ É *Aš-šur ḫa-an-ṭiš* ZI-*ḫa* 96' [x x x]⌜x⌝ GIM LIBIR.RA [x x (x)]

***BAM* 321** (VAT 13690; Assur N4 no. 493)

Tablet:	Single-column tablet in portrait format; collated during the summer of 2015; H 124mm/W 73mm/T 23mm
Content:	Incantation ritual for a man's god and goddess
CDLI no.:	P285403 (photograph)
Bibliography:	*Unedited*
	Köcher 1971: IX and pl. 3–4 no. 321 (copy)
Discussion:	Steinert 2018d: 254
	Böck 2014a: 78–79 note 8

Obv. 1–9	Prayer for a man's god and goddess (DINGIR-*šú u* ᵈ*iš*₈-*tár-šú*)
Obv. 10–17	Fragmentary ritual instruction involving numerous plants
Obv. 18–23	Fragmentary incantation
Obv. 24–26	Fragmentary ritual instruction
Obv. 27–31	Prayer for Nabû and Tašmētu (ᵈAG *u* ᵈ*taš-me-tù*) mentioning a mother (AMA *a-lit-ti-šú*)
Rev. 32–51	Fragmentary ritual instruction mentioning various gods and the temple of Marduk
Rev. 52–55	Colophon:

[(x) x x x x]⸢x x x⸣[(x x)] ^{53} [(x) x x x]⸢x⸣[x x x] MAŠ.MAŠ ⸢É⸣ [*A*]*š*-⸢*šur*⸣ ^{54} [$^{p.d}$*Nabû*$^{?}$-*bi*$^{?}$-*s*]*u*$^{?}$[-*nu*$^{?}$ ⸣]$^{ú?}$MAŠ.MAŠ É *Aš-šur* ^{55} [DUMU $^{p.d}$*Ba-b*]*a*$_{6}$-MU-DÙ ^{lú}Z[ABA]R.DAB.BA *É-šár-r*[*a*]

BAM **333** (A 479; Assur N4 no. 320)

Tablet:	Fragmentary single-column tablet in portrait(?) format; not collated
Content:	Fragment of a mythological incantation
CDLI no.:	P285413 (copy)
Bibliography:	*Unedited*
	Köcher 1971: XI-XII and pl. 18 no. 333 (copy)
Discussion:	*CAD* Š/1: 318

Obv. 1–8	Fragment of a mythological incantation: "When Anu begat the heaven [...], (and) Ea established the (healing) plant's on earth(/in the netherworld?) ..." (ÉN *šu-un-du* ^{d}*A-nu ir-ḫu-u* AN *iš*(?)-[x] ^{d}DIŠ <*ina*> KI-*tí u-kin-nu ša*[*m-mu*])
(*breaks off*)	
Rev. 1'–4'	Colophon:

a-na ṣa-bat e-[*pe-ši*] $^{2'}$ ^{p}*Ki-ṣir*-AN.ŠÁR DUMU $^{p.d}$PA-*b*[*e-sun*] $^{3'}$ ^{lú}MAŠ.MAŠ É AN.[ŠÁR] $^{4'}$ *ḫa-an-ṭiš is-su-ḫa*

BAM **351** (A 260; Assur N4 no. 38)

Tablet:	Single-column tablet in portrait format; not collated
Content:	Prescription for treating an eye illness
CDLI no.:	P285423 (copy)
Bibliography:	Heeßel 2010d: 157–58 (translation)
	Köcher 1971: XIV and pl. 29 no. 351 (copy)
Discussion:	Schuster-Brandis 2008: 105, 107 no. 58, 264
	Scurlock and Andersen 2005: 789
	Fincke 2000: 90–91

Obv.	[Broken]
Rev. 1–6	List of stones
Rev. 7–12	Prescription for the 11 listed stones against an eye illness (*bir-rat* IGI^{II}) where reed wool is plaited and the stones are harrowed thereon, seven wrappings are made and bound (KEŠDA-*su-ma*) to the patient's left hand while reciting the incantation "release the sight" (ÉN IGI.DU$_{8}$ DUḪ) twice
Rev. 13–15	Catch-line; colophon:

ana ṣa-bat DÙ-*ši* ^{p}*Ki-ṣir-Aš-šur* ^{15} *ḫa-an-ṭiš* ZI-*ḫa*

BAM **366** (VAT 13822; Assur N4 no. 307)

Tablet:	Slim tablet with two columns in portrait format; collated during the summer of 2016; H 97mm/W 57mm/T 20mm
Content:	List taking stock of stones availiable in the N4 house
CDLI no.:	P285437 (photograph)
Bibliography:	*Unedited*
	Köcher 1971: XIX and pl. 40–41 no. 366 (copy)
Discussion:	Schuster-Brandis 2008: 61–62 and note 172

Obv. col. i 1–19	Various stones of which the N4 collection had between 6–14 of each
(*Breaks off*)	
Obv. col. ii 1–24	Various stones of which the N4 collection had between 2–5 of each
(*Breaks off*)	
Rev. col. iii 1'–25'	Various stones of which the N4 collection had between 1–2 of each
Rev. col. iv 1'–17'	Various stones of which the N4 collection had 1 of each
Rev. col. iv 18'–23'	A statements concluding the list: "A total of 315 stones (for) 'neck-(amulet(s))' of Marduk, which *are suitable for use*, placed [*in*? ...], the tablets"; colophon:

[x] ^{p}*Ki-ṣir*-[x x] $^{23'}$ [x x x x x(?)]

Beckman and Foster 1988 no. 21 (YBC 7124+7138(+)7141; Assur N4 no. –)

Tablet:	Fragmentary tablet with two columns in portrait(?) format; collated via private photographs
Content:	Unknown incantation ritual
CDLI no.:	P308113; P308127; P308130 (no images)
Bibliography:	*Unedited*
	Beckman and Foster 1988: 4, 23–24 no. 21 (copy)

Obv. col. i 1–26'	Unknown incantation ritual with a longer fragmentary entry of uncertain content
Obv. col. ii	[Broken]
Rev. col. iii 1'–8'	Two fragmentary entries, both possibly mentioning figurines (NU.MEŠ)
Rev. col. iv 1'–4"	Colophon:

[(*completely broken*)] 2' [LIBIR.RA.BI].GIM AB.SAR BA.AN.È.A 3' [(*break of uncertain length*) PKi-ṣir(?)]-⌜AN⌝.ŠÁR lúMAŠ.MAŠ É AN.ŠÁR [(*break of uncertain length, one or more lines broken after col. iv 3'*)] 4" [(*break of uncertain length*)] *la ta-pa*!*-šiṭ*

CT 37 **pl. 24–25** (BM 108861; Assur N4 no. 624)

Tablet:	Tablet with two columns on each side in portrait format; not collated
Content:	Lú lexical list with Sumerian terms and Akkadian readings
CDLI no.:	P366023 (copy)
Bibliography:	Civil 1969: 227–230 (edition)
	Hunger 1968: 71 no. 203 ms F (colophon)
	CT 37 pl. 24–25 (copy)
Discussion:	Meier 1937–39: 246 and note 38

Obv. col. i 1'–17'	Fragmentary entries from a Lú lexical list with Sumerian terms read as *bārû* and *āšipu*
Obv. col. ii	[Broken]
Rev. col. iii 1'–38'+col. iv 1'–30'	Lú lexical list with Sumerian titles and Akkadian translations of professions; individual lines include notes on the pronunciation of Sumerograms
Rev. 31'–34'	Colophon:

[LIBIR.RA.BI].GIM AB.SAR.ÀM BA.AN.È 32' [(DUB P*Ki-ṣi*]*r-Aš-šur* lúMAŠ.MAŠ 33' [(DUMU p.dPA-*be-su-nu*) l]úMAŠ.MAŠ É *Aš-šur* 34' [(DUMU p.d*Ba-ba*$_6$-MU-DÙ) lúZABA]R.DAB.BA *É-šár-r*[*a*] (*Breaks off*)

KAL **4 no.** 7 (VAT 13607+13970+14027; Assur N4 no. –)

Tablet:	Single-column fragment in portrait(?) format; not collated
Content:	Apotropaic *namburbi*-ritual connected to withcraft
CDLI no.:	P480931 (–)
Bibliography:	*CMAwR* 2: 408–418 no. 11.3 ms E (edition)
	Maul and Strauß 2011: 10, 34–35 no. 7, 176–77 (copy and edition)

Obv. 1'–6'	Diagnostic statement with a description to keep bad omens from a man and his house
Obv. 7'–10'	Ritual instruction
Obv. 11'–15'	Prayer for Šamaš

(*Breaks off*)

Rev. 1'–3'	"Ditto" ritual instruction
Rev. 4'–6'	List of days suitable for conducting the ritual to keep witchcraft from coming near a man for the rest of his life ([*a-di*] AL.TI *kiš-pi* NU TE.MEŠ-*šú*)
Rev. 7'–8'	Colophon:

[*ú-ìl-t*]*i šá* ^{p}*Ki*-⸢*ṣir*⸣-*Aš-šur* MAŠ.MAŠ ^{p}*Aš-šur-šá-k*[*ìn*-MU] $^{8'}$ [(x x x x x)]⸢x⸣[(x x)]⸢x⸣ EN ⸢x⸣[(*breaks off*)]

KAL **4 no. 19** (VAT 14005; Assur N4 no. –)

Tablet:	Single-column fragment in portrait(?) format; collated during the summer of 2016
Content:	Fragmentary ritual
CDLI no.:	P499676 (–)
Bibliography:	Maul and Strauß 2011: 13, 48–49, 184 (copy and edition)

Obv.	[Broken]
Rev. 1'–4'	Remains of a ritual instruction possibly describing a figurine thrown into the river ([N]U$^{?}$ *a-na* ÍD ⸢ŠUB⸣-[*di*])
Rev. 5'-lo.e. 8'	Colophon:

[GIM LIBI]R-*šu* [*š*]*à-ṭir ba*-[*ri*] $^{6'}$ [DUB(?) ^{p}*K*]*i-ṣir-Aš-šur* ŠÁMAN.LÁ T[UR] $^{7'}$ [DUMU $^{p.d}$*Nabû-bé-s*]*u-n*[*u*] MAŠ.MAŠ É AN.Š[ÁR] $^{8'}$ [*ḫa-an-ṭiš*] *is-su-ha*

KAL **4 no. 37** (VAT 14006; Assur N4 no. –)

Tablet:	Single-column fragment in portrait(?) format; not collated
Content:	Fragmentary ritual against an evil spirit(?)
CDLI no.:	P499684 (–)
Bibliography:	Maul and Strauß 2011: 17, 85–86, 206 (copy and edition)

Obv. 1–9	Fragmentary ritual instruction
Obv. 10–14	Fragmentary prayer
(*Breaks off*)	
Rev. 1'–6'	Fragmentary ritual instruction providing provisions for a figurine(?), presumably of an evil spirit
Rev. 7'–10'	Colophon:

[(LIBIR.RA.BI.GIM AB.SAR?) B]A.AN.È $^{8'}$ [(x x x x x x) *ša* ^{d}*Nabû* NI]R-*su* $^{9'}$ [DUMU (^{p}x x x x x) MAŠ.MAŠ] É *Aš-šur* $^{10'}$ [DUMU (^{p}x x x x x) MAŠ.MAŠ] É *Aš-šur*

***KAL* 4 no. 41** (VAT 13599; Assur N4 no. –)

Tablet: Single-column fragment in portrait(?) format; collated during the summer of 2016

Content: Ritual possibly for treating *garābu*

CDLI no.: P499688 (–)

Bibliography: Maul and Strauß 2011: 17–18, 90–92, 210 (copy and edition)

Obv. 1–8 Diagnostic statement, possibly describing the illness *garābu*, and a fragmentary ritual instruction where something is thrown into the river (*a-na* ÍD ŠUB-*di*)

Obv. 9–12 Fragmentary ritual instruction preserving three plants

(*Breaks off*)

Rev. 1'–3' Colophon:

[(DUB$^{?}$-*pi*$^{?}$) ^{p}*Ki-ṣi*]*r*-AN.ŠÁR ŠÁMAN.LÁ T[UR] $^{2'}$ [DUMU $^{p.d}$*Nabû-bēssun*(*u*) ^{l}]^{ú}MAŠ.MAŠ É AN.Š[ÁR] $^{3'}$ [DUMU $^{p.d}$*Ba-ba*$_{6}$-MU-DÙ ^{lú}Z]ABAR.DAB.BA *É-š*[*ár-ra*]

***KAL* 7 no. 24** (VAT 7820; Assur N4 no. –)

Tablet: Single-column tablet in portrait format; collated from the photograph in *KAL* 7

Content: A ritual for "entering the palace" (É-gal-ku$_{4}$-ra)

CDLI no.: –

Bibliography: Meinhold 2017: 8, 61–63, 164–165, 194–195 (photograph, copy and edition)

Obv. 1–8, 12–14 Incantations

Obv. 9, 15 Rubrics: "Recitation for entering the palace"

Obv. 10–11 Ritual instructions

(*Breaks off*)

Rev. 1'–3' Fragmentary incantation

Rev. 4' Rubric, same as the above

Rev. 5'–7' Ritual instructions

Rev. 8'–10' Catch-line; colophon:

⌜4$^{?}$-*ú*⌝ *nis-ḫu* GIM SUMUN-*šú* ⌜SAR⌝ [*b*]*a*-⌜*ri*⌝ $^{10'}$ [*ú-il-t*]*i* ^{p}*Ki-ṣir-Aš-šur* [MAŠ.MAŠ(?)]

***KAL* 9 no. 41** (VAT 20444b+VAT 20652; Assur N4 no. –)

Tablet: Single-column tablet in portrait(?) format; not collated

Content: Fragmentary prayer and a brief ritual instruction

CDLI no.: –

Bibliography:	Jakob 2018: 11, 91–92, 212 (copy and edition)
Obv. 1–9+rev. 1'–2'(?)	Fragmentary prayer to various gods concerning transgressions (*gillatu* and *ḫiṭītu*)
Rev. 3'	Ritual instruction: "You re[cite (it)] 3 times in fr[ont of] [(*divinity*)]"
Rev. 4'–5'	Colophon:

[*a-na ṣa-bat*] ⌜*e*⌝*-pe-ši* ᴾ*Ki-ṣir-*[(*breaks off*)] 5' [(x x x x x) *z*]*a-mar* SA[R-*ma*? È (*breaks off*)]

KAL **10 no. 1** (VAT 13760; Assur N4 no. –)

Tablet:	Single-column tablet in portrait(?) format; not collated
Content:	Guidelines for performing a ritual against a "Curse" (*māmītu*)
CDLI no.:	–
Bibliography:	Maul 2019: 71–98 ms A, 389–395 (photograph, copy and edition)

Obv. 1'–18'	Ritual instructions for performing libations for various gods, applying ritual remedies for the patient and a figurine of the "Curse", reciting incantations and sacrificing a sheep for divination
Obv. 19', 20', 21'	Incantation incipits and brief ritual instructions
Obv. 22'–24'	Ritual instructions
Obv. 25'	Incantation incipit and a brief ritual instruction
(*Breaks off*)	
Rev. 1', 2', 3', 4', 5'–6', 7', 8', 9', 10'–11', 12', 13', 14'–15', 16', 17'–18', 19', 20'–21'	Incantation incipits and brief ritual instructions
Rev. 22'–23'	Ritual instructions for the patient ([lú G]IG)
Rev. 24'–27'	Ritual instructions for dealing with the figurine of the "Curse" to release the evil (ḪUL-*š*[*ú* DU$_8$-*ir*])
Rev. 28'–29'	Colophon:

[(x) x x x x x x x x *ana ṣa*]*-bat e-pe-š*[*i* x x x x x (x)] 29' [(x) x ᴾ*Kiṣir-Aššur* DUMU] ⌜p.dAG⌝-*bé-*[*sun*(*u*) x x x x x (x)] (*breaks off*)

KAL **10 no. 4** = ***LKA*** **151+153** (VAT 13618+13627+13858+13886+14056a+14956b+14056c+14057+ 14058(+)14056d; Assur N4 nos. 551 and 556)

Tablet:	Single-column tablet in portrait format; not collated
Content:	Incantations and ritual instructions for releasing a "Curse" (*māmītu*)
CDLI no.:	P414061; P414063 (–; –)

Bibliography:	Maul 2019: 109–129 ms A, 406–413 (photograph, new copy and edition)
	Maul 2010a: 225 (partial new copy)
	Maul 2003: 179 (partial new copy)
	Ebeling 1953a: XIV, 210–212 nos. 151 and 153 (old copies)
Discussion:	Maul 2004: 89 and note 29

Obv. 1–11	Diagnostic statement and ritual instruction
Obv. 12–13, 14–33	Incantations
Obv. 34–35	Ritual instruction
Obv. 36–49, 50–55	Incantations
Obv. 56	Ritual instruction
Obv. 57–rev. 5, rev. 6–20	Incantations
Rev. 21	Ritual instruction
Rev. 22–30	Incantation
Rev. 31	Ritual instruction
Rev. 32–37	Incantation
Rev. 38	Ritual instruction
Rev. 39–44	Incantation
Rev. 45	Ritual instruction
Rev. 46	Rubrick: "Recitation for releasing a "Curse" ([KA.INI]M.MA ⸢NAM⸣.É[RIM.BÚR].⸢RU⸣.DA.KÁM)
Rev. 47–51	Catch-line; colophon:

[GIM SUM]UN-*šú* SAR IGI.KÁR DUB-*pi* ^{p}*K*[*i-ṣ*]*ir-Aššur* ^{lú}*šam-lu-*⸢*ú*⸣ 49 [DUMU ^{p}]$^{\text{.d}}$PA-*bé-su-nu* ^{lú}MAŠ.MAŠ É AN.ŠÁR 50 [DUMU ^{p}]$^{\text{.d}}$*Ba-ba*$_6$-MU-DÙ ^{lú}ZABAR.DAB.BA *É-šár-ra* 51 [*ša ṭuppa šu*]-⸢*a*⸣-*tú* TÙM DINGIR ⸢*ša-me-e*⸣ *qaq-qa-ri* IGI^{II}-*šú lit-*[*ba-lu*]

***KAL* 10 no. 5 = *LKA* 152** (VAT 13646; Assur N4 no. 587)

Tablet:	Single-column tablet in portrait format; not collated
Content:	Incantations and ritual instructions against a "Curse" (*māmītu*)
CDLI no.:	P414062 (–)
Bibliography:	Maul 2019: 109–129 ms B, 414–415 (new copy and edition)
	Hunger 1968: 71 no. 203 ms E (colophon)
	Ebeling 1953a: XIV, 211 no. 152 (old copy)

Obv. 1–11	Diagnostic statement and ritual instruction
Obv. 12–13, 14–(*breaks off*)	Fragmentary Incantations
Rev. 1'–3'	Fragmentary incantation

Rev. 4'	Fragmentary ritual instruction
Rev. 5'–10'	Fragmentary incantation
Rev. 11'	Fragmentary ritual instruction
Rev. 12'	Rubrick: "Recitation [for releasing] a "Cur[se"]" ([K]A.INIM.MA NAM.ÉR[IM.MA.BÚR.RU.DA.KÁM(?)])
Rev. 13'–16'	Catch-line; colophon:

[*k*]*i-ma* SUMUN-*šú šà-ṭir-m*[*a bà-rì*(?)] ^{15} DUB-*pi* ^{p}*Ki-ṣir-Aš-šur* DUMU ⌜^{p}⌝.[^{d}*Nabû-bēssun*(*u*) (*break of uncertain length*)] ^{16} DUMU ^{d}*Ba-*ba_6-M[U-DÙ (*break of uncertain length*)]

KAL 10 **no. 13** (VAT 14283; Assur N4 no. –)

Tablet:	Fragmentary single-column tablet(?) in portrait(?) format; not collated
Content:	Fragmentary instructions for treating a "Curse" (*māmītu*)
CDLI no.:	–
Bibliography:	Maul 2019: 134–136, 435 (photograph and edition)

Obv. 1–12	Fragmentary diagnostic statement and ritual instruction
(*Breaks off*)	
Rev. 1'	[Broken]
Rev. 2'–3'	[Broken]
Rev. 4'–5'	Fragmentary ritual instruction(?)
Rev. 6'–7'	Colophon:

ki-ma SUMUN-⌜*šú ana ṣa*⌝-[*b*]*at* DÙ-*š*[*i* (*ca. five signs*)] $^{7'}$ ⌜*ú*⌝-*ìl*-⌜*ti*⌝ ^{p}⌜*Ki*⌝-[*ṣi*]*r*-AN.ŠÁR [(*ca. four signs*)]

KAR **21** (VAT 8252; Assur N4 no. 135)

Tablet:	Single-column tablet in portrait format; not collated
Content:	Ritual for a man continually seeing ghosts
CDLI no.:	P369006 (copy)
Bibliography:	Scurlock 2006: 187–188 no. 5 ms B, 197–199 no. 10 ms B, 212–213 no. 17, 226–227 no. 21 ms B, 734–735 (edition)
	Scurlock 1988a: 169–178 no. 15–17 ms G, 211–213 ms G no. 55 (edition)
	Hunger 1968: 70 no. 201 ms G (colophon)
	Ebeling 1919a: 38–39 no. 21 (copy)
Discussion:	Seux 1976: 423–424
	Castellino 1955 ms B
	von Soden 1936: 270–71
	Ebeling 1931a: 122, 146–154 no. 30 ms F

Obv. 1–12	Prayer for Šamaš
Obv. 13	Rubric: "(for) one (who) continually sees dead people" (ÚŠ.MEŠ IGI.MEŠ)
Obv. 14–17	Ritual instruction for making figurines
Obv. 18–23	Prayer for Enki
Edge 24	Rubric identical to the one above
Rev. 1–6	Ritual instruction
Rev. 7–10	The incipit of a prayer to Šamaš where the remaining three lines have been erased after being written
Rev. 11–18	"If a man continually sees dead people" (DIŠ NA ÚŠ.MEŠ IGI.MEŠ-⸢*mar*⸣) and a ritual instruction
Rev. 19–22	Catch-line; colophon:

a-na ṣa-bat DÙ-*ši* ᵖ*Ki-ṣir-Aš-šur* ZI

***KAR* 38** (VAT 8240; Assur N4 no. 134)

Tablet:	Single-column tablet in portrait format; not collated
Content:	Apotropaic *namburbi*-ritual connected to improperly executed rituals
CDLI no.:	P369022 (copy)
Bibliography:	Maul 1994: 421–431 ms A with previous references (edition)
	Hunger 1968: 69 no. 198 ms A (colophon)
	Ebeling 1955b: 184–189 (edition)
	Ebeling 1931b: 47–52 (edition)
	Ebeling 1919a: 66–69 no. 38 (copy)
Discussion:	Ebeling 1954a: 5

Obv. 1–8	*namburbi*-ritual for removing any evil connected to improperly executed rituals followed by brief instructions
Obv. 9–23, 32–rev. 10, 18–27	Incantations and prayers
Obv. 24–31, rev. 11–17, 28–39	Ritual instructions
Rev. 40–42	Catch-line; colophon:

a-na mu-še-piš-ú-ti ḫa-an-ṭiš ZI-[*ḫa*?] [42] DUB-*pi* ᵖ[*K*]*i-ṣir-Aš-šur* MAŠ.MAŠ É AN.[ŠÁR]

***KAR* 62** (VAT 8267; Assur N4 no. 104)

Tablet:	Single-column tablet in portrait format; not collated
Content:	Ritual against someone angry
CDLI no.:	P369044 (copy)

Bibliography:	Hunger 1968: 71 no. 203 ms G (colophon)
	Ebeling 1931b: 22–24 (edition)
	Ebeling 1919a: 109–110 no. 62 (copy)
Discussion:	*CMAwR* 1: 289

Obv. 1–20	Incantation
Rev. 1	Rubric: "To appease the angry (one)" (*ana ze-na-a ana* DI$^{!}$-*me*)
Rev. 2–15	Ritual Instruction for producing a figurine and burying it
Rev. 16–18	Colophon:

GIM SUMUN-*šú šà-*[*ṭ*]*ir-*[*m*]*a* È ^{17} *ú-ìl-ti* ^{p}*Ki-ṣ*[*i*]*r-Aš-šur* ^{18} MAŠ.MAŠ É AN.ŠÁR

KAR **63** (VAT 8271; Assur N4 no. 101)

Tablet:	Single-column tablet in portrait format; collated during the summer of 2016; H 105mm/W 64mm/T 21mm
Content:	Ritual connected to anger against a man
CDLI no.:	P369045 (copy)
Bibliography:	Hunger 1968: 69 no. 199 ms A (colophon)
	Ebeling 1931b: 16–20 (edition)
	Ebeling 1919a: 111–112 no. 63 (copy)

Obv. 1–6	Incantation
Obv. 7	Rubric: "If someone is angry with a man" (DIŠ NA *mám-ma* U[GU]-*šú sa-bu-us*)
Obv. 8–18	Ritual instructions
Obv. 19–30	Incantation
(*Breaks off*)	
Rev. 1'–3'	Fragmentary
Rev. 4'–15'	Incantation
Rev. 16'	Rubric: "If they cry out in anger to a man" (DIŠ NA *ra-aʾ-ba-ni-iš i-šá-su-šú*)
Rev. 17'–21'	Ritual instruction
Rev. 22'–25'	Colophon:

(Moved in) *nis-ḫu qí-ta-a-a-ú* $^{23'}$ *ki-ma* SUMUN-*šú* SAR-*ma bà-rì za-mar* ZI-*ḫa* $^{24'}$ *ú-ìl-ti* ^{p}*Ki-ṣir-Aš-šur* MAŠ.MAŠ É *Aš-šur* $^{25'}$ [D]UMU $^{p.d}$PA-*bi-sún* MAŠ.MAŠ É *Aš-šur-ma*

KAR 80 = ***KAL*** **2 no. 8** (VAT 8276; Assur N4 no. 139)

Tablet:	Single-column tablet in portrait format; not collated
Content:	Incantation ritual for treating a *bēl dabābi* causing witchcraft

CDLI no.: P369061 (*KAR* copy)

Bibliography: *CMAwR* 1: 293–305 no. 8.4 ms A, 306–317 no. 8.5 ms B (edition)
Schwemer 2007b: 10, 31–36, 143–147 (new copy and edition with further references)
Hunger 1968: 71 no. 203 ms H (colophon)
Ebeling 1919a: 146–149 no. 80 (copy)
Ebeling 1918: 27–34 (edition)

Discussion: *CMAwR* 1: 51
Scurlock and Andersen 2005: 800
Seux 1976: 396–399
Abusch 1974: 258

Obv. 1–11: Diagnostic statement designating the source of symptoms originating from a *bēl dabābi* causing witchcraft (*kišpu*) followed by brief instructions

Obv. 12–43: Prayer for Šamaš

Rev. 1–14: Partially fragmentary prayer

Rev. 15–19: Ritual instruction

Rev. 20–24: Incantation

Rev. 25–36: Prayer for Šamaš

Rev. 37: Rubric: "*ušburrudû* for burning figurines" (UŠ$_{11}$.BÚR.RU.DA. KAM *ša* NU.MEŠ *qa-li-i*)

Rev. 38–39: Colophon:

[GI]M SUMUN-*šú šà-ṭir-ma ba-rì* DUB-*pi* [p]*Ki-ṣir-Aš-šur* MAŠ.MAŠ É *Aš-šur* 39
[DU]MU [p.d]AG-*be-sun* [lú]ME.ME É AN.[ŠÁR]

KAR **90** (VAT 8250; Assur N4 no. 67)

Tablet: Single-column tablet in portrait format; not collated

Content: Ritual actions connected to *ilī ul īde*

CDLI no.: P369071 (copy)

Bibliography: Ebeling 1931a: 114–128 no. 28 (edition)
Ebeling 1919a: 159–160 no. 90 (copy)

Discussion: Lenzi 2011: 42, 433
Lambert 1974: 269–270

Obv. 1: Heading: "When you perform the ritual of 'My god, I did not know'" (*e-nu-ma né-pe-ši ì-lí ul i-de te-*[*ep-pu-šú*])

Obv. 1–20+rev. 1–15: Ritual instruction

Rev. 16: Brief prescription-like instruction

Rev. 17, 18, 19	"Ditto" prescription-like instructions
Rev. 20	First entry is a statement: "you perform the ritual of *Šurpu* after this" (EGIR-*šú ne-pi-ši šá šur-pa te-pu-uš*); colophon:

a-na ṣa-bat DÙ-*ši* ^{p}*Ki-ṣ*[*ir*-x x]

KAR **171** (VAT 8021; Assur N4 no. 86)

Tablet:	Single-column tablet in landscape format; not collated
Content:	Ritual against a *bēl dabābi*
CDLI no.:	P369139 (copy)
Bibliography:	*Unedited*
	Hunger 1968: 70 no. 201 ms H (colophon)
	Ebeling 1919a: 307 no. 171 (copy)
Discussion:	Labat 1939: 98

Obv. 1–3	Statement of the problem: "If an 'adversary' (*bēl dabābi*) chases a man ..." (DIŠ NA EN DU$_{11}$.DU$_{11}$ *i-ra-da-da-š*[*u*]
Obv. 4–rev. 18	Ritual instruction
Rev. 19	Colophon:

ana ṣa-bat e-pe-ši Ki-ṣir-Aš-šur [Z]I$^{?}$

KAR **230** (VAT 8254; Assur N4 no. 100)

Tablet:	Single-column tablet in portrait format; collated during the summer of 2016; H 95mm/W 52mm/T 20mm
Content:	Incantation ritual used when going to the patient's house
CDLI no.:	P369194 (copy)
Bibliography:	*Unedited*
	Hunger 1968: 71 no. 203 ms I (colophon)
	Ebeling 1920–23: 157–158 no. 230 (copy)
Discussion:	Sections 6.2, 6.2.1, 6.2.2, 6.2.3, and 6.2.4 (treatment and discussion of individual lines)
	Lenzi 2008a: 166–167 (treatment and discussion of individual lines)
	Heeßel 2000: 70 and note 7 (treatment and discussion of individual lines)

Obv. 1–14	Incantation: "Who attacked him (i.e., the patient) and changed his mind ..." (*man-nu im-qut* UGU-*šú-ma ú-*⸢*šá*⸣*-an-ni ṭè-en-šú*), see Section 6.2.1

Obv. 15	Rubric: "The *āšipu* goes to the patient's house" ([lú]MAŠ.MAŠ *ana* É [lú]GIG DU-*ma*)
Obv. 16–rev. 8	Ritual instruction including a statement arguing for the efficiency of the ritual, see Section 6.2.2
Rev. 9–11	Secrecy statement, see Section 6.2.3
Rev. 12–15	Colophon:

GABA.RI KÁ.DINGIR.RA[ki] SAR È [13] *ú-ìl-ti* [P]*Ki-ṣir*-AN.ŠÁR MAŠ.MAŠ [14] DUMU [p.d]AG-[*b*]*e-sún* MAŠ.MAŠ É AN.ŠÁR [15] DUMU [p.d]*Ba-ba*$_6$-MU.DÙ ⸢ZABAR⸣.DAB[.BA *É-šar-ra*]

***KAR* 267** (VAT 8237; Assur N4 no. 69)

Tablet:	Single-column tablet in portrait format; collated during the summer of 2016; H 150mm/W 80mm/T 25mm
Content:	Incantation ritual against ghosts and states of confusion/"fit"
CDLI no.:	P369233 (copy)
Bibliography:	Scurlock 2006: 352–358 no. 119 ms A, 359–364 no. 120 ms A, 737 note 7 (edition) Farber 1987: 260–261 (translation) Hunger 1968: 69 no. 199 ms B (colophon) Ebeling 1931a: 138–42 no. 30 ms C (edition) Ebeling 1920–23: 215–217 no. 267 (copy)
Discussion:	*CMAwR* 2: 132 *CMAwR* 1: 51 Maul 2010a: 205 and note 52 Foster 1996: 554–555 Stol 1993: 42–46 Scurlock 1988b ms A Bottéro 1983: 156 Seux 1976: 416–420 von Soden 1936: 268–270

Obv. 1–2	Diagnostic statement: "If a ghost afflicts a man, stays continu[ously] in (his) body [and cannot be dispelled], and he continually has states of confusion (caused by) a ghost [...]" (DIŠ NA GIDIM$_4$ DAB-*su ina* SU-*šu il-ta-z*[*a-az-ma* NU DU$_8$-*ár*] *ù ḫa-a-a-at-ti* GIDIM$_4$ TUKU.MEŠ [(*4–6 signs*)])
Obv. 3–11	Ritual instruction
Obv. 12–26	Prayer for Šamaš

Obv. 27–30 Prayer for Girra

Obv. 31–38 Statement identifying the problem as a ghost followed by brief instructions

Rev. 1–24 Incantation

Rev. 25–28 Catch-line; colophon:

GIM SUMUN-*šú* SAR *ba-rì ḫa-an-ṭiš na-à*[*s-ḫa*] ^{27} DUB-*pi* ^{p}*Ki-ṣir-Aš-šur* A $^{\mathrm{p.d}}$PA-*bi-s*[*ún* (MAŠ.MAŠ É *Aš-šur*)] ^{28} ^{iti}KIN UD.9$^{\mathrm{(abbreviation)}}$.KÁM *lim-mu* ^{p}*ša*-^{d}PA$^{?}$-[*šu-u*(?)]

KAR **298** (VAT 8228; Assur N4 no. 84)

Tablet: Single-column tablet in portrait format; not collated

Content: Ritual instructions for making figurines intended to protect a man's house, partly taken from the series "To exclude the 'Foot of evil' from a man's house" and "To avert *di'u*-illness, plague and epidemic"

CDLI no.: P369267 (copy)

Bibliography: *CMAwR* 1: 204–245 no. 7.10 ms U, 425–429 11.1 ms B (treatment of individual lines)
Wiggermann 1992: 41–104 text no. 2, 202–203 fig. 10 (treatment and collations of individual lines)
Rittig 1977: 151–174 (edition)
Hunger 1968: 70–71 no. 201 ms I (colophon)
Ebeling 1920–23: 236–240 no. 298 (copy)

Discussion: Steinert 2018d: 267

Obv. 1 Heading: "To prevent the *šēd*[*u*-demon from approach]ing and to block the entry of the enemy (lit.: the foot of evil) into a man's house" (⸢*ana* ^{d}⸣A[LAD$^{?}$ NU TE-*ḫ*]*i ù* ⸢GÌR^{II} MUNUS$^{?}$.ḪUL⸣ *ina* É NA ⸢KUD-*si*⸣)

Obv. 2–11 Instructions for making seven figurines of *apkallu*-sages made of *ēru*-wood (7 NU NUN.ME *ša* ^{giš}MA.NU) with further specifications, and the incantation incipit "Seven pre-eminent sages" (ÉN 7 NUN.ME.MEŠ *a-šá-red-du-tú*)

Obv. 12–14 Instructions for making seven figurines of *apkallu*-sages made of clay with the face of a bird and wings (7 NUN NUN.ME *ša* IM IGI MUŠEN PA.MEŠ) with further specifications, and the incantation incipit "You are the image(s) of sage(s), the guardian(s)" (ÉN *at-tú-nu* NU NUN.ME *ma-ṣa-ri*)

Obv. 15–16, 17–18, 19–20	Instructions for making seven figurines of *apkallu*-sages made of clay with fish scales (BAR KU_6 *ša* IM.GE_6 or BAR KU_6 *ez-ḫu*) with further specifications
Obv. 21–25	Instructions for making seven figurines of the *sebetti* made of tamarisk (gišbi-ni) with further specifications, and the incantation incipit "You are the images of Sebettu, the great gods" (ÉN *at-tú-nu* NU.MEŠ dIMIN.BI DINGIR.MEŠ GAL.MEŠ)
Obv. 26–28	Instructions for making a figurine of Narudda of tamarisk (1-*en* NU d*Na-ru-du* giš*bi-ni*) with further specifications
Obv. 29–32	Instructions for making seven figurines of the weapon-men made of tamarisk (7 NU.MEŠ *šu-ut* gišTUKUL.MEŠ *ša* giš*bi-ni*) with further specifications, and the incantation incipit "You are the images of those holding weapons" (ÉN *at-tú-nu* NU.MEŠ *na-áš* giš!TUKUL)
Obv. 33–37	Instructions for making a figurine of "one cubit is his length" made of tamarisk (1-*en* NU gišŠINIG *ša* 1 KÙŠ *la-an-šú*) with further specifications, and the incantation incipit "You are the image that repels the evil one and the enemy" (ÉN *at-ta ṣal-mu sa-kip lem-nu u a-a-bi*)
Obv. 38–40	Instructions for making a figurine of the god of the house made of tamarisk (NU DINGIR É *ša* gišŠINIG) with further specifications, and the incantation incipit "God of the house, guard your home" (ÉN DINGIR É *ú-ṣur* É-*ka*)
Obv. 41–42	Instructions for making statues of the "Big-weather-beast" made of tamarisk (NU.MEŠ U_4.GAL) with further specifications
Obv. 43–44	Instructions for making figurines with further specifications
Obv. 45–46, 47–48, rev- 1–2	Fragmentary instructions for making figurines with further specifications
Rev. 3	Instructions for making figurines of the *mušḫuššu*-dragon made of clay ([NU].MEŠ MUŠ.ḪUŠ IM) with further specifications
Rev. 4–5	Instructions for making figurine(s) of the "Goat-fish" made of clay ([NU] ⌜SUḪUR⌝.MÁŠ IM) with further specifications

Rev. 6–7	Instructions for making figurines of the "Fish-man" made of clay (NU.MEŠ KU$_6$.LÚ.U$_{19}$.LU IM) with further specifications
Rev. 8	Instructions for making figurines of the "Scorpion-man" made of clay (NU.MEŠ GÍR.TAB.LÚ.U$_{19}$.LU IM) with further specifications
Rev. 9–10, 11–12	Instructions for making figurines with further specifications
Rev. 13	Instructions for making figurines of Lulal made of clay (NU.MEŠ ^{d}LÚ.LÀL IM) with further specifications
Rev. 14	Instructions for making figurines of Latarak made of clay (NU.MEŠ ^{d}*La-ta-rak* IM) with further specifications
Rev. 15–16	Instructions for making figurines of "Lion-man" made of clay (NU.MEŠ UR.MAḪ.LÚ.U$_{19}$.LU) with further specifications
Rev. 17–22	Various instructions for making figurines of pairs of dogs made of clay with further specifications, such as their names
Rev. 23–25	Instructions for making models of boats made of tamarisk ([NU] MÁ.GUR$_8$.MEŠ ^{giš}*bi-ni*) with further specifications
Rev. 26–29	Instructions for making figurines of clay
Rev. 30–35	Ritual instructions for: "[When someone] – the foot (lit.: feet) of evil is permanently bou[nd to him]" ([DIŠ NA] GÌR^{II} MUNUS.ḪUL [KI/EGIR-*š*]*ú*$^{?}$ [*ir*]-*ta-kás*)
Rev. 36–37	Ritual instructions
Rev. 38–40	Ritual instructions for: "To cut off the foot of evil in a man's house" (*ana* GÌR MUNUS.ḪUL *ina* É NA KUD-*si*)
Rev. 41–42	Ritual instructions with an incantation incipit recited against: "If a man's gate is creaking – so that witchcraft not approach that man's house" (DIŠ NA KÁ É-*šú* <*ḫu-*>*ub-bu-ub kiš-pi ana* É NA B[I] {*ina*} NU TE-*e*)
Rev. 43–44	Ritual instructions for burying substances at the outer gate of a house "So that witchcraft not approach a man and his house" (*ana kiš-pi ana* NA *u* É-*šú* NU TE-*e*)
Rev. 45–46	Fragmentary instructions
Lo.e. 48	Colophon:

[(*ana ṣabāt epēši*?)] ^{p}*Ki-ṣir-Aš-šur* MAŠ.MAŠ *za-mar* [ZI-*ḫa*(?)]

KAR 307 (VAT 8917; Assur N4 no. 116)

Tablet:	Single-column tablet in portrait format; not collated
Content:	Mystical text describing aspects of the world and a ritual involving the king
CDLI no.:	P336234 (copy)

Bibliography:	Horowitz 1998: 3–19, 208, 216–217, 223, 226, 243–247, 250, 258, 260, 263, 268, 274, 286, 318–320, 334, 336, 348, 345, 401 pl. 1 (new copy of a select passage and discussion)
	Livingstone 1989: XXIV-XXV, 99–102 no. 39 (edition and discussion)
	Livingstone 1986: 7, 82–85, 94–97, 124–125, 145–148, 233–234, 257, 260 (edition)
	Hunger 1968: 72 no. 206 (colophon)
	Ebeling 1931a: 28–37 no. 7 (edition)
	Ebeling 1920–23: 252–255 no. 307 (copy)
Discussion:	Lenzi 2008a: 173, 216
	Reiner 1995: 21 note 75 with further bibliography

Obv. 1–29	Mythological correlation between objects, animals and substances with individual divine figures; provides a description of a chariot and actors for a ritual (cf. *SAA* 3 no. 38)
Obv. 30–rev. 19	Mythological description of the world
Rev. 20–25	Description of the king's paraphernalia and incense
Rev. 26–31	Secrecy formula, see Sections 6.2.3 and 8.6; colophon:

GIM SUMUN-*šú šà-ṭir-ma ba-rì* ^{28} [(MU?)] (*uninscribed space*) PA-*ṭu-u* GIM SUMUN-*ma* ^{29} [DUB] ^{p}*Ki-ṣir-Aš-šur* MAŠ.MAŠ É AN.ŠÁR A $^{p.d}$PA-*bi-su-nu* ^{30} [^{lú}]MAŠ.MAŠ É AN.ŠÁR ^{31} [DUMU/A $^{p.d}$*B*]*a-ba*$_{6}$-MU-DÙ ZABAR.DAB.BA *É-šár-ra*

KAR **374** (VAT 8008; Assur N4 no. 89)

Tablet:	Single-column tablet in portrait format; not collated
Content:	Incantation ritual connected to divine(?) anger
CDLI no.:	P369341 (copy)
Bibliography:	*Unedited*
	Hunger 1968: 68–69 no. 197 ms A (colophon)
	Ebeling 1920–23: 315–316 no. 374 (copy)
Discussion:	Reiner 1995: 23 note 85
	Maul 1994: 75 note 35

Obv. 1–23 (22–23 on the edge)	Incantation addressing Venus(?): "You have risen, star, you are the first one" (ÉN MUL *tap-pu-ḫa pa-nu-u at-ta*)

Rev. 1'–16' Ritual instruction "(In order) to throw *off* anger" (*ana ru-ub-bi* ŠUB-*di*)

Rev. 17'–19' Colophon:

ki-ma SUMUN-*šú šà-ṭir-ma bà-rì* $^{18'}$ DUB-*pi* ^{p}*Ki-ṣir-Aš-šur* MAŠ.MAŠ É *Aš-šur* $^{19'}$ *ana ṣa-bat* DÙ-*ši za-mar* ZI-*ḫa*

KAV 42 = **George 1992 pl. 37–38** (VAT 8918; Assur N4 no. 138)

Tablet: Tablet with three columns on each side and various layouts on the reverse in portrait format; not collated

Content: Geographical list describing the city of Assur's temples, city gates and ziggurats

CDLI no.: P285518 (old copy)

Bibliography: Parpola 2017: 132–139 no. 49 (edition)
George 1992: 173–184 ms d, pl. 37–38 no. 20 (new copy, edition, and discussion)
Menzel 1981: T 146–166 ms A (edition)
Hunger 1968: 72 no. 207 (colophon)
Schroeder 1920: VIII, 37–39 no. 42 (old copy)

Discussion: Parpola 2017: 49
Ermidoro 2017: XXVII–XXVIII
Pongratz-Leisten 2017: XXXVIII

Obv. col. i–iii 1–119 List of the gods resident in Assur grouped according to temples

Obv. col. iii 120–33 List of the thirteen city gates of Assur

Rev. 1–13 [Broken, but likely contained the beginning of the list below]

Rev. 14–32+left edge List of temples in Assur with Sumerian names explained by Akkadian translations and identified with a divine owner; entries are divided onto three columns (col. iv-vi). One additional entry is placed on the left edge of the tablet, possibly due to lack of space

Rev. 33–35 Section on the three ziggurats of Assur

Rev. 36–40 List of the gates from Sennacherib's extension to the *Ešarra* temple complex

Rev. 41–44 Statement that "the old gates are not copied" (KÁ.MEŠ SUMUN. MEŠ NU SAR); Colophon:

PA-[*t*]*u-u* GIM SUMUN-*ma* ^{43} *šà-ṭír* ^{p}*Ki-ṣir-Aš-šur* ^{lú}MAŠ.MAŠ É AN.ŠÁR ^{44} [DUM]U $^{p.d}$PA-*bé-sún* MAŠ.MAŠ É AN.Š[ÁR]

LKA **40** (VAT 13633; Assur N4 no. 517)

Tablet:	Single-column tablet in portrait format; not collated
Content:	*Šuʾilla*-prayer to Tašmētu
CDLI no.:	P413951 (–)
Bibliography:	*CMAwR* 2: 341–349 no. 9.7 ms C, pl 73 (new copy of the obverse and edition)
	Seux 1976: 294–296 (translation)
	Hunger 1968: 69 no. 199 ms C (colophon)
	Ebeling 1953a: IX, 58–59, 58–59 no. 40 (copy)
	Ebeling 1953c: 24 (edition of the reverse)
Discussion:	Frechette 2012: 263, 273–274
	Meyer 1976: 400, 424

Obv. 1'–12'	[Broken]
Rev. 1'–7'	Fragmentary prayer
Rev. 8'	Rubric: "*Šuʾilla*-prayer (to) Tašmētu" (ŠU.ÍL.LÁ ^{d}*Taš-me-t*[u_4?])
Rev. 9'–11'	Colophon:

[*ki-ma*] SUMUN-*šú šà-ṭir bà-rì ana* DAB DÙ-*ši na-à*[*s-ḫa*] [10'] [DUB]-*pi* ^{p}*Ki-ṣir*-AN.ŠÁR DUMU $^{p.d}$AG-*be-su*[*n* MAŠ.MAŠ É *Aš-šur*] [11'] [DUMU] $^{p.d}$*Ba-*ba_6-MU-DÙ ZABAR.DAB.BA *É-šár-r*[*a*]

LKA **43** (VAT 13631; Assur N4 no. 509)

Tablet:	Single-column tablet in portrait format; collated during the summer of 2016; H 92mm/W 59mm/T 22mm
Content:	*Šuʾilla*-prayer to Madānu
CDLI no.:	P413955 (–)
Bibliography:	Mayer 1976: 394, 459–465 (edition)
	Seux 1976: 316–318 (translation)
	Hunger 1968: 68–69 no. 197 ms B (colophon)
	Ebeling 1953a: IX, 64–65 no. 43 (copy)
Discussion:	Frechette 2012: 170 note 10, 178 note 6, 259
	Ebeling 1953c: 34–35

Obv. 1–rev. 13	Prayer
Rev. 14	Rubric: "*Šuʾilla*-prayer (to) Madānu" (ŠU.ÍL.LÁ ^{d}DI.KUD)
Rev. 15–18	Colophon:

ki-ma SUMUN-*šú šá-ṭir ba-ri* [16] IM ^{p}*Ki-ṣir-aš-šur* ŠÁMAN.LÁ TUR [17] DUMU $^{p.d}$PA-*be-sun* MAŠ.MAŠ É *Aš-šur* [18] *ḫa-an-ṭiš is-su-ḫ*[*a*]

LKA 70(+)***KAR*** 57 (A 81(+)VAT 8261; Assur N4 no. 119)

Tablet:	Tablet with two columns on each side in portrait format; not collated
Content:	Prayers, incantations, and ritual instructions from the Ištar-Dumuzi incantation ritual
CDLI no.:	P413980; P369039 (– ; copy)
Bibliography:	Scurlock 1988a: 354–357 no. 86 ms CCC (treatment of individual lines) Farber 1977: 127–183 text IIA ms b, pl. 14 (edition and collations of *KAR* 57) Hunger 1968: 71 no. 203 ms A (colophon) Ebeling 1953a: x, 92–94 no. 70+ (copy of *LKA* 70) Ebeling 1919a: 94–97 no. 57 (copy of *KAR* 57) Ebeling 1919b: 1–7, 11–14 (treatment of individual lines)
Discussion:	Hecker 2008: 116–122

Obv. col. i 1–2	Heading: "If a man is seized by a ghost, the *sagḫ*[*ulḫazû*-demon] or 'Any evil', and is continually pursued" (DIŠ NA GIDIM DAB-*su* SAG.Ḫ[UL.ḪA.ZA DAB-*su*] *lu mim-ma lem-nu* DAB-*su-m*[*a* UŠ.UŠ-*š*]*ú*?)
Obv. col. i 3–13, 14–27	Ritual instructions
Obv. col. i 28–29+1'–24', col. ii 1–28+1'–9'	Prayer to Ištar
Obv. col. ii 10'	"You recite this thrice before Ištar" (*an-nam ana* IGI ᵈ15 3-*šú* ŠID-*nu*)
Obv. col. ii 11'–25'	Prayer to Ištar
Obv. col. ii 26'	"You recite this thrice before Ištar"
Rev. col. iii 1–7	Prayer to Ištar and Dumuzi
Rev. col. iii 8	"You recite th[is thrice] before Dumuzi" ([*an-na*]*m ana* I[G]I ᵈ*Dumu-zi* [3-*šú*] ŠID-*nu*)
Rev. col. iii 9–23	Prayer to Dumuzi
Rev. col. iii 24	"You recite this thrice before Dumuzi"
Rev. col. iii 25–30+1'–16'	Prayer to the *Anunnaki*-gods
Rev. col. iii 17'	"You recite this thrice before the *Anunnaki*"
Rev. col. iii 18'–24'+ iv 1–4'	Incantation for a ghost
Rev. col. iv 5"–6"	Fragmentary prayer to Dumuzi
Rev. col. iv 7"	"The *maš*[*maššu* recites this thrice before Dumuzi" ([...]-*zi* ˡᵘ́MAŠ.[MAŠ 3-*šú* DU_{11}].GA)
Rev. col. iv 8"–1+"+1'''–7'''	Ritual instruction for the patient (ˡᵘ́GIG)
Rev. col. iv 8'''–12'''	Incantation concerning Ištar

Rev. col. iv 13'''–17'''	Ritual instruction
Rev. col. iv 18'''–22'''	Catch-line; colophon:

GABA.RI URU NINA^{ki} GIM SUMUN-*šú* SAR-*ma ba-rì* $^{19'''}$ IM ^{p}*Ki-ṣi*[*r-Aš-šur*] MAŠ.MAŠ É *Aš-šur* $^{20'''}$ PEŠ $^{p.d}$A[G]-*be-sun* [MA]Š.MAŠ É *Aš-šur* $^{21'''}$ PEŠ $^{p.d}$[*B*]*a-ba*$_6$-MU-DÙ ^{lú}ZABAR.[DAB.B]A $^{22'''}$ (moved in) *É-šár-r*[*a*]

LKA 77 (VAT 13662+13883; Assur N4 no. 559)

Tablet:	Tablet with three columns on each side in portrait format; not collated
Content:	Compendium of Ḫulbazizi incantations
CDLI no.:	P413986 (–)
Bibliography:	Hunger 1968: 71 no. 203 ms B (colophon)
	Ebeling 1953a: x, 106–117 no. 77 (copy)
	Ebeling 1953b (edition)
Discussion:	Maul 2010: 195

Obv. col. i–rev. col. vi 24	At least 30 Ḫulbazizi incantations in Sumerian on the left side with Akkadian translations on the right

Rev. col. vi 25	"Recitation(s) of Ḫulbazizi (lit.: to eradicate evil)" (KA.INIM.MA ḪUL.BA.ZI.Z[I.K]E$_4$)
Rev. col. vi 26–32	Colophon:

[LIB]IR.R[A].BI.GIM SAR BA.AN.È.A ^{27} DUB ^{p}*Ki-ṣir-Aš-šur* ^{lú}MAŠ.MAŠ É *Aš-šur* ^{28} DUMU $^{p.d}$PA-*bi-sún* ^{lú}MAŠ.MAŠ É *Aš-šur* ^{29} [DUMU $^{p.d}$*Ba-ba*$_6$]-⌜MU-DÙ ZABAR.DAB.BA⌝ ^{30} *É-šár-ra* ^{31} MU ^{d}PA MAN DINGIR.DINGIR *lu ta-*[*pa/paq*]*-làḫ/qid* ^{32} MU SAR *la ta-pá-šiṭ*

LKA 83 (VAT 8268; Assur N4 no. 105)

Tablet:	Single-column tablet in landscape (or square) format; not collated
Content:	Ghost incantations with duplicate passages in the substitute king ritual
CDLI no.:	P413992 (–)
Bibliography:	Scurlock 1988: 343–348 no. 83 ms vv (edition and discussion)
	Tsukimoto 1985: 173–178 (edition and discussion)
	Ebeling 1953a: xi, 122 no. 83 (copy)

Obv. 1–12	Incantation concerning a ghost of a recently deceased
Rev. 13–14	Invocation to take omens and evils down to the netherworld

Rev. 15–21	Incantation for a ghost
Rev. 22	Colophon:

ú-ìl-ti ^{p}*Ki-ṣir-Aš-šur* [MAŠ.MAŠ É] *Aš-šur*

LKA **89+*LKA* 90 = CMAwR 2 pl. 34–43** (VAT 13656+13657; Assur N4 no. 523)

Tablet:	Tablet with two columns on each side in portrait format; not collated
Content:	Ghost ritual connected to the netherworld and witchcraft
CDLI no.:	P413998; P413999 (– ; –)
Bibliography:	*CMAwR* 2: 189–210 no. 8.25 ms B, pl. 34–43 (new copy and edition)
	Scurlock 1988a: 351–354 no. 85 ms ZZ, 357–361 no. 87 ms ZZ (treatment of individual lines)
	Hunger 1968: 68–69 no. 197 ms C (colophon)
	Ebeling 1953a: XI, 131–134 no. 89 and 90 (old copy)
Discussion:	Verderame 2008: 56
	Scurlock 2006: 504, 538, 544
	von Soden 1936: 265–266 and note 1
	Ebeling 1931a: 122

Obv. col. i 1'	Fragmentary diagnostic statement
Obv. col. i 2'–26'+col. i 1"–9"	Fragmentary ritual instructions
Obv. col.i 10"–27"+col. ii 1–12	Fragmentary prayer to Šamaš
Obv. col. ii 13	Brief instructions
Obv. col. ii 14–22+col. ii 1'–30'+rev. col. iii 1–9	Prayer to Gilgameš
Rev. col. iii 10–11	Brief ritual instructions
Rev. col. iii 12–30	Prayer to the Anunnaki gods
Rev. col. iii 31	Brief instructions
Rev. col. iii 32–47	Prayer to the "ghosts of my family" (*at-tu-nu* GIDIM *kim-ti-ia*)
Rev. col. iii 48	Brief instructions
Rev. col. iii 49–68+col. iv 1–4	Incantation for a ghost
Rev. col. iv 5–18+col. iv 1'–3'	Incantation concerning *Ḫumuṭ-tabal*
Col. iv 4'–9' (breaks off)	Catch-line; colophon:

LIBIR.RA.BI.GIM AB.SAR.ÀM *bà-rì* $^{6'}$ [DU]B$^{?}$ ^{p}*Ki-ṣir-Aš-šur* ^{lú}DUGUD MAŠ.MAŠ TUR *šá* ^{d}AG GISKIM-*su* $^{7'}$ [DUMU $^{p.d}$]AG-*bi-su-nu* ^{lú}MAŠ.MAŠ É *Aš-šur* $^{8'}$ [DUMU $^{p.d}$*Ba-ba*$_{6}$-M]U-DÙ ^{lú}ZABAR.DAB.BA *É-šár-ra* $^{9'}$ [(x x x x x x?) *ḫa-an-ṭiš*] *na-as-ḫa*

***LKA* 113** (VAT 13710; Assur N4 no. 305)

Tablet:	Single-column tablet in portrait format; not collated
Content:	Apotropaic *namburbi*-ritual against the evil portended by a bow
CDLI no.:	P414022 (–)
Bibliography:	Maul 1994: 207–208 (translation)
	Caplice 1974: 14–15 (translation)
	Hunger 1968: 72 no. 204 (colophon)
	Ebeling 1955a: 137–138 no. 21 (edition)
	Ebeling 1953a: XII, 163 no. 113 (copy)
Discussion:	Reiner 1995: 88 and note 365,
	Maul 1994: 49 note 17, 54 notes 121–125, 55 note 129, 73 notes 13–14, 107 note 6, 204 note 395
	Lambert 1956: 164
	Ebeling 1954a: 4–5

Obv. 1–2	*Namburbi* ritual against the evil portended by any bow (NAM.BÚR.BI ḪUL ^{giš}BAN DÙ.A.BI) and ritual instructions
Obv. 13–17	Fragmentary prayer to uncertain deity
(*Breaks off*)	
Rev. 1'–6'	Colophon:

GABA.R[I (x x x x x x x x?)] $^{2'}$ *aná* KA IM.[GÍD.DA? (x x x x?)] $^{3'}$ GABA.RI ^{giš}*li*$_9$-*u*$_5$$^{?}$ ⸢x⸣[x KA.DI]NGI[R.RA$^{\text{ki?}}$ (x?)] $^{4'}$ DUB-*pi* ^{p}*Ki-ṣir*-[AN].ŠÁR MA[Š.M]AŠ É *Aš-šur*^{ki} $^{5'}$ DUMU $^{\text{p.d}}$PA-*b*[*i*]-*s*[*ún* MAŠ.M]AŠ É *Aš-šur* $^{6'}$ DUMU $^{\text{p.d}}$*B*[*a-ba*$_6$-MU-D]Ù ZABA[R.DA]B.B[A *É-šár*]-*ra*

***LKA* 115** (VAT 13952; Assur N4 no. 286)

Tablet:	Single-column tablet in portrait format; not collated
Content:	Apotropaic *namburbi*-ritual against any observation in a man's house
CDLI no.:	P414024 (–)
Bibliography:	*CMAwR* 2: 427–430 no. 11.5 ms A, pl. 102 (edition)
	Maul 1994: 502–504 (edition)
	Hunger 1968: 71 no. 202 ms C (colophon)
	Ebeling 1954d: 130–132 (edition)
	Ebeling 1953a: XII, 165 no. 115 (copy)
Discussion:	Ebeling 1954a: 3–4

Obv. 1–2	Entry identifying the problem: "If evil omens have appeared in a man's house – so that the evil of the evil omens not approach

the man and his house" (DIŠ *ina* É NA GISKIM.MEŠ ḪUL.MEŠ IGI.MEŠ-*ra ana* ḪUL GISKIM.MEŠ ḪUL.MEŠ *ana* NA *u* É-*šú* NU TE-*e*)

Obv. 3–8 Ritual instructions

Obv. 9–18 Prayer to Išum

(*Breaks off*)

Rev. 1'–6' Fragmentary instructions

Rev. 7'–9' Instruction for producing and administering a potion to ensure "the evil of the signs (and) omens [*will not appear* in [the man's] house" (ḪUL A.MEŠ GISKIM.MEŠ *ina* ⸢É⸣ [(NA NU IGI?)])

Rev. 10'–12' Colophon:

ki-ma la-bi-ri-šú šà-ṭir bà-r[*ì*] 11' *a-na ṣa-bat e-pe-ši* ^{p}*Ki-ṣir-Aš-šur* MAŠ.MAŠ 12' ⸢*ú*⸣-*šaš-ṭir-ma íb-ri*

***LKA* 119** (A 171; Assur N4 no. 234)

Tablet: Single-column tablet in portrait format; not collated

Content: Apotropaic *namburbi*-ritual against contagion by dust from an evil place

CDLI no.: P414028 (–)

Bibliography: Caplice 1974: 19 (translation)
Hunger 1968: 71 no. 203 ms C (colophon)
Ebeling 1954b: 178–181 (edition)
Ebeling 1953a: XII, 169 no. 119 (copy)

Discussion: Maul 1994: 8 note 67, 52 note 86, 90 note 64, 445 note 15

Obv. 1–11 *Namburbi*-ritual to keep evil dust from a bad place away from a man (NAM.BÚR.BI ḪUL SAḪAR.ḪI.A KI.ḪUL-*e ana* NA NU TE-*e* ...) and instructions

Obv. 12–rev. 7 Prayer to Šamaš

Rev. 8–14 Ritual instructions

Rev. 15–18 Colophon:

ki-ma SUMUN-*šú* SAR-*ma ba-rì* 16 [I]M ^{p}*Ki-ṣir-<Aš>-šur* MAŠ.MAŠ É *Aš-šur* 17 DUMU $^{p.d}$AG-*be-su-nu* MAŠ.MAŠ É *Aš-šur* 18 DUMU $^{p.d}$*Ba-*⸢*ba*?⸣-MU-DÙ MAŠ.MAŠ É *Aš-š*[*ur*]

***LKA* 137** (VAT 13958; Assur N4 no. 529)

Tablet: Single-column tablet in portrait format; not collated

Content: A ritual for performing a stone oracle (psephomancy)

CDLI no.: P414046 (–)

Bibliography: Finkel 1995 (edition and discussion)
Horowitz and Hurowitz 1992: 98–106 (edition and discussion)
Hunger 1968: 72 no. 205 (colophon)
Ebeling 1953a: XIII, 186–187 no. 137 (copy)
Discussion: Steinert 2018d: 258
Reiner 1960a: 25 with references

Obv. 1–28 Prayer to Šamaš
Obv. 29 "Recitation for oracular decisions with alabaster and hematite (stones)" ([K]A.INIM.MA EŠ.BAR ^{na4}GIŠ.NU$_{11}$.GAL ^{na4}KUR-*nu*$^{?}$ [x?])
Rev. 1'–4' Fragmentary ritual instructions
Rev. *diagram* A diagram illustrating drawings made on which to thrown the stones
Rev. 5' Fragmentary description
Rev. 6'–10' Colophon:

ki-i pi-i IM.GÍD.DA $^{p.d}$PA-[(x x x x?)] $^{7'}$ MU PA$^{!}$-*ṭu-u* GIM SU[MUN (*ca. three signs*)] $^{8'}$ *ú-ìl-tì* [^{P}]*Ki-ṣir*-AN.[ŠÁR (x x x x x?)] $^{9'}$ DUMU $^{p.d}$PA-*bi-su-nu* MAŠ.MAŠ [É *Aš-šur*] $^{10'}$ DUMU $^{p.d}$*Ba-ba*$_{6}$-MU-DÙ ^{lú}ZABAR.[DAB.BA *É-šár-ra*]

***LKA* 141** (VAT 13603; Assur N4 no. 543)
Tablet: Fragmentary single-column tablet in portrait(?) format; collated during the summer of 2016; H 74mm/W 91mm/T 21mm
Content: Incantation ritual for reconciling a man with his god
CDLI no.: P414050 (–)
Bibliography: *Unedited*
Hunger 1968: 71 no. 203 ms D (colophon)
Ebeling 1953a: XIII, 195–196 no. 141 (copy)
Discussion: Pedersén 1986: 73 no. 543

Obv. 1–3 Fragmentary incantation
Obv. 4–15 Ritual instructions
Obv. 16 Fragmentary line mentioning the god of a house and a man ([...] DINGIR É DINGIR NA KA.INIM.[MA(?) ...])
Obv. 17–20 Fragmentary incantation(?)
(*Breaks off*)
Rev. 1' Fragmentary incantation
Rev. 2' Fragmentary rubric (KA.INI[M.M]A DINGIR LÚ KI LÚ ⸢x⸣[x x x (x)])
Rev. 3'–8' Ritual instruction
Rev. 9'–12' Colophon:

LIBIR.RA.BI.[G]IM AB.SAR.ÀM BA.AN.È [(...?)] $^{10'}$ DUB-*pi* ^{p}*Ki-*[*ṣ*]*ir-Aš-šur* ^{lú}DUGUD MAŠ.MAŠ TUR ⸢*šá*⸣ [...] $^{11'}$ DUMU $^{\text{p.d}}$*Na-bi-um-bi-sún* ^{lú}MAŠ.MAŠ [É *Aš-šur*] $^{12'}$ [DUMU $^{\text{p.d}}$]*Ba-*[*b*]*a*$_6$-MU-DÙ ^{lú}ZABAR.D[AB.BA *É-šár-ra*]

***LKA* 146** (VAT 13716; Assur N4 no. 534)

Tablet:	Single-column tablet in portrait format; not collated
Content:	Mythological incantation and instructions for producing 21 leather bags worn around the neck
CDLI no.:	P414055 (–)
Bibliography:	*Unedited*
	Lenzi 2008a: 122–125 (treatment of individual lines and discussion)
	Lambert 1980 (treatment of individual lines and discussion)
	Ebeling 1953a: XIV, 202–203 no. 146 (copy)
Discussion:	Steinert 2018d: 253
	Lawson 1994: 47–48
	Lambert 1956: 144

Obv. 1–21	Mythological incantation concerning 21 leather bags worn around the neck (*mêlu*) from Ea
Obv. 22–23	Subscript to the incantation
Obv. 24–rev. 15, 16–24	Ritual instructions
Rev. 25–27	Catch-line; colophon:

[GIM] SUMUN-*šú šà-*[*ṭi*]*r bà-rì* ^{27} *ú-ìl-ti* ^{p}*Ki-*[*ṣir-Aššur* $^{(\text{lú})}$]MAŠ.MAŠ

***LKA* 157 = *KAL* 2 no. 25** (VAT 13644; Assur N4 no. 352)

Tablet:	Fragmentary tablet with two columns perhaps in portrait(?) format; collated via the CDLI photograph
Content:	Incantation ritual against witchcraft
CDLI no.:	P414073 (photograph)
Bibliography:	*CMAwR* 1: 256–269 no. 8.2 ms A (edition)
	Schwemer 2007b: 12, 68–71 no. 25, 176–177 (new copy and edition)
	Hunger 1968: 68–69 no. 197 ms D (colophon)
	Ebeling 1953a: XIV, 218–219 no. 157 (copy)
Discussion:	Schwemer 2010b: 130–131

Obv. col. i 1–13 Diagnostic statement with witchcraft performed against a man who "has been fed (bewitched) bread (and) been given (bewitched) beer to drink" ([NA BI *ki*]*š*-⸢*pi*⸣ *ep*-⸢*šu-šú*⸣-*m*[*a*] ^{13} [*ina akalīš*]*u-k*[*u*]*l ina* KAŠ N[A]G)

Obv. col. i 14–20 Fragmentary incantation

Obv. col. i 21–22 Fragmentary ritual instructions

(*Breaks off*)

Obv. col. ii 1'–6' Fragment of an incantation

(*Breaks off*)

Rev. col. iii 1'–17' Prayer to Šamaš

(*Breaks off*)

Rev. col. iv 1'–5' Fragmentary ritual instructions

Rev. col. iv 6'–12' Subscript stating the ritual is against "If witchcraft has been performed (against) an man"; colophon:

[LI]BIR.RA.BI.GIM AB.SAR ⸢BA.AN.È⸣ $^{8'}$ [DUB-*pi*? ^{p}]*Ki-ṣi*[*r-Aš-šur* MAŠ.]⸢MAŠ⸣ É AN.ŠÁR $^{9'}$ [DUMU $^{p.}$]⸢^{d}PA-*bi*⸣-*s*[*ún* M]AŠ.MAŠ É AN.ŠÁR $^{10'}$ D[UMU $^{p.}$]⸢^{d}⸣*Ba-ba*$_6$-MU-[*i*]*b-ni* $^{11'}$ ^{lú}ZABAR.DAB.BA ⸢*É*⸣-*šár-ra* $^{12'}$ *a-na ṣa-bat e*-⸢*pe-ši*⸣ *ḫa-an*-⸢*ṭiš* ZI⸣-[*ḫa*]

N4 A 400 (A 400; Assur N4 no. –)

Tablet: *Unpublished* (single-column tablet in landscape format; not collated)

Content: Incantation and ritual instruction against *maškadu*

CDLI no.: –

Bibliography: *Unpublished*

Discussion: Pedersén 1986: 64

Unpublished Incantation with a rubrick (KA.INIM.MA *maš*-⸢*ka-du u*⸣ x x ZI.GA) followed by ritual instruction

Unpublished Catch-line; colophon:

LIBIR.RA.BI AB.SAR.ÀM BA.AN.È *new line* *ú-ìl-tì* ^{p}*Ki-ṣir*-AN.ŠÁR ^{lú}ŠÁMAN.LÁ TUR *new line* DUMU $^{p.d}$AG-*bi-su-nu* ^{lú}MAŠ.MAŠ É AN.ŠÁR

N4 A 2191 (A 2191; Assur N4 no. –)

Tablet: *Unpublished* (single-column tablet in portrait format; not collated)

Content: Ritual against a ghost

CDLI no.: –

Bibliography: *Unpublished*

Unpublished	Ritual against a ghost, duplicating *BAM* 323
Unpublished	Colophon:

[LIBIR.RA.BI AB.SA]R.ÀM BA.AN.È *new line* [x x x x]⸢x⸣-⸢da$^{?}$⸣-^{d}AMAR.UTU ^{lú}A.ZU *šá* kur [x] *new line* [x x ^{p}*Ki-ṣi*]*r*-^{d}*aš-šur* ^{lú}ŠÁMAN.LÁ [x (x)] *new line* [DUMU $^{p.d}$AG-*bi-s*] *u-ni* ^{lú}MAŠ.MAŠ É ^{d}[*aš-šur*] *new line* [DUMU $^{p.d}$*Ba-ba*$_{6}$-MU-DÙ ^{lú}ZA]BAR.⸢DAB⸣.BA *é-šá*[*r-ra*]

N4 A 2362 (A 2362; Assur N4 no. –)

Tablet:	*Unpublished* (fragment; not collated)
Content:	Unclear due to damage
CDLI no.:	–
Bibliography:	*Unpublished*

Unpublished	Fragmentary
Unpublished	Colophon:

[… ^{p}*Ki-ṣir*-^{d}*aš-š*]*ur* […] *new line* [DUMU $^{p.d}$AG-*bi*]-*sún* ^{lú}MAŠ.[MAŠ É ^{d}*aš-šur*]

N4 A 2727 (A 2727; Assur N4 no. –)

Tablet:	*Unpublished* (single-column tablet in landscape format; not collated)
Content:	Two incantations with ritual instructions
CDLI no.:	–
Bibliography:	*Unpublished*
Discussion:	Pedersén 1986: 60

Unpublished	Two incantations with instructions and the label "tested remedies, which *are suitable for use*(?)" *bulṭī latkūti ša ina qāti šūṣû*. The initial incantation duplicates *BAM* 105 obv. 1–6 against "Anus illness" (see discussion in Section 8.4.1)
Unpublished	Colophon:

ki-ma SUMUN-*šú šà-ṭir-ma ba*-⸢*rì* PA$^{?}$-*ṭu*$^{?}$-*u*$^{?}$ GIM$^{?}$ SUMUN$^{?}$-*ma*$^{?}$⸣ *new line* *ú-ìl-ti* ^{p}*Ki-ṣir-aš-šur* ⸢^{lú}MAŠ.MAŠ TUR⸣ [(x)] *new line* DUMU $^{p.d}$AG-*bi-su-ni* ⸢^{lú}MAŠ.MAŠ É ^{d}⸣[*aš-šur*]

N4 no. 24 (A 378+387; Assur N4 no. 24)

Tablet:	Single-column tablet in landscape format; collated by Daniel Schwemer
Content:	An incantation to calm an infant, baby, or young child (LÚ.TUR.ḪUN.GÁ)
CDLI no.:	–

Bibliography:	Farber 2014: 271–272 (edition) Farber 1989: 24–25, 102–107 3.4. §34 ms l, pl. 13 (copy and edition)

Obv. 1–rev. 15	Lamaštu-themed incantation
Rev. 16	Rubric: "Recitation to calm a child" (KA.INIM.MA L[Ú].TUR ḪUN.GÁ.KE$_4$)
Rev. 17	Colophon:

IM.GÍD.DA ᵖ*Ki-ṣir*-AN.ŠÁR MAŠ.MAŠ TUR \ ŠÁMAN.LÁ (written underneath MAŠ.MAŠ TUR in smaller script)

N4 no. 110 (A 2719; Assur N4 no. 110)

Tablet:	*Unpublished* (single-column tablet in portrait format; collated via unpublished pictures)
Content:	List of cultic materials and a theological commentary
CDLI no.:	–
Bibliography:	*Unpublished*
Discussion:	Section 8.6 and Ch. 8 note 101 Pedersén 1986: 62 no. 110 Ebeling 1954c: 115

Obv. 1	Opening line with unclear content
Obv. 2–28	List of various cultic materials
Obv. 29–31	Lines, each one ruled off individually, likely describing the cultic circumstances of the list above
Rev. 1–24	List of obscure deities related to various gods, e.g., "'The divine fox' (*is*) Nergal of the funerary offe[rings]" (rev. 5: ᵈKA$_5$.A ᵈU.GUR *šá ki-i*[*s-pi*])
Rev. 25–27	Colophon:

[*k*]*i-ma* SUMUN-*šú* SAR-*ma* È PA-*ṭu-u* GIM SUMUN-*m*[*a*] [26] ⌜*ú*⌝-*ìl-ti* ᵖ*Ki-ṣir-Aš*-⌜*šur*⌝ MAŠ.MAŠ É *Aš-šur* [27] [DU]MU ᵖ·ᵈAG-*bi-sun* MAŠ.MAŠ É AN.ŠÁR

N4 no. 175 (A 191; Assur N4 no. 175)

Tablet:	*Unpublished* (single-column tablet in portrait format; collated via unpublished pictures)
Content:	Guidelines for performing the ritual *bīt mēseri*
CDLI no.:	–
Bibliography:	*Unpublished*
Discussion:	Pedersén 1986: 64 no. 175

Obv. 1–rev. 7 “To perform [(*the ritual of*?)] *bīt mēseri*” ([*ne-peš*(?)] ⸢É *me*⸣-*se-ri a*-⸢*na*⸣ *e-pe-š*[*i* (x x)]) followed by ritual instructions, and from obv. 15ff. incipits for which incantations to recite and the associated instructions

Rev. 8–17 “If you perform *bīt mēseri*” ([*š*]*um-ma* É *me-se-ri* DÙ-*u*[*š*]) followed by incipits for which incantations to recite and the associated instructions

Rev. 18–25 Colophon:

GIM SUMUN-*šú šà-ṭir-ma* BA.AN.⸢È⸣ (*erased line before rev. 19*) *{ŠID-*nu*}* ^{19} ⸢*ú*⸣-[*ìl*]-⸢*ti* ^{p}ZÚ.KEŠDA-^{d}*aš-šur*⸣ ^{lú}ŠAB.T[UR (x)] ^{20} DUMU $^{p.d}$AG-*be-sun* ^{lú}MAŠ.MAŠ É (*Babylonian sign form*) *aš-šur* ^{21} DUMU $^{p.d}$*Ba-ba*$_{6}$-MU-*ib-ni* ^{lú}ZABAR.DAB.BA *é-šár-ra* ^{22} *ana* IGI.DU$_{8}$.A-*šú ḫa-an-ṭiš is-su-ḫa* ^{23} [*š*]*á* IR *e-ma a-na* ^{d}AG ŠU^{II}-*su* ÍL-*ú* ^{24} [*s*]*u-up-pi-šu a-a i-šam-mé* ^{25} [MU]D ^{d}AG u ^{d}AMAR.UTU MU SAR *la ta-pa-šiṭ*

N4 no. 224 (A 185; Assur N4 no. 224)

Tablet: *Unpublished* (single-column tablet in portrait format; collated via unpublished pictures)

Content: Apotropaic *namburbi*-ritual against evil portended by a “curse” (*arratu*)

CDLI no.: –

Bibliography: *Unpublished*
Frankena 1960: 174 (transliteration of individual lines)

Discussion: Maul 1994: 445 note 15
Pedersén 1986: 65 no. 224
Ebeling 1954a: 5 (Assur Photo 4148 = A 185)

Obv. 1–3 A *namburbi*-ritual for undoing the evil of various types of *arratu*-curses (obv. 1–3: ⸢*šum*⸣-*ma* LÚ *ar-rat šag-gaš-t*[*i* …] ^{2} *lu ar-rat* ŠEŠ *lu ar-rat* NIN *l*[*u ar-rat* …] ^{3} NAM.BÚR.BI ḪUL *ar*-[*ra-ti šuātu ana pašāri*])

Obv. 4–9 Ritual instruction

Obv. 10–14 Incantation

Obv. 15 Brief instructions

Obv. 16–17 Prayer to Latarak

Obv. 18–19 Brief instructions

Obv. 20–26 Prayer to Marduk

Obv. 27–rev. 17 Long prayer to Marduk

Rev. 18 Damaged rubrick

Rev. 19–21 Ritual instruction

Rev. 22 Further instructions
Rev. 23–30 Final instruction
Rev. 31–33 Colophon:

LIBIR.RA.BI.GIM AB.SAR ⸢IGI.KÁR⸣ [DU]B-*pi* ^{p}*Ki-ṣir-*[*Aš-šur* ^{l}]^{ú}[x x x (x x)] ^{32} AMAR $^{p.d}$PA-*bi-su-nu* ⸢^{lú}⸣[MAŠ.MAŠ É ^{d}*Aš-šur*] ^{33} [AMAR/DUMU(?)] ⸢$^{p.d}$*Ba-ba*$_{6}$-MU-DÙ ^{lú}⸣ZABAR.DAB.BA [*É-šár-ra*]

N4 no. 228 (A 358; Assur N4 no. 228)

Tablet: *Unpublished* (single-column tablet in portrait format; collated via unpublished pictures)
Content: Bilingual Sumerian-Akkadian incantation for washing the mouth of a statue of the king made from various materials
CDLI no.: –
Bibliography: *Unpublished*
Discussion: Pedersén 1986: 65 no. 228

Obv. 1–rev. 9’ Incantation (obv. 1–2: ÉN alan ⸢nam⸣ gal-gal-la abzu-⸢ta bùluĝ-ĝá⸣ ^{2} ⸢*ṣa-lam*⸣ *ši-ma-ti ra-ba-a-te šá ina ap-si-i* \ *ir-bu-u*)
Rev. 10’–11’ “Recitation (for) washing the mouth of a statue of the king (made) of silver, go[ld], copper, bronze, (and) forest wood” (rev. 10’–11’: KA.INIM.MA ALAM LUGAL *šá* ⸢KÙ.BABBAR KÙ⸣.[SI$_{22}$] $^{11’}$ URUDU ZABAR GIŠ.^{giš}TIR.RA KA LUḪ)
Rev. 12’ Colophon:

ana ṣa-bat DÙ-*ši* ^{p}⸢*Ki-ṣir-Aš-šur*⸣ ZI-*ḫa*

N4 no. 237 (A 390+415; Assur N4 no. 237)

Tablet: *Unpublished* (single-column tablet in portrait format; collated via unpublished pictures)
Content: Incantation and prescriptions for treating ghost-induced illness
CDLI no.: –
Bibliography: *Unpublished*
Discussion: Pedersén 1986: 65 no. 237
Scurlock 2006: nos. 179 and 290 for the duplicate text *KAR* 56 by Kiṣir-Nabû

Obv. 1–13 Sumerian prayer to Šamaš
Obv. 14–15 Rubric: “[If a man] is seized by ghosts, and […] ghosts […]” ([…] GIDIM.MEŠ DAB-*su-ma* ^{15} […]⸢x⸣ GIDIM.MEŠ [(x)] ⸢x⸣)

Obv. 16–27+rev. 1–3	Prescription for producing and tying a magical amulet at the patient's temple, reciting an incantation, and anointing the patient(?)
Rev. 4–11	Prescription for anointing a patient in the case "If a man is sized by a ghost"; several new breaks (*ḫe-pí eš-šú*) are noted in the text
Rev. 12–16	Colophon:

[LIBIR.R]A.BI.GIM AB.SAR BA.AN.È ^{13} *ú-il-tì* ^{p}*Ki-ṣir-*⸢^{d}*Aš-šur*⸣ ^{14} ^{lú}ŠÁMAN.LÁ ⸢BÀN⸣.DA ^{15} DUMU $^{\text{p.d}}$AG-*bi-*⸢*su*⸣*-ni* ^{16} ^{lú}MAŠ.MAŠ É ^{d}*Aš-šur*

N4 no. 241 (A 2397; Assur N4 no. 241)

Tablet:	*Unpublished* (single-column tablet in portrait format; collated via unpublished pictures)
Content:	Words and phrases in Sumerian and Akkadian with an unidentified section
CDLI no.:	–
Bibliography:	*Unpublished*
Discussion:	Section 3.7.3 Pedersén 1986: 65 no. 241

Obv. 1–rev. 2	Brief peculiar words and phrases in Sumerian and Akkadian
Rev. 3	A total of previous entires: "Including 18$^{?}$ *explanatory comments*" (EN ⸢18$^{?}$ *ṣa-a-ti*⸣)
Rev. 4–10	Unidentified and badly damaged section
Rev. 11–14	Colophon:

[LIBIR.R]A.BI.GIM AB.SAR BA.AN.È ^{12} [*ú-il-t*]*ì* ^{p}⸢*Ki*⸣*-ṣir-Aš-šur* ⸢ŠÁMAN.LÁ TUR$^{?}$⸣ ^{13} [DUMU $^{\text{p.d}}$A]G-*bi-sún* ^{lú}MAŠ.MAŠ É ⸢AN.ŠÁR⸣ ^{14} [*ḫa*$^{?}$*-a*]*n*$^{?}$-⸢*ṭiš*$^{?}$⸣ *ú-šá-áš-*⸢*ṭir*⸣ *{*ma*}*

N4 no. 254 (Ass. 13955/xy; Assur N4 no. 254)

Tablet:	*Unpublished*
Content:	(*Bīt mēseri*?)
CDLI no.:	–
Bibliography:	*Unpublished*
Discussion:	Pedersén 1986: 65 no. 254

Unknown	Colophon:

(Kiṣir-Aššur, [broken title]?)

N4 no. 289 (A 2743; Assur N4 no. 289)

Tablet:	*Unpublished* (fragmentary single-column tablet in portrait(?) format; collated via unpublished pictures)
Content:	Ritual instructions for performing the ritual "A substitute for Ereškigal"
CDLI no.:	–
Bibliography:	*Unpublished*
Discussion:	Pedersén 1986: 66 no. 289
	Nasrabadi 1999: 41–43 and Tsukimoto 1985: 128–129 for duplicate texts, including *LKA* 79 by Kiṣir-Nabû

Obv. 1–15	Ritual instructions for performing the ritual "For giving a substitute (instead of a) man to Ereškigal" (obv. 1: [*ana pu*]-⸢*ú-ḫi* LÚ *a-na*⸣ [^{d}*Er*]*eš*-⸢*ki-gal* ŠÚM-*ni*⸣)
(*Breaks off*)	
Rev. 1'–4'	Colophon:

LIBIR.RA.BI.GI[M AB.SA]R.⸢ÀM BA.AN.È⸣ $^{2'}$ IM ^{p}*Ki-ṣir*-^{d}*Aš-šur* ^{lú}ŠÁMAN.LÁ BÀN.DA $^{3'}$ DUMU $^{p.d}$AG-*bi-su-nu* ^{lú}MAŠ.MAŠ BAL.TIL^{ki}-*u* $^{4'}$ [DUMU $^{p.}$]⸢^{d}*Ba*⸣-*ba*$_{6}$-MU-DÙ ^{lú}ZABAR.DAB.BA *É-šár-ra*

N4 no. 401 (Ass. 13956/fn; Assur N4 no. 401)

Tablet:	*Unpublished*
Content:	(Literary text?)
CDLI no.:	–
Bibliography:	*Unpublished*
Discussion:	Pedersén 1986: 68 no. 401

Unknown	Colophon:

(Kiṣir-Aššur, [broken title]?)

N4 no. 443 (A 2189; Assur N4 no. 443)

Tablet:	*Unpublished* (single-column tablet in portrait(?) format; not collated)
Content:	Prayer to Girra(?) or another divinity
CDLI no.:	–
Bibliography:	*Unpublished*
Discussion:	Pedersén 1986: 69

Unpublished	Prayer to a divinity, which may be identified as Girra
Unpublished	Colophon:

[*ana ṣa*]*-bat e-pe-ši* ᵖ*Ki-*[*ṣir-*…] *new line* […] ⸢É⸣ *aš-šur za-mar is-*[*su-ḫa*(?) …]

PKTA **pl. 10–11 =** ***SAA*** **20: 234–235** (VAT 8005; Assur N4 no. 98)

Tablet:	Single-column tablet in portrait format; not collated
Content:	Temple service rites for the temples of Assyria
CDLI no.:	–
Bibliography:	Parpola 2017: 100–102 no. 37, 234–235 (new copy and edition)
	Menzel 1981: T 110–112 no. 53 (edition)
	Ebeling 1950: IV, pl. 10–11 (copy)
Discussion:	Ermidoro 2017: XXVI–XXVII
	Pongratz-Leisten 2017: XXXVII, XLI
	Ermidoro 2015: 125–26
	Pongratz-Leisten 2015: 394
	Menzel 1981: 151–153
	van Driel 1969: 60–75, 165

Obv. 1'–8'	Instructions for the Assur temple
Obv. 9'–31'	Instructions for the "House of the god of Nineveh" (É DINGIR *š*[*a*] ⸢NINA[!]⸣[ki])
Rev. 1–23	Various rituals actions before various gods
Rev. 24–25 (*breaks off*)	Colophon:

[LIBIR.RA.BI.GIM *šá-ṭ*]*ir b*[*a*]*-rì* 25 [x x x ᵖ*Ki-ṣi*]*r-*[*Aš-šur* MAŠ.MAŠ] ⸢É AN⸣.Š[ÁR (*breaks off*)]

PKTA **pl. 39–40** (A 155; Assur N4 no. 330)

Tablet:	Slim and fragmentary two-columned vertically oriented tablet; not collated
Content:	Decrees by king Shalmaneser (the 5th?), and perhaps Sennacherib(?), regarding the Aššur temple personnel
CDLI no.:	–
Bibliography:	Parpola 2017: 144–145 no. 51 (edition)
	Menzel 1981: T 18–19 no. 16 (edition)
	Ebeling 1950: IV, pl. 39–40 (copy)
Discussion:	Ermidoro 2017: XXVIII–XXIX
	van Driel 1969: 179–82

Col. i 1–4	"The cup['s$^{?}$...] of the [Assur] temple, which Shalmanessar, king of [Assyria], established" (⸢GÚ⸣.ZI x[x x x (x)] ^{2} *ša* É [^{d}*Aš-šur ša*] ^{3} $^{p.d}$DI-*ma-nu*-MAŠ MAN ⸢KUR⸣ [AŠ] ^{4} *ú-ki-nu*$^{!}$*-u-ni*)
Col. i 5'–ii 17'	Fragmentary list of personnel with titles and connected divinities describing their duties and what they receive
Col. iii 1'	Decree from Sennacherib(?) (^{p}30-[PAB.MEŠ-SU MAN KUR AŠ(?)])
Col. iii 2'–iv 14'	Fragmentary list of personnel with titles and connected divinities describing their duties
Col. iv 15'–17'	Colophon:

⸢GIM⸣ SUMUN-*šú* SAR-*ma* IG[I.KAR(?)]/*b*[*a*$^{!}$*-rì*(?)] $^{16'}$ ⸢ŠU^{II}⸣ ^{p}*Ki-ṣi*[*r-Aš-šur*] $^{17'}$ ⸢MAŠ$^{!}$⸣.MAŠ ⸢É⸣ [AN.ŠÁR]

***RA* 15 pl. 76** ((Unknown); Assur N4 no. 631)

Tablet:	Single-column tablet in portrait format; collated from the copy as the original is considered lost
Content:	Prescriptions for treating snakebites, scorpion stings and a horse illness
CDLI no.:	–
Bibliography:	Appendix 2 (edition) Hunger 1968: 70 no. 200 ms E (colophon) Scheil 1918 (copy and edition)
Discussion:	Steinert 2018d: 276 George 2016: 165 Böck 2011: 697 Stol 2011: 400–402

Obv. 1'–11'	Various prescriptions for simple remedies against snakebites
Obv. 12'–13'	Prescription consisting of seven plants anointed onto the affected area of a snakebite
Obv. 14'–25'	Various prescriptions for simple remedies against scorpion stings
(*Breaks off*)	
Rev. 0'–4'	Fragmentary prescription for pouring medication into the left nostril of a horse(?) ([(x) x x x x] *na-ḫir* 2,30-*šú* DUB-[*ak-ma*])
Rev. 5'–8'	Fragmentary prescription for pouring medication into the left nostril to reach the stomach of an ill horse ([*ina*] ⸢DUG$^{?}$⸣ *zi-ri-qí ana n*[*a*]*-ḫir* 2,30-*šú* DUB-*ak* [*a*$^{?}$]*-na* ANŠE$^{!}$.KUR.RA *ša* bu ḫi DAB-*su* SIG$_5$-*iq*)
Rev. 9'–15'	Catch-line; colophon:

⸢32?⸣-*ú nis-ḫu* GABA.RI ^{giš}*li*$_9$-*u*$_5$$^{?}$ $^{11'}$ DUB-*pi* ^{p}*Ki-ṣir*-AN.ŠÁR$^{!}$ ^{lú}ŠÁMAN$^{!}$.LA$^{!}$ TUR *ša* ^{d}PA *tuk*$^{!}$-*lat-su* $^{12'}$ DUMU $^{p.d}$PA-*bi-sún* ^{lú}MAŠ.MAŠ É *Aš-šur* $^{13'}$ DUMU $^{p.d}$*Ba-ba*$_6$-MU-DÙ ^{lú}ZABAR.DAB.BA *É-šár-ra* $^{14'}$ [MU *šaṭ-r*]*u la ta-pa-šiṭ* NÍG.GIG ^{d}ŠE.NAGA $^{15'}$ [(x) x x] x x x *ni-ṭil* IGI^{II}-*šú li*-⸢*it*⸣-*b*[*al*]

***RA* 40 pl. 116** (Saint-Étienne 60; Assur N4 no. 630)

Tablet:	Single-column tablet in portrait format; collated via the CDLI photograph
Content:	Prescriptions for treating internal illnesses
CDLI no.:	P431342 (photograph)
Bibliography:	Scurlock and Andersen 2005: 48 no. 3.98, 178 no. 8.65, 181 no. 8.81, 184 no. 8.96, 801 (treatment of individual lines) Cadelli 2000: 195 ms D (treatment of individual lines) Millard and Sigrist 1985: 573 Hunger 1968: 70 no. 200 ms F (colophon) Labat and Tournay 1945–46 (copy and edition) Scheil 1921: 16 (treatment of individual lines)

Obv. 1–3	Prescription for a potion against *ašû*, *pašittu*, or *lubāṭu* illness
Obv. 4–7	Prescription intended to induce vomit (BURU$_8$-*ma*), after which the patient eats a hot soup(?) (*baḫ-ra*)
Obv. 8–12	Prescription for dripping fluid onto the tip of the patient's tongue (KIR$_4$ EME-*šú* [*t*]*u-qar-ra-ár*) and pouring medication into his nose via a reed pipette (^{gi}SAG.KUD$^{!}$ DIR-*ma ana na-ḫi-ri-šú* DUB), whereupon the patient drinks beer and vomits (KAŠ.SAG NAG.MEŠ-*ma i-àr-rù*)
Obv. 13–18	Prescription consisting of 11 plants for the lungs (11 Ú.MEŠ ḪAR.[MEŠ$^{?}$]) made into seven pills eaten on an empty stomach (7 *ku-pa-tin-ni* DÙ-*uš* NU *pa-tan* G[U$_7$ (x?)])
Obv. 19–20	Fragmentary prescription for drinking a potion on an empty stomach and administering an enema(?) (*ina* DÚR-*šú* […])
Obv. 21	Fragmentary prescription
(*Breaks off*)	
Rev. 1'–5'	Colophon:

DUB-*pi* ^{p}*Ki-ṣir*-AN.ŠÁR ^{lú}ŠÁ[MAN.LÁ TUR(?)] ^{2} [DUMU $^{p.}$]^{d}AG-*bi-sún* ^{lú}MAŠ.MAŠ ⸢É⸣ [(*Aššur*)] ^{3} ⸢DUMU⸣ $^{p.d}$*Ba-ba*$_6$-MU-DÙ ^{lú}ZABAR.DAB.BA [(*Ešarra*)] ^{4} MU ^{d}AG *u* ^{d}AMAR.UTU *šu-mi šaṭ-rù la ta-pa-*[*šiṭ*] ^{5} *šà* IR ^{d}A[G] ZÀḪ-*šú liq-b*[*i*]

APPENDIX 2

Edition of *RA* 15 pl. 76

Manuscripts

A = *RA* 15 pl. 76
Copy : Scheil 1918 pl. 76.
Edition: Scheil 1918.
Comments: George 2016: 165; Böck 2011: 697; Stol 2011: 400–402.
Content: Mainly one-lined prescriptions against snakebites (obv. 1'–13') and scorpion stings (obv. 14'–25'), plus two fragmentary prescriptions for treating a horse (rev. 0'–4' and 5'–8').

B = *BAM* 42
Copy: Köcher 1963a no. 42.
Edition: Transliteration on the BabMed website; Geller 2014: 18–19 note 26; Heeßel 2010c: 153–54 edited the last part of the text.
Comments: Scurlock 2014: 469–71; Finkel 1999: 213 and note 3.
Content: Prescriptions for illnesses of the airways (obv. 1–12, 13–23, 24–35, 36–41, rev. 42–49, 50–56, 57–60, 61–62) and snakebite (rev. 63–68). Only the relevant prescriptions against snakebite are edited below.

C = *AMT* 92,7
Copy: Thompson 1923 pl. 92 no. 7.
Edition: Transliteration on the BabMed website.
Content: Small fragment containing the remains of three prescriptions, two of which are against snakebite (obv. 6'–7', 8'; cf. obv. 1'–5').

Transliteration

Obverse A

1'

A obv. 1'	[x x x x x x x x x x x x x-*l*]*u*$^{?}$ ⸢GU$_{7}$$^{!?}$⸣-[*ma*$^{?}$ *ina*$^{?}$]-⸢*eš*⸣
B rev. 63	DIŠ NA MUŠ ⸢*iš*⸣-*šuk-šú* ⸢ú$^{?}$⸣*ur-ba*-⸢*ti*⸣ *ta-qàl-lu* GU$_{7}$-*ma né-eš*
C obv. 6'–7'	DIŠ NA MUŠ *iš-šik-šú* SUḪUŠ *ur-ba-ti* [7] *ta-qal-lap* GU$_{7}$-*ma ina-eš*
A+B	If a snake bit a man, you roast an *urbatu*-plant, he eats (it), and he will live (B: he lives).
C	If a snake bit a man, you peel the root of an *urabatu*-plant, he eats (it) and he will live.

2’

A obv. 2’	[DIŠ KI.MIN x x x x x (x)]⸢igi x NAG$^{?}$-*ma* <*ina*> UGU$^{!?}$ *niš*$^{?}$⸣-*ki*-[*šú*] GAR-*an*
B rev. 64	DIŠ NA MUŠ ⸢*iš*⸣-*šuk-šú* [^{ú}]⸢IGI⸣-*lim* ⸢SÚD⸣ *ina* KAŠ NAG-*ma né-eš* DIŠ MIN ^{ú}IGI-*lim ina* UGU *niš-ki-šú* GAR-*an né*-[*eš*]
C obv. 8’	DIŠ KI.MIN ^{ú}IGI-*lim* *ina* KAŠ NAG-*ma ina-eš*
A	[If ditto …] he drinks (it) and places (it) <onto> [his] bite.
B	If a snake bit a man, you crush *imḫur-līm*, he drinks (it) in beer and he lives. If ditto, you place *imḫur-līm* onto his bite, he lives.
C	If ditto he drinks *imḫur-līm* in beer and he will live.

3’

A obv. 3’	[DIŠ KI.MIN x x x x (x)] ⸢^{ú}*kam*$^{?}$-*ka*⸣-[*du*] SÚD$^{!}$ *ana* IGI MAR-*ma ina-eš*
B rev. 65–66a	DIŠ NA MUŠ ⸢*iš*⸣-*šuk-šú* ^{ú}IGI-[*lim* ^{giš}ŠE].NÁ.A GU$_7$-*ma* <*né-eš*> DIŠ MIN ^{ú}*ṣa-ṣu-um-tú* ^{giš}*kám-ka-du* SÚD 66 ⸢x(?) *ana*⸣ IGI M[AR]-*ma*⸣ *né-eš* : →
A	[If ditto], you crush […], (and) *kamkadu*-plant, you anoint (it) onto (the affected area), and he will live.
B	If a snake bit a man, he eats *imḫur*-[*līm*]-plant (and) [*šu*]*nû*-plant, and <he lives>. If ditto, you crush *ṣaṣumtu*-plant (and) *kamkadu*-plant [x] you anoint (it) onto (the affected area), and he lives.

4’

A obv. 4’	DIŠ [KI.MIN] ⸢^{ú}⸣*an-daḫ-šum* SÚD IGI [G]IG *ta-kar-ma ina-eš*
B rev. 66b	DIŠ MIN ⸢^{ú}⸣*an-daḫ-še* SÚD IGI GIG *ta-kar-ma né-eš*
A+B	If ditto, you crush *andaḫšu*-plant, you rub (it) on the surface of the wound, and he will live (B: he lives).

5’

A obv. 5’	DIŠ K[I.MI]N ⸢^{ú}⸣*tar-muš*$_8$ SÚD *ina* KAŠ SAG NAG-*ma ina-eš*
B rev. 67’a	DIŠ MIN ⸢^{ú}⸣[*t*]*ar-muš*$_8$ SÚD *ina* KAŠ [N]AG-*ma né-eš* …
A+B	If ditto, you crush *tarmuš*-plant, he drinks (it) in first-quality beer, and he will live (B: he lives).

6’

A obv. 6’	DIŠ K[I.MI]N ⸢SUḪUŠ⸣ ^{giš}NAM.TAR NÍTAḪ *ina* GÚ-*šú* GAR-*an*
B rev. 68	DIŠ MIN [^{ú}]NAM.TAR NÍTAḪ ⸢ḪÁD$^{?}$.DU$^{?}$⸣ SÚD *ina* DÈ *tu-ṣar-rap-ma né-eš*

A If d[itt]o, you place the root of a male *pillû*-plant around his neck.

B If ditto, you crush *dried*(?) male *pillû*-plant, you burn (it) over coal and he lives.

7’

A obv. 7’ DIŠ K[I.MI]N ^{ú}*bar-ra-qi-tú ina* KAŠ SAG$^{!}$ NAG

A If d[itt]o, he drinks *barraqītu*-plant in first-quality beer.

8’

A obv. 8’ DIŠ K[I.MI]N ^{ú}*el-pe-tu ḫi-mu-ú ana* IGI ZÚ LÁ-⸢*du*⸣

A If d[itt]o, bind *elpetu*-reed (in) a *ḫimû*-wad over the bite.

9’

A obv. 9’ DIŠ K[I.MI]N ^{ú}*ur-ba-tú*$^{!}$ *ḫi-mu-ú ana* IGI ZÚ LÁ-*du*

A If d[itt]o, bind *urbatu*-reed (in) a *ḫimû*-wad over the bite.

10’

A obv. 10’ DIŠ [KI].MIN ^{ú}PA-PA-*a-nu ḫi-mu-ú* GIŠ.NÚ$^{!}$-*šu* NIGIN-⸢*ú*⸣

A If [di]tto, surround his bed with *arariānu*-plant (in) a *ḫimû*-wad.

11’

A obv. 11’ DIŠ [KI].MIN ^{ú}EME.UR.GI$_7$ Ú ZÚ MUŠ *u* UR.GI$_7$ *ina* GÚ$^{!}$-*šú* GAR-*an*

A If [di]tto, “Dog’s tongue”, a plant for the bite of snake and dog, you place around his neck.

12’

A obv. 12’ ⸢^{ú}ŠAKIR$^{?}$⸣ ^{ú}EME.UR.GI$_7$ ^{ú}GAMUN ^{ú}*ur-ba-tú* $^{ú!}$IGI-*lim* ^{ú}*el-pi-tú*

A ⸢*šakirû*$^{?}$⸣-plant, “Dog’s tongue”,-plant *kamūnu*-cumin(?), *urbatu*-plant, “It cures a thousand”-plant, *elpetu*-reed,

13’

A obv. 13’ ⸢^{ú}*kur-ka*⸣-*nu-u* 7 Ú.MEŠ *ni-šik* MUŠ *ina* Ì.GIŠ EŠ.MEŠ

A (and) *kurkānû*-plant: 7 ingredients (for) snake bite, he is anointed (with these) in oil.

14’

A obv. 14’ [DIŠ NA G]ÍR$^{!}$.TAB SÌG$^{!}$-*su* EME.D[I]R [S]AG$^{!}$.DU-*su* KUD-*is* MÚD.MEŠ-*šú* IGI *ziq-ti* EŠ.MEŠ *ina-eš*

A [If a sc]orpion stung a [man], you cut off the head of a lizard, you anoint the surface of the sting (with) its blood, and he will live.

15’

A obv. 15’ [KI.MIN] ZÌ.MEŠ MURUB$_4$ IGI ⸢*ziq*⸣-*ti ki-sir*!-*ma ina-eš*

A [If ditto], block the centre of the surface of the sting (with) flour, and he will live.

16’

A obv. 16’ [KI.MI]N ^{ú}GAMUN SÚD *ina* KAŠ NAG *u* GU$_7$-*ma ina-eš*

A [If ditt]o, you crush *kamūnu*-cumin(?), he drinks (it) in beer and he eats (it), and he will live.

17’

A obv. 17’ [KI.MIN] ⸢*ru-pu*⸣-*uš-ti* GUD!? IGI *ziq-ti* EŠ-*ma ina-eš*

A [If ditto], you anoint the surface of the sting (with) ox saliva, and he will live.

18’

A obv. 18’ [MUŠ].⸢DÍM.GURUN⸣.NA SAG.DU-*su* KUD!-*is* MÚD.MEŠ IGI *ziq-ti* EŠ.MEŠ DIDA GU$_7$!

A You cut off the head of a *pizallūru*-gecko, you anoint the surface of the sting (with) the blood, (and) he eats! *billatu*-substance.

19’

A obv. 19’ [x]⸢x⸣ ú me ti šá ⸢še?⸣ ri 7-*šú* ⸢nu?⸣ li ⸢iḫ? x(?)⸣ tu *ina-eš*

A [...] ..., seven times, [x] ..., (and) he will live

20’

A obv. 20’ [(x)]⸢x⸣ ⸢me?⸣ *ta-šá-ḫal* GEŠTIN ZÌ.M[EŠ?] ⸢NÍG⸣.LÁ GAR-⸢*an*⸣ *ina-eš*

A You sieve [...], (in) wine (and) *flour*? you apply (it as) a poultice, (and) he will live.

21’

A obv. 21’ [(x) x x x x(?)] SÚD *ina* KAŠ S[A]G NAG-*ma ina-eš*

A [...] you crush [...], he drinks (it) in first-q[ual]ity beer, and he will live.

22’

A obv. 22’ [x x x(?)] ⸢SÚD⸣ *ina* KAŠ SAG! NAG *ina* Ì.GIŠ ŠÉŠ-*ma* ⸢GÚ? x?⸣[x (x)]

A [...(?)] you crush [...], he drinks it in first-quality beer, he is anointed with oil and the neck(?) [...].

23’

A obv. 23’ [x x x x]⌜x⌝ SÚD!? *ina* KAŠ NAG *ina* Ì.GIŠ ŠÉŠ-*su* [x] ⌜diš⌝ [x (x)]

A [...(?)] you *crush*(?) [...], he drinks (it) in beer, you anoint him with oil, [...].

24’

A obv. 24’ [x x x x(?) *ina* KAŠ(?)] NAG *ina* Ì.GIŠ ŠÉ[Š-*su-ma ina-eš*(?)]

A [...], he drinks [(it) in beer(?)], you anoi[nt him] with oil, [(and he will live?)].

25’

A obv. 25’ [x x x x x x(?) *ina*?] ⌜KAŠ NAG *ina* Ì⌝[.GIŠ ŠÉŠ-*su-ma*(?) *ina-eš*(?)]

A [...], he drinks (it) [in] beer, [you anoint him(?)] with oil, [(and he will live?)].

Reverse A

0’

A rev. 0’ [x x x x x x x(?)]⌜x⌝[x x x(?)]

A [...]

1’

A rev. 1’ [x x x x x(?)] ⌜x sag⌝ ḫa [x x x x(?)]

A [...]

2’

A rev. 2’ [x x (x) x x] ⌜šu⌝ si bi ⌜x⌝ [x x x (x)]

A [...]

3’

A rev. 3’ [x x x x]⌜x⌝-*tu a-ḫa-meš tu*-[x x x x]

A [...] together you [...]

4’

A rev. 4’ [x x (x) x x] *na-ḫir* 2,30-*šú* DUB-[*ak-ma ina-eš*(?)]

A [...] you pour it into its left nostril [(and it will live?)].

5’

A rev. 5’ [x x x]⌜x⌝-*e* SUḪUŠ ú[...]

A [...] root of [...]-plant

6’

A rev. 6’ [x(?)] SÚD *ina* KAŠ *lu ina* GEŠTIN GAZ$^{?}$

A [x(?)] you pound, you pulverize(?) (this) in beer or in wine,

7’

A rev. 7’ [*ina*] ⌜DUG$^{?}$⌝ *zi-ri-qí ana n*[*a*]-*ḫir* 2,30-*šú* DUB-*ak*

A You pour (it) into its left nostril [*via*] a “*stomach tube*”,

8’

A rev. 8’ [*a*$^{?}$]-*na* ANŠE$^{!}$.KUR.RA *ša* bu ḫi DAB-*su* SIG$_{5}$-*iq*

A It is good [f]or a horse that is seized (by) *bu ḫi*.

Colophon

A rev. 9’ DIŠ NA$^{!}$ ŠÀ-*šú* E$_{11}$$^{!}$ *ù ú*$^{!}$-*rad* ŠÀ-*ba-šú* E$_{11}$ *a-lam*$^{?}$

A If a man’s$^{!}$ stomach rises (to vomit) and *settles*$^{!}$, (and) his stomach (after having) settled *rises*(?) (again)

A rev. 10’ ⌜32$^{?}$⌝-*ú nis-ḫu* GABA.RI ^{giš}*le-ʾi*

A 32nd(?) extract, copy of a writing-board,

A rev. 11’ DUB-*pi* ^{p}*Ki-ṣir*-AN.ŠÁR$^{!}$ ^{lú}ŠÁMAN$^{!}$.LA$^{!}$ TUR *ša* ^{d}PA *tuk*$^{!}$-*lat-su*

A Tablet of Kiṣir-Aššur, the *šamallû ṣeḫru* whose trust is Nabû,

A rev. 12’ DUMU $^{p.d}$PA-*bi-sún* ^{lú}MAŠ.MAŠ É *Aš-šur*

A Son of Nabû-bēssunu, *mašmaš bīt Aššur*,

A rev. 13’ DUMU $^{p.d}$*Ba-ba*$_{6}$-MU-DÙ ^{lú}ZABAR.DAB.BA *É-šár-ra*

A Son of Bāba-šuma-ibni, *zabardabbû*-priest of the *Ešarra*-temple.

A rev. 14’ [MU *šaṭ-r*]*u la ta-pa-šiṭ* NÍG.GIG ^{d}ŠE.NAGA

A Do not erase the written name, (it is) a taboo of Nisaba,

A rev. 15’ [(x) x x] x x x *ni-ṭil* IGI^{II}-*šú li*-⌜*it*⌝-*b*[*al*]

A […], may [DN] take aw[ay] his eyesight!

General Observations

Ms A was copied by Kiṣir-Aššur and is not duplicated exactly in either of the other mss. As such, it serves as the main manuscript for this edition. It was copied, transliterated, and translated in Scheil 1918. However, Scheil's copy is problematic in several places (see the commentary below). Unfortunately, Scheil provided no inventory number, collection name, or other indications as to the location of the tablet. Consequently, it is currently considered lost and Scheil's copy is the basis for my emendations of what I assume must be incorrectly copied signs. As the majority of the incorrect signs appear to have either too many or too few strokes, it is possible that Scheil copied the tablet according to a picture without further collation. Furthermore, it is difficult to interpret whether the right edge on the obverse and reverse was the slightly damaged edge of the tablet or if ms A broke off from a multi-columned tablet. I assume that the manuscript was single-columned. For further discussion of this text, see Section 3.5 and Chapter 4.

The obverse of ms A contains prescriptions related to applying or anointing various substances onto bites and stings or drinking and eating certain potions or substances. Although several plants remain unidentified, it is possible that the effect of applying these various plants could in some instances induce diffusion so that the venom would be (partially) extracted from the bite/sting. Note that some of the same plants used in individual prescriptions in ms A-C against snakebite are also used in the single potion (*mašqītu*) consisting of 13 plants that are drunk in wine against snakebite in *BAM* 176 (see Geller 2014: 18 note 26).

The translation of prescriptions ending in (verbal form)-*ma* TI/*ina-eš* are translated as "he (drinks/eats/etc.) …, and he will live", although it should be noted that Scurlock has argued that these constructions designate "a subordinate 'if' clause" (Scurlock and Andersen 2005: xvi with further references). I have left this possible distinction out of the translations, as it would make the content too confusing.

Ms A has dividing lines after obv. 11' and 13', which separate the entry in obv. 12'–13'. This entry is the only prescription on the obverse that is longer than a single line. Ms A breaks off after obv. 25'. The beginning of the reverse of ms A is broken. Dividing lines occur after rev. 4' and rev. 8'. The colophon in obv. 9'–15' breaks off after rev. 15', although it remains uncertain if more lines once existed.

Two plant lists, *CT* 14 pl. 23 (K. 9283) and *STT* 92, which list ingredients, maladies, and methods for administering the drugs, partially duplicate individual lines of ms A. Both plant lists are unedited, although see Böck 2014a: 156 for *STT* 92. *CT* 14 pl. 23 generally contains Babylonian sign forms. Of note, both lists provide the lines on ms A obv. 7'–11' in roughly the same order with infinitive verbal forms (see below). It therefore seems that the lines in ms A originally originated from a plant list.

Commentary

Obverse

1' Ms A is difficult to reconstruct, as there are few readable signs. It is possible that the line duplicated ms B rev. 63, which is taken as the basis for comparison. Geller (2014: 18 note 26) reads SUḪUŠ instead of ⌜ú?⌝. Heeßel (2010c: 154) only reads *urbatu*, which is followed here. Furthermore, in ms C the root (SUḪUŠ) of the *urbatu*-plant is peeled (*qalāpu*), see CAD (Q: 58–59).

The verb *našāku* ordinarily has the thematic vowels *a*/*u* and it is rarely attested with *i*/*i* (CAD N/2: 53–54; CDA: 244; *AHw*: 758). Ms C has /i/ as the thematic vowel, which indicates the verb had undergone a change (see Kouwenberg 2010: 77–78; von Soden 1995: 141 §87d). The passage from ms C is one of the only instances quoted in the CAD.

For the *urbatu*-plant, see obv. 9'.

1'–6' Ms B ends the prescriptions with the stative *né-eš* rather than ms A's more common *ina-eš* from *nêšu* "to live, stay alive, recover" (CAD N/2: 197–98). BAM 42 was excavated in the N4 collection and copied by a certain Aššur-šākin-šumi without a title and with a broken tablet designation. For Aššur-šākin-šumi, see Fadhil 2018; Maul and Strauß 2011: 34–35, 104–108, 120–122; Maul 2010a: 216 note 101. There does not appear to be a copying statement in the colophon. According to Finkel (1999: 213 note 3), the snake treatments were added in a smaller hand, perhaps as an "afterthought". For the overlap between these two tablets, see Section 3.5.1.

2' Obv. 2' in ms A may have combined the two individual prescriptions found in ms B rev. 64. Ms A contains the instructions NAG?-*ma* and GAR-*an*, which match the individual instructions in the two prescriptions found in ms B rev. 64. If this interpretation is correct, ms A should also contain the phrase *ina* UGU before *niš-ki-šú*. However, the remaining wedges do not entirely support this, and I therefore transliterate <*ina*> ⌜UGU?⌝.

The plant used in ms B-C is ^{ú}IGI-*lim* called *imḫur-līm* "it cures a thousand (illnesses)" and is associated with the *errû*-colocynth(?) (CAD I-J: 118–19; see *CMAwR* 2: 511; *CMAwR* 1: 470). *Imḫur-līm* is described in *Šammu šikinšu* as having the tendrils of the *qiššû*-gourd, the seed of the *ḫurātu*-plant, a bitter as well as soft root, and red-golden offshoots (see Stadhouders 2012: 4 §23–24, 8 §14; Stadhouders 2011: 10 §23–24, 19 §14). It can be used against every kind of sore and "'the Furious One', a deputy (*šanû*) of Adad" (ibid.; see also BAM 379 col. ii 55' in Stadhouders 2012: 16; Stadhouders 2011: 35). The plant is listed in the "Dreckapotheke" section of Uruanna as "dust from the tracks of a wolf", line 23: ... [SAḪA]R *ki-bi-is* UR.BAR.RA (Rumor 2017: 7, 26 line 23). *Imhur-līm* also appears in BAM 1 col. i 58 col. ii 50 (Attia and Buisson 2012: 27–28; CAD T: 62).

The plant list *STT* 92 col. i 5 probably had a similar entry: Ú IGI-*lim* : Ú ZÚ [MUŠ : x x x x x x x x(?)], "The plant *imḫur-līm* : a plant (for) [snake] bite [...]".

3' Ms A is very fragmentary, but may duplicate the second prescription in ms B rev. 65–66a. Both prescriptions in ms B rev. 65–66a are quoted for reference. The addition in ms B rev. 65 of <*né-eš*> follows Heeßel (2010c: 154).

The reconstruction [^{giš}ŠE].NÁ.A in ms B seems to fit the line, and is also followed by Heeßel (2010c: 154) and Geller (2014: 18 note 26). The *šunû*-plant was likely a shrub or perhaps a "chaste tree" (*CAD* Š/3: 309–10; see also Freedman 2017: 137 line 51', 138 line 74'; *CMAwR* 2: 514; *CMAwR* 1: 236, 473 with further references). In Uruanna's "Dreckapotheke" section, *uḫūlu qarnānû* is equated with the names *šunû* and *baltu* (Rumor 2017: 20, 31 line 115; see also *CMAwR* 1: 473; Geller 2005: 3). In the pharmacological-therapeutic compendium *BAM* 1, the *šunû*-plant can be crushed in oil and anointed onto the affected area to treat an illness ([DA]B *šá-da-ni*, possibly a type of fever, see Bácskay 2018: 146ff.), and the root can be crushed into oil and drunk in good beer against *suālu*-cough or *ḫaḫḫu*-phlegm (Attia and Buisson 2012: 26 col. i 40, 27 col. ii 31, 28 col. ii 44, 30 col. iv 14).

The *ṣaṣumtu*-plant in ms B rev. 65 is connected to the healing goddess Gula and is stated in Uruanna to be her plant (Böck 2014a: 158–59; see also *CAD* Ṣ: 116; *AHw*: 1987; *CMAwR* 2: 514). The plant is unidentified, but according to *BAM* 1 it is effective against *ḫimiṭ ṣēti* if drunk in good beer and anointed onto the affected area, against *ašû*-illness if drunk in good beer, and it can be crushed into hot ghee and anointed onto the affected area (Attia and Buisson 2012: 26 col. i 49, 27 col. ii 3 and col. ii 19; see also *CMAwR* 1: 234, 472). In Uruanna's "Dreckapotheke" section, the plant is referred to as "the head of a black raven" and "wool of a virgin ewe" (Rumor 2017: 19, 22, 30 line 103, 31 line 123). Another pharmacological text describes the plant as a drug "for keeping vermin out of a man's house. You put it in water and sprinkle the house with it" (Stadhouders 2012: 17 col. iv 20–21; Stadhouders 2011: 37 col. iv 20–21). It was believed to be effective to deter wild animals (Böck 2014a: 162–163, 168). The *ṣuṣumtu*-plant's name may refer to something going out (*waṣû*), perhaps indicating some excreta (see Böck 2014a: 159). These excreta could be from the plant itself or perhaps the wound once the plant was applied.

The *kamkadu*-plant in ms B rev. 65 is unidentified (see *CAD* K: 123–24; *CMAwR* 2: 511; Geller 2014: 84; *CMAwR* 1: 470; Kinnier-Wilson 2005: 47). In sufficient quantities, the plant was considered a bad omen and the 59th tablet of *Šumma ālu* line 35 states: "If *kamkadu*-plant becomes thick, that field will be abandoned" (see also the 55th tablet line 5; Freedman 2017: 99, 103, 126). The "Dreckapotheke" section of Uruanna refers to the plant as "an *išqippu*-earthworm" or perhaps *išqippu*-bird (Rumor 2017: 5, 25 line 8; see CAD I–J: 261). The second interpretation is perhaps more plausible as in BAM 1 the plant is placed on a wound against the problem "spur(?) of the bird" (*ḫi-dar* MUŠEN, CAD Ḫ: 194; see Attia and Buisson 2012: 28 col. ii 54).

4' The *andaḫšu* was perhaps "a bulbous spring vegetable" (CAD A/2: 112–13) or an "alliaceous plant or variety of crocus" (*CMAwR* 1: 468; see *CMAwR* 2: 508 with references). In comparison, OB texts mention the plant in relation to aromatics (Middeke-Conlin 2014: 26, 39). The plant is used in a prescription against chest pains (Maul and Strauß 2011: 101–102 col. ii' 5'), as well as a phylactery against *ummu*-fever (Bácskay 2017: 51). The *andaḫšu*-plant occurs in BAM 1, which states it could be drunk against *suālu*-cough or *šīqu*-illness (Attia and Buisson 2012: 27 col. ii 33 and col. ii 40). An omen in the 55th tablet of *Šumma ālu* refers to someone growing the plant in a field: "If ditto ((someone) grows) *andaḫšu*-plant ditto (in a field), an enemy will carry off his equipment; ill health will be in store for him" (Freedman 2017: 101 line 62').

The writing GIG refers to *simmu* "skin eruption, lesion" (CAD S: 276–78; Böck 2014a: 22–24). This is the only prescription in ms A and C referring to the bite as a *simmu*.

For the final verbal form, see also CAD K: 239–240.

5' The *tarmuš*-plant is possibly a species of *lupine* (see CAD T: 238–39; *CMAwR* 2: 515; *CMAwR* 1: 473 with references). The plant is also used in BAM 1 col. ii 52 (Attia and Buisson 2012: 28). The "Dreckapotheke" section of Uruanna lists the plant as "fat of a male pig mottled with red", "fat from the kidneys of a white pig mottled with red", and "dust from the footstep of a *ḫannu*(?)-man" (Rumor 2017: 11, 28 line 51).

Ms B rev. 67' comprises two entries. The second half of the line does not appear in ms A. Geller (2014: 18–19 note 26) reads ms B rev. 67'b as follows: DIŠ MIN ^{giš}*mi*-URU$_4$-*iš*-^{giš}MÁ-*ra*$^!$ *ina* Ù-*šú* GAR.GAR-*ma né-eš*, "If ditto, you keep applying *mirišmara* during his sleep, and he will get better" (see Heeßel 2010c: 154).

6' The *pillû*-plant is often interpreted as "mandrake", although this remains uncertain. Recently, Kinnier Wilson has suggested the plant may have been a species of mistletoe (see discussion with further references in CAD P: 376–77; *CMAwR* 2: 513; *CMAwR* 1: 471; Kinnier Wilson 2011: 5–10). The plant is regularly attested in a "male" variant that is also the one used in mss A and B. However, only ms A prescribes using the root of the plant. The *pillû*-plant is among a few select plants that demand certain attention when pulled out of the ground (see Böck 2014a: 158 and note 84 with further references). The ambivalent nature of the plant can be read in an entry in the 59th tablet of *Šumma ālu* line 26: "If *pillû*-tree(?) grows(?), the people's health will not be good" (Freedman 2017: 126). In Uruanna's "Dreckapotheke" section, the *pillû*-plant is referred to as "black (spot/hair?) from the (upper) leg of a donkey" or the "nail of a black dog" (Rumor 2017: 10, 27 lines 44–45; see also ibid.: 18, 30 line 94). The plant has a wide range of uses (e.g., Scurlock 2014: 400, 436, 478, 494, 519, 526–27, 541, 547; cf. Attia and Buisson 2012: 26 col. i 1, 30 col. iv 2).

The reading ⸢ḪÁD$^{?}$.DU$^{?}$⸣ remains tentative. Heeßel (2010c: 154) interpreted this as an instruction to the reader similar to SÚD (see also Geller 2014: 18–19 note 26). I read this as an adjective, which is also a possibility with this Sumerogram, as the process of drying would have taken too long in relation to the presumed immediate use of such a prescription.

The plant list *CT* 14 pl. 23 obv. 9 may also prescribe the root of the *pillû*-plant, to be placed around the neck of the patient: [Ú SUḪU]Š$^{??}$ NAM.TAR.⸢RA⸣ : Ú ZÚ MUŠ : *ina* GÚ-*šú* GAR-*an*, "[…] *pillû*-plant : a plant (for) snakebite : you place (it) around his neck".

7' The plant *barraqītu* seems to be attested exclusively in connection to snakebites and there are therefore relatively few references to it (see *CAD* B: 113). An alternative name listed in Uruanna for this plant is *zarraštu*, which is only attested lexically (*CAD* Z: 69).

In this and the following lines in ms A and the partial duplicate *CT* 14 pl. 23 (see below), the sign ZÚ is written for "bite" *nišku*. This word is normally written ZÚ.KUD for *našāku* literally "to split the teeth" (Borger 2004: 256; see *CAD* N/2: 281–82).

7'–11' The lines in ms A are partly duplicated in the traditional plant list format in *CT* 14 pl. 23 and *STT* 92. The plant lists contain the same elements and method of administering the drugs as ms A. Interestingly, ms A obv. 6'–13' do not contain the statement that the patient will recover, nor do such statements occur in the plant lists. This information supports that the entries in ms A were originally partly derived from a plant list. The row of entries is almost the same in all three manuscripts:

CT 14 pl. 23 obv. 10 [Ú *bar*]-*ra-qi-tú* : Ú ZÚ MUŠ : *ina* KAŠ.SAG NAG-*ú*
STT 92 col. i 10' [Ú] *bar-ra-q*[*ú*$^{?}$-*tú*] : Ú ZÚ [MUŠ : x x x x x]
[The plant *bar*]*raqītu* : a plant (for) snakebite : drink (it) in first-quality beer.

CT 14 pl. 23 obv. 6 [Ú *el-p*]*e-tú* : Ú KA MUŠ : *ḫi-mu-ú ana* IGI ZÚ [LÁ-*du*]
STT 92 col. i 6 Ú *el-*[*p*]*e-tú* : Ú ZÚ M[UŠ : x x x x x x x x]
The plant *elpetu* : a plant (for) snakebite: [bind (it in)] a *ḫimû*-wad over the bite.

CT 14 pl. 23 obv. 7 [Ú *ur-b*]*a-tú* : Ú ZÚ MUŠ : *ḫi-mu-ú ana* IGI ZÚ LÁ-[*du*]
STT 92 col. i 7 Ú *u*[*r-b*]*a-tú*$^{!}$: Ú ZÚ [MUŠ : x x x x x x x x]

The plant *urbatu* : a plant (for) snakebite : bind (it in) a *ḫimû*-wad over the bite.

CT 14 pl. 23 obv. 8 [^{ú}PA-PA]-⌜*a*⌝-*nu* : Ú ZÚ MUŠ : *ḫi-mu-ú* GIŠ.NÚ-[(*šú*) NIGIN-*ú*]

STT 92 col. i 8 Ú [PA-P]A-*a-nu* : Ú ZÚ [MUŠ : x x x x x x x x]

The plant *arariānu* : a plant (for) snakebite : [surround his] bed (with it in) a *ḫimû*-wad.

CT 14 pl. 23 obv. 11 [^{ú}EM]E.UR$^{!}$.GI$_{7}$: Ú ZÚ MUŠ *u* UR.GI$_{7}$: LÚ *šu-ku-lu u* NAG-*u*

STT 92 col. i 11 [Ú EM]E.UR.[GI$_{7}$] : Ú ZÚ MUŠ [x x x x x x x x x x]

[… "Dog]'s tongue" : a plant for the bite of snake and dog : make the man consume and drink (it).

It is possible that *STT* 92 col. i 11 should be restored according to *CT* 14 pl. 23 obv. 11, see Böck 2014a: 156.

For the translation of the infinitives, see below.

8'–10' The verbal forms in these lines in ms A are marked as infinitives, but translated as imperatives or precatives, e.g., NAG-*ú* "drink, he shall drink", LÁ-*du* "bandage, he shall bandage". This form of the infinitive is referred to as the "heischenden Infinitiv" by von Soden (1995: 252 §150*), and occurs instead of the "Heischendes Präsens" in some briefer recipes or pharmacological works (ibid.: 127, 252; see Aro 1961: 28–29 and note 1). As stated above, such forms in prescriptions seem to be rare, thereby stessing the relationship between the plant lists *CT* 14 pl. 23 as well as *STT* 92 and ms A.

8' The ingredient *elpetu* was likely a reed and is translated "rush, reed" (*CAD* E: 108–109) or "cattail rush" (Scurlock 2018: 528). It is also listed in *Malku* as *nīmu* (Hrůša 2010: 62, 186), which is likely also a "rush" (*CAD* N/2: 235). The *elpetu*-reed could possibly be used to weave baskets, which fits the context of a "wad" (see *CAD* E: 109). Medically, the plant is not well attested. The plant seems to have caught fire easily and to have grown in places, which could be flooded (Scurlock 2018: 530, 532, 535). It is described in Uruanna as the "bed of Ištar" and having a red top (ibid.: 351 and note 19, 534 and notes 29 and 31). Furthermore, it is possible that the plant was believed to dry up excess fluid (ibid.: 533).

This prescription and the following two (ms A obv. 8'–10') make use of a so-called *ḫimû* that is interpreted as a "wad made of reeds, used against snake bite" (*CAD* Ḫ: 193–94). The majority of references therefore seem to originate from ms A and the plant list *CT* 14 pl. 23. According to the *CAD* (Ḫ: 194), it is possible that the word refers to "a specific form or arrangement in which certain sedge-like plants were used" (see Thompson 1949: 10 note 3).

According to this interpretation, the plant used must have been bound to form the "wad", which is the favoured translation in *CAD* (U-W: 212b): "to be bound in a wad over the bite".

9' The *urbatu* is translated as a "rush, reed", *CAD* (U-W: 211–212). A related term may also refer to an illness or a certain *urbatu*-worm (see Scurlock and Andersen 2005: 82–83). Several plants are listed against this worm in *Šammu šikinšu* (Stadhouders 2012: 8 §6, 10 § 27'; Stadhouders 2011: 17 §6, 22 §27'). The *urbatu*-reed has the "Dreckapotheke" name "papyrus" in Uruanna (Rumor 2017: 24, 32 line 138). An incantation continuously referring to the "red *urbatu*" and "red river/water" may have been used for draining an abscess and afterwards bandaging a wound (Scurlock 2014: 441–443). In the case of a venomous snakebite, it is important to attempt to remove as much venom as possible. Therefore, references to an ingredient used in relation to draining unwanted fluids fits the context. The *urbatu*-worm is also listed in a series of maladies in a Gula healing incantation (Böck 2014a: 108–109, 179 and note 78). Note that an *urbatu*-worm, possibly a tapeworm, is listed as a diagnosis in several prescriptions in the N4 manuscript *BAM* 159 col. ii 25–48 (see ibid.: 109; Scurlock 2014: 495–98). It is also in this manuscript that we later find the two prescriptions for horses in *BAM* 159 col. v 33–47 (see below), which mirrors the situation in ms A, in which horse prescriptions are found on the reverse.

10' The reading of PA-PA-*a-nu* appears to be the otherwise unknown *arariānu*-plant (*CAD* A/2: 232–33). In Uruanna's "Dreckapotheke" section, the plant is referred to as "dog saliva" (Rumor 2017: 23, 31 line 133). This name may explain why this plant was listed immediately before the "dog's tongue"-plant in the following entry.

The bed and the bedroom were places of privacy in which the patient was frequently located (e.g., Stol 1997: 408; van der Toorn 1996: 60–61). Therefore, the plant may have been used here to surround the bed in order to ensure that further evil could not befall the patient, but at the same time to treat the area in which the patient was located. Although the plant could be used medically, the *CAD* (A/2: 233) cites a use "for conciliating one's god", which may partially explain the effect of the plant, namely to ensure a benign relationship with the divine power who possibly sent the snake that bit the patient.

It is unclear how a *ḫimû*-wad could be used to surround a bed. The other possible solution is to translate "to wrap (up)" (*CAD* L: 73), although this does not solve the problem.

11' The plant *lišān kalbi* "dog's tongue" may be another name for the *buʾšānu*-plant derived from *baʾāšu* "to smell bad, stink" (Böck 2014a: 157–58, 166–68, 173). In Uruanna's "Dreckapotheke" section, the *lišān kalbi*-plant is called "bat's head", and it is also the name for the *armēdu*-plant and in some instances the *nikiptu*-plant (Rumor 2017: 5, 9–10, 25 line 9, 27 line 38 and 42). *Šammu šikinšu* describes the plant as having leaves "wide open" and "red" (Böck 2014a: 157; Stadhouders 2012: 10 §28'; Stadhouders 2011: 22 §28'). Perhaps it can be identified with the modern "hound's tongue" *Cynoglossum* (*CMAwR* 2: 512; *CMAwR* 1: 471 with references). The plant was considered "Gula's/Ninigizibara's dog" and therefore directly connected to the healing goddess (Böck 2014a: 167). It was widely applicable against many varied symptoms and illnesses (ibid.: 140–56, 174–75). The plant is listed in Uruanna as a plant against snakebite (ibid.: 156). In *BAM* 1, *lišān kalbi* is listed numerous times and various parts of the plant are used. These parts can be used in a potion against, e.g., *suālu*-cough, *ḫaḫḫu*-phlegm or *amurriqānu*-jaundice (Attia and Buisson 2012: 27 col. ii 35, 28 col. ii 45+ col. ii 60+ col. iii 20, 29 col. iii 42).

12'–13' This is the only prescription that covers more than one line on the obverse of ms A. It includes plants used individually in several of the preceding lines in ms A obv. 12'–13', except for one plant that does not seem to occur in the previous prescriptions, namely the partially reconstructed *šakirû*-plant. The sign was copied by Scheil (1918: 75–76) as ⸢KA⸣. The ŠAKIR sign is close to KA, and this plant is listed in Uruanna as a plant against snakebite (*ni-šik* MUŠ). Therefore, the reconstruction is plausible (see *CAD* Š/1: 168).

The *šakirû*-plant is unidentified, but may be related to "henbane" (*CMAwR* 2: 514; see *CMAwR* 1: 472; *CAD* Š/1: 167–68). The name was also part of a plant called ᵘ̇ŠAKIR ᵈ*Šá-maš* that is equated with another unknown plant called *pīru*-plant in Uruanna (*CAD* P: 420), and provided with the "Dreckapotheke" name "tongue of a *tiqqû*-ox" (Rumor 2017: 13, 20 line 62). Perhaps accidentally, bull saliva was used against a scorpion sting in ms A obv. 17' (see below). Note also that the Sumerogram ŠAKIR is listed as part of plant names in Uruanna, read as PA-PA-*a-nu*, which was used in ms A in obv. 10' (see *STT* 391 obv. 16–17). Various plants resembling the *šakirû*-plant were listed as useful against horse colic (*kīs libbi*), *bennu*-epilepsy, and *maškadu*-illness (i.e., abdominal pains and motoric problems) in *Šammu šikinšu* (Stadhouders 2012: 3 §15'–17', 4 §25'; Stadhouders 2011: 8–9 §15'–17', 11 §25'). A possible variant of horse colic was treated in ms A on the reverse (see below).

The *kurkānû*-plant is unidentified (see *CMAwR* 2: 512; *CMAwR* 1: 471 with references). The plant could be used against, e.g., *aḫḫāzu*- and *amurriqānu*-jaundice (Böck 2014a: 125 note 106), renal and rectal problems, and possibly also against *maškadu*-illness (Geller 2005: 42–43, 46–47, 88–89, 162–63, 190–91, 202–207, 236–37, 258–59). Uruanna's "Dreckapotheke" section provides *kurkānû* with the name "dust of the latrine" (Rumor 2017: 20, 30 line 108).

The writing *u ina* in ms A is peculiar and cannot be explained. It may be due to a mistake by Kiṣir-Aššur, or the copy may be incorrect. I have chosen to emend the line and remove the {*u*}.

It is unclear if EŠ.MEŠ in these lines and ms A obv. 14’ and 18’ denotes a variant of a G-stem or a Gtn- or D-stem of *pašāšu* (see CAD P: 247–49). It is translated as a G-stem throughout this edition (ibid.: 247).

14’ From this line in ms A until the text breaks, the focus shifts from snakebites to scorpion stings. There is an accompanying change in the preserved ingredients, among which the blood of certain reptiles and the saliva of a bull are used (see below).

The *ṣurāru* (EME.DIR and EME.ŠID) is an unspecified lizard (CAD Ṣ: 254–56; see George 2016: 165; Freedman 2006a: 166 and note for line 1, 204 and note for line 1). Although lizards are attested in medicinal prescriptions, they are not frequently used (see George 2016: 167; Scurlock 2014: 407–8, 410–12, 415–16, 452, 464, 525–26, 534, 546, 675, 677; Geller 2005: 40–41, 100–101; CAD Ṣ: 255). They were considered ominous and appear in the 32nd tablet of *Šumma ālu* (CAD Ṣ: 254–55; see Freedman 2006: 164–189). The 33rd tablet of *Šumma ālu* contains omens concerning the *pizallūru*-gecko (MUŠ.GIM.GURUN.NA) (Freedman 2006a: 202–213). Such ominous entries appearing consecutively as *ṣurāru* and *pizallūru* are also observed in the first subseries of Sa-gig (Heeßel 2001–02: 32–33). The blood of the *pizallūru*-gecko is also used in ms A obv. 18’, and the appearance of these ingredients together may have been influenced by the order expressed in the omen series.

The reason for applying the blood of lizards and, later in ms A obv. 18’, of geckos to a scorpion sting may result from the gecko’s, and perhaps also the lizard’s, ability to kill certain scorpions and even tolerate their venom (Zlotkin et al. 2003). If this is true of the various species used in these prescriptions, it may have been believed that the blood of an animal that was capable of overcoming the venom and defeating the powerful and venomous scorpion provided the user with the same effect. An omen in *Šumma ālu* refers to the ominous event of a gecko killing a snake in a man’s house (Freedman 2006a: 208–209 line 75’).

For “the surface of the sting” (*pan ziqti*), see CAD Z: 132; CAD P: 89–90.

15’ The application of flour may relate to the application of dough onto scorpion stings elsewhere (see George 2016: 165 with further references). However, the reasoning behind applying flour may not have been exactly the same, as it is possible that flour was supposed to absorb fluid or blood from the wound and thereby symbolize the extraction of the venom.

The imperative *ki-sir!-ma* likely stems from *kesēru* “to block, dam a river, make a pavement” (CAD K: 313–314), although the only medical example quoted in the CAD relates to tampons in the nose. Similar use of the imperative in prescriptions is observed in, e.g., OB medical texts, see George 2016: 166. Another possibility would be to read *ke-sir*$^{!}$*-ma* as a stative where the plural ZÌ.MEŠ is treated as a collective singular ("flour blocks …"). It is difficult to account for another verb, such as *kaṣāru*.

16' The *kamūnu* (GAMUN) is possibly a type of cumin (CAD K: 131–32 with references). It was considered to be a benign plant, and an entry in the 55th tablet of *Šumma ālu* states: "If ditto ((someone) grows) *kamūnu* ditto (in a field), he will prevail over his adversary; he will be happy" (Freedman 2017: 101 line 63', 106). The ingredient is called "bat wing" in Uruanna's "Dreckapotheke" section (Rumor 2017: 16, 29 line 84). A variant called "*kamūnu* of tamarisk" is named "*gabû*-stone" (ibid.: 12, 28 line 53). Note that another term *kamūnu* refers to a fungus, although it is referred to with a different Sumerogram (UZU.DIR; CAD K: 133; see SAA 13 no. 71). The entries in Uruanna spell the word phonetically or use the Sumerogram ^{ú}GAMUN$^{(\text{sar})}$. In the latter examples, the entries must refer to the plant.

For this line, see also George 2016: 165.

17' Saliva (*rupuštu*) appears to be frequently attested in connection to bulls/oxen (*alpu*) in various treatments (CAD R: 415; see also George 2016: 165). Although bull saliva may have had certain therapeutic qualities, a connection between thick bull saliva, semen and potency motifs in scorpion incantations (*araḫḫi*-incantations; see Cooper 1996) likely provide a conceptual overlap that explain the possible magical abilities of this substance. Furthermore, at least in humans, scorpion venom may cause excessive salivation (see Section 4.1.2). For bull saliva in connection to potency, see also Scurlock 2014: 548, 550. See also the OB manuscript *BAM* 393 obv. 19–20, which contains a related entry utilizing bull saliva against a scorpion sting.

18' The line does not appear to begin with KI.MIN, and probably should be restored as: [MUŠ.DÍ]M.GURUN.NA for a *pizallūru*- or *pizallurtu*-gecko (George 2016: 165; see Freedman 2006a: 204 note for line 1 with further references). It remains uncertain if this term refers to a coded plant (Böck 2011: 697). It should be noted that *šammu šikinšu* lists the *lišān kalbi* "Dog's tongue"-plant, which is mentioned in other prescriptions in this text as a plant upon which the *pizallūru*-gecko lies (CAD L: 209 with references; see also notes for line 11' above). For the possible reasoning behind applying the blood of a gecko, see the commentary to ms A obv. 14' above.

The ingredient *billatu* (DIDA) seems to be a dry substance used in relation to the preparation of (instant) beer and it can be crushed and eaten in medical texts (CAD B: 228; see *CMAwR* 2: 509 and *CMAwR* 1: 54, 469 with references). As there is no mention of a fluid into which the *billatu* can be mixed, the final sign should be read GU$_7^!$. This differs slightly from the translation by Böck (2011: 697) of this line: "If a scorpion has stung a man, cut the head of a *pizallurtu*-gecko and smear the blood on the wound, (the patient) should drink instant beer".

The line ends somewhat abruptly without the expected *ina-eš*.

19' The signs in Scheil's copy can be grouped and read in numerous ways. There does not appear to be enough room to reconstruct [DIŠ KI.MIN]. The line is difficult to make sense of, regardless how the signs are read. A reading IM.ŠÚ could designate *imšukku* "a clay cover" (CAD I-J: 138–39). In at least one instance, a LB ritual for a dog bite rubs the wound with clay and fashions a dog from the clay afterwards (Finkel 1999: 219–221). The statement 7-*šú* likely indicates an action repeated seven times. The sign after 7-*šú* appears to be NU, BE, or PAB, although the interpretation remains uncertain. Presumably, the final signs spell out a verbal form that cannot be properly reconstructed. This verbal form may have been a precative (*li-*...).

20' The initial ingredient that is sieved (*šaḫālu*) cannot be properly read, but could be ⸢ú!⸣LAL! for *ašqulālu* (see CAD A/2: 452–53).

The transliteration becomes highly uncertain after GEŠTIN. The next signs look like lu ⸢x?⸣ lal and thereafter GAR-⸢*an*⸣ *ina-eš*. It is difficult to make sense of these signs in their current state, but it is possible the LU actually comprised ZÌ and a broken MEŠ. The reading ⸢NÍG⸣.LÁ GAR-⸢*an*⸣ in ms A obv. 20' was established in the CAD (N/2: 49). The sentence was likely abbreviated, but one would expect a preposition and another verbal form, such as *balālu*. Finally, we should expect GAR-⸢*an*⸣-*ma ina-eš*.

21' George (2016: 165) notes this line among the entries in the text that administer the potion by mouth alone.

22'–24' The final prescriptions on the obverse of ms A, alongside ms A obv. 16' and 18', are the only prescriptions on the obverse that employ more than one method of application (see George 2016: 165).

22' The final instruction after the patient is anointed (ŠÉŠ-*ma*) cannot be properly read. The first sign may be GÚ for "neck" (*kišādu*). If this is correct, one would expect a pronominal suffix referring to the patient. However, this does not seem to be the case.

23' The first readable sign is MAR for *eqû* "to smear, anoint" or *zakû* "to winnow, scatter". However, as the line later continues ŠÉŠ-*su* "you anoint him", it is questionable if the initial sign is MAR. I have emended the sign to a SÚD to accommodate a crushed ingredient drunk in beer and placed in oil for anointing the patient.

Reverse

4' This line is quoted in the CAD (N/1: 137b') as: *ana na-ḫir šumēlišu tašappak*, "you pour it into his left nostril". A similar method of application with a specified vessel is listed in ms A rev. 7'. The only parallels that use the specific "left nostril", beside ms A rev. 7' below, are from *BAM* 159 col. v 36: *ina na-ḫir* GÙB-*šú* DUB-*ak-ma* TI (see Parys 2014: 34; Scurlock 2014: 498–99) and various plant lists (see Stol 2011: 400). As a result, the "irrational" left nostril was only used in prescriptions in relation to horses (387–99, 391–93, 400–402). Combined with the discussion by Stol (2011: 400–402) of the following prescription for an ill horse in ms A, the prescription in ms A rev. 0'–4' most likely also relates to a horse. As a result, the third person pronominal suffix has been translated "it" to reflect the horse. See Sections 3.5.2 and 4.4.3 for discussions of these lines.

5'–8' Treated in Stol 2011: 40–402. He translates the passage as: "Du wirst […], Wurzel der Pflanze […] pulverisieren, in Bier order Wein feinstoßen(?), (…) mit einer …-Röhre in sein linkes Nasenloch gießen. [F]ür ein Pferd, (…) (*ša* BU ḪI LU SU), ist es gut."

Stol (2011: 387–92) also treated a comparable prescription found on *BAM* 159 col. v 33–36 (see Parys 2014: 23, 34–35, 60–61; Scurlock 2014: 498–99) that is quoted here for comparison: ^{ú}*zi-im*-KÙ.BABBAR ^{ú}*zi-im*-KÙ.GI ^{ú}*ár-zal-lá* 34 ^{ú}SAR-A.ŠÀ ^{ú}*el-lat*-A.ŠÀ ^{ú}⸢*ka-su*⸣-*u* 35 ^{ú}TUR.A.NI SUḪUŠ ^{ú}TUR.A.NI 8 Ú *ki-is* ŠÀ-*bi* 36 *šá* ANŠE.KUR.RA *i-na* GEŠTIN SUR *ina na-ḫir* GÙB-*šú* DUB-*ak-ma* TI, "(list of ingredients), 8 plants for horse *kīs libbi* (colic). You pour it into its left nostril in pressed wine and it will recover". See also *STT* 93 obv. 35'–37'; *BAM* 309 col. i' 1'–4'.

6' The majority of horse treatments use GEŠTIN SUR "pressed" or "drawn wine" (CAD Ṣ: 63–64; e.g., *BAM* 159 col. v 36; *CT* 14 pl. 41 Rm. 362 lines 1'–5'; Stol 2011: 388, 393; Scurlock 2014: 498–99), but this does not appear to be the case in this prescription.

The description that the ingredients are first "pounded, crushed" *sâku* (SÚD) and thereafter "crushed in" a fluid *ḫašālu* (GAZ) are also found in the second horse prescription in *BAM* 159 col. v 37–47 (Stol 2011: 394; see Parys 2014: 23, 34–35, 60–61; Scurlock 2014 498–99). Stol (2011: 394) translates these verbal forms as: "… wirst du pulverisieren (und) zusammen mit … wirst du (es) zerstoßen(?)", and Scurlock (2014: 499) translates: "you grind … you crush (everything) with …".

7' The medicament is administered through a DUG *ziriqi*, possibly to be translated as a "stomach tube" (Stol 2011: 401–2 and notes 257–58 with references). CAD (Z: 134) interprets it as a sort of pipette, von Soden as "Ton-pipette" (*AHw*: 1532), and Stol (Stol 2011: 401–2 and notes 257–58) translates it as "…-Röhre".

The DUG designates it as a clay object comparable to various fluid containers (ibid.: 401 and note 256). Stol stresses the uniqueness of the instrument, as this is the only example (cf. *BAM* 159 discussed in Parys 2014: 23 and Böck 2009a: 117 and notes 56–57). This method for treating horse colic is also attested in the Ugaritic hippiatric texts (Cohen and Sivan 1983: 9–10, 16–17 with references) and the method is still applied today (e.g., Lopes et al. 2004: 696, 702). See the discussion in Sections 3.5.2 and 4.4.3.

Similarly to the method of application in ms A rev. 4', this mixture is administrated into the "left nostril" of the horse (see above).

8' This line is problematic and the copy is probably wrong. Scheil's copy and translation read: [*i*]-*na* GEŠTIN KUR.RA *ṭa-bu ḫi-ṭu-su* SIG$_5$-*iq*, "avec du bon vin de montagne, - son point se calmera" (Scheil 1918: 77, 79). The GEŠTIN KUR.RA is quoted in the *CAD* (K: 205) as "mountain wine", a type of wine exclusively attested in this text. As a result, Stol (2011: 400–401 and note 251) argued convincingly via the parallel prescription in *BAM* 159 col. v 33–36 (see above) that this line was incorrectly copied and should read: ANŠE$^{!}$.KUR.RA *ša* ..., with the remaining sentence relating to the horse's illness being cured (SIG$_5$-*iq*) with the prescription.

Stol proposed that the doubtful signs after *ša*, which read BU ḪI LU SU, could describe the illness afflicting the horse. The end of the sentence can therefore be read: *ša* ... DAB-*su* SIG$_5$-*iq*, i.e., "to make well that which has seized it (i.e., the horse)". Stol (2011: 401 and note 254) suggested reading the signs bu-ḫi as *qíd-ḫi* for a relatively unknown illness *qidḫu* "Entzündung"(?) that is perhaps read *saḫḫu*(?) (*AHw*: 921; *CAD* Q: 251; *CDA*: 289). Another reading suggested by Stol (2011: 401 note 254) is *sír-ḫi* for *ṣir-ḫi* spelling the poorly attested illness *ṣirḫu* "Fieberglut" from the verb *ṣarāḫu* "to heat, scorch" (*CAD* Ṣ: 98; *AHw*: 1083; see *ṣiriḫtu* "inflammation", in *CAD* Ṣ: 207; *AHw*: 1104–5). This illness, however, is attested as an animal illness in a *namburbi*-ritual edited by Caplice (1970: 120 line 64; see also Stol 2011: 383), who translated *ṣirḫu* as "dirge", a well-attested similar word (*CAD* Ṣ: 205–6) derived from another similar verb *ṣarāḫu* "to sing a lamentation" (see *CAD* Ṣ: 99–100). Both meanings could fit the presumed colic-like state of the horse that this prescription aimed to cure. Some illnesses affecting the *libbi* "stomach, abdomen, heart", and possibly also the illness *kīs libbi*, were connected to depressed emotional states (Cadelli 2000: 363–65, 372–73; see Parys 2014: 4–5; Chalendar 2013: 14–17; Steinert 2012: 232–33; Böck 2010a: 69; cf. note 205). Furthermore, *kīs libbi* could potentially turn into *māmītu* (Scurlock and Andersen 2005: 508) and, by extension, the illness could produce fever. If the spelling here was supposed to designate *ṣirḫu*, both verbs *ṣarāḫu* "to heat" and "to sing a lamentation" could fit the symptoms of this presumably colic-like illness.

9' The catch-line is difficult to read. Scheil (1918: 77, 79–80) read it as follows with modified readings of Sumerograms: DIŠ NA$_4$ (alt.: TAK, for NA(?)) ŠÀ-*šú* È *ù* RAT RAT ŠÀ-*ba-šú* È *a-rik*(?), "Si quelqu'un son intérieur se soulève et que la douleur soulève son cœur …". The copy shows NA$_4$ instead of NA (cf. Scheil 1918: 77, 80). As a result, it is possible that several signs in this line were incorrectly copied. Similar copying mistakes occur throughout Scheil's copy, e.g., in rev. 11' and several emendations are suggested here.

The *ù* over *u* for a conjunction seems unusual in this context, and syntactically we would expect E$_{11}$-*ma* instead of *u*. It is not impossible that *ù* marked an alternative to the first verbal form (von Soden 1995: 212 §117c) or maybe a disjunctive statement, although this would ordinarily be spelled *ū lū* (ibid.: 258). This cannot be properly explained, and the sign cannot be emended to fit the context better at present. I translate *ù* as "and", but the spelling may have had a different function.

Scheil recognized that the catch-line was connected to the inners (ŠÀ) rising (E$_{11}$) (Scheil 1918: 77, 79). As the word "stomach" *libbu* (ŠÀ) and the sign for "to go up/go down" *elû*/*warādu* (E$_{11}$) are mentioned twice in the catch-line, it is likely that it quotes a symptom description concerned with nausea. However, such diagnoses often use a verb related to vomiting, such as *arû* (Scurlock and Andersen 2005: 126–28; Cadelli 2000: 337; see, e.g., CAD A/2: 316; CAD E: 121; CAD P: 208–9). No mention of vomit is made in this catch-line. A number of signs in the line cannot be properly read without emendation. Scheil read RAT RAT over the emended *ú*$^{!}$-*rad*, and *a-rik*(?) as the final two signs. The first of the final signs is *a*, but the last sign is unclear. I have emended it to ⌜*lam*$^{?}$⌝. By emending RAT RAT to *ú*$^{!}$-*rad* and *a-rik*(?) to *a-lam*$^{?}$ it is possible to provide each instance of È with its opposite meaning, i.e. "if a man's$^{!}$ stomach rises (to vomit) and *settles*$^{!}$, (and) his stomach (after having) settled *rises*(?) (again)". This would provide a description of continuing states of nausea. However, this interpretation is not without problems. Verbal forms of *elû* with initial *a*- are only attested as imperatives and second person singular forms, and these mainly stem from OB examples (see CAD E: 116). As a result, the spelling cannot be explained here, but I fail to see other interpretations.

The catch-line remains without duplicates or parallels.

10' According to Scheil's copy, the number reads ⌜32$^{?}$⌝. However, the two wedges after 30 are written horizontally instead of vertically. Although this writing is attested, it does not occur on the few other examples of numbered *nisḫus* from Kiṣir-Aššur (see Section 9.2.3).

11' Kiṣir-Aššur's name and a number of signs after the name cannot be read properly on Scheil's copy. Scheil also failed to make proper sense of the line and transliterated ^{p}*Ki-ṣir* (dingir) rab-gan-me DUMU *ša* ^{d}PA *ba-laṭ-su*. Hunger

(1968: 70) transliterated the name as ^{p}*Ki-ṣir-*^{d}DÌM.ME.TUR and emended the ending correctly as *ša* ^{d}PA *tuk-lat-su* (*BAK* 200 ms E). The best transcription of the Sumerogram in the name appears to be *Lamaštu*, although this reading makes little sense and the copy does not support Hunger's transliteration. I suggest emending most of the signs and reading: ^{p}*Ki-ṣir*-AN.ŠÁR$^{!}$ ^{lú}ŠÁMAN$^{!}$.LÁ$^{!}$ TUR *ša* ^{d}PA *tuk*$^{!}$*-lat-su*. This produces a regular spelling of Kiṣir-Aššur's name, and furthermore provides him with a title that most likely existed on the original tablet, although this cannot be checked.

14' The final phrase, NÍG.GIG ^{d}ŠE.NAGA, is only attested in this Kiṣir-Aššur colophon. However, colophons with NÍG.GIG DN are attested (see Hunger 1968: 163 with references), albeit rarely with Nisaba. Ms A is quoted in CAD (I–J: 56) as: "do not efface [the tablet], it is a sin against Nisaba". Nisaba was originally a goddess of grain and writing, but lost importance after the OB period, although she continued to be connected to Nabû and to be referenced in the scribal arts (Michalowski 1998–2001: 575, 578–79; see CAD N/2: 273). Due to Nisaba's role as a goddess of writing and her association with Nabû, she was presumably a learned substitute for Nabû. She was occasionally addressed in NA sources, e.g., in a compendium of *šu'illa*-prayers from the Nabû temple in Kalḫu (CTN 4 no. 168), a Sumerian mythical tale (Civil and Lambert 1983), and the Akkadian disputation-like poem known as "Nisaba and wheat" attested at Ḫuzirina and perhaps Assur (Jiménez 2017: 65–68; Lambert 1996: 168–75).

15' Hunger (1968: 70) suggested reconstructing: [*ša itabbalu* DN] IGI^{II}-*šú li-*[*it-bal*] based on comparative examples from other copyists (see Hunger 1968: 177–78 with examples). In the remaining signs copied by Scheil we should therefore expect a divine name, but at present this cannot be reconstructed. Alternatively, the line could be reconstructed as: [*šá* IM UR$_{5}$]-⸢*tú* TÙM $^{d?}$NAGA$^{!?}$⸣ aš(?) IGI^{II}-*šú li-*⸢*it*⸣*-b*[*al*], "[the one who] removes [th]is [tablet], let Nisaba [x] take aw[ay] his eyes" (see the N4 manuscript *BAM* 1 in Attia and Buisson 2012: 30 col. iv 31; Hunger 1968: 79 no. 234 line 6). This would, however, ruin the current reading *ni-ṭil*, which is most likely correct. None of the comparable examples listed by Hunger contain a preposition such as *ina*, and the alternative interpretation must be considered unlikely.

Bibliography

Abusch, T.

1974 “Mesopotamian Anti-Witchcraft Literature: Texts and Studies Part I: The Nature of Maqlû: Its Character, Divisions and Calendrical Setting”, *JNES* 33/2, pp. 251–262.

2002 *Mesopotamian Witchcraft: Toward a History and Understanding of Babylonian Witchcraft Beliefs and Literature* (Ancient Magic and Divination 5; Leiden, Boston, and Köln: Brill and STYX)

2008 “The Witch’s Messages: Witchcraft, Omens, and Voodoo-Death in Ancient Mesopotamia”, in: R. J. van der Spek (ed.), *Studies in Ancient Near Eastern World View and Society Presented to Marten Stol on the Occasion of his 65th Birthday, 10 November 2005, and his Retirement from the Vrije Universiteit Amsterdam* (Bethesda: CDL Press), pp. 53–95.

2015 *The Witchcraft series Maqlû* (Writings from the Ancient World 37; Atlanta: SBL Press)

2016 *The Magical Ceremony Maqlû: A Critical Edition* (Ancient Magic and Divination 10; Leiden and Boston: Brill)

Abusch, T. and D. Schwemer

2011 *Corpus of Mesopotamian Anti-Witchcraft Rituals Volume One* (Ancient Magic and Divination 8/1; Leiden and Boston: Brill)

Abusch. T., D. Schwemer, M. Luukko and G. van Buylaere

2016 *Corpus of Mesopotamian Anti-Witchcraft Rituals Volume Two* (Ancient Magic and Divination 8/2; Leiden and Boston: Brill)

Al-Rawi, F. N. H.

2000 “Cuneiform Inscriptions in the Collections of the John Rylands Library, University of Manchester”, *Iraq* 62, pp. 21–63.

Al-Rawi, F. N. H. and A. R. George

1990 “Tablets from the Sippar Library. II. Tablet II of the Babylonian Creation Epic”, *Iraq* 52, pp. 149–157.

1994 “Tablets from the Sippar Library. III. Two Royal Counterfeits”, *Iraq* 56, pp. 135–148.

2006 “Tablets from the Sippar Library XIII: ‘*Enūma Anu Ellil* XX’”, *Iraq* 68, pp. 23–57.

Alirol, E., S. K. Sharma, H. S. Bawaskar, U. Kuch, F. Chappuis

2010 “Snake Bite in South Asia: A Review”, *PLOS Neglected Tropical Diseases* 4/1, pp. 1–9.

Alster, B. and J. van Dijk

1972 “A Sumerian Incantation against Gall”, *OrNS* 41/3, pp. 349–358.

Ambos, C.

2007 "Types of Ritual Failure and Mistakes in Ritual in Cuneiform Sources", in: U. Hüsken (ed.), *When Rituals Go Wrong: Mistakes, Failure, and the Dynamics of Ritual* (Studies in the History of Religions 115; Leiden and Boston: Brill), pp. 25–47.

2010 "Ritual Healing and the Investiture of the Babylonian King", in: W. S. Sax, J. Quack and J. Weinhold (eds.), *The Problem of Ritual Efficacy* (Oxford: Oxford University Press), pp. 17–44.

2013a *Der König im Gefängnis und das Neujahrsfest im Herbst: Mechanismen der Legitimation des Babylonischen Herrschers im 1. Jahrtausend v. Chr. und ihre Geschichte* (Dresden: ISLET-Verlag)

2013b "Rites of Passage in Ancient Mesopotamia: Changing Status by Moving through Space: *Bīt rimki* and the Ritual of the Substitute King", in: C. Ambos and L. Verderame (eds.), *Apporaching Rituals in Ancient Cultures* (Pisa and Rome: Fabrizio Serra Editore), pp. 39–54.

Andrae, W.

1910 "Aus den Berichten Dr. W. Andraes aus Assur", *MDOG* 44, pp. 28–40.

1938 *Das Wiedererstandene Assur* (Leipzig: J. C. Hinrichs Verlag)

Angsanakul, J. and V. Sitprija

2013 "Scorpion Venoms, Kidney and Potassium", *Toxicon* 73, pp. 81–87.

Annus, A.

2002 *The God Ninurta in the Mythology and Royal Ideology of Ancient Mesopotamia* (State Archives of Assyria Studies 14; Helsinki: The Neo-Assyrian Text Corpus Project)

Annus, A. and A. Lenzi

2010 *Ludlul Bēl Nēmeqi. The Standard Babylonian Poem of the Righteous Sufferer* (State Archives of Assyria Cuneiform Texts 7; Helsinki: The Neo-Assyrian Text Corpus Project)

Anonymous

1981 "Excavations in Iraq, 1979–80", *Iraq* 43, pp. 167–198.

1987 "Excavations in Iraq, 1985–86 (Plate XLVII)", *Iraq* 49, pp. 231–251 and pl. 47.

Arbøll, T. P.

2018a "Tracing Mesopotamian Medical Knowledge: A Study of *maškadu-* and Related Illnesses", in: G. van Buylaere, M. Luukko, D. Schwemer and A. Mertens-Wagschal (eds.), *Sources of Evil. Studies in Mesopotamian Exorcistic Lore* (Ancient Magic and Divination 15; Leiden and Boston: Brill), pp. 261–284.

2018b "Kiṣir-Aššur's name and Title in Writing", *N.A.B.U.* 2018/2, note no. 50, pp. 80–83.

2019 "A Newly Discovered Drawing of a Neo-Assyrian Demon in *BAM* 202 Connected to Psychological and Neurological Disorders", *JMC* 33, pp. 1–31.

Forthcoming "A New Look at Eels and their Use in Mesopotamian Medicine", submitted to: L. Recht and C. Tsouparopoulou (eds.), *Animal Encounters in the Ancient Near East* (McDonald Institute Monograph Series; Cambridge: McDonald Institute for Archaeological Research)

Aro, J.

1961 *Die Akkadischen Infinitivkonstruktionen* (Studia Orientalia Edidit Societas Orientalis Pennica 26; Helsinki: Suomalaisen Kirjallisuuden Kirjapaino Oy Helsinki)

Ashley, F. H., A. E. Waterman-Pearson and H. R. Whay

2005 "Review Article: Behavioural Assessment of Pain in Horses and Donkeys: Application to Clinical Practice and Future Studies", *Equine Veterinary Journals* 37/6, pp. 565–575.

Al-Asmari, A. K. and A. A. Al-Saif

2003 "Scorpion Sting Syndrome in a General Hospital in Saudi Arabia", *Saudi Medical Journal* 25/1, pp. 64–70.

Attia, A.

2000 "A propos de la signification de šer'ânu dans les textes médicaux mésopotamiens: une question d'anatomie", *Historie des Sciences Médicales* 34/1, pp. 47–56.

Attia, A. and G. Buisson

2003 "Edition de texte 'Si le crane d'un home contient de la chaleur, deuxième tablette'", *JMC* 2003/1, pp. 1–24.

2012 "BAM 1 et consorts en transcription", *JMC* 19, pp. 22–51.

Attinger, P.

2008 "La medicine mésopotamienne", *JMC* 11–12, pp. 1–96.

Avalos, H.

1995 *Illness and Health Care in the Ancient Near East: The Role of the Temple in Greece, Mesopotamia, and Israel* (Harvard Semitic Monographs 54; Atlanta: Scholars Press)

2007 "Epilepsy in Mesopotamia Reconsidered", in: I. L. Finkel and M. J. Geller (eds.), *Disease in Babylonia* (Cuneiform Monographs 36; Leiden and Boston: Brill), pp. 131–136.

Bácskay, A.

2017 "The Natural and Supernatural Aspects of Fever in Mesopotamian Medical Texts", in: S. Bhayro and C. Rider (eds.), *Demons and Illness from Antiquity to the Early-Modern Period* (Leiden and Boston: Brill), pp. 39–52.

2018 *Therapeutic Prescriptions against Fever in Ancient Mesopotamia* (Alter Orient und Altes Testament 447; Münster: Ugarit-Verlag)

Bácskay, A. and K. Simkó

2012 "Leitfaden der Beschwörungskunst, Some Remarks on a Well-known Text", *N.A.B.U.* 2012/3, note no. 52, pp. 67–70.

Baker, H. D.

2000 *The Prosopography of the Neo-Assyrian Empire. Volume 2, Part I: Ḫ-K* (Helsinki: The Neo-Assyrian Text Corpus Project)

2001 *The Prosopography of the Neo-Assyrian Empire. Volume 2, Part II: L-N* (Helsinki: The Neo-Assyrian Text Corpus Project)

2011 *The Prosopography of the Neo-Assyrian Empire. Volume 3, Part II: Š-Z* (Helsinki: The Neo-Assyrian Text Corpus Project)

2017 *The Prosopography of the Neo-Assyrian Empire. Volume 4/I. Index of Professions* (Helsinki: The Neo-Assyrian Text Corpus Project)

Bawaskar, H. S. and P. H. Bawaskar

2012 "Scorpion Sting: Update", *Journal of the Association of Physicians of India* 60, pp. 46–55.

Bär, J.

2003 "Walter Andrae – Ein Wegbereiter der modernen Archäologie. Grabungstechnik, Dokumentation, naturwissenschaftliche Analysen und Alltag", in: J. Marzahn and B. Salje (eds.), *Wiedererstehendes Assur: 100 Jahre deutsche Ausgrabungen in Assyrien* (Mainz: Verlag Philipp von Zabern), pp. 45–52.

Beaulieu, P.-A.

1992 "New Light on Secret Knowledge in Late Babylonian Culture", *ZA* 82, pp. 98–111.

1997 "The Cult of AN.ŠÁR/Aššur in Babylonia after the Fall of the Assyrian Empire", *SAAB* 11, pp. 55–73.

2000 "The Descendants of Sîn-lēqi-unninni", in: J. Marzahn and H. Neumann (eds.), *Assyriologica et Semitica: Festschrift für Joachim Oelsner anläßlich seines 65. Geburtstages am 18. Februar 1997* (Alter Orient und Altes Testament 252; Münster: Ugarit-Verlag), pp. 1–16.

2003 *The Pantheon of Uruk During the Neo-Babylonian Period* (Cuneiform Monographs 23; Leiden and Boston: Brill and Styx)

2007a "Late Babylonian Intellectual Life", in: G. Leick (ed.), *The Babylonian World* (New York and London: Routledge), pp. 473–484.

2007b "The Social and Intellectual Setting of Babylonian Wisdom Literature", in: E. J. Clifford (ed.), *Wisdom Literature in Mesopotamia and Israel* (Atlanta: Society of Biblical Literature), pp. 3–19.

2010 "The Afterlife of Assyrian Scholarship in Hellenistic Babylonia", in: J. Stackert, B. N. Porter and D. P. Wright (eds.), *Gazing on the Deep: Ancient Near Eastern Studies in Honor of Tzvi Abusch* (Bethesda: CDL Press), pp. 1–18.

Becker, A.

1993 *Uruk. Kleinfunde I. Stein* (Ausgrabungen in Uruk-Warka Endberichte 6; Mainz: Verlag Philipp von Zabern)

Beckman, G. and B. R. Foster

1988 "Assyrian Scholarly Texts in the Yale Babylonian Collection", in: E. Leichty, M. deJ. Ellis and P. Gerardi (eds.), *A Scientific Humanist: Studies in Memory of Abraham Sachs* (Occasional Publications of the Samuel Noah Kramer Fund 9; Philadelphia: The University Museum), pp. 1–26.

Bell, C.

1997 *Ritual. Perspectives and Dimensions* (Oxford and New York: Oxford University Press)

Beltramini, A., K. Milojevic and D. Pateron

2017 "Pain Assessment in Newborns, Infants, and Children", *Paediatric Annals* 46/10, pp. 387–395.

Bergeson, P. S. and J. C. Shaw

2001 "Are Infants Really Obligatory Nasal Breathers?", *Clinical Pediatrics* 40, pp. 567–569.

Biggs, R. D.

1967 *ŠÀ.ZI.GA. Ancient Mesopotamian Potency Incantations* (Texts from Cuneiform Sources 2; Locust Valley: J. J. Augustin Publisher)

1987–90 "Medizin. A", in: D. O. Edzard (ed.), *Reallexikon der Assyriologie und Vorderasiatischen Archäologie. Siebter Band* (Berlin and New York: Walter de Gruyter), pp. 623–629.

1995 "Medicine, Surgery, and Public Health in Ancient Mesopotamia", in: J. M. Sasson (ed.), *Civilizations of the Ancient Near East. Volume III* (New York: Charles Schribner's Sons and Simon & Schuster MacMillan), pp. 1911–1924.

van Binsbergen, W. and F. Wiggermann

1999 "Magic in history. A Theoretical Perspective, and its Application to Ancient Mesopotamia", in: T. Abusch and K. van der Toorn (eds.), *Mesopotamian Magic: Textual, Historical, and Interpretative Perspectives* (Ancient Magic and Divination 1; Groningen: STYX Publications), pp. 3–34.

Black, J. A.

1985 "*Nasāhu* 'to copy'", *RA* 79, pp. 92–93.

Black, J. A. and W. J. Tait

1995 "Archives and Libraries in the Ancient Near East", in: J. M. Sasson (ed.), *Civilizations of the Ancient Near East vol. IV* (New York: Charles Schribner's Sons and Simon & Schuster MacMillan), pp. 2197–2209.

Borger, R.

1957–71 "Geheimwissen", in: E. Weidner and W. von Soden (eds.), *Reallexikon der Assyriologie und Vorderasiatischen Archäologie. Dritter Band* (Berlin and New York: Walter de Gruyter), pp. 188–191.

1967 [1956] *Die Inschriften Asarhaddons Königs von Assyrien* (Archiv für Orientforschung Beiheft 9; Osnabrück: Biblio-Verlag) [Archiv für Orientforschung Beiheft 9; Graz: Archiv für Orientforschung]

1969 "Die Erste Teiltafel der zi-pà Beschwörungen (ASKT 11)", in: W. Röllig (ed.), *lišān mitḫurti. Festschrift Wolfram Freiherr von Soden zum 19. VI. 1968 gewidmet von Schülern und Mitarbeitern* (Alter Orient und Altes Testament 1; Neukirchen-Vluyn: Verlag Butzon & Bercker Kevelaer and Neukirchener Verlag des Erziehungsvereins Neukirchen-Vluyn) pp. 1–22.

1970a "Neues Material zu ASKT Nr. 11", *WdO* 5/2, pp. 172–175.

1970b "Bemerkungen zu den akkadischen Kolophonen", *WdO* 5/2, pp. 165–171.

1973 "Die Weihe eines Enlil-Priesters", *BiOr* 30/1, pp. 163–176 and pls. 5–7.

1974 "Die Beschwörungsserie Bīt mēseri und die Himmelfahrt Henochs", *JNES* 33/2, pp. 183–196.

1994 "The Incantation Series *Bīt Mēseri* and Enoch's Ascension to Heaven", in: R. S. Hess and D. T. Tsumura (eds.), *I Studied Inscriptions from Before the Flood. Ancient Near Eastern, Literacy, and Linguistic Approaches to Genesis 1–11* (Sources for Biblical and Theological Study 4; Winona Lake: Eisenbrauns), pp. 224–233.

1996 *Beiträge zum Inschriftenwerk Assurbanipals: Die Prismenklassen A, B, C = K, D, E, F, G, H, J und T sowie andere Inschriften* (Weisbaden: Harrassowitz Verlag)

2004 *Mesopotamisches Zeichenlexikon* (Alter Orient und Altes Testament 305; Münster: Ugarit-Verlag)

Bottéro, J.

1983 "Les morts et l'au-delà dans les rituels en accadien contre l'action des 'revenants'", *ZA* 73, pp. 153–203.

1985 *Mythes et Rites de Babylone* (Genève and Paris: Slatkine and Champion)

1987–90 "Magie", in: E. Weidner and W. von Soden (eds.), *Reallexikon der Assyriologie und Vorderasiatischen Archäologie. Siebter Band* (Berlin and New York: Walter de Gruyter), pp. 200–234.

1995 *Textes culinaires Mésopotamiens. Mesopotamian Culinary Texts* (Mesopotamian Civilizations 6; Winona Lake, Indiana: Eisenbrauns)

Boyer, P.

2002 [2001] *Religion Explained. The Human Instincts that Fashion Gods, Spirits and Ancestors* (London: Vintage Books) [New York: Basic Books]

Boyer, L., A. Alagón and A. Theodorou

2009 "Antivenom for Children with Neurotoxicity from Scorpion Stings. The Authors Reply", *The New England Journal of Medicine* 361/6, p. 632.

Böck, B.

2000 *Die Babylonisch-Assyrische Morphoskopie* (Archiv für Orientforschung Beiheft 27; Wien: Selbstverlag des Instituts für Orientalistik der Universität Wien)

2001 "Ein 'anatomisches Bildwörterbuch'", *Aula Orientalis* 19, pp. 163–172.

2002 "Physiognomie und Schicksal? Oder wie der altmesopotamische Mensch mit einem durch ein physiognomisches Omen angekündigtes Unheil umgegangen sein mag", *Sefarad* 62, pp. 241–57.

2003 "When You Perform the Ritual of 'Rubbing'": On Medicine and Magic in Ancient Mesopotamia", *JNES* 62/1, pp. 1–16.

2007 *Das Handbuch Muššu'u "Einreibung": Eine Serie sumerischer und akkadischer Beschwörungen aus dem 1. Jt. vor Chr.* (Biblioteca del Próximo Oriente Antiguo; Madrid: Consejo Superior de Investigaciones Científicas)

2008 "Babylonisch-assyrische Medizin in Texten und Untersuchungen: Erkrankungen des uro-genitalen Traktes, des Enddarmes und des Anus", *WZKM* 98, pp. 295–346.

2009a "On Medical Technology in Ancient Mesopotamia", in: A. Attia and G. Buisson (eds.), *Advances in Mesopotamian Medicine from Hammurabi to Hippocrates: Proceedings of the International Conference "Oeil malade et mauvais oeil," Collège de France, Paris, 23rd June 2006* (Cuneiform Monographs 37; Leiden and Boston: Brill), pp. 105–128.

2009b "Diagnose im Alten Mesopotamien. Überlegungen zu Grenzen und Möglichkeiten der Interpretation keilschriftlicher diagnosticher Texte", *OLZ* 104, pp. 381–398.

2009c "*Proverbs* 30:18–19 in the Light of Ancient Mesopotamian Cuneiform Texts", *Sefarad* 69/2, pp. 263–279.

2010a "Innere Krankheiten", in: B. Janowski and D. Schwemer (eds.), *Texte aus der Umwelt des Alten Testaments. Neue Folge. Band 5. Texte zur Heilkunde* (Gütersloh and München: Gütersloher Verlagshaus), pp. 69–77.

2010b "Epilepsie, Schlagenfall und Lähmung", in: B. Janowski and D. Schwemer (eds.), *Texte aus der Umwelt des Alten Testaments. Neue Folge. Band 5. Texte zur Heilkunde* (Gütersloh and München: Gütersloher Verlagshaus), pp. 90–98.

2010c "Krankheiten der Extremitäten und unteren Körperhälfte", in: B. Janowski and D. Schwemer (eds.), *Texte aus der Umwelt des Alten Testaments. Neue Folge. Band 5. Texte zur Heilkunde* (Gütersloh and München: Gütersloher Verlagshaus), pp. 99–106.

2010d "Pharmakologische Texte", in: B. Janowski and D. Schwemer (eds.), *Texte aus der Umwelt des Alten Testaments. Neue Folge. Band 5. Texte zur Heilkunde* (Gütersloh and München: Gütersloher Verlagshaus), pp. 163–168.

2011 "Sourcing, Organizing, and Administering Medicinal Ingredients", in: K. Radner and E. Robson (eds.), *The Oxford Handbook of Cuneiform Culture* (Oxford: Oxford University Press), pp. 690–705.

2014a *The Healing Goddess Gula: Towards an Understanding of Ancient Babylonian Medicine* (Culture and History of the Ancient Near East 67; Leiden, Boston: Brill)

2014b "Die Hymne *Ninisina A* Z. 30–42 mit einem Exkurs über ša$_3$, 'Bauch, Magen-Darm-Trakt' als Sitz der Gefühle", in: L. Kogan, N. Koslova, S. Loesov and S. Tischchenko (eds.), *Studies in Sumerian Language and Literature: Festschrift für Joachim Krecher* (Babel und Bibel 8; Winona Lake, Indiana: Eisenbrauns), pp. 101–122.

In press "Gedanken zu dem Drogen-Inventar aus Assur – KADP 36 (VAT 8903)", in: S. Maul (ed.), *Assur-Forschungen 2* (Wiesbaden: Harrassowitz)

Böhme, S.

2010 "Eigentümerwechsel im 'Haus des Beschwörungspriesters' von Assur gegen Ende der 2. Hälfte des 7. Jahrhunderts", in: Y. Hazırlayan and Ş. Dönmez (eds.), *Veysel Donbaz'a Sunulan Yazılar. DUB.SAR É.DUB.BA.A. Studies Presented in Honour of Veysel Donbaz* (Istanbul: Yayinlari), pp. 35–39.

Brisch, N.

2015 "Recovering the World's Oldest Language" [Review], ⟨http://marginalia.lareviewofbooks.org/nicole-brisch/⟩ (accessed 07/08/2017).

Brosius, M. (ed.)

2003 *Ancient Archives and Archival Traditions. Concepts of Record-Keeping in the Ancient World* (Oxford: Oxford University Press)

van Buren, E. D.

1937–39 "The Scorpion in Mesopotamian Art and Religion", *AfO* 12, pp. 1–28.

Burke, P.

2008 *What is Cultural History?* (Cambridge: Polity Press)

Cadelli, D. S.

1997 "Lrsque l'enfant paraît … malade", KTEMA 22, pp. 11–33.

2000 *Recherche sur la Médecine Mésopotamienne. La série šumma amêlu suâlam maruṣ* (Paris: Université De Paris I Panthéon-Sorbonne)

Cagni, L.

1969 *l'Epopea di Erra* (Studi Semitici 34; Rome: Istituto di Studi del Vicino Oriente, Università di Roma)

1970 *Das Erra-Epos Keilschrifttext* (Studia Pohl 5; Rome: Pontificium Institutum Biblicum)

Cancik-Kirschbaum, E. and J. Kahl

2018 *Erste Philologien* (Tübingen: Mohr Siebeck)

Caplice, R.

1965 "Namburbi Texts in the British Museum. I", *OrNS* 34, pp. 105–131 and pls. 15–18.

1967 "Namburbi Texts in the British Museum. III", *OrNS* 36, pp. 273–298 and pls. 58–62.

1970 “Namburbi Texts in the British Museum IV”, *OrNS* 39, pp. 111–151 and pls. 1–9.

1974 *The Akkadian Namburbi Texts: An Introduction* (Sources from the Ancient Near East 1; Los Angeles: Undena Publications)

Castellino, G.

1955 “Rituals and Prayers against ‘Appearing Ghosts’”, *OrNS* 24, pp. 240–274.

Cavigneaux, A.

1981 *Textes scolaires du temple de Nabû Ša Harê vol. I* (Baghdad: Republic of Iraq, Ministry of Culture & Information, State Organization of Antiquities & Heritage)

1996 “Un colophon de type *Nabû ša Ḫarê*”, *Acta Sumerologica* 18, pp. 22–29.

1999a “*Nabû ša ḫarê* und die Kinder von Babylon”, in: J. Renger (ed.), *Babylon: Focus Mesopotamischer Geschichte, Wiege Früher Gelehrsamkeit, Mythos in der Moderne* (Colloquien der Deutschen Orient-Gesellschaft 2; Saarbrücken: SDV Saarbrücker Druckerei und Verlag), pp. 385–391.

1999b “A Scholar’s Library in Meturan?”, in: T. Abusch and K. van der Toorn (eds.), *Mesopotamian Magic: Textual, Historical, and Interpretative Perspectives* (Ancient Magic and Divination 1; Groningen: STYX Publications), pp. 253–276.

Cavigneaux, A. and B. K. Ismail

1998 “Eine zweisprachige Hymne aus dem Haus des Beschwörungspriesters”, *Acta Sumerologica* 20, pp. 1–11.

Cesaretli, Y. and O. Ozkan

2010 “Snakebites in Turkey: Epidemiological and Clinical Aspects Between the Years 1995 and 2004”, *The Journal of Venomous Animals and Toxins including Tropical Diseases* 16/4, pp. 579–586.

Chalendar, V.

2013 “‘Un aperçu de la neuropsychiatrie assyrienne’: Une édition du texte BAM III-202”, *JMC* 21, pp. 1–60.

Charpin, D.

2010a *Reading and Writing in Babylon* [Translated by J. M. Todd] (Cambridge and London: Harvard University Press)

2010b *Writing, Law, and Kingship in Old Babylonian Mesopotamia* [Translated by J. M. Todd] (Chicago and London: University of Chicago Press)

Chippaux, J.-P. and M. Goyffon

2008 “Epidemiology of Scorpionism: A Global Appraisal”, *Acta Tropica* 107, pp. 71–79.

Civil, M.

1974 “Medical Commentaries from Nippur” *JNES* 33/3, pp. 329–338.

Civil, M. (ed.)

1969 *The Series lú = ša and Related Texts* (Materialien zum Sumerischen Lexikon 12; Rome: Pontificium Institutum Biblicum)

2004 *The Series DIRI = (w)atru* (Materialien zum Sumerischen Lexikon 15; Rome: Pontificium Institutum Biblicum)

Civil, M. and W. G. Lambert

1983 "Enlil and Ninlil: The Marriage of Sud", *JAOS* 103/1, pp. 43–66.

Clancier, P.

2009 *Les bibliothèques en Babylonie au Ier millénaire av. J.-C.* (Alter Orient und Altes Testament 363; Münster: Ugarit-Verlag)

2014 "Teaching and Learning Medicine and Exorcism at Uruk During the Hellenistic Period", in: A. Bernard and C. Proust (eds.), *Scientific Sources and Teaching Contexts Throughout History: Problems and Perspectives* (Boston Studies in the Philosophy and History of Science 301; Heidelberg, New York and London: Springer), pp. 41–68.

Cohen, C.

1983 "The Ugaritic Hippiatric Texts and *BAM* 159", *JANES* 15, pp. 1–12.

Cohen, C. and D. Sivan

1983 *The Ugaritic Hippiatric Texts: A Critical Edition* (American Oriental Series 9; New Haven, Connecticut: American Oriental Society)

Cohen, M. E.

1988 *The Canonical Lamentations of Ancient Mesopotamia. Volume 1–2* (Potomac: Capital Decisions Limited)

1993 *The Cultic Calendars of the Ancient Near East* (Bethesda, Maryland: CDL Press)

Cohen, Y.

2016 "Sheep Anatomical Terminology in the *šumma immeru* Omen Series and Additional Texts", in: J. C. Fincke (ed.), *Divnitation as Science* (Winona Lake, Indiana: Eisenbrauns), pp. 79–92.

Cohen, Y. and S. Kedar

2011 "Teacher-Student Relationships: Two Case Studies", in: K. Radner and E. Robson (eds.), *The Oxford Handbook of Cuneiform Culture* (Oxford: Oxford University Press), pp. 229–247.

Collins, T. J.

1999 *Natural Illness in Babylonian Medical Incantations Volume I-II* (Dissertation; Chicago: The University of Chicago)

Cooper, J. S.

1996 "Magic and M(is)use: Poetic Promiscuity in Mesopotamian Ritual", in: M. E. Vogelzang and H. L. J. Vanstiphout (eds.), *Mesopotamian Poetic Language: Sumerian and Akkadian* (Cuneiform Monographs 6; Groningen: STYX Publications), pp. 47–57.

2009 "Wind and Smoke: Giving up the Ghost of Enkidu, Comprehending Enkidu's Ghosts", in: M.-C. Poo (ed.), *Rethinking Ghosts in World Religions* (Studies in the History of Religions 123; Leiden and Boston: Brill), pp. 23–32.

Couto Ferreira, E.

2009 *Etnoanatomía y partonomía del cuerpo humano en sumerio y acadio: El léxico Ugu-mu* (Dissertation; Barcelona: Pompeu Fabra University)

2017 "'Let me be your canal': some thoughts on agricultural landscape and female bodies in Sumero-Akkadian sources", in: L. Feliu, F. Karahashi, and G. Rubio (eds.), *The First 90 Years. A Sumerian Celebration in Honor of Miguel Civil* (Studies in Ancient Near Eastern records 12; Boston and Berlin: De Gruyter), pp. 54–69.

2018 "Putting Theory into Practice: Kiṣir-Aššur's Expertise between Textual Knowledge and Practical Experimentation", in: S. V. Panayotov and L. Vacín (eds.), *Mesopotamian Medicine and Magic. Studies in Honor of Markham J. Geller* (Ancient Magic and Divination 14; Leiden and Boston: Brill), pp. 149–166.

Curtis, J. E., H. McCall, D. Collon and L. al-Gailani Werr (eds.)

2008 *New Light on Nimrud – Proceedings of the Nimrud Conference 11th–13th March 2002* (London: British Institute for the Study of Iraq and The British Museum)

Da Riva, R.

2014 "Assyrians and Assyrian Influence in Babylonia (626–539 BCE)", in: S. Gaspa, A. Greco, D. M. Bonacossi, S. Ponchia and R. Rollinger (ed.), *From Sources to History. Studies on Ancient Near Eastern Worlds and Beyond. Dedicated to Giovanni Battista Lanfranchi on the Occasion of His 65th Birthday on June 23, 2014* (Alter Orient und Altes Testament 412; Münster: Ugarit-Verlag), pp. 99–125.

Dalley, S.

2013 *The Mystery of the Hanging Garden of Babylon: An Elusive World Wonder Traced* (Oxford: Oxford University Press)

Dalley, S. and J. N. Postgate

1984 *The Tablets from Fort Shalmaneser* (Cuneiform Texts from Nimrud 3; Oxford: British School of Achaeology in Iraq)

Davis, N. Z.

1985 [1983] *The Return of Martin Guerre* (Middlesex, New York, Victoria, Ontario and Auckland: Penguin Books) [Harvard: Harvard University Press]

Dehesa-Davila, M., A. C. Alagon and L. D. Possani

1995 "Clinical Toxicology of Scorpion Stings", in: J. Meier and J. White (eds.), *Handbook of Clinical Toxicology of Animal Venoms and Poisons* (Boca Raton, New York, London, and Tokyo: CRC Press), pp. 221–238.

Deller, K., F. M. Fales and L. Jakob-Rost

1995 "Neo-Assyrian Texts from Assur. Private Archives in the Vorderasiatisches Museum of Berlin", *SAAB* 9/1–2, pp. 3–137.

Delnero, P.
2012 *The Textual Criticism of Sumerian Literature* (The Journal of Cuneiform Studies Supplemental Series 3; Boston: American Schools of Oriental Research)

Dhorme, E.
1923 *L'emploi métaphorique des noms de parties du corps en hébreu et en akkadien* (Paris: Librairie Orientaliste Paul Geuthner)

van Dijk, J.
1983 *Lugal UD ME-LÁM-bi NIR.GÁL: Le récit épique et didactique des Travaux de Ninurta, du Déluge et de la Nouvelle Création. Texte, traduction et introduction. Tome II: Introduction à la reconstruction du texte Inventaire des Textes. Partition, copies des originaux* (Leiden: E. J. Brill)

van Dijk, J., A. Goetze and M. I. Hussey
1985 *Early Mesopotamian Incantations and Rituals* (Yale Oriental Series 11; New Haven and London: Yale University Press)

Donbaz, V. and S. Parpola
2001 *Neo-Assyrian Legal Texts in Istanbul* (Studien zu den Assur-Texten 2; Saarbrücken: SDV Saarbrücker Druckerei und Verlag)

van Driel, G.
1969 *The Cult of Aššur* (Assen: van Gorcum & Comp. N. V. and Dr. H. J. Prakke & H. M. G. Prakke)

Durand, J.-M.
1982 *Documents cunéiformes de la IVe section de l'Ecole Pratique des Hautes Etudes Tome I. Catalogue et copies cunéiforms* (Genève, Paris: Librairie Droz)

Ebeling, E.
1915 "Assyrische Beschwörungen", ZDMG 69/1, pp. 89–103.
1918 *Quellen zur Kenntnis der babylonischen Religion I* (Mitteilungen der Vorderasiatischen Gesellschaft 23/1; Lepzig: J. C. Hinrichs'sche Buchhandlung)
1919a *Keilschrifttexte aus Assur Religiösen Inhalts. Erster Band* (Leipzig: J. C. Hinrichs'sche Buchhandlung)
1919b *Quellen zur Kenntnis der babylonischen Religion II* (Mitteilungen der Vorderasiatischen Gesellschaft 23/2; Lepzig: J. C. Hinrichs'sche Buchhandlung)
1920–23 *Keilschrifttexte aus Assur religiösen Inhalts. Zweiter Band* (Leipzig: J. C. Hinrichs'sche Buchhandlung)
1931a *Tod und Leben nach den Vorstellungen der Babylonier* (Berlin and Leipzig: Walter de Gruyter & Co.)

1931b "Aus dem Tagewerk eines assyrischen Zauberpriesters", *Mitteilungen der Altorientalischen Gesellschaft* 5/3, pp. 1–52.

1950 *Parfümrezepte und kultische Texte aus Assur* (Roma: Pontificium Institutum Biblicum)

1951 *Bruchstücke einer mittelassyrischen Vorschriftensammlung für de Akklimatisierung und Trainierung von Wagenpferden* (Deutche Akademie der Wissenschaften zu Berlin Institut für Orientforschung 7; Berlin: Akademie-Verlag)

1953a *Literarische Keilschrifttexte aus Assur* (Berlin: Akademie-Verlag)

1953b "Samlungen von Beschwörungsformeln teils in sumerisch-akkadischer, teils in sumerischer oder akkadischer Sprache", *ArOr* 21, pp. 357–423.

1953c *Die Akkadische Gebetsserie "Handerhebung"* (Deutsche Akademie der Wissenschaften zu Berlin Institut für Orientforschung 20; Berlin: Akademie-Verlag)

1954a "Beiträge zur Kenntnis der Beschwörungsserie Namburbi", *RA* 48/1, pp. 1–15.

1954b "Beiträge zur Kenntnis der Beschwörungsserie Namburbi", *RA* 48/4, pp. 178–191.

1954c "Kultische Texte aus Assur", *OrNS* 23, pp. 114–128.

1954d "Beiträge zur Kenntnis der Beschwörungsserie Namburbi", *RA* 48/3, pp. 130–141.

1955a "Beiträge zur Kenntnis der Beschwörungsserie Namburbi (*suite*)", *RA* 49/3, pp. 137–148.

1955b "Beiträge zur Kenntnis der Beschwörungsserie Namburbi (*suite*)", *RA* 49/4, pp. 178–192.

van der Eijk, P.

2008 "The Role of Medicine in the Formation of Early Greek Thought", in: P. Curd and D. W. Graham (eds.), *The Oxford Handbook of Presocratic Philosophy* (Oxford: Oxford University Press), pp. 385–412.

Eilers, W.

1933 "Ein verkannter medizinischer Keilschrifttext", *Sudhoffs Archiv für Geschichte der Medizin* 26/4, pp. 318–328.

Eisenberg, L.

1977 "Disease and Illness. Distinctions Between Professional and Popular Ideas of Sickness", *Culture, Medicine and Psychiatry* 1, pp. 9–23.

Elman, Y.

1975 "Authoritative Oral Tradition in Neo-Assyrian Scribal Circles", *JANES* 7, pp. 19–32.

Ember, C. R. and M. Ember (eds.)

2004 *Encyclopedia of Medical Anthropology. Health and Illness in the World's Cultures* (New York, Boston, Dordrecht, London, and Moscow: Kluwer Academic and Plenum Publishers)

Epping, J. and J. N. Strassmaier
1891 "Neue babylonische Planeten-Tafeln. III", ZA 6, pp. 217–244.
Ermidoro, S.
2015 *Commensality and Ceremonial Meals in the Neo-Assyrian Period* (Studi orientali 3; Venezia: Edizioni Ca'Foscari)
2017 "The Nature and Content of the Corpus", in: S. Parpola (ed.), *Assyrian Royal Rituals and Cultic Texts* (State Archives of Assyria 20; Helsinki: The Neo-Assyrian Text Corpus Project), pp. XV–XXX.
Fadhil, A.
1998 "Der Prolog des Codex Hammurapi in einer Abschrift aus Sippar", in: Anonymous (ed.), *XXXIVème Rencontre Assyriologique Internationale* (Ankara: Türk Tarih Kurumu Basimevi), pp. 717–729 and pls. 211–213.
Fadhil, A. A.
2012 *Eine kleine Tontafelbibliothek aus Assur (Ass. 15426)* (Dissertation; Heidelberg: Heidelberg University)
2018 "IM 148516 – Ein neues Abwehrzauberritual vor dem Mondgott", ZA 108/2, pp. 192–202.
Fadhil, O., M. A. Salim and I. M. Abd
2009 *Key Biodiversity Survey of Central and Western Iraq* (Sulaimani: Nature Iraq)
Faist, B.
2007 *Alltagstexte aus neuassyrischen Archiven und Bibliotheken der Stadt Assur* (Studien zu den Assur-Texten 3; Wiesbaden: Harrassowitz Verlag)
Farber, W.
1977 *Beschwörungsrituale an Ištar und Dumuzi: attī Ištar ša ḫarmaša Dumuzi* (Wiesbaden: Franz Steiner Verlag GMBH)
1987 "Rituale und Beschwörungen in akkadischer Sprache", in: W. Farber, H. M. Kümmel and W. H. P. Römer, *Rituale und Beschwörungen I* (Texte aus der Umwelt des Alten Testaments 2; Gütersloh: Gütersloher Verlagshaus Gerd Mohn), pp. 212–281.
1989 *Schlaf, Kindchen, Schlaf! Mesopotamische Baby-Beschwörungen und –Rituale* (Mesopotamian Civilizations 2; Winona Lake: Eisenbrauns)
1990a "Magic at the Cradle: Babylonian and Assyrian Lullabies", *Anthropos* 85, pp. 139–148.
1990b "*Mannam lušpur ana Enkidu*: Some New Thoughts about an Old Motif", JNES 49/4, pp. 299–321.
1995 "Witchcraft, Magic, and Divination in Ancient Mesopotamia", in: J. M. Sasson (ed.), *Civilizations of the Ancient Near East. Volume III* (New York: Charles Schribner's Sons and Simon & Schuster MacMillan), pp. 1895–1909.
2004 "How to Marry a Disease: Epidemics, Contagion, and a Magic Ritual Against the 'Hand of the Ghost'", in: H. F. J. Horstmanshoff and M. Stol (eds.), *Magic*

and Rationality in Ancient Near Eastern and Graeco-Roman Medicine (Leiden, Boston: Brill), pp. 117–132.

2014 *Lamaštu: An Edition of the Canonical Series of Lamaštu Incantations and Rituals and Related Texts from the Second and First Millennia B.C.* (Mesopotamian Civilizations 17; Winona Lake, Indiana: Eisenbrauns)

Feldt, L.

2015 "Monstrous Figurines from Mesopotamia. Textuality, Spatiality and Materiality in Rituals and Incantations for the Protection of Houses in First-Millennium Aššur", in: D. Boschung and J. N. Bremmer (eds.), *The Materiality of Magic* (Morphomata 20; Paderborn: Wilhelm Fink), pp. 59–96.

Fet, V., W. D. Sissom, G. Lowe and M. E. Braunwalder

2000 *Catalog of the Scorpions of the World (1758–1998)* (New York: The New York Entomological Society)

Fincke, J.

2000 *Augenleiden nach keilschriftlichen Quellen: Untersuchungen zur altorientalischen Medizin* (Würzburger medizinhistorische Forschungen 70; Würzburg: Verlag Königshausen & Neumann)

2001 "Der Assur-Katalog der Serie *enūma anu enlil* (EAE)", *OrNS* 70, pp. 19–39.

2003–04 "The Babylonian Texts of Nineveh. Report on the British Museum's *Ashurbanipal Library Project*", *AfO* 50, pp. 111–149.

2004 "The British Museum's Ashurbanipal Library Project", *Iraq* 66, pp. 55–60.

2017 "Assyrian Scholarship and Scribal Culture in Kalḫu and Nineveh", in: E. Frahm (ed.), *A Companion to Assyria* (Hoboken and Chichester: Wiley Blackwell), pp. 378–397.

Finkbeiner, U. and B. Pongratz-Leisten

1992 "Beispiele altorientalischer Städte. Residenzen des Assyrischen Reiches. Assur: 1 : 4.000", in: H. Gaube and W. Röllig (eds.), *Tübinger Atlas des Vorderen Orients. Karten zu Teil B: Geschichte* (Wiesbaden: Reichert Verlag), pl. IV 21.

Finkel, I. L.

1988 "Adad-apla-iddina, Esagil-kīn-apli, and the Series SA.GIG", in: E. Leichty, M. deJ. Ellis and P. Gerardi (eds.), *A Scientific Humanist: Studies in Memory of Abraham Sachs* (Occasional Publications of the Samuel Noah Kramer Fund 9; Philadelphia: The University Museum), pp. 143–159.

1991 "*Muššu'u, Qutāru*, and the Scribe Tanittu-Bēl", *Aula Orientalis* 9, pp. 91–104.

1995 "In Black and White: Remarks on the Assur Psephomancy Ritual", *ZA* 85, pp. 271–276.

1999 "On Some Dog, Snake and Scorpion Incantations", in: T. Abusch and K. van der Toorn (eds.), *Mesopotamian Magic: Textual, Historical, and Interpretative Perspectives* (Ancient Magic and Divination 1; Groningen: STYX Publications), pp. 213–250.

2000 "On Late Babylonian Medical Training", in: A. R. George and I. L: Finkel (eds.), *Wisdom, Gods and Literature: Studies in Assyriology in Honour of W. G. Lambert* (Winona Lake, Indiana: Eisenbrauns), pp. 137–223.

2011 "Drawings on Tablets", *Scienze dell'Antichità* 17, pp. 337–344.

Foster, B. R.

1991 "On Authorship in Akkadian Literature", *Annali* 51, pp. 17–32.

1996 *Before the Muses: An Anthology of Akkadian Literature. Volume I–II* [Second Edition] (Bethesda: CDL Press)

2002 "Animals in Mesopotamian Literature", in: B. J. Collins (ed.), *A History of the Animal World in the Ancient Near East* (Handbuch der Orientalistik 64; Leiden, Boston, and Köln: Brill), pp. 271–288.

Frahm, E.

1998 "Anmerkungen zu den *ālu*-Kommentaren aus Uruk", *N.A.B.U.* 1998/1, note no. 11, pp. 13–14.

1999 "Nabû-zuqup-kēnu, das Gilgameš-Epos und der Tod Sargons II.", *JCS* 51, pp. 73–90.

2004 "Royal Hermeneutics: Observations on the Commentaries from Ashurbanipal's Libraries at Nineveh", *Iraq* 66, pp. 45–50.

2010a "Reading the Tablet, the Exta, and the Body: The Hermeneutics of Cuneiform Signs in Babylonian and Assyrian Text Commentaries and Divinatory Texts", in: A. Annus (ed.), *Divination and Interpretation of Signs in the Ancient World* (Oriental Institute Seminars 6; Chicago: The Oriental Institute of the University of Chicago), pp. 93–142.

2010b "The Latest Sumerian Proverbs", in: S. C. Melville and A. L. Slotsky (eds.), *Opening the Tablet Box. Near Eastern Studies in Honor of Benjamin R. Foster* (Culture and History of the Ancient Near East 42; Leiden and Boston: Brill), pp. 155–184.

2011a *Babylonian and Assyrian Text Commentaries: Origins of Interpretation* (Guides to the Mesopotamian Textual Record 5; Münster: Ugarit-Verlag)

2011b "Keeping Company with Men of Learning: The King as Scholar", in: K. Radner and E. Robson (eds.), *The Oxford Handbook of Cuneiform Culture* (Oxford: Oxford University Press), pp. 508–532.

2015 "Commentary on Udug-hul 2–4 (CCP 2.2.2)", ⟨http://ccp.yale.edu/P413991⟩ (accessed 27/03/2017).

2018a "The Exorcist's Manual: Structure, Language, *Sitz im Leben*", in: G. van Buylaere, M. Luukko, D. Schwemer and A. Mertens-Wagschal (eds.), *Sources of Evil. Studies in Mesopotamian Exorcistic Lore* (AMD 15; Leiden and Boston: Brill), pp. 9–47.

2018b "Commentary on Tummu bītu, Šurpu 2 (CCP 2.1.C)", ⟨http://ccp.yale.edu/P470058⟩ (accessed 14/03/2017).

Frahm, E. (ed.)
2017 *A Companion to Assyria* (Hoboken and Chichester: Wiley Blackwell)
Frahm, E., M. Frazer and E. Jiménez
2013a "Commentary on Tummu bītu, Maqlû 1–2 (CCP 2.1.A)", ⟨http://ccp.yale.edu/P461111⟩ (accessed 14/03/2017).
2013b "Commentary on Enūma Anu Enlil 20 (CCP 3.1.20.A)", ⟨http://ccp.yale.edu/P394833⟩ (accessed 11/08/2017).
Frahm, E., E. Jiménez and M. Frazer
2016 "Commentary on Marduk's Address, Muššu'u, and Udughul (CCP 2.2.1.A.b)", ⟨http://ccp.yale.edu/P430865⟩ (accessed 25/02/2017).
Frame, G. and A. George
2005 "The Royal Libraries of Nineveh: New Evidence for King Ashurbanipal's Tablet Collecting", *Iraq* 67, pp. 265–284.
Frame, G. and C. Waerzeggers
2011 "The Prebend of Temple Scribe in First Millennium Babylonia", ZA 101, pp. 127–151.
Frankena, R.
1960 "Erica Reiner, *Šurpu, A Collection of Sumerian and Akkadian Incantations*" [Review], *BiOr* 17/3, pp. 172–174.
Frechette, C. G.
2012 *Mesopotamian Ritual-prayers of 'Hand-lifting' (Akkadian Šuillas): An Investigation of Function in Light of the Idiomatic Meaning of the Rubric* (Alter Orient und Altes Testament 379; Münster: Ugarit-Verlag)
Freedman, S. M.
1998 *If a City is Set on a Height: The Akkadian Omen Series Šumma Alu ina Mēlê Šakin Volume 1: Tablets 1–21* (Occasional Publications of the Sumuel Noah Kramer Fund 17; Philadelphia: The University Museum)
2006a *If a City is Set on a Height: The Akkadian Omen Series Šumma Alu ina Mēlê Šakin Volume 2: Tablets 22–40* (Occasional Publications of the Sumuel Noah Kramer Fund 19; Philadelphia: The University Museum)
2006b "BM 129092: A commentary on Snake Omens", in: A. K. Guinan, M. deJ. Ellis, A. J. Ferrara, S. M. Freedman, M. T. Rutz, L. Sassmannshausen, S. Tinney and M. W. Waters, *If a Man Builds a Joyful House: Assyriological Studies in Honor of Erle Verdun Leichty* (Cuneiform Monographs 31; Leiden, Boston: Bill), pp. 149–166.
2017 *If a City is Set on a Height: The Akkadian Omen Series Šumma Alu ina Mēlê Šakin Volume 3: Tablets 41–63* (Winona Lake: Eisenbrauns)
Freydank, H.
2001 "*lēʾāni* 'Holztafeln' – eine Grundlage der mittelassyrischen Verwaltung", in: T. Richter, D. Prechel and J. Klinger (eds.), *Kulturgeschichten. Altorientalistische*

Studien für Volkert Haas zum 65. Geburtstag (Saarbrücken: Saarbrücker Druckerei und Verlag), pp. 103–111.

Fronzaroli, P.

2005 "A Veterinary Prescription Found at Ebla (TM.75.G.1645)", in: L. Kogan, N. Koslova, S. Loesov, and S. Tishchenko (eds.), *Memoriae Igor M. Diakonoff. Babel und Bibel 2* (Orientalia et Classica 8; Winona Lake, Indiana: Eisenbrauns), pp. 89–99.

Frymer-Kensky, T.

1983 "The Tribulations of Marduk. The So-called 'Marduk Ordeal Text'", *JAOS* 103/1, pp. 131–141.

Gabbay, U.

2016 *The Exegetical Terminology of Akkadian Commentaries* (Culture and History of the Ancient Near East 82; Leiden, Boston: Brill)

Gabbay, U. and E. Jiménez

2019 "Cultural Imports and Local Products in the Commentaries from Uruk. The Case of the Gimil-Sîn Family", in: C. Proust and J. Steele (eds.), *Scholars and Scholarship in Late Babylonian Uruk* (Why the Sciences of the Ancient World Matter 2; Cham: Springer), pp. 53–88.

Gaines, A. D. and R. Davis-Floyd

2004 "Biomedicine", in: C. R. Ember and M. Ember (eds.), *Encyclopedia of Medical Anthropology. Health and Illness in the World's Cultures* (New York, Boston, Dordrecht, London, and Moscow: Kluwer Academic and Plenum Publishers), pp. 95–109.

Geers, F. W.

1926 "A Babylonian Omen Text", *The American Journal of Semitic Languages and Literature* 43/1, pp. 22–41.

Gehlken, E.

2005 "Childhood and Youth, Work and Old Age in Babylonia – a Statistical Analysis", in: H. D. Baker and M. Jursa (eds.), *Approaching the Babyonian Economy. Proceedings of the START Project Symposium held in Vienna, 1–3 July 2004* (Alter Orient und Altes Testament 330; Münster: Ugarit-Verlag), pp. 89–120.

Gelb, I. J.

1954 "Two Assyrian King Lists", *JNES* 13/4, pp. 209–230.

Geller, M. J.

1990 "Astronomy and Authorship", *BSOAS* 53/2, pp. 209–213.

1999 "Freud and Mesopotamian Magic", in: T. Abusch and K. van der Toorn (eds.), *Mesopotamian Magic: Textual, Historical, and Interpretative Perspectives* (Ancient Magic and Divination 1; Groningen: STYX Publications), pp. 49–55.

2000 "Incipits and Rubrics", in: A. R. George and I. L: Finkel (eds.), *Wisdom, Gods and Literature: Studies in Assyriology in Honour of W. G. Lambert* (Winona Lake, Indiana: Eisenbrauns), pp. 225–258.

2001–02 "West Meets East: Early Greek and Babylonian Diagnosis", *AfO* 48–49, pp. 50–75.

2004 "Anus and Kidneys", JMC 4, pp. 1–8.

2005 *Renal and Rectal Disease Texts* (Die babylonisch-assyrische Medizin in Texten und Untersuchungen 7; Berlin and New York: De Gruyter)

2007a "Phlegm and Breath – Babylonian Contributions to Hippocratic Medicine", in: I. L. Finkel and M. J. Geller (eds.), *Disease in Babylonia* (Cuneiform Monographs 36; Leiden, Boston: Brill), pp. 187–199.

2007b "Incantations within Akkadian Medical Texts", in: G. Leick (ed.), *The Babylonian World* (New York and London: Routledge), pp. 389–399.

2007c "Médicine et magie: l'*asû*, l'*âšipu* et le *mašmâšu*", JMC 9, pp. 1–8.

2007d "Textes médicaux du Louvre, nouvelle edition AO 11447, AO 7760 et AO 66774. Première partie", JMC 10, pp. 4–18.

2010 *Ancient Babylonian Medicine: Theory and Practice* (Chichester: Wiley-Blackwell)

2012 "Y a-t-il une medicine sans magie en Mésopotamie?", JMC 20, pp. 43–52.

2014 *Melothesia in Babylonia: Medicine, Magic, and Astrology in the Ancient Near East* (Science, Technology, and Medicine in Ancient Cultures 2; Boston, Berlin, Munich: De Gruyter)

2015 "Encyclopaedias and Commentaries", in: J. C. Johnson (ed.), *In the Wake of the Compendia: Infrastructural Contexts and the Licensing of Empiricism in Ancient and Medieval Mesopotamia* (Science, technology, and Medicine in Ancient Cultures 3; Boston and Berlin: De Gruyter), pp. 31–45.

2016 *Healing Magic and Evil Demons: Canonical Udug-hul Incantations* (Die babylonisch-assyrische Medizin in Texten und Untersuchungen 8; Boston, Berlin: De Gruyter)

2018a "A Babylonian Hippocrates", in: U. Steinert (ed.), *Assyrian and Babylonian Scholarly Text Catalogues* (Die babylonisch-assyrische Medizin in Texten und Untersuchungen 9; Boston and Berlin: De Gruyter), pp. 42–54.

2018b "The Exorcist's Manual (KAR 44)", in: U. Steinert (ed.), *Assyrian and Babylonian Scholarly Text Catalogues* (Die babylonisch-assyrische Medizin in Texten und Untersuchungen 9; Boston and Berlin: De Gruyter), pp. 292–312.

Geller, M. J. and S. L. Cohen

1995 "Kidney and urinary tract disease in ancient Babylonia, with translations of the cuneiform sources", *Kidney International* 47, pp. 1811–1815.

Geller, M. J. and S. V. Panayotov

In press *Mesopotamian Eye Disease Texts* (Die Babylonisch-assyrische Medizin in Texten und Untersuchungen 10; Boston and Berlin: De Gruyter)

George, A. R.

1988 "Three Middle Assyrian Tablets in the British Museum", *Iraq* 50, pp. 25–37.

1991 "Babylonian Texts from the Folios of Sidney Smith. Part Two: Prognostic and Diagnostic Omens, Tablet I", *RA* 85, pp. 137–163 and figs. 1–5.

1992 *Babylonian Topographical Texts* (Orientalia Lovaniensia Analecta 40; Belgium: Uitgeverij Peeters Leuven)

1993a *House Most High: The Temples of Ancient Mesopotamia* (Mesopotamian Civilizations 5; Winona Lake, Indiana: Eisenbrauns)

1993b "W. Farber: Schlaf, Kindchen, schlaf! Mesopotamische Baby-Beschwörungen und -Rituale" [Review], *JNES* 52/4, pp. 298–300.

1999 "The Dogs of Ninkilim: Magic against Field Pests in Ancient Mesopotamia", in: H. Klengel and J. Renger (eds.), *Landwirtschaft im Alten Orient. Ausgewählte Vorträge der XVL. Recontre Assyriologique Internationale Berlin, 4.–8.7.1994* (Berliner Beiträge zum Vorderen Orient 18; Berlin: Dietrich Reimer Verlag), pp. 291–299.

2003 *The Babylonian Gilgamesh Epic: Introduction, Critical Edition and Cuneiform Texts Volume I–II* (Oxford: Oxford University Press)

2003–04 "P. D. Gesche: Schulunterricht in Babylonien im ersten Jahrtausend v. Chr." [Review], *AfO* 50, pp. 403–406.

2007 "The Epic of Gilgameš: Thoughts on Genre and Meaning", in: J. Azize and N. Weeks (eds.), *Gilgameš and the World of Assyria. Proceedings of the Conference Held at Mandelbaum House, The University of Sydney, 21–23 July 2004* (Ancient Near Eastern Studies Supplement 21; Leuven, Paris, and Dudley: Peeters), pp. 37–65.

2009 *Babylonian Literary Texts in the Schøyen Collection* (Cornell University Studies in Assyriology and Sumerology 10; Bethesda, Maryland: CDL Press)

2010 "The colophon of MS 5007", in: M. Civil, *The Lexical Texts in the Schøyen Collection* (Cornell University Studies in Assyriology and Sumerology 12; Bethesda, Maryland: CDL Press), pp. 274–279.

2013 "The Poem of Erra and Ishum: A Babylonian Poet's View of War", in: H. Kennedy (ed.), *Warfare and Poetry in the Middle East* (London and New York: I. B. Tauris), pp. 39–71.

2015 "On Babylonian Lavatories and Sewers", *Iraq* 77, pp. 75–106.

2016 *Mesopotamian Incantations and Related Texts in the Schøyen Collection* (Cornell University Studies in Assyriology and Sumerology 32; Bethesda: CDL Press)

Gesche, P. D.

2001 *Schulunterricht in Babylonien im ersten Jahrtausend v. Chr.* (Alter Orient und Altes Testament 275; Münster: Ugarit-Verlag)

Gilbert, A. S.

2002 "The Native Fauna of the Ancient Near East", in: B. J. Collins (ed.), *A History of the Animal World in the Ancient Near East* (Handbuch der Orientalistik 64; Leiden, Boston, and Köln: Brill), pp. 3–78.

Ginzburg, C.

1980 *The Cheese and the Worms. The Cosmos of a Sixteenth-Century Miller* [Translated by J. Tedeschi and A. Tedeschi] (Baltimore: The Johns Hopkins University Press)

1985 *The Enigma of Piero* [Translated by M. Ryle and K. Soper] (London: Verso)

1990 *Myth, Emblems, Clues* [Translated by J. Tedeschi and A. C. Tedeschi] (London: Hutchinson Radius)

2012 *Threads and Traces. True False Fictive* [Translated by A. C. Tedeschi and J. Tedeschi] (Berkeley, Los Angeles, and London: University of Califonia Press)

2015 "Microhistory and world history", in: J. H. Bentley, S. Subrahmanyam and M. E. Wiesner-Hanks (eds.), *The Cambridge World History. Volume VI. The Construction of a Global World, 1400–1800 CE. Part 2: Patterns of Change* (Cambridge: Cambridge University Press), pp. 446–473.

Ginzburg, C. and C. Poni

1991 "The Name and the Game: Unequal Exchange and the Historiographic Marketplace", in: E. Muir and G. Ruggiero (eds.), *Microhistory and the Lost Peoples of Europe* (Baltimore and London: The Johns Hopkins University Press), pp. 1–10.

Glassner, J.-J.

2005 "L'aruspice mésopotamien et le regard de l'anatomiste", *JMC* 6, pp. 22–33.

Gleerup, K. B., B. Forkman, C. Lindegaard and P. H. Andersen

2015 "An Equine Pain Face", *Veterinary Anaesthesia and Analgesia* 42, pp. 103–114.

Golz, D.

1974 *Studien zur altorientalischen und griechischen Heilkunde. Therapie – Arzneibereitung – Rezeptstruktur* (Sudhoffs Archiv 16; Wiesbaden: Franz Steiner Verlag GMBH)

Gonçalves, S., V. Julliand and A. Leblond

2002 "Risk Factors Associated with Colic in Horses", *Vet. Res.* 33, pp. 641–652.

Göçmen, B., H. Arikan, Y. Özbel, A. Mermer, K. Çiçek

2006 "Clinical, Physiological and Serological Observations of a Human Following a Venomous Bite by *Macrovipera lebetina Lebetina* (Reptilia: Serpentes)", *Acta Parasitologica Turcica* 30/2, pp. 158–162.

Grayson, A. K. and J. Novotny

2012 *The Royal Inscriptions of Sennacherib, King of Assyria (704–681 BC), Part 1* (The Royal Inscriptions of the Neo-Assyrian Period 3/1; Winona Lake: Eisenbrauns)

Gregory, B. S.

1999 "Is Small Beautiful? Microhistory and the History of Everyday Life", *History and Theory* 38/1, pp. 100–110.

Gries, H.

2017 *Der Assur-Tempel in Assur. Das assyrische Hauptheiligtum im Wandel der Zeit. Teil 1–2* (Wissenschaftliche Veröffentlichungen der Deutschen Orient-Gesellschaft 149; Wiesbaden: Harrassowitz Verlag)

Guinan, A.

1996 "Left/Right Symbolism in Mesopotamian Divination", *SAAB* 10/1, pp. 5–10.

2002 "A Severed Head Laughed: Stories of Divinatory Interpretation", in: L. Ciraolo and J. Seidel (eds.), *Magic and Divination in the Ancient World* (Ancient Magic and Divination 2; Leiden, Boston, and Köln: Brill and Styx), pp. 7–40.

2014 "Laws and Omens: Obverse and Inverse", in: J. C. Fincke (ed.), *Divination in the Ancient Near East. A Workshop on Divination Conducted during the 54th Rencontre Assyriologique Internationale, Würzburg, 2008* (Winona Lake: Eisenbrauns), pp. 105–122.

Guinan, A. and E. Leichty

2008 "Tasteless Tablets", in: van der Spek (ed.), *Studies in Ancient Near Eastern World View and Society Presented to Marten Stol on the Occasion of his 65th Birthday, 10 November 2005, and his Retirement from the Vrije Universiteit Amsterdam* (Bethesda, Maryland: CDL Press), pp. 49–50.

Gurney, O. R.

1935 "Babylonian Prophylactic Figures and Their Rituals", *Annals of Archaeology and Anthropology* 22, pp. 31–96 and pls. 11–14.

1956 "The Sultantepe Tablets (Continued) V. The Tale of the Poor Man of Nippur", *Anatolian Studies* 6, pp. 145–164.

Gurney, O. R. and J. J. Finkelstein

1957 *The Sultantepe Tablets I* (Occasional Publications of the British Institute of Archaeology at Ankara 3; London: The British Institute of Archaeology at Ankara)

Habeeb, I. N. and N. Rastegar-Pouyani

2016 "Georgraphical Distribution of the Snakes of Iraq", *Mesopotamia Environmental Journal* 2/3, pp. 67–77.

Haller, A.

1954 *Die Gräber und Grüfte von Assur* (Wissenschaftliche Veröffentlichungen der Deutschen Orient-Gesellschaft 65; Berlin: Verlag Gebr. Mann)

Hallo, W. W.

1962 "New Viewpoints on Cuneiform Literature", *IEJ* 12, pp. 13–26.

2008 "MUL.APIN and the Names of Constellations", in: van der Spek (ed.), *Studies in Ancient Near Eastern World View and Society Presented to Marten Stol on the Occasion of his 65th Birthday, 10 November 2005, and his Retirement from the Vrije Universiteit Amsterdam* (Bethesda, Maryland: CDL Press), pp. 235–253.

Harkins, T.
2012 "Venemous Snakes of Iraq and Kuwait", ⟨http://www.med.navy.mil/sites/nmcphc/documents/program-and-policy-support/chppmsnakebrf.pdf⟩ (accessed 22/08/2017).

Haussperger, M.
1997 "Die mesopotamische Medizin und ihre Ärzte aus heutiger Sicht", ZA 87, pp. 196–218.
1999 "Das 'Fachbuch' der Erkrankungen der Atmungsorgane", ZA 89, pp. 165–200.
2000 "Einige Anmerkungen zum 'Fachbuch der Abdominalerkrankungen'", in: R. Dittmann, B. Hrouda, U. Löw, P. Matthiae, R. Mayer-Opificius and S. Thürwächter (eds.), *Variatio Delectat. Iran und der Westen. Gedenkschrift für Peter Calmeyer* (Alter Orient und Altes Testament 272; Münster: Ugarit-Verlag), pp. 343–346.
2002 "Die Krankheiten des Verdauungstraktes", *WdO* 32, pp. 33–73.

Hecker, K.
1977 "Tradition und Originalität in der altorientalischen Literatur", *Archív Orientální* 45, pp. 245–258.
2008 "Rituale und Beschwörungen", in: B. Janowski and G. Wilhelm (eds.), *Texte aus der Umwelt des Alten Testaments. Neue Folge. Band 4. Omina, Orakel, Rituale und Beschwörungen* (Gütersloh and München: Gütersloher Verlagshaus), pp. 61–127.

Heeßel, N. P.
2000 *Babylonisch-assyrische Diagnostik* (Alter Orient und Altes Testament 43; Münster: Ugarit-Verlag)
2001–02 "'Wenn ein Mann zum Haus des Kranken geht …': Intertextuelle Bezüge zwischen der Serie *šumma ālu* und der zweiten Tafel der Serie SA.GIG", *AfO* 48–49, pp. 24–49.
2002a *Pazuzu. Archäologische und philologische Studien zu einem altorientalischen Dämon* (Ancient Magic and Divination 4; Leiden, Boston, and Köln: Brill and Styx)
2002b "Ein neubabylonisches Rezept zur Berauschung und Ausnüchterung", in: C. Wunsch (ed.), *Mining the Archives. Festschrift for Christopher Walker on the Occasion of His 60th Birthday 4 October 2002* (Babylonische Archive 1; Dresden: Islet), pp. 99–107.
2006 "Der verschwiegene Unterschied: Die Geschlechterdifferenz in medizinischen Texten aus dem Alten Mesopotamien", in: B. Heininger and R. Lindner (eds.), *Krankheit und Heilung: Gender – Religion – Medizin* (Berlin: LIT Verlag), pp. 9–24.
2007a *Divinatorische Texte I: Terrestrische, teratologische, physiognomische und oneiromantische Omina* (Keilschrifttexte aus Assur literarischen Inhalts 1; Wiesbaden: Harrassowitz Verlag)

2007b “The Hands of the Gods: Disease Names, and Divine Anger”, in: I. L. Finkel and M. J. Geller (eds.), *Disease in Babylonia* (Cuneiform Monographs 36; Leiden, Boston: Brill), pp. 120–130.

2008a “Astrological Medicine in Babylonia”, in: A. Akasoy, C. Burnett and R. Yoeli-Tlalim (eds.), *Astro-Medicine: Astrology and Medicine, East and West* (Firenze: SISMEL – Edizioni del Galluzzo), pp. 1–16.

2008b “Warzen, beulen und narben. Eine Sammlung medizinischer rezepte und physiognomischer beobachtungen aus Assur gegen geischtsmale”, in: van der Spek (ed.), *Studies in Ancient Near Eastern World View and Society Presented to Marten Stol on the Occasion of his 65th Birthday, 10 November 2005, and his Retirement from the Vrije Universiteit Amsterdam* (Bethesda, Maryland: CDL Press), pp. 161–171.

2009 “The Babylonian Physician Rabâ-ša-Marduk. Another Look at Physicians and Exorcists in the Ancient Near East”, in: A. Attia and G. Buisson (eds.), *Advances in Mesopotamian Medicine from Hammurabi to Hippocrates: Proceedings of the International Conference “Oeil malade et mauvais oeil,” Collège de France, Paris, 23rd June 2006* (Cuneiform Monographs 37; Leiden and Boston: Brill), pp. 13–28.

2010a “Neues von Esagil-kīn-apli. Die ältere Version der physiognomischen Omenserie *alamdimmû*”, in: S. M. Maul and N. P. Heeßel (eds.), *Assur-Forschungen: Arbeiten aus der Forschungsstelle ”Edition literarischer Keilschrifttexte aus Assur” der Heidelberger Akademie der Wissenschaften* (Wiesbaden: Harrassowitz Verlag), pp. 139–188.

2010b “Einleitung zu Struktur und Entwicklung des Corpus der therapeutischen Texte”, in: B. Janowski and D. Schwemer (eds.), *Texte aus der Umwelt des Alten Testaments. Neue Folge. Band 5. Texte zur Heilkunde* (Gütersloh and München: Gütersloher Verlagshaus), pp. 31–35.

2010c “Diverse Therapien, gemischte Texte und Sammeltafeln”, in: B. Janowski and D. Schwemer (eds.), *Texte aus der Umwelt des Alten Testaments. Neue Folge. Band 5. Texte zur Heilkunde* (Gütersloh and München: Gütersloher Verlagshaus), pp. 153–156.

2010d “Gebinde mit Amulettsteinen und anderen therapeutischen Substanzen”, in: B. Janowski and D. Schwemer (eds.), *Texte aus der Umwelt des Alten Testaments. Neue Folge. Band 5. Texte zur Heilkunde* (Gütersloh and München: Gütersloher Verlagshaus), pp. 157–164.

2011 “‘Sieben Tafeln aus sieben Städten’ – Überlegungen zum Prozess der Serialisierung von Texten in Babylonien in der zweiten Hälfte des zweiten Jahrtausends v. Chr.”, in: E. Cancik-Kirschbaum, M. Van Ess and J. Marzahn (eds), *Babylon. Wissenskultur in Orient und Okzident* (Topoi Berlin Studies of the Ancient World 1; Berlin and Boston: De Gruyter), pp. 171–196.

2012 *Divinatorische Texte II. Opferschau-Omina* (Keilschrifttexte aus Assur literarischen Inhalts 5; Wiesbanden: Harrassowitz Verlag)

2014 "Amulette und 'Amulettform': Zum Zusammenhang von Form, Funktion und Text von Amuletten im Alten Mesopotamien", in: J. F. Quack and D. C. Luft (eds.), *Erscheinungsformen und Handhabungen heiliger Schriften* (Materielle Textkulturen 5; Berlin, München, and Boston: De Gruyter), pp. 53–77.

2017 "Assyrian Scholarship and Scribal Culture in Ashur", in: E. Frahm (ed.), *A Companion to Assyria* (Hoboken and Chichester: Wiley Blackwell), pp. 368–377.

2018 "A New Medical Therapeutic Text on Rectal Disease", in: S. V. Panayotov and L. Vacín (eds.), *Mesopotamian Medicine and Magic. Studies in Honor of Markham J. Geller* (Ancient Magic and Divination 14; Leiden and Boston: Brill), pp. 310–342.

Heffron, Y.

2014 "Revisiting 'Noise' (*rigmu*) in *Atra-ḫasīs* in Light of Baby Incantations", *JNES* 73/1, pp. 83–93.

Helle, S.

2018 "The Role of Authors in the 'Uruk List of Kings and Sages': Canonization and Cultural Contact", *JNES* 77/2, pp. 219–234.

Herrero, P.

1984 *La Thérapeutique Mésopotamienne* (Paris: Editions Recherche sur les civilisations)

Holcombe, S. J., F. J. Derksen and N. E. Robinson

2007 "Electromyographic Activity of the *Palatinus* and *Palatopharyngeus* Muscles in Exercising Horses", *Equine Veterinary Journal* 39/5, pp. 451–455.

Holma, H.

1911 *Die Namen der Körperteile im Assyrisch-Babylonischen. Eine lexikalisch-etymologische Studie* (Helsinki and Leipzig: Soumalaisen Tiedeakatemian Kustantama and August Priest)

Horowitz, W.

1998 *Mesopotamian Cosmic Geography* (Mesopotamian Civilizations 8; Winona Lake, Indiana: Eisenbrauns)

Horowitz, W. And V. A. Hurowitz

1992 "Urim and Thummim in Light of a Psephomancy Ritual from Assur (*LKA* 137)", *JANES* 21, pp. 95–115.

Howard, M.

1955 "Technical Description of the Ivory Writing-Boards from Nineveh", *Iraq* 17/1, pp. 14–20.

Hrůša, I.

2010 *Die akkadische Synonymenliste malku = šarru: Eine Textedition mit Übersetzung und Kommentar* (Alter Orient und Altes Testament 50; Münster: Ugarit-Verlag)

2015 *Ancient Mesopotamian Religion: A Descriptive Introduction* [Translated by M. Tait] (Münster: Ugarit-Verlag)

Hruška, B.

1974 "Zur letzten Bearbeitung des Erraepos", *Archív Orientální* 42, pp. 354–365.

Hunger, H.

1968 *Babylonische und assyrische Kolophone* (Alter Orient und Altes Testament 2; Neukirchen-Vluyn: Verlag Butzon & Bercker Kevelaer and Neukirchener Verlag des Erziehungsvereins Neukirchen-Vluyn)

1992 *Astrological Reports to Assyrian Kings* (State Archives of Assyria 8; Helsinki: Helsinki University Press)

Hunger, H. and D. Pingree

1989 *MUL.APIN: An Astronomical Compendium in Cuneiform* (Archiv für Orientforschung Beiheft 24; Horn: Verlag Ferdinand Berger & Söhne Gesellschaft M. B. H.)

1999 *Astral Sciences in Mesopotamia* (Handbuch der Orientalistik 44; Leiden, Boston, and Köln: Brill)

Huntsman, R. J., N. J. Lowry and K. Sankaran

2008 "Nonepileptic motor phenomena in the neonate", *Paediatric Child Health* 13/8, pp. 680–684.

Hussein, M. M.

2016 *Nimrud: The Queens' Tombs* [Translated by M. Altaweel] (Baghdad and Chicago: Iraqi State Board of Antiquities and Heritage and The Oriental Institute of the University of Chicago)

Huxley, M.

2000 "The Gates and Guardians in Sennacherib's Addition to the Temple of Assur", *Iraq* 62, pp. 109–138.

Hyman, P., P. J. Milla, M. A. Benninga, G. P. Davidson, D. F. Fleisher, and J. Taminiau

2006 "Childhood Functional Gastrointestinal Disorders: Neonate/Toddler", *Gastroenterology* 130, pp. 1519–1526.

Ismail, B.

1982 "Neuere Tontafelfunde im Irak", in: H. Hirsch, *Vorträge gehalten aus der 28. Rencontre Assyriologique Internationale in Wien 6.-10. Juli 1981* (Archiv für Orientforschung Beiheft 19; Horn: Verlag Ferdinand Berger & Söhne Gesellschaft M.B.H.), pp. 198–200.

Izre'el, S.

2001 *Adapa and the South Wind: Language Has the Power of Life and Death* (Mesopotamian Civilizations 10; Winona Lake: Eisenbrauns)

Jacobsen, T.

1989 "The lil$_2$ of ^{d}En-lil$_2$", in: H. Behrens, D. Loding and M. T. Roth (eds.), *DUMU-E$_2$-DUB-BA-A: Studies in Honor of Åke W. Sjöberg* (Occasional Publications of the Samuel Noah Kramer Fund 11; Philadelphia: The University Museum), pp. 267–276.

Jakob, S.

2003 *Mittelassyrische Verwaltung und Sozialstruktur: Untersuchungen* (Cuneiform Monographs 29; Leiden, Boston: Brill and Styx)

2018 *Ritualbeschreibungen und Gebete III* (Keilschrifttexte aus Assur literarischen Inhalts 9; Wiesbanden: Harrassowitz Verlag)

Al Jadir, W.

1998 "Decouverte d'une bibliotheque dans le temple de la Ville de Sippar (Abu Habbah)", in: Anonymous (ed.), *XXXIV*[ème] *Rencontre Assyriologique Internationale* (Ankara: Türk Tarih Kurumu Basimevi), pp. 707–715 and pls. 207–209.

Jastrow, M.

1913 "An Assyrian Medical Tablet in the Possession of the College of Physicians", *Transactions of the College of Physicians of Philadelphia*, pp. 365–400.

Jean, C.

2006 "*La magie néo-Assyrienne en contexte: Recherches sur le metier d'exorciste et le concept d'āšipūtu* (State Archives of Assyria Studies 17; Helsinki: The Neo-Assyrian Text Corpus Project)

Jiménez, E.

2014a "New Fragments of Gilgamesh and Other Literary Texts from Kuyunjik", *Iraq* 76, pp. 99–122.

2014b "Commentary on Therapeutic (én munus ù-tu-ud-da-a-ni) (CCP 4.2.A.a)", ⟨http://ccp.yale.edu/P459066⟩ (accessed 19/06/2017).

2015 "Commentary on Sagig 13 and 12 (CCP 4.1.13.B)", ⟨http://ccp.yale.edu/P294665⟩ (accessed 01/12/2016).

2017 *The Babylonian Disputation Poems* (Culture and History of the Ancient Near East 87; Leiden and Boston: Brill)

Johnson, J. C.

2014 "Towards a Reconstruction of SUALU IV: Can we Localize K 2386+ in the Therapeutic Corpus?", *JMC* 24, pp. 11–38.

2015 "Depersonalized Case Histories in the Babylonian Therapeutic Compendia", in: J. C. Johnson (ed.), *In the Wake of the Compendia. Infrastructural Contexts and the Licensing of Empiricism in Ancient and Medieval Mesopotamia* (Science, Technology, and Medicine in Ancient Cultures 3; Boston, Berlin: De Gruyter), pp. 289–315.

2018 "Towards a New Perspective on Babylonian Medicine: The Continuum of Allegoresis and the Emergence of Secular Models in Mesopotamian Scientific Thought", in: U. Steinert (ed.), *Assyrian and Babylonian Scholarly Text Catalogues* (Die babylonisch-assyrische Medizin in Texten und Untersuchungen 9; Boston and Berlin: De Gruyter), pp. 55–88.

In press *Gastrointestinal Disease and Its Treatment in Ancient Mesopotamia* (Die Babylonisch-assyrische Medizin in Texten und Untersuchungen 11; Boston and Berlin: De Gruyter)

Jordan, J.

1908 "Aus den Berichten aus Assur", *MDOG* 38, pp. 26–44.

Joyner, C.

1999 *Shared Traditions. Southern History and Folk Culture* (Urbana, Chicago and Springfield: University of Illinois Press)

Jursa, M.

1999 *Das Archiv des Bēl-rēmanni* (Publications de l'Institut historique-archéologique néerlandais de Stamboul 86; Leiden: Nederlands Historisch-Arhcaeologisch Instituut te Istanbul)

Kämmerer, T. R.

1995 "Die erste Pockendiagnose stammt aus Babylonien", *Ugarit-Forschungen* 27, pp. 129–168.

Kedar, S.

2014 "Apprenticeship in the Neo-Babylonian Period: A Study of Bargaining Power", in: L. Marti (ed.), *La famille dans le Proche-Orient ancient: réalités, symbolismes, et images. Proceedings of the 55th Rencontre Assyriologique Internationale at Paris 6–9 July 2009* (Winona Lake, Indiana: Eisenbrauns), pp. 537–546.

Kinnier Wilson, J. V.

1962 "The Nimrud Catalogue of Medical and Physiognomical Omina", *Iraq* 24/1, pp. 52–62.

1965 "An Introduction to Babylonian Psychiatry" in: H. G. Güterbock and T. Jacobsen (eds.), *Studies in Honor of Benno Landsberger on His Seventy-fifth Birthday April 21, 1965* (AS 16; Chicago: The University of Chicago Press), pp. 289–298.

1966 "Leprosy in Ancient Mesopotamia", *RA* 60, p. 47–58.

1996 "Diseases of Babylon: an examination of selected texts", *Journal of the Royal Society of Medicine* 89, pp. 135–140.

2005 "Notes on the Assyrian Pharmaceutical Series Uru.an.na: *maštakal*", *JNES* 64/1, pp. 45–51.

2011 "A Journey through the Prescriptions", *JMC* 17, pp. 1–24.

Kinnier Wilson, J. V. and E. H. Reynolds

2007 "On Stroke and Facial Palsy in Babylonian Texts", in: I. L. Finkel and M. J. Geller (eds.), *Disease in Babylonia* (Cuneiform Monographs 36; Leiden and Boston: Brill), pp. 67–99.

Kleinman, A.

1980 *Patients and Healers in the Context of Culture. An Exploration of the Borderland between Anthropology, Medicine, and Psychiatry* (Comparative

Studies of Health Systems and Medical Care 3; Berkeley and Los Angeles: University of California Press)
1998 "Experience and Its Moral Modes: Culture, Human Conditions, and Disorder", *The Tanner Lectures on Human Values April 13–16, 1998*, ⟨https://tannerlectures.utah.edu/_documents/a-to-z/k/Kleinman99.pdf⟩ (accessed 25/02/2020)

Klengel-Brandt, E.
1968 "Apotropäische Tonfiguren aus Assur", *Forschungen und Berichte* 10, pp. 19–37 and pls. 1–10.
1975 "Eine Schreibtafel aus Assur", *Altorientalische Forschungen* 3, pp. 169–171 and pl. 21.

Koch(-Westenholz), U. S.
1995 *Mesopotamian Astrology: An Introduction to Babylonian and Assyrian Celestial Divination* (CNI Publications 19; Copenhagen: Museum Tusculanum Press)
1999 "The Astrological Commentary *Šumma Sîn ina tāmartīšu* Tablet 1", *Res Orientales* 12, pp. 149–165.
2000 *Babylonian Liver Omens: the Chapters Manzāzu, Padānu and Pān tākalti of the Babylonian Extispicy Series mainly from Aššurbanipal's Library* (CNI Publications 25; Copenhagen: Museum Tusculanum Press)
2005 *Secrets of Extispicy. The Chapter Multābiltu of the Babylonian Extispicy Series and Niṣirti bārûti Texts Mainly from Aššurbanipal's Library* (Alter Orient und Altes Testament 326; Münster: Ugarit-Verlag)
2010 "Three Strikes and You're Out! A View on Cognitive Theory and the First-Millennium Extispicy Ritual", in: A. Annus (ed.), *Divination and Interpretation of Signs in the Ancient World* (Oriental Institute Seminars 6; Chicago: The Oriental Institute of the University of Chicago), pp. 43–60.
2011 "Sheep and Sky: Systems of Divinatory Interpretation", in: K. Radner and E. Robson (eds.), *The Oxford Handbook of Cuneiform Culture* (Oxford: Oxford University Press), pp. 447–469.
2013 "Nils Heeßel, Divinatorische Texte I … Nils Heeßel, Divinatorische Texte II" [Review], *ZA* 103, pp. 241–244.
2015 *Mesopotamian Divination Texts: Conversing with the Gods. Sources from the First Millennium BCE* (Guides to the Mesopotamian Textual Record 7; Münster: Ugarit-Verlag)
Unpublished "The *āšipu* – Healer and Diviner?", ⟨https://www.academia.edu/591778/The_Ashipu_-_Healer_and_Diviner⟩ (accessed 04/06/2017).

Kouwenberg, N. J. C.

2010 *The Akkadian Verb and Its Semitic Background* (Languages of the Ancient Near East 2; Winona Lake, Indiana: Eisenbrauns)

Köcher, F.

1949 *Beschwörungen gegen die Dämonin Lamaštu*, ⟨http://echo.mpiwg-berlin.mpg.de/ECHOdocuView?mode=imagepath&url=/mpiwg/online/permanent/library/Q56UUN4X/pageimg⟩ (accessed 04/06/2017) (Dissertation; Berlin: University of Berlin)

1955 *Keilschrifttexte zur assyrisch-babylonischen Drogen- und Pflanzenkunde* (Deutsche Akademie der Wissenschaften zu Berlin Institut für Orientforschung 28; Berlin: Akademie-Verlag)

1963a *Die babylonisch-assyrische Medizin in Texten und Untersuchungen I: Keilschrifttexte aus Assur 1* (Berlin: Walter de Gruyter & Co.)

1963b *Die babylonisch-assyrische Medizin in Texten und Untersuchungen II: Keilschrifttexte aus Assur 2* (Berlin: Walter de Gruyter & Co.)

1964 *Die babylonisch-assyrische Medizin in Texten und Untersuchungen III: Keilschrifttexte aus Assur 3* (Berlin: Walter de Gruyter & Co.)

1971 *Die babylonisch-assyrische Medizin in Texten und Untersuchungen IV: Keilschrifttexte aus Assur 4, Babylon, Nippur, Sippar, Uruk und unbekannter Herkunft* (Berlin: Walter de Gruyter & Co.)

1978 "Spätbabylonische medizinische Texte aus Uruk: Seriengestaltung der medizinisch-therapeutischen Texte. Ein erstes Zeugnis babylonischer Krankheitstheorie. 'Hand eines Totengeistes': Symptombeschreibungen und Diagnosen", in: C. Habrich, F. Marguth and J. H. Wolf (eds.), *Medizinische Diagnostik in Geschichte und Gegenwart: Festschrift für Heinz Goerke zum sechzigsten Geburtstag* (München: Werner Fritsch), pp. 17–39

1980a *Die babylonisch-assyrische Medizin in Texten und Untersuchungen V: Keilschrifttexte aus Nineveh 1* (Berlin, New York: Walter de Gruyter)

1980b *Die babylonisch-assyrische Medizin in Texten und Untersuchungen VI: Keilschrifttexte aus Nineveh 2* (Berlin, New York: Walter de Gruyter)

1995 "Ein Text medizinischen Inhalts aus dem neubabylonischen Grab 405", in: R. M. Boehmer, F. Pedde, and B. Salje, *Uruk. Die Gräber* (Ausgrabungen in Uruk-Warka Endberichte 10; Mainz: Verlag Philipp von Zabern), pp. 203–217.

Kolev, R. K.

2013 *The Babylonian Astrolabe: The Calendar of Creation* (State Archives of Assyria Studies 22; Helsinki: The Neo-Assyrian Text Corpus Project)

Kottak, C. P.

2010 *Window on Humanity. A Concise Introduction to Anthropology* (New York: McGraw-Hill)

Kraus, F. R.

1947 "Die Istanbuler Tontafelsammlung", *JCS* 1/2, pp. 93–119.

Krebernik, M.

1984 *Die Beschwörungen aus Fara und Ebla: Untersuchungen zur ältesten keilschriftlichen Beschwörungsliteratur* (Texte und Studien zur Orientalistik 2; Hildesheim, Zürich, and New York: Georg Olms Verlag)

2007 "Richtergott(heiten)", in: M. P. Streck (ed.), *Reallexikon der Assyriologie und Vorderasiatischen Archäologie. Band 11 5./6. Lieferung* (Berlin and New York: Walter de Gruyter), pp. 354–361.

Krecher, J.

1957–71 "Glossen", in: E. Weidner and W. von Soden (eds.), *Reallexikon der Assyriologie. Dritter Band* (Berlin and New York: Walter de Gruyter), pp. 431–440.

Küchler, F.

1904 *Beiträge zur Kenntnis der Assyrisch-Babylonischen Medizin* (Leipzig: J. C. Hinrichs'sche Buchhandlung)

Labat, R.

1939 *Hémérologies et Ménologies d'Assur* (Paris: Librairie d'Amérique et d'Orient Adrien-Maisonneuve)

1951 *Traité dkkadien de diagnostics et prognostics médicaux I–II* (Collection de Travaux de l'Académie Internationale d'Historie des Sciences 7; Paris and Leiden: Academie Internationale d'Historie des Sciences and Brill)

1952 "Henry E. Siegerist: A History of Medicine, Vol. I: Primitive and Archaic Medicine" [Review], *JCS* 6, pp. 128–133.

1959 "Le premier chapitre d'un précis médical assyrien", *RA* 53, pp. 1–18.

Labat, R. and J. Tournay

1945–46 "Un texte médical inédit", *RA* 40/3, pp. 113–122.

Lafont, B.

1987 "zabar-dab$_5$, *zab/mardabbum*", *N.A.B.U.* 1987/4, note no. 94, pp. 51–52.

Lambert, W. G.

1956 "Erich Ebeling, Literarische Keilschrifttexte aus Assur" [Review], *Bibliotheca Orientalis* 13/3, pp. 143–146.

1957 "Ancestors, Authors, and Canonicity", *JCS* 11/1, pp. 1–14.

1957–58 "A Part of the Ritual for the Substitute King", *AfO* 18, pp. 109–112 and pl. 10.

1959 "The Sultantepe Tablets. A Review Article" [Review], *RA* 53, pp. 119–138.

1962 "A Catalogue of Texts and Authors", *JCS* 16/3, pp. 59–77.

1967 "The Gula Hymn of Bulluṭsa-rabi", *OrNS* 36, pp. 105–132 and pls. 8–23.

1974 "Dingir.šà.dib.ba Incantations", *JNES* 33/4, pp. 367–322.

1980 "The Twenty-One 'Poultices'", *Anatolian Studies* 30, pp. 77–83.

1989 "The Laws of Hammurabi in the First Millennium", in: M. Lebeau and P. Talon (eds.), *Reflets des deux fleuves: Volume de mélanges offerts À A. Finet* (Akkadica Supplementum 6; Leuven: Peeters), pp. 95–98.

1996 [1960] *Babylonian Wisdom Literature* (Winona Lake: Eisenbrauns) [Oxford: Oxford University Press]

2007 *Babylonian Oracle Questions* (Mesopotamian Civilizations 13; Winona Lake, Indiana: Eisenbrauns)

2008 "The Classification of Incantations", in: R. D. Biggs, J. Myers and M. T. Roth (eds.), *Proceedings of the 51st Rencontre Assyriologique Internationale Held at the Oriental Institute of the University of Chicago July 18–22, 2005* (Studies in Ancient Oriental Civilization 62; Chicago: The Oritental Institute of the University of Chicago), pp. 93–97.

2013 *Babylonian Creation Myths* (Mesopotamian Civilizations 16; Winona Lake, Indiana: Eisenbrauns)

Lambert, W. G. and A. R. Millard

1969 *Atra-ḫasīs: The Babylonian Story of the Flood* (Oxford: Oxford University Press)

Landsberger, B.

1926 "Die Eigenbegrifflichkeit der Babylonischen Welt", *Islamica* 2, pp. 355–372.

1934 *Die Fauna des Alten Mesopotamien nach der 14. Tafel der Serie ḪAR-ra = ḫubullu* (Abhandlungen der philologisch-historischen Klasse der Sächsischen Akademie der Wissenschaften 6; Leipzig: Verlag von S. Hirzel)

1960 *MSL VIII/1. The Fauna of Ancient Mesopotamia. First Part. Tablet XIII* (Materialien zum Sumerischen Lexikon 8/1; Rome: Pontificium Institutum Biblicum)

1962 *MSL VIII/2. The Fauna of Ancient Mesopotamia. Second Part. ḪAR-ra = ḫubullu Tablets XIV and XVIII* (Materialien zum Sumerischen Lexikon 8/2; Rome: Pontificium Institutum Biblicum)

1976 *The Conceptual Autonomy of the Babylonian World* [Translated by T. Jacobsen, B. Foster and H. von Siebenthal] (Monographs on the Ancient Near East 1/4; Malibu: Undena Publications)

Landsberger, B. (ed.)

1967 *ḪAR-ra = ḫubullu Tablet XV and related texts* (Materialien zum Sumerischen Lexikon 9; Rome: Pontificium Institutum Biblicum)

Landsberger, B. and T. Jacobsen

1955 "An Old Babylonian Charm Against *merḫu*", *JNES* 14/1, pp. 14–21.

Langdon, S.

1917 "Assyrian Grammatical Texts", *RA* 14/2, pp. 75–86.

Lapinkivi, P.

2010 *The Neo-Assyrian Myth of Ištar's Descent and Resurrection* (*SAACT* 6; Winona Lake, Indiana: Eisenbrauns)

Lawson, J. N.

1994 *The Concept of Fate in Ancient Mesopotamia of the First Millennium* (Wiesbaden: Harrassowitz Verlag)

Leichty, E.

1964 "The Colophon", in: Anonymous (ed.), *From the Workshop of the Chicago Assyrian Dictionary. Studies Presented to A. Leo Oppenheim June 7, 1964* (Chicago: The Oriental Institute of the University of Chicago), pp. 147–154.

1970 *The Omen Series Šumma izbu* (Texts from Cuneiform Sources 4; New York: J. J. Augustin Publisher)

2011 *The Royal Inscriptions of Esarhaddon, King of Assyria (680–669 BC)* (The Royal Inscriptions of the Neo-Assyrian Period 4; Winona Lake: Eisenbrauns)

Leick, G.

2003 [1994] *Sex and Eroticism in Mesopotamian Literature* (London and New York: Routledge) [London and New York: Routedge]

Lenzi, A.

2008a *Secrecy and the Gods: Secret Knowledge in Ancient Mesopotamia and Biblical Israel* (State Archives of Assyria Studies 19; Helsinki: The Neo-Assyrian Text Corpus Project)

2008b "The Uruk List of Kings and Sages and Late Mesopotamian Scholarship", *JANER* 8/2, pp. 137–169.

2011 *Reading Akkadian Prayers & Hymns: An Introduction* (Ancient Near East Monographs 3; Atlanta: The Society of Biblical Literature)

Lepore, J.

2001 "Historians Who Love Too Much: Reflections on Microhistory and Biography", *The Journal of Amerian History* 88/1, pp. 129–144.

Levi, G.

1991 "On Microhistory", in: P. Burke (ed.), *New Perspectives on Historical Writing* (Cambridge: Polity Press), pp. 93–113.

Lieberman, S. J.

1990 "Canonical and Official Cuneiform Texts: Towards an Understanding of Assurbanipal's Personal Tablet Collection", in: T. Abusch, J. Huehnergard and P. Steinkeller (eds.), *Lingering Over Words: Studies in Ancient Near Eastern Literature in Honor or William L. Moran* (Atlanta: Scholars Press), pp. 305–336.

Lifshitz, M., H. Kastel, I. Harman-Boehm

2002 “*Cerastes cerastes* Envenomation in an 18 Year Old Female: a Case Report”, *Toxicon* 40, pp. 1227–1229.

Lincoln, B.

2003 *Holy Terrors. Thinking about Religion after September 11* (Chicago and London: The University of Chicago Press)

Livingstone, A.

1986 *Mystical and Mythological Explanatory Works of Assyrian and Babylonian Scholars* (Oxford: Oxford University Press)

1989 *Court Poetry and Literary Miscellanea* (State Archives of Assyria 3; Helsinki: Helsinki University Press)

2007 “Ashurbanipal: Literate or Not?”, ZA 97, pp. 98–118.

Lock, M. and V.-K. Nguyen

2010 *An Anthropology of Biomedicine* (Malden, Oxford, and Chichester: Wiley-Blackwell)

Lopes, M. A. F., N. A. White, L. Donaldson, M. V. Crisman and D. L. Ward

2004 “Effects of Enteral and Intravenous Fluid Therapy, Magnesium Sulphate, and Sodium Sulphate on Colonic Contents and Feces in Horses”, *American Journal of Veterinary Research* 65/5, pp. 695–704.

Loud, G. and C. B. Altman

1938 *Khorsabad. Part II. The Citadel and the Town* (Oriental Institute Publications 40; Chicago and Illinois: The University of Chicago Press)

Löhnert, A.

2007 “The Installation of Priests According to Neo-Assyrian Documents”, SAAB 16, pp. 273–286.

Lucas, S. M. and J. Meier

1995 “Biology and Distribution of Scorpions of Medical Importance”, in: J. Meier and J. White (eds.), *Handbook of Clinical Toxicology of Animal Venoms and Poisons* (Boca Raton, New York, London, and Tokyo: CRC Press), pp. 205–219.

Lundström, S.

2009 *Die Königsgrüfte im Alten Palast von Assur* (Wissenschaftliche Veröffentlichungen der Deutschen Orient-Gesellschaft 123; Wiesbaden: Harrassowitz Verlag)

Læssøe, J.

1953 “Literacy and Oral Tradition in Ancient Mesopotamia”, in: Anonymous (ed.), *Studia Orientalia Ioanni Pedersen* (Copenhagen: Einar Munksgaard), pp. 205–218.

1955 *Studies on the Assyrian Ritual and Series bît rimki* (København: Ejnar Munksgaard)

MacGinnis, J. D. A. P.

1989 "Some Inscribed Horse Troughs of Sennacherib", *Iraq* 51, pp. 187–192.

2002 "The Use of Writing Boards in the Neo-Babylonian Temple Administration at Sippar", *Iraq* 64, pp. 217–236.

Macgregor, S. L.

2012 *Beyond Hearth and Home: Women in the Public Sphere in Neo-Assyrian Society* (State Archives of Assyria Studies 21; Helsinki: The Neo-Assyrian Text Corpus Project)

Machinist, P.

1978 *The Epic of Tukulti-Ninurta I. A Study in Middle Assyrian Literature* (Dissertation; Yale: Yale University)

1983 "Rest and Violence in the Poem of Erra", *JAOS* 103/1, pp. 221–226.

MacLeod, R.

2010 [2000] "Introduction: Alexandria in History and Myth", in: R. MacLeod (ed.), *The Library of Alexandria. Centre of Learning in the Ancient World* (London and New York: I. B. Tauris & Co Ltd) [London and New York: I. B. Tauris & Co Ltd], pp. 1–18.

Magnússon, S. G. and I. M. Szijártó

2013 *What is Microhistory? Theory and Practice* (New York: Routledge)

Mallowan, M. E. L.

1954 "The Excavations at Nimurd (Kalḫu)", *Iraq* 16/1, pp. 59–114.

Matouš, L.

1933 *Die lexikalischen Tafelserien der Babylonier und Assyrer in den Berliner Museen. I. Gegenstandslisten* (*Serie ḪAR-ra = ḫubullu*) (Berlin: Staatlichen Museen zu Berlin Vorderasiatische Abteilung)

Mattern, S. P.

2013 *The Prince of Medicine: Galen in the Roman Empire* (Oxford: Oxford University Press)

Maul, S. M.

1988 *"Herzberuhigungsklagen". Die sumerisch-akkadischen eršaḫunga-Gebete* (Wiesbaden: Otto Harrassowitz)

1994 *Zukunftsbewältigung: Eine Untersuchung altorientalischen Denkens anhand der babylonisch-assyrischen Löserituale* (*Namburbi*) (Baghdader Forschungen 18; Mainz: Verlag Philipp von Zabern)

1998 "*tikip santakki mala bašmu … Anstelle eines Vorwortes*", in: S. M. Maul (ed.), *Festschrift für Rykle Borger zu seinem 65. Geburtstag am 24. Mai 1994. tikip santakki mala bašmu …* (Cuneiform Monographs 10; Groningen; STYX Publications), pp. xii–xvii.

1999a "Der assyrische König – Hüter der Weltordnung", in: K. Watanabe (ed.), *Priests and Officials in the Ancient Near East* (Heidelberg: Universitätsverlag C. Winter), pp. 201–214.

1999b "How the Babylonians Protected Themselves against Calamities Announced by Omens", in: T. Abusch and K. van der Toorn (eds.), *Mesopotamian Magic: Textual, Historical, and Interpretative Perspectives* (Ancient Magic and Divination 1; Groningen: STYX Publications), pp. 123–129.

2000 "Die Frühjahrsfeierlichkeiten in Aššur", in: A. R. George and I. L: Finkel (eds.), *Wisdom, Gods and Literature: Studies in Assyriology in Honour of W. G. Lambert* (Winona Lake, Indiana: Eisenbrauns), pp. 389–420.

2003 "Wie die Bibliothek eines assyrischen Gelehrten wiedersteht" in: J. Marzahn and B. Salje (eds.), *Wiedererstehendes Assur: 100 Jahre deutsche Ausgrabungen in Assyrien* (Mainz: Verlap Philipp von Zabern), pp. 175–182.

2004 "Die 'Lösung von Bann': Überlegungen zu altorientalischen Konzeptionen von Krankheit und Heilkunst", in: H. F. J. Horstmanshoff and M. Stol (eds.), *Magic and Rationality in Ancient Near Eastern and Graeco-Roman Medicine* (Leiden and Boston: Brill), pp. 79–95.

2009 "Die Lesung der Rubra DÙ.DÙ.BI und KÌD.KÌD.BI", *OrNS* 78/1, pp. 69–80.

2010a "Die Tontafelbibliothek aus dem sogenannten 'Haus des Beschwörungspriesters'", in: S. M. Maul and N. P. Heeßel (eds.), *Assur-Forschungen: Arbeiten aus der Forschungsstelle "Edition literarischer Keilschrifttexte aus Assur" der Heidelberger Akademie der Wissenschaften* (Wiesbaden: Harrassowitz Verlag), pp. 198–228.

2010b "Rituale zur Lösung des 'Banns'", in: B. Janowski and D. Schwemer (eds.), *Texte aus der Umwelt des Alten Testaments. Neue Folge. Band 5. Texte zur Heilkunde* (Gütersloh and München: Gütersloher Verlagshaus), pp. 135–146.

2013 "Ein altorientalischer Pferdesegen – Seuchenprophylaxe in der assyrischen Armee", *ZA* 103/1, pp. 16–37.

2017 "Assyrian Religion", in: E. Frahm (ed.), *A Companion to Assyria* (Hoboken and Chichester: Wiley Blackwell), pp. 336–358.

2018 "'Ninurta-Duft' oder: Von den Vorsichtsmaßnahmen, die ein mesopotamischer Heiler ergreifen sollte, bevor er einen erkrankten Patienten aufsuchte", *ZA* 108/2, pp. 175–191.

2019 *Bannlösung (nam-érim-búr-ru-da). Die Therapie eines auf eidliche Falschaussage zurückgeführten Leidens. Teil 1–2* (Keilschrifttexte aus Assur literarischen Inhalts 10; Wiesbaden: Harrassowitz Verlag)

Maul, S. M. and R. Strauß

2011 *Ritualbeschreibungen und Gebete I* (Keilschrifttexte aus Assur literarischen Inhalts 4; Wiesbaden: Harrassowitz Verlag)

May, N. N.

2017 "The Connection of Neo-Assyrian Scholars to the Temple Officialdom: Some Evidence, Mostly from Colophons", *N.A.B.U.* 2017/2, note no. 54, pp. 96–101.

2018 "Exorcists and Physicians at Assur: More on their Education and Interfamily and Court Connections", ZA 108/1, pp. 63–80.

Mayer, W.

1983 "Sargons Feldzug gegen Urartu – 714 v. Chr. Text und Übersetzung", MDOG 115, pp. 65–132.

Mayer, W.

1976 *Untersuchungen zur Formensprache der Babylonischen "Gebetsbeschwörungen"* (Studia Pohl 5; Rome: Biblical Institute Press)

1994 "Akkadische Lexikographie: 'CAD' Š$_1$" [Review], *OrNS* 63/2, pp. 111–120.

1999 "Das Ritual *KAR* 26 mit dem Gebet 'Marduk 24'", *OrNS* 68/2, pp. 145–163.

Mayer, W. And W. H. van Soldt

1991 "Akkadische Lexikographie: *CAD* S" [Review], *OrNS* 60/2, pp. 109–120.

McCabe, A.

2007 *A Byzantine Encyclopaedia of Horse Medicine: The Sources, Compilation, and Transmission of the Hippiatrica* (Oxford: Oxford University Press)

Meier, G.

1937–39 "Kommentare aus dem Archiv der Tempelschule in Assur", *AfO* 12, pp. 237–246 and pls. 13–14.

1939 "Lexikalische Bemerkungen", *OrNS* 8, pp. 301–305.

1941–44 "Die zweite Tafel der Series *bīt mēseri*", *AfO* 14, pp. 139–152.

Meinhold, W.

2009 *Ištar in Aššur: Untersuchung eines Lokalkultes von ca. 2500 bis 614 v.Chr.* (Alter Orient und Altes Testament 368; Münster: Ugarit Verlag)

2017 *Ritualbeschreibungen und Gebete II* (Keilschrifttexte aus Assur literarischen Inhalts 7; Wiesbaden: Harrassowitz Verlag)

Melville, S. C.

2004 "Neo-Assyrian Royal Women and Male Identity: Status as a Social Tool", *Journal of the American Orient Society* 124/1, pp. 37–57.

Menzel, B.

1981 *Assyrische Tempel. Band I–II* (Studia Pohl 10/I–II; Rome: Biblical Institute Press)

Meyer, J.-W.

1987 *Untersuchungen zu den Tonlebermodellen aus dem Alten Orient* (Alter Orient und Altes Testament 39; Neukirchen-Vluyn: Verlag Butzon & Bercker Kevelaer, Neukirchener Verlag Neukirchen-Vluyn)

Michalowski, P.

1981 "Carminative Magic: Towards an Understanding of Sumerian Poetics", ZA 71/1, pp. 1–18.

1990 "Presence at the Creation", in: T. Abusch, J. Huehnergard and P. Steinkeller (eds.), *Lingering Over Words: Studies in Ancient Near Eastern Literature in Honor or William L. Moran* (Atlanta: Scholars Press), pp. 381–396.

1998–2001 "Nisaba. A", in: D. O. Edzard (ed.), *Reallexikon der Assyriologie und Vorderasiatischen Archäologie. Neunter Band* (Berlin and New York: Walter de Gruyter), pp. 575–79.

1999 "Commemoration, Writing, and Genre in Ancient Mesopotamia", in: C. S. Kraus (ed.), *The Limits of Historiography. Genre and Narrative in Ancient Historical Texts* (Leiden, Boston, and Köln: Brill), pp. 69–90.

2003 "The Libraries of Babel. Text, Authority, and Tradition in Ancient Mesopotamia", in: G. J. Dorleijn and H. L. J. Vanstiphout (eds.), *Cultural Repertoires. Structure, Function and Dynamics* (Leuven, Paris, and Dudley: Peeters), pp. 105–129.

Middeke-Conlin, R.

2014 "The Scents of Larsa: A Study of the Aromatics Industry in an Old Babylonian Kingdom", *CDLJ* 2014:1, pp. 1–53.

van de Mieroop, M.

2006 "Karen Radner: Die Macht des Namens" [Review], *ZA* 96, pp. 273–276.

2016 *Philosophy Before the Greeks. The Pursuit of Truth in Ancient Mesopotamia* (Princeton and Oxford: Princeton University Press)

Miglus, P. A.

1996 *Das Wohngebiet von Assur. Stratigraphie und Architektur* (Wissenschaftliche Veröffentlichungen der Deutschen Orient-Gesellschaft 93; Berlin: Gebr. Mann Verlag)

2000 "Die letzten Tage von Assur und die Zeit danach", *Isimu* 3, pp. 85–99.

2006 "Qal'at Širqāṭ (Assur)". in: M. P. Streck (ed.), *Reallexikon der Assyriologie und Vorderasiatischen Archäologie. Band 11 1./2. Lieferung* (Berlin and New York: Walter de Gruyter), pp. 146–152.

Millard, A.

1994 *The Eponyms of the Assyrian Empire 910–612 BC* (State Archives of Assyria Studies 2; Helsinki: The Neo-Assyrian Text Corpus Project)

Millard, A. R. and M. Sigrist

1985 "Catalogue des tablettes cunéiformes du Couvent Saint-Étienne", *Revue Biblique* 92, pp. 570–576.

Monroe, M. W.

2019 "Looking Through the Cracks: Tracing Damage in Textual History", *MAARAV* 23, pp. 115–135 and pl. 8.

Muir, E.

1991 "Introduction: Observing Trifles", in: E. Muir and G. Ruggiero (eds.), *Microhistory and the Lost Peoples of Europe* [Translated by E. Branch] (Baltimore and London: The Johns Hopkins University Press), pp. vii–xxviii.

Müller-Karpe, M., M. Kunter and M. Schultz
2008 "Results of the Palaeopathological Investigations on the Royal Skeletons from Nimrud", in: J. E. Curtis, H. McCall, D. Collon and L. al-Gailani Werr (eds.): *New Light on Nimrud – Proceedings of the Nimrud Conference 11th–13th March 2002* (London: British Institute for the Study of Iraq and The British Museum), pp. 141–148.

Myer, C. F.
1975 *The Use of Aromatics in Ancient Mesopotamia* (Dissertation; Pennsylvania: University of Pennsylvania)

Nadali, D. and L. Verderame
2014 "Experts at War. Masters Behind the Ranks of the Assyrian Army", in: H. Neumann, R. Dittmann, S. Paulus, G. Neumann and A. Schuster-Brandis (eds.), *Krieg und Frieden im Alten Vorderasien. 52e Renconctre Assyriologique Internationale. International Congress of Assyriology and Near Eastern Archaeology. Münster, 17.-21. Juli 2006* (Alter Orient und Altes Testament 401; Münster: Ugarit-Verlag), pp. 553–566.

Nasrabadi, B. M.
1999 *Untersuchungen zu den Bestattungssitten in Mesopotamien in der Ersten Hälfte des Ersten Jahrtausends v. Chr.* (Baghdader Forschungen 23; Mainz: Verlag Philipp von Zabern)

Neugebauer, O.
1969 *The Exact Sciences in Antiquity* (New York: Dover Publications, Inc.)

Noegel, S. B.
2007 *Nocturnal Ciphers: The Allusive Langauge of Dreams in the Ancient Near East* (American Oriental Series 89; New Haven, Connecticut: American Oriental Society)

Nougayrol, J.
1972 "Textes Religieux (II)", *RA* 66/2, pp. 141–145.

Novotny, J.
2014 *Selected Royal Inscriptions of Assurbanipal* (State Archives of Assyria Cuneiform Texts 10; Helsinki: The Neo-Assyrian Text Corpus Project)

Nutton, V.
2004 *Ancient Medicine* (London and New York: Routledge)

Oates, J.
1991 "The Fall of Assyria (635–609 B.C.)", in: J. Boardman, I. E. S. Edwards, N. G. L. Hammond and E. Sollberger (eds.), *The Cambridge Ancient History. Second Edition. Volume III Part 2* (Cambridge: Cambridge University Press), pp. 162–193.

Oppenheim, A. L.
1960 "Assyriology – Why and How?", *Current Anthropology* 1/5, pp. 409–423.

1967 *Letters from Mesopotamia. Offifical, Buisness, and Private Letters on Clay Tablets from Two Millennia* (Chicago and London: The University of Chicago Press)

1977 [1964] *Ancient Mesopotamia. Portrait of a Dead Civilization* (Chicago and London: The University of Chicago Press) [Chicago: The University of Chicago Press]

Oppenheim, A. L. And L. F. Hartman

1945 "The Domestic Animals of Ancient Mesopotamia According to the XIIIth Tablet of the Series ḪAR.RA = *ḫubullu*", *JNES* 4/3, pp. 152–177.

Ornan, T.

2002 "The Queen in Public: Royal Women in Neo-Assyrian Art", in: S. Parpola and R. M. Whiting (eds.)., *Sex and Gender in the Ancient Near East. Proceedings of the 47th Rencontre Assyriologique Internationale, Helsinki, July 2–6, 2001. Part II* (Helsinki: The Neo-Assyrian Text Corpus Project), pp. 461–477.

Oshima, T.

2014: *Babylonian Poems of Pious Sufferers. Ludlul Bēl Nēmeqi and the Babylonian Theodicy* (Orientalische Religionen in der Antike 14; Tübingen: Mohr Siebeck)

Ossendrijver, M.

2011 "Exzellente Netzwerke: Die Astronomen von Uruk", in: G. J. Selz and K. Wagensonner (eds.), *The Empirical Dimension of Ancient Near Eastern Studies* (Wien: LIT Verlag), pp. 631–644.

Panayotov, S. V.

2013 "A Ritual for a Flourishing Bordello", *Bibliotheca Orientalis* 20, pp. 286–310 and figs. 1–4.

2015 "Loretz, *Hippologia Ugaritica. Das Pferd in Kultur, Wirtschaft, Kriegführung und Hippiatrie Ugarits: Pferd, Esel und Kamel in biblischen Texten. Mit einem Beitrag von M. Stol über Pferde, Pferdekrankheiten und Pferdemedizin in altbabylonischer Zeit*" [Review], *Bibliotheca Orientalis* 72, pp. 484–489.

2016 *"Die Lampe am Krankenbett". Untersuchungen zu altorientalischen Gebeten an den Lichtgott Nuska* (Cuneiform Digital Library Preprints 4; Heidelberg: Heidelberg University)

2018a "Magico-medical Plants and Incantations on Assyrian House Amulets", in: G. van Buylaere, M. Luukko, D. Schwemer and A. Mertens-Wagschal (eds.), *Sources of Evil. Studies in Mesopotamian Exorcistic Lore* (Ancient Magic and Divination 15; Leiden and Boston: Brill), pp. 192–222.

2018b "Notes on the Assur Medical Catalogue with Comparison to the Nineveh Medical Encyclopaedia" in: U. Steinert (ed.), *Assyrian and Babylonian*

Scholarly Text Catalogues (Die babylonisch-assyrische Medizin in Texten und Untersuchungen 9; Boston and Berlin: De Gruyter), pp. 89–120.

Parpola, S.

1983a *Letters from Assyrian Scholars to the Kings Esarhaddon and Assurbanipal Part II: Commentary and Appendices* (Alter Orient und Altes Testament 5/2; Neukirchen-Vluyn; Verlag Butzon & Bercker Kevelaer and Neukirchener Verlag Neukirchen-Vluyn)

1983b "Assyrian Library Records", *JNES* 42/1, pp. 1–29.

1986 "The Royal Archives of Nineveh", in: K. R. Veenhof (ed.), *Cuneiform Archives and Libraries. Papers read at the 30e Rencontre Assyriologique Internationale. Leiden, 4–8 July 1983* (Publications de l'Institut historique-archéologique néerlandais de Stamboul 57; Leiden: Nederlands Historisch-Archaeologisch Instituut te Istanbul), pp. 223–236.

1987 "The Forlorn Scholar", in: F. Rochberg-Halton (ed.), *Language, Literature, and History: Philological and Historical Studies Presented to Erica Reiner* (American Oriental Series 67; New Haven: Amerian Oriental Society), pp. 257–278.

1993 *Letters from Assyrian and Babylonian Scholars* (State Archives of Assyria 10; Helsinki: Helsinki University Press)

1997 *Assyrian Prophecies* (State Archives of Assyria 9; Helsinki: Helsinki University Press)

Parpola, S. (ed.)

2017 *Assyrian Royal Rituals and Cultic Texts* (State Archives of Assyria 20; Helsinki: The Neo-Assyrian Text Corpus Project)

Parpola, S. and K. Watanabe

1988 *Neo-Assyrian Treaties and Loyalty Oaths* (State Archives of Assyria 2; Helsinki: Helsinki University Press)

Parys, M.

2014 "Édition d'un texte médical thérapeutique retrouvé à Assur (BAM 159)", *JMC* 23, pp. 1–88.

Payne, E.

2010 "A New Addition to the Musical Corpus", in: S. C. Melville and A. L. Slotsky (eds.), *Opening the Tablet Box. Near Eastern Studies in Honor of Benjamin R. Foster* (Culture and History of the Ancient Near East 42; Leiden and Boston: Brill), pp. 291–300.

Payton, R.

1991 "The Ulu Burun Writing-Board Set", *Anatolian Studies* 41, pp. 99–106.

Pearce, L. E.

1993 "Statements of Purpose: Why the Scribes Wrote", in: M. E. Cohen, D. C. Snell and D. B. Weisberg (eds.), *The Tablet and the Scroll: Near Eastern Studies in Honor of William W. Hallo* (Bethesda, Maryland: CDL Press), pp. 185–193.

Pearce, L. and L. Doty

2000 "The Activities of Anu-bēlšunu, Seleucid Scribe", in: J. Marzahn and H. Neumann (eds.), *Assyriologica et Semitica: Festschrift für Joachim Oelsner anläßlich seines 65. Geburtstages am 18. Februar 1997* (Alter Orient und Altes Testament 252; Münster: Ugarit-Verlag), pp. 331–42.

Pedersén, O.

1985 *Archives and Libraries in the City of Assur: A Survey of the Material from the German Excavations Part I* (Uppsala: Almqvist & Wiksell)

1986 *Archives and Libraries in the City of Assur: A Survey of the Material from the German Excavations Part II* (Uppsala: Almqvist & Wiksell)

1987 "Private Archives in Assur", *SAAB* 1/1, pp. 43–52.

1998 *Archives and Libraries in the Ancient Near East 1500–300 B.C.* (Bethesda, Maryland: CDL Press)

Pientka(-Hinz), R.

2004 "Aus der Wüste ins Schlafzimmer – Der Skorpion", in: C. Nicolle (ed.), *Nomades et Sédentaires dans le Proche-Orient Ancien: Compte rendu de la XLVIe Rencontre Assyriologique Internationale (Paris, 10–13 juillet 2000)* (Amurru 3; Paris: Éditions Recherche sur les Civilisations), pp. 389–404.

2009 "Schlange. A", in: *Reallexikon der Assyriologie und Vorderasiatischen Archäologie. Band 12 3/4* (Berlin and New York: Walter de Guyter), pp. 202–18.

Plantholt, I. S.

2014 "A New Look at the Kassite Medical Letters, and an Edition of Šumu-libši Letter N 969", *ZA* 104/2, pp. 171–181.

In press "Visible Death and Audible Distress: The Personification of Death (*Mūtu*) and Associated Emotions as Inherent Conditions of Life in Akkadian Sources", in: J. Llop and S.-W. Hsu (eds.), *The Expression of Emotions in Ancient Egypt and Mesopotamia* (Culture and History of the Ancient Near East; Leiden and Boston: Brill)

Ponchia, S. and M. Luukko

2013 *The Standard Babylonian Myth of Nergal and Ereškigal: Introduction, Cuneiform Text and Transliteration with a Translation, Glossary and Commentary* (State Archives of Assyria Cuneiform Texts 8; Winona Lake: Eisenbrauns)

Pongratz-Leisten, B.

1999 *Herrschaftswissen in Mesopotamien. Formen der Kommunikation zwischen Gott und König im 2. und 1. Jahrtausend v. Chr.* (State Archives of Assyria Studies 10; Helsinki: The Neo-Assyrian Text Corpus Project)

2015 *Religion and Ideology in Assyria* (Studies in Ancient Near Eastern Records 6; Boston and Berlin: De Gruyter)

2017 "The Assyrian State Rituals: Re-invention of Tradition", in: S. Parpola, *Assyrian Royal Rituals and Cultic Texts* (State Archives of Assyria 20; Helsinki: The Neo-Assyrian Text Corpus Project), pp. XXXI–LXXV.

Postgate, J. N.

1992 *Early Mesopotamia. Society and Economy at the Dawn of History* (London and New York: Routledge)

Potts, D. T.

2010 [2000] "Before Alexandria: Libraries in the Ancient Near East", in: MacLeod, R. (ed.), *The Library of Alexandria. Centre of Learning in the Ancient World* (London and New York: I. B. Tauris) [London and New York: I. B. Tauris & Co Ltd], pp. 19–34.

Prechel, D.

1996 *Die Gottin Ishara. Ein Beitrag zur altorientalischen Religionsgeschichte* (Abhandlungen zur Literatur Alt-Syrien-Palästinas und Mesopotamiens 11; Münster: Ugarit-Verlag)

Preusser, C.

1954 *Die Wohnhäuser in Assur* (Wissenschaftliche Veröffentlichungen der Deutschen Orient-Gesellschaft 64; Berlin: Verlag Gebr. Mann)

Radner, K.

1995 "The Relation Between Format and Content of Neo-Assyrian Texts", in: R. Mattila (ed.), *Nineveh, 612 BC. The Glory and Fall of the Assyrian Empire* (Helsinki: Helsinki University Press), pp. 63–77.

1997 *Die Neuassyrischen Privatrechtsurkunden als Quelle für Mensch und Umwelt* (State Archives of Assyria Studies 6; Helsinki: The Neo-Assyrian Text Copus Project)

1998 *The Prosopography of the Neo-Assyrian Empire. Volume 1, Part I: A* (Helsinki: The Neo-Assyrian Text Corpus Project)

1999a *The Prosopography of the Neo-Assyrian Empire. Volume 1, Part II: B-G* (Helsinki: The Neo-Assyrian Text Corpus Project)

1999b *Ein Neuassyrisches Privatarchiv der Tempelgoldschmiede von Assur* (Studien zu den Assur-Texten 1; Saarbrücken: SDV Saarbrücker Druckerei und Verlag)

2005 *Die Macht des Namens: Altorientalische Strategien zur Selbsterhaltung* (SANTAG 8; Wiesbaden: Harrassowitz Verlag)

2009 "The Assyrian King and his Scholars: The Syro-Anatolian and the Egyptian Schools", in: M. Luukko, S. Svärd and R. Mattila (eds.), *Of God(s), Trees, Kings, and Scholars: Neo-Assyrian and Related Studies in Honour of Simo Parpola* (Studia Orientalia 106; Helsinki: Finnish Oriental Society), pp. 221–238.

2011 "Royal Decision-Making: Kings, Magnates, and Scholars", in: K. Radner and E. Robson (eds.), *The Oxford Handbook of Cuneiform Culture* (Oxford: Oxford University Press), pp. 358–379.

2017a "Assur's 'Second Temple Period'. The Restoration of the Cult of Aššur, c. 538 BCE", in: C. Levin and R. Müller (eds.), *Herrschaftslegitimation in vorderorientalischen Reichen der Eisenzeit* (Orientalische Religionen in der Antike 21; Tübingen: Mohr Siebeck), pp. 77–96.

2017b "Economy, Society, and Daily Life in the Neo-Assyrian Period", in: E. Frahm (ed.), *A Companion to Assyria* (Hoboken and Chichester: Wiley Blackwell), pp. 209–228.

Reade, J.

1986 "Archaeology and the Kuyunjik archives", in: K. R. Veenhof (ed.), *Cuneiform Archives and Libraries. Papers read at the 30e Rencontre Assyriologique Internationale. Leiden, 4–8 July 1983* (Publications de l'Institut historique-archéologique néerlandais de Stamboul 57; Leiden: Nederlands Historisch-Archaeologisch Instituut te Istanbul), pp. 213–222.

Rebahi, H., H. Nejmi, T. Abouelhassan, K. Hasni and M. Samkaoui

2014 "Severe Envenomation by *Cerastes cerastes* Viper: An Unusual Mechanism of Acute Ischemic Stroke", *Journal of Stroke and Cerebrovascular Diseases* 23/1, pp. 169–172.

Reed, C. A. and H. Marx

1959 "A Herpetological Collection from Northeastern Iraq", *Transactions of the Kansas Academy of Science (1903–)* 62/1, pp. 91–122.

Reiner, E.

1958 *Šurpu: A Collection of Sumerian and Akkadian Incantations* (Archiv für Orientforschung Beiheft 11; Osnabrück: Biblio Verlag)

1960a "Fortune-Telling in Mesopotamia", *JNES* 19/1, pp. 23–35.

1960b "Plague Amulets and House Blessings", *JNES* 19/2, pp. 148–155.

1961 "The Etiological Myth of the 'Seven Sages'", *OrNS* 30/1, pp. 1–11.

1987 "Magic Figurines, Amulets, and Talismans", in: A. E. Farkas, P. O. Harper, and E. B. Harrison (eds.), *Monsters and Demons in the Ancient and Medieval Worlds. Papers Presented in Honor of Edith Porada* (Mainz: Verlag Philipp von Zabern), pp. 27–36.

1995 *Astral Magic in Babylonia* (Transactions of the American Philosophical Society 85/4; Philadelphia: The American Philosophical Society)

Reiner, E. and M. Civil

1967 "Another Volume of Sultantepe Tablets" [Review], *JNES* 26/3, pp. 177–211.

Ritter, E. K.

1965 "Magical-expert (=*āšipu*) and Physician (=*asû*). Notes on Two Complementary Professions in Babylonian Medicine", in: H. G. Güterbock and T. Jacobsen (eds.), *Studies in Honor of Benno Landsberger on His Seventy-fifth Birthday April 21, 1965* (Assyriological Studies 16; Chicago: The University of Chicago Press), pp. 299–321.

Rittig, D.

1977 *Assyrisch-babylonische Kleinplastik magischer Bedeutung vom 13.-6. Jh. v. Chr.* (Münchener Vorderasiatische Studien 1; München: Verlag Uni-Druck München)

Robson, E.

2008 "Mesopotamian Medicine and Religion: Current Debates, New Perspectives", *Religion Compass* 2/4, pp. 455–483.

2011a "The Production and Dissemination of Scholarly Knowledge", in: K. Radner and E. Robson (eds.), *The Oxford Handbook of Cuneiform Culture* (Oxford: Oxford University Press), pp. 557–576.

2011b "Empirical Scholarship in the Neo-Assyrian Court", in: G. J. Selz and K. Wagensonner (eds.), *The Empirical Dimension of Ancient Near Eastern Studies* (Wien: LIT Verlag), pp. 603–630.

2013 "Reading the Libraries of Assyria and Babylonia", in: J. König, K. Oikonomopoulou and G. Woolf (eds.), *Ancient Libraries* (Cambridge: Cambridge University Press), pp. 38–56.

2014 "Tracing Networks of Cuneiform Scholarship with Oracc, GKAB, and Google Earth", in: M. T. Rutz and M. M. Kersel (eds.), *Archaeologies of Texts: Archaeology, Technology, and Ethics* (Oxford and Philadelphia: Oxbow Books), pp. 142–163.

2019 *Ancient Knowledge Networks. A Social Gepgraphy of Cuneiform Scholarship in First-Millennium Assyria and Babylonia* (London: UCL Press)

Rochberg(-Halton), F.

1984 "Canonicity in Cuneiform Texts", *JCS* 36/2, pp. 127–144.

1987 "The Assumed 29th *Aḫû* Tablet of *Enūma Anu Enlil*", in: F. Rochberg-Halton (ed.), *Language, Literature, and History: Philological and Historical Studies Presented to Erica Reiner* (American Oriental Series 67; New Haven: Amerian Oriental Society), pp. 327–350.

1988 *Aspects of Babylonian Celestial Divination: The Lunar Eclipse Tablets of Enūma Anu Enlil* (Archiv für Orientforschung Beiheft 22; Horn: Verlag Ferdinand Berger & Söhne Gesellschaft M.B.H.)

2004 *The Heavenly Writing. Divination, Horoscopy, and Astronomy in Mesopotamian Culture* (Cambridge: Cambridge University Press)

2010 "'If P, then Q': Form and Reasoning in Babylonian Divination", in: A. Annus (ed.), *Divination and Interpretation of Signs in the Ancient World* (Oriental Institute Seminars 6; Chicago: The Oriental Institute of the University of Chicago), pp. 19–28.

2011 "Observing and Describing the World Through Divination and Astronomy", in: K. Radner and E. Robson (eds.), *The Oxford Handbook of Cuneiform Culture* (Oxford: Oxford University Press), pp. 618–636.

2015 "The Babylonians and the Rational", in: J. C. Johnson (ed.), *In the Wake of the Compendia: Infrastructural Contexts and the Licensing of Empiricism in Ancient and Medieval Mesopotamia* (Science, Technology, and Medicine in Ancient Cultures 3; Boston and Berlin: De Gruyter), pp. 209–246.

2016 *Before Nature. Cuneiform Knowledge and the History of Science* (Chicago and London: The University of Chicago Press)

2018 "The Catalogues of *Enūma Anu Enlil*", in: U. Steinert (ed.), *Assyrian and Babylonian Scholarly Text Catalogues* (Die babylonisch-assyrische Medizin in Texten und Untersuchungen 9; Boston and Berlin: De Gruyter), pp. 121–136.

Roth, M.

1995 *Law Collections from Mesopotamia and Asia Minor* (Writings from the Ancient World 6; Atlanta: Scholars Press)

Röllig, W.

1987–90 "Literatur", in: D. O. Edzard (ed.), *Reallexikon der Assyriologie und Vorderasiatischen Archäologie. Siebter Band* (Berlin and New York: Walter de Gruyter), pp. 35–66.

Rumor, M.

2017 "The 'AŠ section' of Uruanna III in *Partitur*", *JMC* 29, pp. 1–34.

Rutz, M.

2011 "Threads for Esagil-kīn-apli: The Medical Diagnostic-Prognostic Series in Middle Babylonian Nippur", *ZA* 101, pp. 294–308.

Saggs, H. W. F.

1975 "Historical Texts and Fragments of Sargon II of Assyria. 1. The 'Aššur Charter'", *Iraq* 37/1, pp. 11–20.

Salin, S.

2015 "When Disease 'Touches', 'Hits', or 'Seizes' in Assyro-Babylonian Medicine", *KASKAL* 12, pp. 319–336.

2016 "Transmission and Interpretation of Therapeutic Texts. *Šumma amēlu muḫḫašu umma ukāl*: A Case Study", *Distant Worlds Journal* 1, pp. 117–132.

Sallaberger, W.

2007 "Benno Landsbergers 'Eigenbegrifflichkeit' in wissenschaftsgeschichtlicher Perspektive", in: C. Wilcke (ed.), *Das geistige Erfassen der Welt im Alten Orient. Beiträge zu Sprache, Religion, Kultur und Gesellschaft* (Wiesbaden: Harrassowitz Verlag), pp. 63–82.

Sallaberger, W. and F. H. Vulliet

2005 "Priester. A. I", in: D. O. Edzard and M. P. Strck (eds.), *Reallexikon der Assyriologie und Vorderasiatischen Archäologie. Band 10 7./8. Lieferung* (Berlin and New York: Walter de Gruyter), pp. 617–640.

Scheil, V.

1918 "Notules", *RA* 15, pp. 75–86.

1921 "Catalogue de la Collection Eugène Tisserant", *RA* 18/1, pp. 1–33.

Schmidtchen, E.

2018 "The Edition of Esagil-kīn-apli's Catalogue of the Series *Sakikkû* (SA.GIG) and *Alamdimmû*", in: U. Steinert (ed.), *Assyrian and Babylonian Scholarly Text Catalogues* (Die babylonisch-assyrische Medizin in Texten und Untersuchungen 9; Boston and Berlin: De Gruyter), pp. 313–334.

Schramm, W.

2001 *Bann, Bann! Eine sumerisch-akkadische Beschwörungsserie* (Göttinger Arbeitshefte zur Altorientalischen Literatur 2; Göttingen: Seminar für Keilschriftforschung)

2008 *Ein Compendium sumerisch-akkadischer Beschwörungen* (Göttinger Beiträge zum Alten Orient 2; Göttingen: Universitätsverlag Göttingen)

Schroeder, O.

1920 *Keilschrifttexte aus Assur verschiedenen Inhalts* (Keilschrifttexte aus Assur Verschiedenen Inhalts; Leipzig: J. C. Hinrichs'sche Buchhandlung)

Schuster-Brandis, A.

2008 *Steine als Schutz- und Heilmittel: Untersuchung zu ihrer Verwendung in der Beschwörungskunst Mesopotamiens im 1. Jt. v. Chr.* (Alter Orient und Altes Testament 46; Münster: Ugarit-Verlag)

Schutte, A. J.

1976 "Carlo Ginzburg", *The Journal of Modern History* 48/2, pp. 296–315.

Schwemer, D.

2007a *Abwehrzauber und Behexung: Studien zum Schadenzauberglauben im alten Mesopotamien* (Wiesbanden: Harrassowitz Verlag)

2007b *Rituale und Beschwörungen gegen Schadenzauber* (Keilschrifttexte aus Assur literarischen Inhalts 2; Wiesbaden: Harrassowitz Verlag)

2010a "'Forerunners' of *Maqlû*. A New *Maqlû*-related Fragment from Assur", in: J. Stackert, B. N. Porter and D. P. Wright (eds.), *Gazing on the Deep. Ancient Near Eastern and Other Studies in Honor of Tzvi Abusch* (Bethesda: CDL Press), pp. 201–220.

2010b "Therapien gegen Geistern oder von Hexerei verursachte Leiden", in: B. Janowski and D. Schwemer (eds.), *Texte aus der Umwelt des Alten Testaments. Neue Folge. Band 5. Texte zur Heilkunde* (Gütersloh and München: Gütersloher Verlagshaus), pp. 123–134.

2011 "Magic Rituals: Conceptualization and Performance", in: K. Radner and E. Robson (eds.), *The Oxford Handbook of Cuneiform Culture* (Oxford: Oxford University Press), pp. 418–446.

2015 "The Ancient Near East", in: D. J. Collins (ed.), *The Cambridge History of Magic and Witchcraft in the West* (Cambridge: Cambridge University Press), pp. 17–51.

2017 *The Anti-Witchcraft Ritual Maqlû: The Cuneiform Sources of a Magic Ceremony from Ancient Mesopotamia* (Wiesbaden: Harrassowitz Verlag)

Scurlock, J. A.

1988a *Magical Means of Dealing with Ghosts in Ancient Mesopotamia* (Dissertation; Chicago: The University of Chicago)

1988b "KAR 267//BMS 53: A Ghostly Light on *bīt rimki*?", *Journal of the American Oriental Society* 108/2, pp. 203–209.

1997 "Ghosts in the Ancient Near East: Weak or Powerful?", *Hebrew Union College Annual* 68, pp. 77–96.

1999 "Physician, Exorcist, Conjurer, Magician: A Tale of Two Healing Professionals", in: T. Abusch and K. van der Toorn (eds.), *Mesopotamian Magic: Textual, Historical, and Interpretative Perspectives* (Ancient Magic and Divination 1; Groningen: STYX Publications), pp. 69–79.

2002a "Animals in Ancient Mesopotamian Religion", in: B. J. Collins (ed.), *A History of the Animal World in the Ancient Near East* (Handbuch der Orientalistik 64; Leiden, Boston, and Köln: Brill), pp. 361–388.

2002b "Some Thoughts on Ancient Mesopotamian Magic and Religion", *BiOr* 59, pp. 468–482.

2006 *Magico-Medical Means of Treating Ghost-Induced Illnesses in Ancient Mesopotamia* (Ancient Magic and Divination 3; Leiden and Boston: Brill and Styx)

2014 *Sourcebook for Ancient Mesopotamian Medicine* (Writings from the Ancient World 36; Atlanta, Georgia: SBL Press)

2018 "*Elpetu*-Rush, Inanna and the Flood: A Tale of Human Ingratitude", in: S. V. Panayotov and L. Vacín (eds.), *Mesopotamian Medicine and Magic. Studies in Honor of Markham J. Geller* (Ancient Magic and Divination 14; Leiden and Boston: Brill), pp. 528–536.

Scurlock, J. A. and B. R. Andersen

2005 *Diagnoses in Assyrian and Babylonian Medicine: Ancient Sources, Translations, and Modern Medical Analyses* (Urbana and Chicago: University of Illinois Press)

Seidl, U. and W. Sallaberger

2005–06 "Der 'Heilige Baum'", *AfO* 51, pp. 54–74.

Selz, G. J.

2014 "Plant Metaphors: On the Plant of Rejuvenation", in: S. Gaspa, A. Greco, D. M. Bonacossi, S. Ponchia and R. Rollinger (ed.), *From Sources to History. Studies on Ancient Near Eastern Worlds and Beyond. Dedicated to Giovanni Battista Lanfranchi on the Occasion of His 65th Birthday on June 23, 2014* (Alter Orient und Altes Testament 412; Münster: Ugarit-Verlag), pp. 655–667.

Seux, M.-J.

1976 *Hymnes et prières aus dieux de Babylonie et d'Assyrie* (Paris: Les Éditions du Cerf)

Shalita, E. A. and R. D. Wells

2007 "Treatment of Yellow Scorpion (*Leiurus quinquestriatus*) Sting: A Case Report", *Journal of the American Pharmacists Association* 47/5, pp. 616–619.

Siddall, L. R.

2013 *The Reign of Adad-nīrārī III: An Historical and Ideological Analysis of an Assyrian King and His Times* (Cuneiform Monographs 45; Leiden, Boston: Brill)

Simon, Z. B.

2015 "Microhistory: In General", *Journal of Social History*, pp. 237–248.

Sjöberg, Å. W.

1972 "In Praise of the Scribal Art", *JCS* 24/4, pp. 126–131.

1973 "Der Vater und sein missratener Sohn", *JCS* 25/3, pp. 105–169.

Smith, J. Z.

2004 *Relating Religion. Essays in the Study of Religion* (Chicago and London: The University of Chicago Press)

von Soden, W.

1936 "Bemerkungen zu den von Ebeling in 'Tod und Leben' Band I bearbeiteten Texten", *ZA* 43, pp. 251–276.

1995 *Grundriss der Akkadischen Grammatik* [Third Edition] (Analecta Orientalia 33; Rome: Editrice Pontificio Istituto Biblico)

Sofer, S.

1995 "Scorpion envenomation", *Intensive Care Med* 21, pp. 626–628.

Sofer, S., E. Shahak and M. Gueron

1994 "Scorpion Envenomation and Antivenom Therapy", *The Journal of Pediatrics* 124/6, pp. 973–978.

Stadhouders, H.

2011 "The Pharmacopoeial Handbook *Šammu šikinšu* – An Edition", *JMC* 18, pp. 3–51.

2012 "The Parhamcopoeial Handbook *Šammu šikinšu* – A Translation", *JMC* 19, pp. 1–21.

2013 "A Time to Rejoice: The Egalkura Rituals and the Mirth of Iyyar", in: L. Feliu, J. Llop, A. Millet Albà and J. Sanmartín (eds.), *Time and History in the Ancient Near East: Proceedings of the 56th Rencontre Assyriologuqe Internationale at Barcelona 26–30 July 2010* (Winona Lake, Eisenbrauns), pp. 301–323.

Stadhouders, H. and S. V. Panayotov

2018 "From Awe to Audacity. Stratagems for Apporaching Authorities Successfully: The Istanbul Egalkura Tablet A 373", in: S. V. Panayotov and L. Vacín (eds.), *Mesopotamian Medicine and Magic. Studies in Honor of Markham J. Geller* (Ancient Magic and Divination 14; Leiden and Boston: Brill), pp. 623–697.

Starr, I.

1983 *The Rituals of the Diviner* (Bibliotheca Mesopotamica 12; Malibu: Undena Publications)

1990 *Queries to the Sungod: Divination and Politics in Sargonid Assyria* (State Archives of Assyria 4; Helsinki: Helsinki University Press)

Steinert, U.

2012 *Aspekte des Menscheins im Alten Mesopotamien: Eine Studie zu Person und Identität im 2. und 1. Jt. v. Chr.* (Cuneiform Monographs 44; Leiden, Boston: Brill)

2015 "'Tested' Remedies in Mesopotamian Medical Texts: a Label for Efficacy Based on Empirical Observation?", in: J. C. Johnson (ed.), *In the Wake of the Compendia: Infrastructural Contexts and the Licensing of Empiricism in Ancient and Medieval Mesopotamia* (Science, Technology, and Medicine in Ancient Cultures 3; Boston and Berlin: De Gruyter), pp. 103–145.

2016 "Körperwissen, Tradition und Innovation in der babylonischen Medizin", *Paragrana* 25, pp. 195–254.

2018a "Catalogues, Texts, and Specialists: Some Thoughts on the Aššur Medical Catalogue and Mesopotamian Healing Professions", in: G. van Buylaere, M. Luukko, D. Schwemer and A. Mertens-Wagschal (eds.), *Sources of Evil. Studies in Mesopotamian Exorcistic Lore* (Ancient Magic and Divination 15; Leiden and Boston: Brill), pp. 48–132.

2018b "Introduction: Catalogues, Corpora and Canons in Mesopotamian Scholarship", in: U. Steinert (ed.), *Assyrian and Babylonian Scholarly Text Catalogues* (Die babylonisch-assyrische Medizin in Texten und Untersuchungen 9; Boston and Berlin: De Gruyter), pp. 7–24.

2018c "Catalogues, Texts and Specialists: Some Thoughts on the Assur Medical Catalogue, Mesopotamian Medical Texts and Healing Professions", in: U. Steinert (ed.), *Assyrian and Babylonian Scholarly Text Catalogues* (Die babylonisch-assyrische Medizin in Texten und Untersuchungen 9; Boston and Berlin: De Gruyter), pp. 158–202.

2018d "The Assur Medical Catalogue (AMC)", in: U. Steinert (ed.), *Assyrian and Babylonian Scholarly Text Catalogues* (Die babylonisch-assyrische Medizin in Texten und Untersuchungen 9; Boston and Berlin: De Gruyter), pp. 203–208, 219–291.

Steinert, U. (ed.)

2018e *Assyrian and Babylonian Scholarly Text Catalogues* (Die babylonisch-assyrische Medizin in Texten und Untersuchungen 9; Boston and Berlin: De Gruyter)

Steinert, U., S.V. Panayotov, M.J. Geller, E. Schmidtchen, J.C. Johnson

2018 "AMC Text Edition", in: U. Steinert (ed.), *Assyrian and Babylonian Scholarly Text Catalogues* (Die babylonisch-assyrische Medizin in Texten und Untersuchungen 9; Boston and Berlin: De Gruyter), pp. 209–219.

Steinert, U. and L. Vacín

2018 "BM 92518 and Old Babylonian Incantations for the 'Belly'", in: S.V. Panayotov and L. Vacín (eds.), *Mesopotamian Medicine and Magic. Studies in Honor of Markham J. Geller* (Ancient Magic and Divination 14; Leiden and Boston: Brill), pp. 698–744.

Stevens, K.

2013 "Secrets in the Library: Protected Knowledge and Professional Identity in Late Babylonian Uruk", *Iraq* 75, pp. 211–253.

Stol, M.

1987–88 "Leprosy. New Light from Greek and Babylonian Sources", *JEOL* 30, pp. 22–31.

1991–92 "Diagnosis and Therapy in Babylonian Medicine", *JEOL* 32, pp. 42–65.

1993 *Epilepsy in Babylonia* (Cuneiform Monographs 2; Groningen: STYX Publications)

1997 "Avalos, Hector – Illness and Health Care in the Ancient Near East: the Role of the Temple in Greece, Mesopotamia and Israel" [Review], *Bibliotheca Orientalis* 54, pp. 406–410.

2000 *Birth in Babylonia and the Bible: Its Mediterranean Setting* (Cuneiform Monographs 14; Groningen: STYX Publications)

2004–05 "Pflanzenkunde", in: D.O. Edzard and M.P. Streck (eds.), *Reallexikon der Assyriologie und Vorderasiatischen Archäologie. Band 10 5./6.-7./8. Lieferung* (Berlin and New York: Walter de Gruyter), pp. 503–6.

2006 "The Digestion of Food According to Babylonian Sources", in: L. Battini and P. Villard (eds.), *Médecine et médecins au Proche-Orient ancien. Actes du colloque international organisé à Lyon les 8 et 9 novembre 2002, Maison de l'Orient et de la Méditerranée* (BAR Internaltion Series 1528; Oxford: Archaeopress), pp. 103–119.

2007a “Fevers in Babylonia”, in: I. L. Finkel and M. J. Geller (eds.), *Disease in Babylonia* (Cuneiform Monographs 36; Leiden and Boston: Brill), pp. 1–39.

2007b “Remarks on some Sumerograms and Akkadian Words”, in: M. T. Roth, W. Farber, M. W. Stolper and P. Von Beschtolsheim (eds.), *From the Workshop of the Chicago Assyrian Dictionary Volume 2: Studies Presented to Robert D. Biggs June 4, 2004* (Assyriological Studies 27; Chicago: The Oriental Institute of the University of Chicago), pp. 233–242.

2009a “Insanity in Babylonian Sources”, *JMC* 13, pp. 1–12.

2009b “‘To be ill’ in Akkadian: The Verb *Salā’u* and the Substantive *Sili’tu*”, in: A. Attia and G. Buisson (eds.), *Advances in Mesopotamian Medicine from Hammurabi to Hippocrates* (Cuneiform Monographs 37; Leiden and Boston: Brill), pp. 29–46.

2011 “Pferde, Pferdekrankheiten und Pferdemedizin in altbabylonischer Zeit”, in: O. Loretz, *Hippologia Ugaritica: Das Pferd in Kultur, Wirtschaft, Kriegführung und Hippiatrie Ugarits. Pferd, Esel und Kamel in biblischen Texten* (Alter Orient und Altes Testament 386; Münster: Ugarit-Verlag), pp. 363–402.

Szijártó, I. M.

2013a “Introduction: Against Simple Truths”, in: S. G. Magnússon and I. M. Szijártó, *What is Microhistory? Theory and Practice* (New York: Routledge), pp. 1–12.

Sørensen, J.

2007 *A Cognitive Theory of Magic* (Lanham, New York, Toronto and Plymouth; Altamira Press)

2013 “Magic Reconsidered: Towards a Scientifically Valid Concept of Magic”, in: B.-C. Otto and M. Stausberg (eds.), *Defining Magic. A Reader* (Sheffield and Bristol: Equinox), pp. 229–242.

Talon, P.

2003 “The Use of Glosses in Neo-Assyrian Letters and Astrological Reports”, in: P. Marrassini (ed.), *Semitic and Assyriological Studies Presented to Pelio Fronzaroli by Pupils and Colleagues* (Wiesbaden: Harrassowitz Verlag), pp. 648–665.

Tanret, M.

2011 “Learned, Rich, Famous, and Unhappy: Ur-Utu of Sippar”, in: K. Radner and E. Robson (eds.), *The Oxford Handbook of Cuneiform Culture* (Oxford: Oxford University Press), pp. 270–287.

Taylor, J. H.

2011 “Tablets as Artefacts, Scribes as Artisans”, in: K. Radner and E. Robson (eds.), *The Oxford Handbook of Cuneiform Culture* (Oxford: Oxford University Press), pp. 5–31.

Thompson, R. C.
1923 *Assyrian Medical Texts* (London, Edinburgh, Glasgow, Copenhagen, New York, Toronto, Melbourne, Cape Town, Bombay, Calcutta, and Madras: Humphrey Milford and Oxford University Press)
1949 *A Dictionary of Assyrian Botany* (London: The British Academy)
Thureau-Dangin, F.
1912 *Une relation de la huitième campagne de Sargon (714 av. J.-C.)* (Textes cunéiformes du Louvre 3; Paris: Librairie Paul Geuthner)
du Toit, J. S.
1998 "Ancient Near Eastern Collection Development: Reappraising the Problematic Nature of the Description of Ancient Library and Archival Practices", in: J. Prosecký (ed.), *Intellectual Life of the Ancient Near East. Papers Presented at the 43rd Rencontre assyriologique internatinale Prague, July 1–5, 1996* (Prague: Oriental Institute), pp. 389–396.
Too, Y. L.
2010 *The Idea of the Library in the Ancient World* (Oxford: Oxford University Press)
van der Toorn, K.
1985 *Sin and Sanction in Israel and Mesopotamia* (Studia Semitica Neerlandica 22; Assen, Maastricht: van Gorcum)
1996 *Family Religion in Babylonia, Syria and Israel: Continuity and Change in the Forms of Religious Life* (Studies in the History and Culture of the Ancient Near East 7; Leiden, New York, and Köln: E. J. Brill)
2007 *Scribal Culture and the Making of the Hebrew Bible* (Cambridge and London: Harvard University Press)
Tsukimoto, A.
1985 *Untersuchungen zur Totenpflege (kispum) im alten Mesopotamien* (Alter Orient und Altes Testament 216; Neukirchen-Vluyn: Verlag Butzon & Bercker Kevelaer, Neukirchener Verlag Neukirchen-Vluyn)
1999 "'By the Hand of Madi-Dagen, the Scribe and *Apkallu*-Priest' – A Medical Text from the Middle Euphrates Region", in: K. Watanabe (ed.), *Priests and Officials in the Ancient Near East* (Heidelberg: Universitätsverlag C. Winter), pp. 187–200.
Unger, E.
1928 "Aššur, Stadt", in: E. Ebeling and B. Meissner (eds.), *Reallexikon der Assyriologie. Erster Band* (Berlin and Leipzig: Walter de Gruyter and Co.), pp. 170–195 and pls. 20–30.
Unschuld, P. U.
1980 *Medizin in China: Eine Ideengeschichte* (Munich: Verlag C. H. Beck)
2009 *What Is Medicine? Western and Eastern Approaches to Healing* [Translated by K. Reimers] (Berkeley, Los Angeles and London: University of California Press)

Vanstiphout, H. L. J.

1986 "Some Thoughts on Genre in Mesopotamian Literature", in: K. Hecker and W. Sommerfeld (eds.), *Keilschriftliche Literaturen. Ausgewählte Vorträge der XXXII. Rencontre Assyriologique Internationale Münster, 8.–12.7.1985* (Berliner Beiträge zum Vorderen Orient 6; Berlin: Dietrich Reimer Verlag), pp. 1–11.

1999 "'I Can Put Everything in Its Right Place'. Generic and Typological Studies as Strategies for the Analysis and Evaluation of Mankind's Oldest Literature", in: B. Roest and H. Vanstiphout (eds.), *Aspects of Genre and Type in Pre-modern Literary Cultures* (Groningen: STYX Publications), pp. 79–99.

Veenhof, K. R.

1986a "Cuneiform Archives. An introduction", in: K. R. Veenhof (ed.), *Cuneiform Archives and Libraries. Papers read at the 30e Rencontre Assyriologique Internationale. Leiden, 4–8 July 1983* (Publications de l'Institut historique-archéologique néerlandais de Stamboul 57; Leiden: Nederlands Historisch-Archaeologisch Instituut te Istanbul), pp. 1–36.

Veenhof, K. R. (ed.)

1986b *Cuneiform Archives and Libraries. Papers read at the 30e Rencontre Assyriologique Internationale. Leiden, 4–8 July 1983* (Publications de l'Institut historique-archéologique néerlandais de Stamboul 57; Leiden: Nederlands Historisch-Archaeologisch Instituut te Istanbul)

Veldhuis, N.

1990 "The Heart Grass and Related Matters", *Orientalia Lovaniensia Periodica* 21, pp. 27–44.

1995–96 "On Interpreting Mesopotamian Namburbi Rituals" [Review], *AfO* 42–43, pp. 145–154.

1999 "The Poetry of Magic", in: T. Abusch and K. van der Toorn (eds.), *Mesopotamian Magic: Textual, Historical, and Interpretative Perspectives* (Ancient Magic and Divination 1; Groningen: STYX Publications), pp. 35–48.

2003 "On the Curriculum of the Neo-Babylonian School" [Review], *JAOS* 123/3, pp. 627–633.

2010 "The Theory of Knowledge and the Practice of Celestial Divination", in: A. Annus (ed.), *Divination and Interpretation of Signs in the Ancient World* (Oriental Institute Seminars 6; Chicago: The Oriental Institute of the University of Chicago), pp. 77–92.

2014 *History of the Cuneiform Lexical Tradition* (Guides to the Mesopotamian Textual record 6; Münster: Ugarit-Verlag)

Verderame, L.

2008 "La Formazione dell'Esperto (*ummânu*) nel Periodo Neo-Assiro", *Historiae* 5, pp. 51–67.

2012 “A Bibliography of Ancient Mesopotamian Medicine”, *JMC* 20, pp. 1–42.

2013 “Means of Substitution: The Use of Figurines, Animals, and Human Beings as Substitutes in Assyrian Rituals”, in: C. Ambos and L. Verderame (eds.), *Approaching Rituals in Ancient Cultures* (Rivista Degli Studi Orientali Nuova Serie 86 Supplement no. 2; Pisa and Rome: Fabrizio Serra Editore), pp. 301–323.

2014 “A Glimpse into the Activities of Experts (*ummânu*) at the Assyrian Royal Court”, in: S. Gaspa, A. Greco, D. M. Bonacossi, S. Ponchia and R. Rollinger (ed.), *From Sources to History. Studies on Ancient Near Eastern Worlds and Beyond. Dedicated to Giovanni Battista Lanfranchi on the Occasion of His 65th Birthday on June 23, 2014* (Alter Orient und Altes Testament 412; Münster: Ugarit-Verlag), pp. 713–728.

2018 “Ninmaḫ and Her Imperfect Creatures: The Bed Wetting Man and Remedies to Cure Enuresis (*STT* 238)”, in: S. V. Panayotov and L. Vacín (eds.), *Mesopotamian Medicine and Magic. Studies in Honor of Markham J. Geller* (Ancient Magic and Divination 14; Leiden and Boston: Brill), pp. 779–800.

Villard, P.

1997 “L’éducation d’Assurbanipal”, *KTEMA* 22, pp. 135–149.

1998 “Kiṣir-Aššur et la bibliothèque de Nineve”, *N.A.B.U.* 1998/1, note no. 16, p. 19.

2007 “Quelques notes sur le clergé d’Aššur à la fin de l’époque néoassyrienne”, *Akh Purattim* 2, pp. 321–334.

Virolleaud, Ch.

1912 *L’Astrologie Chaldéenne. Second Supplément. Texte Cunéiforme (1re Partie)* (Paris: Librairie Paul Geuthner)

Volk, K.

1999 “Kinderkrankheiten nach der Darstellung babylonisch-assyrischer Keilschrifttexte”, *OrNS* 68/1, pp. 1–30.

Waetzoldt, H.

1974 *Das Schreiberwesen in Mesopotamien nach den Texten aus neusumerischer Zeit (ca. 2164–2003 v. Chr.)* (Habilitation; Heidelberg: Heidelberg University)

1989 “Der Schreiber als Lehrer in Mesopotamien”, in: J. G. Prinz von Hohenzollern and M. Liedtke (eds.), *Schreiber, Magister, Lehrer. Zur Geschichte und Funktion eines Berufsstandes* (Bad Heilbrunn: Verlag Julius Klinkhardt), pp. 33–50.

Wagensonner, K.

2011 “A Scribal Family and its Orthographic Peculiarities: On the Scientific Work of a Royal Scribe and his Sons”, in: G. J. Selz and K. Wagensonner (eds.), *The Empirical Dimension of Ancient Near Eastern Studies* (Wien: LIT Verlag), pp. 645–701.

2014a “A Note on the Colophon of VAT 9487”, *CDLN* 2014: 19.

2014b “nam-dub-sar-ra a-na mu-e-pad$_3$-da-zu … De l’apprentissage et l’éducation des scribes médio-assyriens”, in: L. Marti (ed.), *La famille dans le Proche-Orient ancient: réalités, symbolismes, et images. Proceedings of the 55th Rencontre Assyriologique Internationale at Paris 6–9 July 2009* (Winona Lake, Indiana: Eisenbrauns), pp. 457–467.

Walker, C. B. F.

1980 "Some Mesopotamian Inscribed Vessels", *Iraq* 42/1, pp. 84–86.

Walker, C. and M. Dick

2001 *The Induction of the Cult Image in Ancient Mesopotamia. The Mesopotamian Mīs Pî Ritual* (State Archives of Assyria Literary Texts 1; Helsinki: The Neo-Assyrian Text Corpus Project)

Watanabe, C. E.

2002 *Animal Symbolism in Mesopotamia. A Contextual Approach* (Wiener Offene Orientalistik 1; Wien: Institut für Orientalistik der Universität Wien)

Warrell, D. A.

1995 "Clinical Toxicology of Snakebite in Africa and the Middle East/Arabian Peninsula", in: J. Meier and J. White (eds.), *Handbook of Clinical Toxicology of Animal Venoms and Poisons* (Boca raton, New York, London, and Tokyo: CRC Press), pp. 433–492.

Wasserman, N.

1996 "An Old-Babylonian Medical Text against the *kurārum* Disease", *RA* 90, pp. 1–5.

2012 "*Maškadum* and Other Zoonotic Diseases in Medical and Literary Akkadian Sources", *Bibliotheca Orientalis* 69, pp. 426–436.

Watson, R. and W. Horowitz

2011 *Writing Science before the Greeks: A Naturalistic Analysis of the Babylonian Astronomical Treatise MUL.APIN* (Culture and History of the Ancient Near East 48; Leiden and Boston: Brill)

Watson, W. G. E.

2004 "Akkadian Loanwords in Ugaritic: the Hippiatric Texts", in: C. McCarthy and J. F. Healey (eds.), *Biblical and Near Eastern Essays. Studies in Honour of Kevin J. Cathcart* (London and New York: T&T Clark International), pp. 240–257.

Wee, J. Z.

2012 *The Practice of Diagnosis in Mesopotamian Medicine: With Editions of Commentaries on the Diagnostic Series Sa-gig* (Dissertation; Yale: Yale University)

2015 "Phenomena in Writing", in: J. C. Johnson (ed.), *In the Wake of the Compendia: Infrastructural Contexts and the Licensing of Empiricism in Ancient and Medieval Mesopotamia* (Science, Technology, and Medicine in Ancient Cultures 3; Boston and Berlin: De Gruyter), pp. 247–287.

2016 "A Late Babylonian Astral Commentary on *Marduk's Address to the Demons*", *JNES* 75/1, pp. 127–167.

Weidner, E. F.
1937–39 "Neue Bruchstücke des Berichtes über Sargons achten Feldzug", *AfO* 12, pp. 144–148.
1952–53 "Die Bibliothek Tiglatpilesers I.", *AfO* 16, pp. 197–215.
Wessel, M. A., J. C. Cobb, E. B. Jackson, G. S. Harris, A. C. Detwiler
1954 "Paroxysmal Fussing in Infancy, Sometimes Called 'Colic'", *Pediatrics* 14/5, pp. 421–435.
Westbrook, R.
2003 "The Character of Ancient Near Eastern Law", in: R. Westbrook (ed.), *A History of Ancient Near Eastern Law* (Handbuch der Orientalistik 72/1; Leiden and Boston: Brill), pp. 1–90.
Westenholz, Aa.
2007 "The Graeco-Babyloniaca Once Again", ZA 97, pp. 262–313.
Westenholz, J. G.
2010 "The Tale of Two Little Organs: The Spleen and the Pancreas", *JMC* 15, pp. 2–24.
Westenholz, J. G. and M. Sigrist
2006 "The Brain, the Marrow and the Seat of Cognition in Mesopotamian Tradition", *JMC* 7, pp. 1–10.
2008 "The Measure of Man: The Lexical Series Ugu-mu", in: R. D. Biggs, J. Myers and M. T. Roth (eds.), *Proceedings of the 51st Rencontre Assyriologique Internationale Held at the Oriental Institute of the University of Chicago July 18–22, 2005* (Studies in Ancient Oriental Civilization 62; Chicago: The Oriental Institute of the University of Chicago), pp. 221–230.
Wiggermann, F. A. M.
1992 *Mesopotamian Protective Spirits: The Ritual Texts* (Cuneiform Monographs 1; Groningen: STYX & PP Publications)
1993–97 "*Mušḫuššu*", in: D. O. Edzard (ed.), *Reallexikon der Assyriologie und Vorderasiatischen Arhcäologie. Achter Band* (Berlin and New York: Walter de Gruyter), pp. 455–462.
1997 "Transtigridian Snake Gods", in: I. L. Finkel and M. J. Geller (eds.), *Sumerian Gods and Their Representations* (Cuneiform Monographs 7; Groningen: STYX Publications), pp. 33–55.
2000 "Lamaštu, Daughter of Anu. A Profile", in: M. Stol, *Birth in Babylonia and the Bible: Its Mediterranean Setting* (Cuneiform Monographs 14; Groningen: STYX Publications), pp. 217–252.
2007a "The Four Winds and the Origins of Pazuzu", in: C. Wilcke (ed.), *Das geistige Erfassen der Welt im Alten Orient: Sprache, Religion, Kultur und Gesellschaft* (Wiesbaden: Harrassowitz Verlag), pp. 125–165.

2007b “Some Demons of Time and their Functions in Mesopotamian Iconography”, in: B. Groneberg and H. Spieckermann (eds.), *Die Welt der Götterbilder* (Beihefte zur Zeitschrift für die alttestamentliche Wissenschaft 376; Berlin, New York: Walter de Gruyter), pp. 102–116.

2008 “A Babylonian Scholar in Assur”, in: van der Spek (ed.), *Studies in Ancient Near Eastern World View and Society Presented to Marten Stol on the Occasion of his 65th Birthday, 10 November 2005, and his Retirement from the Vrije Universiteit Amsterdam* (Bethesda, Maryland: CDL Press), pp. 203–234.

2010 “The Image of Dumuzi. A Diachronic Analysis”, in: J. Stackert, B. N. Porter and D. P. Wright (eds.), *Gazing on the Deep. Ancient Near Eastern and Other Studies in Honor of Tzvi Abusch* (Bethesda, Maryland: CDL Press), pp. 327–350.

2011 “The Mesopotamian Pandemonium. A Provisional Census”, *SMSR* 77/2, pp. 298–322.

Wilhelm, G.

1979 “Ein neues Lamaštu-Amulett”, *ZA* 69, pp. 34–40.

Winter, U.

2012 [1983] *Frau und Göttin. Exegetische und ikonographische Studien zum weiblichen Gottesbild im Alten Israel und in dessen Umwelt* (Jerusalem and Tübingen: SLM Press and Tobiaslib) [Orbis Biblicus et Orientalis 53; Fribourg and Göttingen: Academic Press and Vandenhoeck & Ruprecht]

Wiseman, D. J.

1955 “Assyrian Writing-Boards”, *Iraq* 17/1, pp. 3–13.

Worthington, M.

2003 “A Discussion of Aspects of the UGU Series”, *JMC* 2, pp. 2–13.

2005 “Edition of UGU 1 (=BAM 480 etc.)”, *JMC* 5, pp. 6–43.

2006 “Edition of BAM 3”, *JMC* 7, pp. 18–48.

2007 “Addenda and Corrigenda to ‘Edition of UGU 1 (= BAM 480 etc.)’ and ‘Edition of BAM 3’”, *JMC* 9, pp. 43–46.

2012 *Principles of Akkadian Textual Criticism* (Studies in Ancient Near Eastern Records 1; Boston and Berlin: De Gruyter)

Wu, Y.

2001 “Rabies and Rabid Dogs in Sumerian and Akkadian Literature”, *Journal of the American Oriental Society* 121/1, pp. 32–43.

Wyplosz, J.

2006 “Quelques reflexions sur l’aruspice mésopotamien et le regard de l’anatomiste”, *JMC* 8, pp. 24–28.

Young, A.
1982 "The Anthropologies of Illness and Sickness", *Annual Review of Anthropology* 11, pp. 257–285.
Zamazalová, S.
2011 "The Education of Neo-Assyrian Princes", in: K. Radner and E. Robson (eds.), *The Oxford Handbook of Cuneiform Culture* (Oxford: Oxford University Press), pp. 313–328.
Zernecke, A. E.
2008 "Warum sitzt der Skorpion unter dem Bett? Überlegungen zur Deutung eines altorientalischen Fruchtbarkeitssymbols", *Zeitschrift des Deutschen Palästina-Vereins (1953-)* 124/2, pp. 107–127.
Zgoll, A.
2004 *Die Kunst des Betens: Form und Funktion, Theologie und Psychagogik in babylonisch-assyrischen Handerhebungsgebeten an Ischtar* (Alter Orient und Altes Testament 308; Münster: Ugarit-Verlag)
Ziegler, N.
2005 "Les vaisseaux sanguins et *Enûma eliš* VI: 5", *JMC* 5, pp. 4–5.
Zilberg, P. and W. Horowitz
2016 "A Medico-Magical Text from the Otago Tablets, Dunedin New Zealand", *ZA* 106/2, pp. 175–184.
Zimmern, H.
1915–16 "Zu den 'Keilschrifttexten aus Assur religiösen Inhalts'", *ZA* 30, pp. 184–228.
Zlotkin, E., T. Milman, G. Sion and Y. L. Werner
2003 "Predatory behaviour of gekkonid lizards, *Ptyodactylus* spp., towards the scorpion *Leiurus quinquestriatus hebraeus*, and their tolerance of its venom", *Journal of Natural History* 37, pp. 641–646.
De Zorzi, N.
2011 "The Omen Series *Šumma izbu*: Internal Structure and Hermeneutic Strategies", *KASKAL* 8, pp. 43–75.
2014 *La Serie Teratomantica Šumma izbu. I-II* (History of the Ancient Near East Monographs 15; Padova: S.A.R.G.O.N. Editrice e Libreria)
Zucconi, L. M.
2007 "Mesopotamian Healers as Diviners", *JMC* 10, pp. 19–33.

Indices

Numbers by themselves refer to page numbers; numbers following n. refer to a footnote on the relevant page; numbers following n. and connected with + refer to several footnotes on the same page; letters (e.g., a, b, c, d) following n. refer to notes in relation to a table on the relevant page.

General Index

Note that references to personal names, divine names and geographical names are selective.

Index of Select Texts Discussed

Index of Select Akkadian and Sumerian Words and Phrases Discussed